THE

GUIDING SYMPTOMS

OF OUR

MATERIA MEDICA

BY

C. HERING, M. D.

VOLUME VI.

PHILADELPHIA:

PUBLISHED BY THE ESTATE OF CONSTANTINE HERING,

112 and 114 North Twelfth Street.

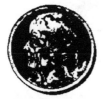

Author's Mark.

PRESS OF GLOBE PRINTING HOUSE, PHILADELPHIA.

PREFACE.

IN giving Volume VI to the profession, we recognize that our labor has been one of unusual pleasure and satisfaction, for it contains, besides a large number of valuable medicines, LACHESIS TRIGONOCEPHALUS, the pet child of Dr. Hering.

We quote a circular he issued in 1878, addressed "To All Friends of Lachesis :"

"Be it known that next 28th of July it will be fifty years since the first trituration and first dilution in alcohol of the snake poison Trigonocephalus Lachesis was made.

"We intend to celebrate that day by closing a collection of reports, consisting of provings, toxicological effects, cures, characteristics, corroborations, etc., etc. Quotations from books or journals where *Lachesis* has been mentioned are solicited, since it is possible that some may have escaped the author's notice.

"In the life of the author the order of the Parcæ or Fates has been reversed. Atropos, the inevitable, who cuts the thread, came to him first when a little boy in the form of a caterpillar on his father's grapevine and gave the incentive to the study of natural history.

"Then came Lachesis, the disposer of destinies; and Clotho comes last and holds the distaff while the author spins the fabric of symptoms.

"The son and daughter of *Lachesis*, by name *Psorinum* and *Lyssinum*, heretofore called *Hydrophobinum*, are receiving a careful revision and will be printed before long. The several brothers and sisters of *Lachesis* are waiting to be acknowledged and proved, particularly the Naja of East India, and the

Lance viper of Martinique. We do not even have a complete collection of the effects of the bite of any of these snakes.

"The *Lachesis Jubilee* could not be better celebrated than by sending contributions to such a collection; also cured cases, provings, etc., etc., all of which will be gratefully acknowledged by the author and embodied in the monograph.

"CONSTANTINE HERING."

To all who responded to the invitation (their names are printed in the list of Clinical Authorities heading *Lachesis*) the editors return thanks in the name of the author, who did not live to publish his monograph.

In collecting the clinically verified symptoms of *Lac Caninum* and *Lac Defloratum*, remedies that are fast growing in usefulness and popularity, we are indebted for valuable assistance to Drs. S. Swan, of New York, and E. W. Berridge, of London, besides others in the profession.

CHARLES G. RAUE,
CALVIN B. KNERR, } *Editors.*
CHARLES MOHR,

GUIDING SYMPTOMS

OF OUR

MATERIA MEDICA.

HEPAR SULPH. CALC.

Sulphuret of Lime.   *Ca. S.*

Introduced by Hahnemann, who used the white interior of oyster shells and pure flowers of sulphur, from which are prepared the triturations.

Provings by Hahnemann, Stapf, etc. See Allen's Encyclopedia, vol. 4, p. 572.

CLINICAL AUTHORITIES.—*Mania with scabies*, Sztaraveszki, Hom. Clinics, vol. 1, p. 56; *Affection of mind*, Dulac, Med. Inv., vol. 9, p. 145; Raue's Rec., 1873, p. 45; *Headaches*, Simmons, Organon, vol. 2, p. 66; *Sensitiveness of scalp*, Chase, Organon, vol. 3, p. 377; *Eruption about ears*, Edgar, Organon, vol. 3, p. 98; *Iritis with hypopyon*, Hills, Raue's Rec., 1873, p. 70; *Kerato-iritis*, Payr, Raue's Rec., 1870, p. 107; *Hypopyon* (3 cases), Gallavardin, Calcutta Jour., vol. 1, p. 274; Farrington, Korndœrfer, Raue's Rec., 1872, p. 75; Bicking, Rück. Kl. Erf., vol. 1, p. 254; *Epithelioma of cornea*, Hills, Trans. Am. Inst. Hom., 1872, p. 521; *Herpes cornea*, Raue's Rec., 1871, p. 58; *Ophthalmia argenti*, Rück. Kl. Erf., vol. 1, p. 271; (6 cases), Gallavardin, Calcutta Jour., vol. 1, p. 274; *Traumatic ophthalmia*, Caspari, B. J. H., vol. 6, p. 366; *Catarrhal inflammation of eyes*, Knorre, B. J. H., vol. 6, p. 364; *Inflammation of eyes*, Schreter, B. J. H., vol. 6, p. 365; *Scrofulous inflammation of eyes*, Tülff, Kallenbach, Gross, Rück. Kl. Erf., vol. 5, p. 125; Bicking, Allg. Kl. Erf., vol. 1, p. 268; *Inflammation of lids*, Griesselich, B. J. H., vol. 6, p. 364; *Itching of ears after scarlatina* (2 cases), Walker, Raue's Rec., 1874, p. 91; *Coryza, ozœna*, Kafka, Raue's Rec., 1870, p. 124; Boyce, B. J. H., vol. 34, p. 494; Chargé, Rück. Kl. Erf., vol. 1, p. 397; *Affection of nose*, Starr, Hom. Clinics, vol. 3, p. 17; *Scrofulous inflammation of nose*, Sattorordin, Calcutta Journ., vol. 1, p. 274; *Affection of cheek*, Bathig, Hom. Clinics, vol. 1, p. 171; *Affection of inferior maxillary*, Ostrom, Times Retros., 1875, p. 19; *Parotitis*, Sircar, Raue's Rec., 187, p. 87; *Tonsillitis*, Wurmb, Hirsch, Rück. Kl. Erf., vol. 5, p. 239;

❚❚Fainting from slightest pains; evenings.

³ Inner Head. ❚Aching in forehead: as if bruised; like a boil; from midnight till morning.

❙❙Burrowing headache in frontal region as if an abscess were forming.

❙❙Violent headache, at night, as if forehead would be torn out, with general heat, without thirst.

❚Headache with a feeling as if eyes would be drawn back into head.

❚Tensive, aching pain above nose.

❚Headache over eyes pressing down upon eyes.

❙❙Pressure and drawing in temples by day.

❚Painful throbbing in r. temple.

❚Aching in vertex, with palpitation of heart, in evening.

❚Stitches in head, when stooping; sensation as if skull would burst, waking him at night.

❚Sticking headache.

❚Hammering sensation in head.

❚Burrowing, sharp headache, neuralgic in character.

❚Boring headache: at root of nose, every morning; in r. temple, from without inwards; < from motion or stooping.

❚Pressure in head, semi-lateral, as from a plug or dull nail, at night, and when waking in morning; < when moving eyes and on stooping; > when rising and from binding head up tight.

❚❚Constant pressive pain in one-half of brain, as from a plug or nail.

❚Wabbling as of water in brain.

❚Sense of swashing in head.

❚Headache when shaking head.

❚Headache > by tying something tightly around head.

❚Dull headache every morning in bed, > after rising.

❚Morning headache, < from every concussion.

❚Lancinating headache, > when walking in open air.

❚❚Headache from abuse of mercury.

❚Traumatic cerebritis, in infants and children, with spasms.

❙❙Pulse-like stitches in lower portion of occiput.

❚Pressive pain externally right of occiput, gradually extending to nape, throat and shoulder blades.

❚Severe stitches in occiput and both temples, as if a plug or nail were being driven in.

⁴ Outer Head. ❚Head bent backward, with swelling below larynx; violent pulsation of carotids, rattling breathing.

❚Sensitiveness of scalp to touch, with burning and itching in morning after rising (after abuse of mercury).

❚Extreme sensitiveness of scalp, could hardly bear to comb her hair or have anything touch the head.

❙❙Disposed to take cold from uncovering head.
❙Burning itching on scalp, from forehead to occiput.
❙Nightly pain in skull bones.
❙Nodosities on head, sore to touch, > by covering head warmly and from sweat.
❙Painful tumors on head; sebaceous tumors inflamed and ready to discharge.
❙Boils on head and neck, very sore on contact.
❙Falling off of hair, with very sore, painful pimples, and large bald spots on scalp.
❙Loss of hair following mercurialization or chronic headache.
❙Cold, clammy perspiration, smelling sour, principally on head and face, with aversion to being uncovered; < from least exercise and during night; > from warmth and when at rest.
❙Fissured eruption behind and on both ears, exuding a thick, gluey secretion, which mats hair; resents with force an attempt to place finger on head; utter abhorrence to be bathed, during which she would scream and fight.
❙❙Humid eruptions: feel sore; of fetid odor; itching violently on rising in morning; burning and feeling sore on scratching; scabs easily torn off, leaving a raw, bleeding surface.
❙Favus, extending to nape of neck or face.

'Sight and Eyes. ❙Photophobia.
❙Objects appear to be red.
❙Feeling of blindness before eyes on rising and standing up after sitting bent over.
❙Sight becomes dim when reading.
❙Eyes become dim, cannot see well in evening by candle light.
❙Anæsthesia of retina, the result of looking at an eclipse; sees a light spot in centre of field of vision, surrounded by a dark ring, and again by a lighter ring, all of which were constantly turning and changing into various colors, especially green; < coming into room from bright sunlight; feeling as if eyes were being pulled back into head, with photophobia; vision $\frac{21}{100}$; field of vision very much contracted.
❙Flickering before eyes; pupils dilated and insensible to light; after abuse of mercury.
❙❙Inflammation of ciliary body.
❙Purulent capsulitis after extraction of cataract.
❙Prolapsus iridis.
❙Iritis with hypopyon or associated with small abscesses in iris (suppurative iritis).

∎Anterior chamber about half filled with pus; eye sensitive to light and air, and must be covered; no syphilitic origin. θIritis with hypopyon.

∎After injury to eye, violent inflammation; sclerotica looks like raw beef; light intolerable; feeling as of sand in eye; in anterior chamber a collection of pus apparently about two lines in diameter; meditates suicide, especially in evening. θHypopyon.

∎Onyx.

∎Cornea dim, opaque and bulging, with a blister-like elevation, as large as end of knitting needle, in centre, forming base of an open ulcer; hypopyon; fever with pressing, burning, bruised pain in eyes, extending into head. θHypopyon.

∎For three months l. cornea so hazy that iris could hardly be seen, and for two months r. cornea had gradually become involved from periphery toward centre; both corneæ opaque and vision lost; considerable pain in eyes and head, with iritis; great ciliary injection and excessive dread of light; lachrymation; no history of syphilis.

∎Severe inflammation in cornea and iris of l. eye; cornea ulcerated superficially, much ciliary injection, pupil contracted, iris sluggish, great photophobia and lachrymation, much pain extending from eye into corresponding side of head, < at night, especially about 2 or 3 A.M.; seat of pain in head, as well as eye, quite sore to touch; lids considerably swollen and slight discharge. θKerato-iritis.

∎Kerato-iritis with ulceration of cornea, hypopyon, sensitiveness to air and touch.

∎Ulcers and abscesses of cornea, especially for deep sloughing form and when hypopyon is present; intense photophobia; profuse lachrymation; great redness of cornea and conjunctiva, even chemosis; pains severe, of a throbbing, aching, stinging character; > from warmth, so that he constantly wishes to keep eye covered; < from any draught of air; at night or in evening lids often swollen, spasmodically closed and very sensitive to touch, or may be red, swollen and bleed easily upon opening.

∎Sclerotic violet red, cornea dim; great photophobia and lachrymation; lower lids swollen. θUlceration of cornea.

∎Recurring ulceration of cornea in ophthalmia scrofulosa.

∎Torpid ulceration of cornea; where there is a want of lachrymal secretion.

∎Red, vascular, elevated ulcer, like a piece of red flesh, at margin of cornea.

∎Opacities of cornea.

❚Acute aggravation of pannus, which tends toward ulceration, especially in mercurialized subjects.
┃┃Epithelioma of cornea.
❚Herpes conjunctivæ bulbi; enlarged veins, run nearly horizontally towards cornea, and terminating in little blisters near edge of cornea; < from crying.
❚Eyes very red, great photophobia, lids red and swollen, with burning pain in affected parts. θOphthalmia.
❚Inflammation of eyes and lids; sore to touch; lachrymation.
❚Catarrhal inflammation and blenorrhœa of eyes; lids inflamed, excoriated, running, as if corroded, especially at inner canthus; internal surface of lids, especially of lower, of deep red color and inflamed; heat, especially in morning on waking; pain, as of a burn, smarting, itching in lids; lids and angles agglutinated in morning by purulent mucus; conjunctiva red, traversed by large vessels; photophobia; in evening, vision of colored and dim halos around candle, with pressive pain forcing her to shut eyes occasionally.
❚Inflammation of eye, small ulcer on l. cornea; eyeballs slightly swollen; eyes closed by swelling at night, and discharging much purulent mucus; hair fell off profusely, leaving bald places on scalp; scabs on head, face and neck, painful when touched; itching in scalp; frequent calls to stool, with difficult evacuations; sour smelling sweat at night; peevish, fretful humor.
❚Violent pain over r. eyebrow; excessive lachrymation of l. eye; photophobia alternating with unusually clear and distinct vision in dark part of room; everything appearing illuminated; at times objects appeared red; l. pupil much dilated, not sensitive even to strong light; r. pupil normal; conjunctiva reddened from canthi, but not on cornea; sensation as if eyes projected; painful pressure in eyeball as if bruised; acute bruised pain on slightest touch. θForeign body in eye.
┃┃Purulent conjunctivitis with profuse discharge and excessive sensitiveness to air and touch.
❚Catarrhal conjunctivitis after inflammatory stage has passed.
❚Scrofulous inflammation of eyes, especially in phlegmatic, fat, large bellied children, with fine white skin, light hair, thick neck and swollen glands, subject to eruptions and ulcerations of skin.
❚Chronic inflammation of eyes, with great photophobia, lachrymation and mucous discharge; formation of ulcers with pressing, burning pains as if eyes were bruised.
❚Symptomatic forms of chronic catarrh of conjunctiva with

infarction of Meibomian glands and purulent secretion, in scrofulous subjects.

❚Stitches in the eyes.

❚Pressure in eyes, especially on moving them, with redness.

❚Eyes ache from bright daylight, when moving them.

❙❙Pain in eye at each step.

❚Eyeballs sore to touch; pain as if they would be drawn back into head.

❚Pressing pain in eyeballs, feel bruised when touched.

❚Pressure in eyes as from sand.

❚Eyes are protruded. *θ*Croup.

❚Dacryo-cystitis and orbital cellulitis, especially if pus has formed and there is great sensitiveness to touch, with throbbing pain; prevents formation of pus or accelerates its discharge.

❚Inflammation of lachrymal sac after pus has formed; blenorrhœa, with great sensitiveness to touch and to cold, with profuse discharge.

❚Lachrymal duct closed by an exudative swelling; constant lachrymation; had existed a long time.

❙❙Burning pains in bones above orbits.

❚Smarting pain in external canthus, with accumulation of hardened mucus.

❙❙Cutting pain in outer canthus.

❙❙Anchylops

❚Redness, inflammation and swelling of upper lid, with pain more pressing than sticking.

❚Redness, inflammation and swelling of upper lid, with pressive pain.

❚Lids closed in morning on waking, cannot open them for a long time.

❚Blepharophthalmia when Meibomian glands are involved, and when little pimples surround the inflamed eye.

❚After frequent straining of eyes, inflammation of glands of both eyelids; lids swollen, palpebral conjunctiva inflamed, erysipelatous; at outer canthi lids as if corroded and ulcerated; secretion of glands increased; eyes agglutinated in morning; every effort and light cause pain.

❚Upper lid margins unevenly rounded, swollen and red; tough mucus in lashes and canthi; scleral conjunctiva injected with red vessels running towards cornea, where they form little vesicles with turbid secretion; lachrymation; pain in evening, agglutination in morning; r. eye worse; small pimples or little furuncles on face, or elsewhere, in complication with tinea.

❚Acute phlegmonous inflammation of lids, which tends toward suppuration; lids swollen, tense and shining, as if erysipelas had invaded them, with throbbing, aching, stinging pain and sensitiveness to touch; pains < cold, > warmth.

❚Blepharitis; after the first stage, when suppuration threatens; lids inflamed, throbbing, aching, stinging, very sensitive to touch; ameliorated by heat.

❚Chronic ciliary blepharitis complicated with swelling of Meibomian glands, or ulcers and swellings on margin of lid, which are painful in evening and upon touch.

❚Palpebral tumors.

❙❙Spasmodically closed eyelids (at night).

❚Eczema palpebrarum, where scabs are thick and honeycombed.

❚❚Little pimples surround inflamed eyes.

⁶ Hearing and Ears. ❚Whizzing and throbbing in ears, with hardness of hearing.

❚Cracking in ear when blowing nose.

❚Darting pain in ears.

❚Increase of earwax.

❚Discharge of fetid pus from ears.

❚Canal filled with white, cheesy, bloody pus, and surrounding skin scurfy and irritated; little pustules in meatus and auricle, wherever pus touched; hemorrhage from slightest touch; > from hot applications, cannot bear anything cold.

❚Itching of ears, green discharge; liquid wax.

❚Itching in ears.

⁷ Smell and Nose. ❙❙Hyperæsthesia of smell.

❚Sense of smell acute, also with vertigo.

❚Loss of smell.

❚Nosebleed (after singing).

❚On blowing nose unpleasant sensation in l. side of nose with whizzing and snapping in ear.

❚Blowing nose causes a raw feeling in side of nose.

❚The nose feels sore as if bruised.

❙❙Contractive sensation in nose.

❚Itching in nose, causing sneezing.

❚Nose stopped up in morning.

❚Febrile fluent coryza if it gets dry, especially with scrofulous and rachitic children; hoarseness, or hollow, croupy cough.

❚Heat and burning in nose; ulcerative pain in nostrils; drawing pain in nose passing into eyes, becoming a smarting there; pain lasts far into night; annoying occlusion of nostrils; crusts and scabs; interior of nose painful and sensitive to air and touch.

❚Fluent coryza, with continual necessity to blow nose, which yields a thin, badly smelling slime; sometimes yellowish, sticky matter drops out of one nostril.

Coryza, with inflammatory swelling cf nose, painful like from a boil; also with cough.

Blowing of offensive mucus from nose.

Mucus from posterior nares mixed with blood.

Nasal discharge thick and purulent, sometimes tinged with blood.

Offensive smelling discharge from nose, which is swollen and red; scabs in nose; loss of smell; eyes inflamed, lids red, excoriated and burning, as if raw; photophobia.

Violent pain in bony part of nose with thick muco-purulent discharge from one nostril; > in dry weather; < on approach of rain, or in changeable weather; after abuse of mercury.

Four years ago discharge of bone as large as pea from l. nostril, preceded by severe neuralgic pains in region of l. orbit, followed by discharge of mucus, which, after a few months became very profuse and purulent; dizziness and headache.

Scurfy formation in r. half of nose, extending down upon lip with a deep fissure, very sore and sensitive to touch.

Scrofulous inflammation of nose with loss of sense of smell.

Scrofulous coryza with formation of crusts and painful inflammation of alæ nasi.

Ozæna scrofulosa.

Bones of nose painful to touch.

Sore pain on dorsum of nose, when touching it.

Inflammation (redness and heat) of nose.

⁸ **Upper Face.** Yellow color of face, with blue rings around eyes.

Yellowness of face and skin.

Heat and fiery redness of face.

Heat of face, night and morning, on waking at 7 P.M.

Erysipelatous color of face.

Chronic neuralgia of face, extending in streaks into temple, ear, alæ nasi and upper lip; particularly if < in open air, and > wrapping up warmly.

Spasmus facialis, especially if caused by diseased bones or teeth.

Hard swollen cheek, and upon it an outgrowth size of walnut, as hard as cheek.

Pains in malar bones, < from touch, extending to ears and temples, < in fresh air, and > by wrapping up face; at same time coryza, hoarseness, much sweating and rheumatic pains

Bones of face painful to touch.

Erysipelatous swelling of cheeks in morning.

Nettlerash eruption on face.

❚Humid herpes, especially on face.
❚Eruptions scurfy and very painful to touch.
❚Crusty pimples on face of young people.
❚Boils very painful to touch.
❚Lupoid ulceration of face, intolerance of touch, every
    breath of air caused pain.
⁹ **Lower Face.** ❚❚Great swelling of upper lip, painful to
    touch, but otherwise only tense.
❚Sore smarting pimple on vermilion border of upper lip.
❚Middle of lower lip cracked.
❚Eruption, with sensation of heat in corners of mouth.
❚Ulcer at corner of mouth.
❚Hydroa around mouth. θTertian ague.
❚Itching around mouth.
❚Red, itching spot beneath lower lip, soon becoming cov-
    ered with many yellow blisters, which change to a scurf.
❚Boils on lips and chin, very painful to touch.
❙❙White blisters on lips, chin and neck.
❚Itching pimples on chin.
❚Acute inflammation of r. parotid gland; threatened sup-
    puration; a few pimples appeared on face
❚High fever, eyes inflamed and half open; involuntary
    discharges from bowels and bladder; great restlessness.
    θParotitis after scarlet fever.
❚Fungous growth on inferior maxillary, with necrosis.
¹⁰ **Teeth and Gums.** ❚Throbbing pain as if blood were en-
    tering tooth, or a drawing pain; pains < after eating
    and in a warm room, or at night.
❚Toothache in all teeth, immediately after drinking cold
    things, or opening mouth.
❚Toothache, < in warm room, and when biting teeth
    together.
❚Hollow teeth feel too long and painful.
❚Loose molar teeth; mouth sore; breath offensive; small
    aphthæ on gums and roof of mouth.
❚Looseness of teeth; gums tender.
❚❚Gums and mouth very painful to touch, bleed easily.
❚Gums ulcerated, tender and painful.
❚❚Mercurio-syphilitic diseases of gums.
¹¹ **Taste and Tongue.** Taste: putrid; sour; metallic; bitter;
    of rotten eggs in morning.
❚Bitterness in back of throat, with natural taste of food.
❚Coating on back of tongue resembling dry clay.
❚Tip of tongue very painful, and feels sore.
❚❚Hasty speech.
¹² **Inner Mouth.** ❚Offensive odor from mouth, as from disor-
    dered stomach, which he himself notices.
❚White aphthous pustules on inside of lips and cheeks and
    on tongue.

ⁱⁱThrush < on inside of lower lip.

▌Ulcers on gums and in mouth, base resembling lard.

¹⁵ **Throat.** ▌Elongated flabby uvula, with tickling sensation in back of throat and enlargement and inflammation of mucous follicles.

ⁱⁱRoughness of fauces.

▌Swollen tonsils and hard glandular swellings on neck, with sticking, when swallowing, coughing, breathing, or turning neck.

▌Sore throat; tonsils so much swollen as to leave no opening visible; pulse high, about 100; intense pain, could neither speak, move nor swallow; extreme uneasiness. θQuinsy.

▌Tonsils enlarged, red; throat and pharynx raw, and studded over with enlarged reddish follicles; could not venture out in slightest damp without being in fear of inflammation of throat, which at last produced a nervous sort of terror of being choked; incapacitated from work, as the damp from the clay affects him with hoarseness and irritability of chest.

▌Tonsillitis recurring regularly every two or three years; difficult deglutition; severe pain; r. tonsil particularly red and swollen; twenty days after beginning of attack pus is discharged.

▌▌Chronic tonsillitis, especially when accompanied by hardness of hearing.

▌Dryness of throat.

▌Scraping in throat when swallowing saliva.

▌Scraping sore throat, impeding speech but not swallowing.

▌Smarting, rawness and scraping in throat, < swallowing solid food.

▌Violent pressure in throat, believes that it is quite constricted and that she must suffocate.

▌Pain in throat, on swallowing, as from an intense swelling; sensation as if he had to swallow over a swelling.

▌A feeling in throat as of a plug of mucus or an internal swelling at entrance of throat.

▌Sticking in throat, extending to ear on turning head.

▌▌Sticking in throat as from a splinter, on swallowing, extending towards ear on yawning.

▌Stitches in throat, extending to ear, < when swallowing food.

▌Sore ulcerative pain in throat as of a splinter, very severe from afternoon to midnight, preventing sleep.

▌▌Sensation as if a fish bone or splinter were sticking in throat.

ⁱHawking up of mucus.

▌After violent inflammation of throat when there still remains some redness, dryness and swelling of mucous membranes.

¹⁴ **Appetite, Thirst. Desires, Aversions.** ıı Unusual hunger in forenoon.

ıı Excessive thirst from morning till evening.

ı Craving for condiments, sour, highly flavored, pungent articles.

ıı Great desire for vinegar.

ı Longing: for acids; wine; sour and strong tasting things.

ı Appetite for something at times, and when he gets it he does not like it.

ı Aversion to fat.

¹⁵ **Eating and Drinking.** ıı Strong and comfortable feeling after a meal.

ıı Child seems to be better after eating.

ı Heaviness and pressure in stomach after moderate eating.

ıı Hasty speech and hasty drinking.

Better from tobacco.

¹⁶ **Hiccough, Belching, Nausea and Vomiting.** ı Constant sensation of water rising in œsophagus, as if she had eaten sour things

ıı Eructations frequent, odorless and tasteless.

ı Fetid eructations, with sensation of burning in throat.

ı Eructations after eating.

ı Hot, sour regurgitation of food.

ı Heartburn.

ı Inclination to vomit, with flow of saliva from mouth.

ıı Frequent but momentary attacks of nausea.

ı Attacks of nausea, with coldness and paleness.

ı Vomiting of green, acrid water.

ı Sour vomiting.

Vomiting of bile, in morning, after long, violent retching.

ıı Vomiting every morning.

¹⁷ **Scrobiculum and Stomach.** ıı A feeling of hard body in epigastrium, immediately followed by hæmoptysis.

ı Tension across pit of stomach; is obliged to loosen his clothes, and then cannot tolerate sitting.

ı Empty sinking feeling of stomach, > by eating.

ıı Pressure in stomach after moderate eating, as if lead were in it.

ı Pressure and pain in stomach, > by eating, eructation, and by passing flatus.

ı Frequent desire to loosen clothing about stomach after a meal.

ı Dull aching pain in stomach after moderate eating.

ı Stomach painful when walking, as if it hung loose.

ıı Drawing pain from region of stomach to back.

ı Burning in stomach.

∎Gnawing in stomach, as from acids, which also rise up into throat.

∎Acrid feeling in stomach during digestion.

∎Distension of pit of stomach, has to loosen clothing.

∎Swelling and pressure in region of stomach.

∎Stomach frequently and easily disordered.

∎Stomach inclined to be out of order; longing for sour or strong tasting things.

∎Indigestion with burning pain in stomach and up œsophagus, palpitation of heart when pain is severe.

∎Indigestion characterized by eructation of quantities of wine, especially in nervous persons, with craving for condiments.

∎Dyspepsia of herpetic and hemorrhoidal subjects, with flatulency and even tympanitis.

[18] **Hypochondria.** ∣∣Sticking in hepatic region when walking.

∎Stitches: in region of liver; in region of spleen, when walking.

∎Hepatitis with jaundice, stools white or greenish.

∎Frequent bilious attacks especially in Spring and Autumn; engorgement of liver with jaundice; lassitude, inability for work, want of appetite and obstinate constipation; everything, even cold water, has a bitter taste; skin and sclerotic yellow; urine dark; stools whitish; over-fatigue or chill in damp weather brings on attacks of white, frothy diarrhœa; exposure to rays of July sun followed by intense colic which was > by copious and perfectly white stools; paroxysms of ungovernable irritability; enlargement of l. lobe of liver; in Autumn attacks are accompanied by great sexual weakness; is extremely sensitive in change of weather to rain; predicts the approach of rain; very sensitive to damp winds.

∎Liver enlarged, extending two or three inches beyond ribs; every kind of food disagrees; chronic constipation; skin dirty yellow, like the hue of malignant disease; uterus enlarged and anteverted with congestion of ovaries; coitus intolerable; ovum could not be retained. θAfter abuse of mercury.

∎Hepatogenous jaundice, mercurial history.

∎Chronic engorgement of liver.

∎∎Hepatic abscesses.

∎During inflammatory process in cirrhosis of liver.

[19] **Abdomen.** ∎∎Abdomen distended, tense.

∎Abdomen swollen and somewhat tender.

∎Rumbling in abdomen.

∣∣Fermentation above navel, with eructation of hot air.

∎Sensation of soreness, as if bruised, in abdomen, morning.

∎Contractive pain in abdomen.

ı ıSpasmodic contraction in abdomen.

ıCutting pains in abdomen.

ıClawing in umbilical region, extending from both sides
of abdomen towards middle, and sometimes up to pit of
stomach, causing nausea, with anxious heat of cheeks,
by paroxysms; almost like the effects of taking cold, or
the preliminaries of menstruation.

ıColic, with dry, rough cough.

ı ıDeep, circumscribed swelling in ileo-cæcal region; lies
on back, with r. knee drawn up.

ı ıDecreased peristaltic motion.

ıMesenteric tubercles.

ıChronic abdominal affections.

ı ıSwelling and suppuration of inguinal glands.

²⁰ **Stool and Rectum.** ıStools: white and fetid, child has a
sour smell; sour smelling and whitish; clay colored;
green, slimy, of sour smell; light yellow fecal; greenish;
black; thin or papescent; watery; undigested; painless.

Diarrhœa: < during day; after eating, and after drinking
cold water; with colic; with every cutting of teeth; in
morning; colliquative.

ı ıCholera infantum from irritation of teeth, chiefly with
morning aggravation.

ıDysenteric stools; difficult evacuation of soft stool or of
bloody mucus with tenesmus.

ıChronic diarrhœa: after abuse of mercury or quinine;
after suppression of scabies.

ı ıStools soft, yet passed with great exertion.

ı ı Difficult expulsion of a small quantity of soft excrement
with great efforts and tenesmus.

ıSluggishness and inactivity of bowels, in consequence of
which abdominal muscles must bear down in order to
effect an evacuation.

ıConstipation: stools hard and dry; with eruption in bend
of elbows, or in popliteal space, from congestion and in-
action of rectum.

Before stool: pinching in abdomen.

During stool: abdominal pain, straining, pressing, rumbling and nauseous feeling in abdomen; succus prostaticus; heat in hands and cheeks; inclination to lie down.

After stool: sore pain in anus and sanious secretion; soreness of rectum with ichor; tympanitis; obstruction of
nose.

ıBurning in rectum, swelling of anus.

ı ıCreeping in rectum.

ıPromotes speedy suppuration in periproctitis, the swelling being hard and inflamed.

ıProlapsus of rectum, which protruded at every stool about

two inches, with slight oozing of blood; bowel very
difficult to return; engorgement of veins but no distinct
piles; mercurial history.
❙Hemorrhoids from engorgement of liver, with great ab-
dominal distress; preventing abdominal respiration.
❙Hemorrhoids with engorged liver from abuse of mercury.
❙Inflammation and suppuration of hemorrhoidal tumors.
❙Hemorrhage from rectum, with soft stool.
❙Sweat on perineum.

²¹ Urinary Organs. ❙Pain in kidneys with constant urging
to urinate, later purulent sediment in urine; emaciated;
renal region sensitive to slightest touch; incessant, painful urging to urinate, voiding of few drops of purulent
urine; violent fever with unquenchable thirst; colliquative diarrhœa and night sweats. *θ*Kidney disease.
❙Croupous nephritis passing into suppurative stage, with
fever, chills, alternating with burning heat.
❙Albuminuria accompanying and following diphtheria.
❙Enuresis; hot, acrid discharge; head thrown back during sleep.
❙❙Micturition impeded; is obliged to wait awhile before
urine passes, and then it flows slowly.
❙❙Weakness of bladder; urine drops vertically down, is
obliged to wait awhile before any passes.
❙Urine passed tardily and without force, feels as if bladder
could not be emptied thoroughly.
❙❙Is never able to finish urinating; it seems as though
some urine always remains behind in bladder.
❙Painful micturition.
❙Urine: dark red and hot; bloody; sharp, burning, corroding prepuce and pudenda; dark yellow, scalding
whilst discharged; brown red, the last drops mixed with
blood; blood red; pale, clear, on standing, turbid and
thick, and deposits a white sediment; pale, with floccu-
lent, muddy sediment; milky, turbid, even while pass-
ing, with a white sediment.
❙Greasy pellicle on urine, or glistening with various colors.
During urination: sensation in r. shoulder-blade as if
something were running or creeping.
 ❙❙Burning and soreness in urethra.
Stitches in urethra.
❙Inflammation and redness of orifice of urethra.
❙Discharge of mucus from urethra.
❙Wetting the bed at night.

²² Male Sexual Organs. ❙Sexual desire increased, but erec-
tions feeble.
 ❙❙Diminished sexual instinct; feeble erections.
❙Nocturnal emissions; sudden appearance of furuncles;

attacks of blindness during day; waterbrash, with brown coated tongue.

❙Discharge of prostatic fluid, also after micturition and during hard stool.

❙Prostatitis.

❙Discharge of mucus from urethra.

❙Ulcer similar to a chancre, externally on prepuce.

❙Chancres not painful but disposed to bleed readily.

❙Easily bleeding chancres with lardaceous edges and fetid discharge.

❙Chancres secreting watery pus with diffuse borders and red bottoms, elevated above surface.

❙Mercurialized chancres.

❙Itching on penis and at frænum preputii.

❙Phimosis with discharge of pus, accompanied by throbbing.

❙Figwarts, smelling like old cheese or herring brine.

❙Herpes præputialis; small vesicles in groups, whitish, with red bases, and intolerable itching of parts; eruption exceedingly sensitive to touch.

❙Long standing hydrocele; large swelling of scrotum, containing dark, thick fluid; throbbing in scrotum.

❙Large bubo, stony hard, in r. groin. θSyphilis.

❙Bubo in l. groin as large as a hen's egg, stony hard.

❙❙Buboes after mercurial treatment.

❙Scrofulous buboes.

❙❙Humid soreness on genitals, scrotum, and folds between scrotum and thigh.

❙Secondary syphilis.

❚ **Female Sexual Organs.** ❙Uterus enlarged and anteverted, with congestion of ovaries; coitus intolerable; frequent abortions.

❙Uterine ulcers, with bloody suppuration, smelling like old cheese; edges of ulcer sensitive, frequently a pulsative sensation in ulcers.

❙Metritis, with burning, throbbing pains.

❙Congestion of blood to uterus.

❙Hemorrhage from uterus.

❙Menorrhagia, in women with chapped skin and rhagades of hands and feet.

❙Menses delayed and too scanty.

Before menses: constricting headache.

During menses: itching of vulva.

❙❙Discharge of blood between menses.

❙Discharge of white, yellowish, or discolored pus, attended with fetid smell, particularly when occasioned by scrofulous leucorrhœa, or after repeated attacks.

❙Leucorrhœa, with smarting of vulva.

ǀǀPruritus pudendi during menses.

ǀMastitis in hysterical and nervous patients; pain as if in bones of arms and thighs; suppuration preceded by frequent crawls in affected part, which remains hard, with scanty discharge.

ǀScirrhous ulcer on mamma, with stinging burning of edges, smelling like old cheese.

ǀMuch itching, or little pimples around ulcer on mammæ.

ǀItching nipples.

²⁴ **Pregnancy. Parturition. Lactation.** ǀǀFrequent momentary attacks of nausea.

ǀMammæ swollen, not sensitive to touch, but she cannot walk up or down stairs.

ǀCancer of breast, with stinging burning of edges; smells like old cheese.

ǀLittle pimples, or smooth ulcers, surround scirrhous, or principal ulceration.

²⁵ **Voice and Larynx. Trachea and Bronchia.** ǀWeakness of organs of speech and of chest, she cannot speak aloud.

ǀHoarseness, roughness in throat.

ǀObstinate hoarseness; scraping in throat causing rough, barking cough; voice toneless, weak; scarcely audible in evening; pale swelling of tonsils and uvula; lassitude in limbs.

ǀHoarseness, grating, irritation in larynx or lower part of fauces; mucous râles.

ǀǀSensation of down in larynx.

ǀScraping in larynx.

ǀPressure beneath larynx, immediately after supper, as if something were sticking in throat.

ǀPain in one spot of larynx, < by pressure, speech, cough and breathing.

ǀǀSensitiveness of larynx to cold air.

ǀWheezing in larynx, and painfulness of a small spot in larynx.

ǀSudden attacks of suffocation; child looks anxiously about and attempts to cry without being able to do so; loud, whistling inspiration; face dark red; lips bluish; bends head back and gasps for breath; after attacks have lasted ten minutes, they end with a whistling, crowing sound, and are followed by hoarseness.

ǀSpasmodic croup; violent fever, face indicating great anguish; weeping; restless; cough hoarse and rough without sputa.

ǀLies with head thrown back, buried in pillow, face swollen, neck stretched; mucous and sibilant râles; clucking noise in glottis; respiration noisy; cough loud and harsh, with distinct croupy tone; exhaustion; pulse 140, hard and full. *θ*Croup.

∎Assumes a sitting posture, on account of anxiety which sets in when lying down; somnolence, with restless tossing about; respiration snoring, hoarse, whistling, and often so short and oppressed that he starts from sleep with violent, dry, hoarse cough, which causes retching; grasps at larynx, in the greatest fear; begins to cry; red face, protruding eyes, and frequent throwing back of head; after several minutes the paroxysms again return; frequent drinking; great heat; sweat; pulse quick and hard; hasty speech; frequent passages of dark urine. *θ*Croup.

∎Respiration somewhat whistling; on every inspiration great retraction of diaphragm, abdominal muscles and ribs, so that a large concavity is formed; hoarse cough, occasionally croupy in tone; voice hoarse, at times entirely lost; clammy sweat on head, rest of body dry and hot; color of face changing constantly; pulse hard, cannot be counted; tossing about, or sits up hastily. *θ*Croup.

∎Croup with great dryness of larynx and respiratory passages, whistling respiration, dry cough with ineffectual retching, nothing but a slight quantity of frothy saliva being discharged; cough ending with a short sneeze.

∎Lies upon his mother's arm with head thrown back, mouth open, bluish redness of face, protruding eyes; body bathed in sweat; fearful anxiety and dyspnœa; cannot speak. *θ*Croup.

∎Frequently recurring paroxysms of violent croupy cough with great dyspnœa, grasps at larynx; great thirst; pulse 120; respiration anxious and noisy. *θ*Croup.

∎∎Croup after exposure to dry, cold wind, with swelling below larynx; great sensitiveness to cold air; red face, high fever, hoarseness and rattling of moist mucus, which child is unable to get rid of, but still little or no difficulty in breathing; after midnight or towards morning; sensation as if there was a fishbone in throat, or of internal swelling, when swallowing.

∎Croup: with deep, rough, barking cough, hoarseness or loss of voice with slight suffocating spasms, some rattling of mucus; with swelling below larynx; with great sensitiveness to cold air or water; cough < before midnight, or toward morning.

∎Croupy cough, with continual hoarseness.

∎Catarrhal croup with or without fever.

∎Croup, when panaritiæ, anginæ, urticaria or erysipelas prevail.

❙Light attacks of croup in teething children.

❚Violent attacks of croup from time to time, as if suffocation or vomiting would ensue.

❚After influenza violent attack of croup; restless; tossing back of head; anxious, sawing, metallic cough.

❚Violent respiratory efforts, during which chest scarcely moves; anxious throwing back of head; convulsive twitchings; irritation of gums and Schneiderian membrane; vomiting of mucus, mixed with portions of membrane. θCroup.

❚Much green mucus in larynx.

❚Severe laryngeal catarrh, with roughness and pain in upper part of throat; sensation as of a clot of mucus or internal swelling when swallowing; stitches and pain extending from ear to ear.

❚Laryngeal catarrh, grafted on an organism of tubercular disposition; scanty, tenacious, muco-purulent secretion, with difficulty of expectoration; hoarseness remains some time.

❚Acute catarrh of larynx and bronchi with tickling and roughness in larynx, and hoarseness or aphonia; also acute catarrh of lungs with scratching, tickling sensation in air tubes, pressure and heaviness under sternum, and frequent, dry, tearing cough; rough, whistling, respiratory sounds, indicating a dry condition of mucous membranes; such inflammations are usually of long duration; constant oppression of chest and irritation to cough, which become < by long continued and fatiguing coughing, finally gasping for breath, and expectorating very little sputa; < sitting and bending over, must lean back or get up and walk about; < breathing cool air.

❚After catching cold, cough next day, tickling and dryness in air passages, followed by hoarseness and finally aphonia; redness and swelling of posterior wall of pharynx; rough, whistling sound in trachea, extending to large bronchi; larynx and trachea sensitive to touch; on forced inspiration stitching in larynx and cough.

❚Chronic tracheitis (the beginning of tracheal or laryngo-tracheal phthisis); voice hoarse, and if exerted for any length of time accompanied by stitching pain in larynx; in morning on rising, severe cough with stitching pain in larynx and scanty expectoration of mucus; when walking, particularly against wind, and when eating warm food, stitching and burning in throat; no fever.

❚Tracheal and bronchial inflammation in children, with continual fever and headache, difficult, short, anxious breathing, hoarse voice, violent, dry, painful, alternating rough and hollow sounding cough, < by eating and drinking anything cold, by cold air, talking or crying.

^x Respiration. ▮Breathing: rattling; anxious, wheezing; frequent deep breaths, like after running; anxious, short,
wheezing, threatening to suffocate; must bend head
back and sit up.

Involuntary deep inspirations.

▮Attacks of asthma, awaking patient from sleep, face becomes blue, saliva increased; sensation as of dust in
lungs; smoking and throwing head back >; after attack, expectoration frothy.

▮Difficult respiration, preventing sleep at night; whistling,
wheezing, with copious mucous expectoration; just as
he has fallen asleep is aroused and startled by threatened suffocation; must get up to relieve dyspnœa; >
during day. θAsthma after suppressed eruption of skin.

▮Suffocative attacks, compelling him to raise himself up
and bend the head backwards.

ı ıDyspnœa.

^x Cough. ▮Spasmodic cough in paroxysms, with titillation in
larynx and efforts of vomiting.

▮Violent, deep cough, consisting of several impulses which
strike painfully against larynx and occasion retching.

▮Almost uninterrupted cough, from tickling in upper part
of l. side of throat, < talking and stooping, constantly
getting < till late in evening, and then suddenly
ceasing.

▮Titillation, as from dust in throat, inducing cough, which
is deep, wheezing; expectoration only in morning of
mucus, bloody or like pus, generally tasting sour or
sweet.

▮Chronic laryngeal cough, very distressing, especially at
night, compelling her to spring up in bed, from a feeling
of choking or suffocation.

▮Deep, dry cough, with obstructed breathing on inspiring,
and pain in top of chest at every cough.

▮Dry cough, < taking deep inspiration, or speaking any
length of time; roughness in throat; pressure under
sternum; difficult respiration; pressive headache.

▮Suffocative cough, simply caused by tightness of breath.

ı ıSubdued cough from oppression of chest.

▮Dry cough with tightness of chest and sore throat.

▮Deep, dull, whistling cough, in evening without, in morning with expectoration of masses of mucus, purulent
and bloody, sour, or of a sweet taste and offensive odor.

▮Deep, dry, wheezing, hoarse cough; bloody, pus-like, mucous expectoration; rheumatic pains in limbs and joints;
pulse hard, full, acelerated, and at times intermitting;
symptoms < at night and from cold air; > by wrapping up and keeping warm. θChest troubles succeeding repelled itch.

▮Cough so aggravated by deep breathing that it caused vomiting.

▮Troublesome hacking cough as soon as he was about to fall asleep, continuing all night, coughs even on shutting eyes; > during sleep; < 1 P.M. to 1 A.M. θTyphoid.

▮Dry, nervous cough all night.

▮▮Paroxysms of cough, as from taking cold, with excessive sensitiveness of nervous system, as soon as slightest portion of body becomes cold.

▮Coughs when any part of body is uncovered.

▮Cough < from exposure to chilly night air, and from drinking cold water.

▮Paroxysms of dry cough, in evening.

▮Hacking cough, immediately after eating.

▮The child cries when coughing.

▮Cough with expectoration during day, no expectoration at night.

▮▮Croup or cough from exposure to dry West wind.

▮▮Croupy cough, with rattling in chest, but without expectoration.

▮Rattling, choking, moist cough, depending on an organic or catarrhal basis; < towards morning and after eating.

▮Cough: croupish, hoarse; scraping, rough; suffocative; loose and choking; with bloody expectoration; whooping, croupish sound, pain in larynx, choking from mucus in larynx, < in morning; spasmodic; deep, wheezing; deep and dry; deep, dull, whistling; hacking; dry, nervous; barking, after measles.

Cough caused by: limb getting cold; eating or drinking; anything cold; cold air; lying in bed; talking; crying; drinking.

During cough: stitches, burning and swelling in throat; burning in chest and stomach; catching of breath; nausea, retching, vomiting; reverberation in head, throbbing in forehead and temples; dulness; sneezing; chills; anxiety and bending backwards of body in lying.

After cough: sneezing; crying.

▮▮Cough < from evening till midnight.

▮Abundant expectoration of tenacious mucus with relief to the rattling breathing.

▮Dirty yellowish, purulent, badly smelling expectoration.

²⁸ **Inner Chest and Lungs.** ▮Sensation as if hot water were floating in chest; as of drops of hot water in l. chest.

▮▮Soreness in chest.

▮▮Shattering shocks and soreness in chest. .

▮Weakness of chest; cannot talk, from weakness.

▮Spasmodic constriction of chest, after talking.

❙❙Stitching pain in r. side of chest, in direction of back.
❙❙Tenacious mucus in chest.
❙Constant rattling of mucus in chest of infants, threatening suffocation at times.
❙Extreme emaciation, skin cadaverous and dry, countenance of yellowish hue, eyes deeply sunken in sockets, dull and feverish; tongue dry and yellow in middle; thirst, disgust for food, distended epigastrium; hard stool; urine scanty, brownish red; night sweats; alternations of rigor and heat; pulse small, 136; sleeplessness on account of stitches in anterior, inferior and posterior part of chest to shoulder-blade; cough, internal uneasiness, fearful disposition; delirium of frightened character; great inclination to cry; lies immovable on r. side, with knees drawn up to chest; on r. hip-joint commencing bedsore; great fear of being touched, as every movement causes pain in chest, cough and dyspnœa; r. side of chest, arched like a barrel from axilla downwards; intercostal spaces prominent, motionless during respiration; dull sound to percussion; entire absence of respiratory sounds and vocal fremitus; dull sound on percussion over large surface at base of heart; heart's sounds and impulse diminished. θPleuritis with plastic exudation.
❙Pleurisy, croupous exudation, with a yellow or yellowish-brown tint in face, in scrofulous and lymphatic persons.
❙Pleurisy with fibrinous exudation.
❙Diaphragmitis (after *Bryon*.), in fibrinosis; promotes resorption.
❙❙Bronchitis.
❙On r. side of chest in nipple line, in fifth intercostal space, dull percussion sound and weak respiratory murmur; after coughing and profuse expectoration, there was on that place tympanitic percussion sound and bronchial breathing; other portions of chest revealed catarrhal symptoms; expectoration of dirty yellowish masses, badly smelling; respiration accelerated; no fever; cough < in morning. θBronchial catarrh.
❙Bronchitis from repelled eruptions.
❙Subacute catarrhal processes; characterized by incipient collection of glutinous, sticky mucus in air cells, giving rise to violent and suffocative paroxysms of coughing, often attended by retching preceding its expulsion.
❙❙Habitual bronchial catarrhs, with loud rattling of mucus.
❙Chronic catarrh of scrofulous subjects, especially when morbid process shows a tendency to invade pulmonary vesicles.

ꙥGreat emaciation; slight hectic fever; constantly troubled by cough, sometimes spasmodic, with purulent and fetid expectoration, diarrhœa and loss of appetite; r. side of thorax considerably hollowed, with perfectly empty sound on percussion, and intense bronchial respiration and slight râles; l. side abnormally bulging. θPleuro-pneumonia.

ꙥPneumonia, mild suppurative stage, extending only over small part of a lung, with lentescent fever.

ꙥPneumonia, during stage of resolution.

ꙥChronic pneumonia, with profuse purulent expectoration.

ꙥꙥPulmonary abscess; empyema; pyothorax.

ꙥPain in r. occipital protuberance; fluent, acrid, nasal coryza, swelling at root of nose, upper eyelid, upper lip; white ulcers in mouth; uvula elongated, pale; appetite for fat meat and sweet food; thirst for cold water at night; stomach distended after eating; eructations of fluid, then of food; more at night; constipation alternating with diarrhœa; cough constant, moist; moist râles in l. lung; feeble, vesicular respiration; upper part of l. side of thorax dilated backward; curvature of spine between shoulders; agonizing dyspnœa, could not lie in a recumbent position; cough constant from 12 M. till morning; sleeps with head thrown back, restless; the least exposure aggravates all the symptoms. θEmphysema.

ꙥBronchiectasia.

ꙥIn tuberculosis when there is oppression of breathing; periodic stitches; cough before midnight and in morning, dry at first but finally accompanied by a serous expectoration containing small flocculi; occasionally patient will spring up and after coughing expectorate a mass as large as a pea which when crushed between fingers emits a carrion-like odor; in affected parts (particularly upper portions of chest) faint respiratory murmur, with percussion dulness.

ꙥTubercles of lungs in herpetic patients, especially after suppression of exanthems, in scrofulous and in hemorrhoidal subjects.

²⁹ **Heart, Pulse and Circulation.** ꙥPalpitation, with fine stitches in heart and l. half of chest.

ꙞꙞAnxious feeling of debility about heart with palpitation. θHypertrophy.

ꙥDyspnœa, pain in neck, faintness and inability to recline; dry, nervous cough, commencing towards evening and lasting all night. θAngina pectoris.

ꙥSequelæ of angina pectoris; dyspnœa after attack; dry, nervous cough from evening all through night; pain in

neck after attack; faintness and inability to recline after
attack.

I Pulse hard, full, accelerated; at times intermitting.

⁵⁰ **Outer Chest.** I Tettery eruption on chest.

I Suppurating pimples on sternum.

I I Ulcer on last rib of r. side.

⁵¹ **Neck and Back.** I Violent pulsation of carotids.

I Hard, glandular swellings around neck.

I Carbuncle on back of neck; surrounding tissues highly
inflamed and extremely sensitive to touch.

I Carbuncle on l. side of back, extending from upper border of scapula downward about six inches, surrounded
by small pustules; pus offensive and scanty; pain intense, depriving him of sleep; great weakness and prostration.

I Drawing between scapulæ.

Great weakness in whole of spine.

I Sensation as if bruised, in small of back and thighs.

I I Sharp pressure and pain, as from bruises; in small of
back and lumbar vertebra, especially in region of sacro-
iliac symphysis, extending into lower limbs; the pain is
felt when sitting, standing or lying, and causes a sort
of limping when walking.

I Stitches and rheumatic pains in back.

I Blood boils on the back.

I I Red tubercle on r. buttock.

I I Boil on buttock.

⁵² **Upper Limbs.** I I Pain in shoulder as if a weight were resting on it.

I Suppuration of axillary glands.

I Offensive sweat in axillæ.

I Tearing in arms, extending toward the suppuration in
breast.

I I Pain as if bruised in os humeri.

I Encysted tumor or steatoma at point of elbow.

I Violent itching in bend of elbow.

I I Intensely violent itching in bends of elbows, on hands,
wrists and in palms.

I Carbuncle, size of silver half-dollar, on forearm; very
painful, with three spots, like boils, near it.

Swelling of r. hand.

I I Itching, with rough, dry, shrivelled or scaling skin on
hands.

I I Itching in palms.

I Red and hot swelling of joints of hands and fingers.

Swelling of fingers of both hands, with stiffness, while
lying.

I Cold perspiration of hands.

❚Fingers as if dead.

❚Tingling in tips of fingers.

❚Corrosive blister on thumb, stinging when pressed.

❚Thumb livid; violent throbbing, cutting, burning pain; lymphatics inflamed; lump in axilla.

❚Whitlow in palmar surface of ungual phalanx of r. thumb; skin yellow, matter could be seen and felt under it; throbbing, burning pain; cannot bear weight of poultice; pain kept her awake.

❚Inside of r. thumb swollen, livid, with beating, cutting, burning pain, so violent that it drove her to madness.

❚Whitlow on middle finger of r. hand; severe throbbing pain in last joint; hard, red, swollen state of pulp; lymphatics of arm inflamed, lump in axilla; fever and irritation.

❚❚Whitlow; violent, throbbing, "gathering pain;" accelerates suppuration.

❚Whitlows occurring every winter for several years.

❚Panaritium.

❚After injury, suppuration of middle joint of r. index finger; whole finger involved in phlegmonous inflammation.

❚Superficial erysipelatous inflammation around root of nail.

❚Onychia.

³³ **Lower Limbs.** ❚Left hip pains as if sprained, when walking in open air.

❚❚Buttocks and posterior thighs painful when sitting.

❚Hip disease, suppurative stage, patient wants to be tightly covered.

❚Caries of hip-joint.

❚Sensation of soreness in thighs.

❚❚Bruised pain in anterior muscles of thighs.

❚Raised, flat, purplish swelling on l. thigh; it had a doughy feel for a space larger than a silver dollar; small openings; pus ichorous; for a considerable distance around was red, swollen and painful, with two prominent, indurated and painful spots, like boils; pain intense, no sleep for several nights; when this had healed, a second carbuncle, or at least a flat, purplish and painful swelling showed itself, about six inches from first, which *Hepar* healed without suppuration.

❚Carbuncle of r. thigh, nearly three inches in diameter; had it for a week; exceedingly painful and leg swollen; no evidence of boils or pustules; several openings and centre looking gangrenous.

❚Knee pains as if bruised.

❚❚Swelling of knee.

❚Severe pains in lower extremities; pain described as a

terrible corroding itching "as from salt water;" both legs
swollen round ankles, with watery discharge; color of
legs either red or bluish.

ı ıCramp in calves.

ıSwelling of feet around ankles, with difficult breathing.

ıAfter catching cold, pains in foot as after taking a misstep; pains occasionally wander up to thigh; no redness
nor swelling; depression of mind.

ıTickling in soles of feet.

ıCramps: in soles and toes.

ıPricking in both heels.

ı ıColdness of feet.

ıCracked skin of feet.

ıTingling in toes.

ıBurning, stinging pains in toes.

ıViolent stitch extending into great toe.

³⁴ Limbs in General. ıWeakness in limbs; they feel bruised.

ıDrawing pains in limbs, especially in morning, when
awaking.

ıMercurial rheumatism, especially in scrofulous subjects;
tearing and shooting in limbs and joints, < at night,
especially during a chill; excessive nervous excitability,
so that all impressions on body or mind cause internal
trembling.

ıRheumatic pains in limbs and stitches in joints.

ıDry, herpetic eruption in bends of joints, greatly itching.

ıChapped skin and rhagades of hands and feet.

ıThe limb upon which the ulcer has healed cannot bear
its own weight by suspension.

ıContinued dull itching of soles of feet and palms of hands.

³⁵ Rest. Position. Motion. Rest: cold perspiration >.

Lies immovably on r. side with knees drawn up to chest.

Side on which he lies becomes painfully sore, must change
his position.

Lies with head thrown back to escape suffocation.

Lying in bed: causes cough; pain in back and limbs.

Lies on back with r. knee drawn up.

Inclination to lie down.

Inability to recline; could not lie in recumbent position.

Head thrown back, sitting up >.

Sitting: cannot tolerate it from tension of stomach; acute
catarrh of larynx <; pain in back and limbs; buttocks
and posterior thighs pain; falls asleep.

Stooping: stitches in head; boring headache <; pressure
in head <; cough < from tickling in throat.

Standing up after sitting bent over: feeling of blindness.

Rising: pressure in head >; feeling of blindness; great
difficulty from feeling of stiffness of limbs.

Moving: pressure in eyes; headache during fever.

Shaking head: headache.

From slightest motion: sweats easily.

Every movement: causes pain in chest.

Walking: stomach painful; stitches in region of liver; >
catarrh of larynx; against wind, itching and burning
in throat; pain in thigh, back. and lower limbs; causes
limping; in open air l. hip pains.

Cannot walk up and down stairs.

Exercise: cold perspiration <; attacks of debility <.

Springs up in bed: from cough.

Child throws itself about unconsciously.

³⁶ **Nerves.** ❚Disinclination for mental or bodily exertion.

❚Oversensitiveness to pain; fainting from slight pains.

Every impression upon body or mind is followed by trem-
ulousness.

Nervous trembling.

❚Excessive nervousness from abuse of mercury.

❚Trembling weakness, after tobacco smoking.

❚Daily attacks of indescribable sudden debility, commencing with a chilly and creeping sensation in r. leg,
traveling slowly upward to chest, with profuse perspiration on head; suddenly and soon after a feeling of
weakness, as if he was dying, with trembling of limbs
so that he is unable to stand or sit; consciousness retained; attack lasts two or three hours, when strength
gradually returns, coupled with a dull, pressing headache about vertex, which continues for some hours; <
in Summer, after cooling rains, and after bodily exertions and walking; about every four months scabby
eruption, moist at base, of yellowish color, on scalp and
forehead, as far down as eyes, and sometimes on chest.

❚General exhaustion.

❚Paroxysms of fainting in evening, preceded by vertigo.

❚Coldness of head, chiefly forehead; severe headaches, with
sensation of weight at back of eyeballs, and a feeling as
though eyes would be drawn back into head; stiffness
of nape of neck; on rising from seat great difficulty from
a feeling of stiffness of limbs; pain in bottom of back,
around waist, also around shoulders and nape of neck;
numbness of r. arm and hand; burning sensation from
pit of stomach to throat and ears, > by eating; fixed
coldness at pit of stomach, felt occasionally when burning sensation was not present; fatigue from least exercise. θSpinal irritation.

❚Cramp in l. hand which becomes spasmodically closed,
with formication and creeping up arm, extending to
throat, with sensation as if something was sticking there

and that he would choke; face bluish red; mouth drawn
to l. side; complete consciousness; after half-hour,
another, less violent attack, accompanied by tickling in
arm and paralysis of l. side; after four weeks a very
violent attack occurred followed by complete paralysis
of arms and legs, so that he could not move; lameness
of tongue, speech unintelligible. *θ*After suppressed
eruption and abuse of mercury.

▮Traumatic convulsions, caused by excessive pressure on
brain during delivery; trismus of newborn babes.

▮Paralysis from suppressed eruptions, or after mercurial
poisoning.

³⁷ Sleep. So sleepy and fatigued, in evening, that he falls
asleep while sitting.

Great, irresistible inclination to sleep in evening; must lie
down immediately after supper and sleeps till morning.

▮Sleepiness during day, < toward evening, with frequent,
almost spasmodic yawning.

| |Restless, soporous slumber, with head bent backwards.

▮Side on which he lies at night becomes painfully sore;
must change his position.

| |Fright during sleep.

▮Starts from sleep, feeling as if about to suffocate.

| |Violent starts, when falling asleep.

| |Loss of sleep after midnight.

| |Excess of thoughts prevent sleep, after midnight.

| |Wakes at night, with erection and desire to urinate.

| |Dreams: anxious; of fire.

³⁸ Time. Morning: vertigo; on awakening pressure in head
as from a nail; burning and itching of scalp; violent
itching of humid eruption on head; heat in eyes on
awaking; lids and angles agglutinated; lids closed;
nose stopped up; heat of face; erysipelatous swelling
of cheeks; putrid taste; excessive thirst from morning
till evening; vomiting of bile; sensation of soreness in
abdomen; chronic tracheitis; expectoration only; rattling, choking moist cough <; croupy cough <;
eczema. <.

2 A.M.: chill.

Day: pressing and drawing in temples; diarrhœa; attacks
of blindness; dyspnœa >; cough with expectoration;
sleepiness; chill; sweats easily; restless; stools <.

From 4 P.M. all night: heat, delirium, thirst.

From 4 to 8 P.M.: febrile chill.

7 P.M.: heat of face.

8 P. M.: violent chill.

Evening: great anxiety; vertigo with nausea; fainting;
aching in vertex; meditates suicide; lids swollen; pain

in eyes; swellings on lids painful; voice almost inaudible; cough < till late; deep whistling cough; dry cough; cough < till midnight; cough commencing toward evening and lasting all night; irresistible inclination to sleep.

Night: violent headache; sensation as if skull would burst wakes him; pressure in head; cold perspiration <; photophobia and lachrymation <, about 2 or 3 A.M.; lids swollen; vision of colored and dim halos around candle; eyes closed by swelling; sour smelling sweat; spasmodically closed eyelids; pain in nose lasts far into night; heat of face; toothache <; wetting bed; difficult respiration prevents sleep; chronic laryngeal cough; deep wheezing cough <; dry, nervous cough; thirst for cold water; eructations <; wakes with erection and desire to urinate; febrile chill; pain <; dry heat of body; sweat; sleepless; restless; pains in tumors <; burning and throbbing in ulcers.

Midnight: aching in forehead till morning; croup < before; cough constant from 12 M. till morning; loss of sleep after midnight; excess of thought prevents sleep; sweat before midnight.

³⁰ Temperature and Weather. Exquisite sensitiveness to open air.

Better from warmth; desire to be warmly covered, even during hot weather or in a warm place; < from wrapping up warmly.

❙❙Cannot bear to be uncovered; coughs when any part of body is uncovered.

❙❙Ailments from West or Northwest wind (dry, cold wind), or soon after it; improved by warmth.

❙❙Great chilliness in open air.

❙Extremely sensitive to cold air; must be wrapped up to face even in hot weather; cannot bear to be uncovered.

Warmth: cold perspiration >; pains in eyes >; ears >; neuralgia >; pains in malar bones >; toothache <; cough >; chilliness >; nettlerash >.

Covering head warmly: > soreness of head.

Patient with hip disease wants to be warmly covered.

Summer: attacks of debility <.

Dry weather: pain in nose >.

Air: eyes sensitive; eyes < from draught; interior of nose painful and sensitive.

Open air: lancinating headache >; neuralgia of face <; pains in malar bones <; l. hip pains as if bruised when walking; sensitive to; great chilliness in open air.

Least exposure < all symptoms; chill returns.

Dampness: < throat; overfatigue or chill in damp weather brings on attacks of white frothy diarrhœa.

On approach of rain: pains in nose <.
Damp winds: sensitive to.
After cooling rains: attacks of debility <.
Changeable weather: pain in nose <.
Cool air: acute catarrh of larynx <; cough <.
Cold: pain in eyes <; **great** sensitiveness; cough <; any
   part of body exposed causes cough; skin very sensitive;
   pains in tumors.
Cold air: deep, wheezing cough <; least draught causes
   catarrh.
Cold drink: causes toothache; cough <; causes cough.
Dry, cold wind: causes croup.
Exposure to chilly night: cough <.

⁴⁰ Fever. ❙❙Sensitiveness to open air, with chilliness and frequent nausea.
   ❙Great chilliness in open air; must get to warm stove;
   heat feels agreeable but does not relieve.
   ❙❙Desire to be covered even in a warm room.
   ❙Internal chill, with weariness and soreness in all the
   limbs.
   ❙Internal shivering from below upwards.
   ❙Violent shaking chill with chattering of teeth, icy cold-
   ness and paleness of face, hands and feet, unconscious-
   ness and coma.
   ❙Violent chill every morning, at 6 or 7 o'clock, without
   subsequent heat.
   ❙Chill during day, alternating with heat and photophobia.
   ❙Excessive shivering followed by feverishness.
   ❙Chill at 2 A.M., with febrile shivering and hot, dry skin.
   ❙Febrile chill from 4 to 8 P.M., or in night, could not get
   warm, with aggravation of all complaints; without sub-
   sequent heat.
   ❙Pain < during febrile chill at night.
   ❙Nightly chill in bed, with aggravation of all complaints.
   ❙❙Nettlerash, with violent itching and stinging, disap-
   pears as heat begins.
   ❙Burning, febrile heat, with almost unquenchable thirst,
   distressing headache and slight delirium, lasting from
   4 P.M. all night, without chilliness.
   ❙Violent fever with flushing heat in face and head.
   ❙Dry heat of body at night, with sweaty hands, which can-
   not tolerate being uncovered.
   ❙Dry burning heat, with redness of face and violent thirst,
   all night.
   ❙Fever blisters around mouth during pyrexia.
   ❙During heat larynx much affected, hoarse, weak voice.
   ❙❙Morning fever preceded by bitter taste in mouth, re-
   turning twice a day.
   ❙❙Fever, without chill, 4 P.M., lasting all night.

▮Heat very slight in comparison with chill.
▮Flushes of heat, with sweat.
▮Patient sweats easily from least exertion and turns pale, afterwards burning redness of face and heat and dryness of palms of hands.
▮Sweats easily during day, from every exertion of mind or after slight motion.
▮▮Sweats easily, by every, even slight motion.
▮Frequent breaking out of sweat over body, only momentary and without heat.
▮Sweat on perineum, groins and inside of thighs.
▮▮Cold, clammy, frequently sour, offensive smelling sweat.
▮Night or morning sweat, with thirst.
▮Sweats day and night, without relief; or first can't sweat at all, and then sweats profusely.
▮Profuse, sour smelling sweat at night.
▮▮Sweat before midnight.
▮Itching nettlerash precedes paroxysm; chill of three hours' duration followed by heat; during fever headache when moving; loss of consciousness preceded by vertigo; bitter taste in mouth; white coated tongue; vomiting of food; pain and rumbling in abdomen; then follows sweat which covers whole body; thirst in all stages. *θ*Tertian ague.
▮Paroxysm preceded by an itching urticaria; chill; fever with thirst, diarrhœa, rumbling in abdomen, bilious vomiting, formication in arms and dark urine; by the time fever has passed eruption has disappeared. *θ*Quotidian ague.
▮One hour before chill, thirst; after chill, fine, stinging nettlerash, with bleeding at nose, bitter taste in mouth, and greenish diarrhœa; chill followed by heat with sweat and discharge of reddish urine; during termination of latter stage eruption disappeared; during apyrexia great debility, yellow color of face. *θ*Tertian intermittent.
▮Chill generally in evening, preceded by bitter taste in mouth; itching, stinging nettlerash before and during chill, when he constantly desires to be covered; sweat and from the least uncovering chill again.
▮Violent chill, 8 P.M., with chattering of teeth; hands and feet cold; followed by heat with perspiration, especially on chest and forehead, with slight thirst.
▮After catching cold, heat and sweat, with thirst; pain in l. hypochondrium and arm; sweats again at night. *θ*Tertian ague.
▮Pain in limbs, then sweat with thirst, followed by shaking chill with thirst; after chill belching, bitter taste, yellow tongue. *θ*Tertian intermittent fever.

❙Chill, then thirst; one hour later, much heat, with interrupted sleep. θIntermittent.

Apyrexia never clear, constitutional symptoms always present.

Type: simple, quotidian; period the same every day.

❙Hectic fever with intermittent paroxysms.

❙Catarrhal fever; general exhaustion, with great sensitiveness of skin to touch and to slightest cold; constant chilliness, with sore throat, as if raw, painful on swallowing saliva; muscles of nape of neck, especially at sides beneath ears very painful to touch; dry cough; no appetite; no thirst; sleepless the whole night, with groaning and moaning.

❙Scarlatina preceded by cerebral symptoms and parotitis; restlessness day and night; mouth could not be opened, eyes injected and half open; continuous fever; involuntary evacuations; temperature low; child throws itself about unconsciously; dysuria; puffing under lower eyelids.

❙Scarlet fever with hydrops and albumen in urine; convulsions, bloated face; nosebleed.

❙After scarlet fever, anasarca and ascites; urine suppressed; tongue clean; next day convulsions followed by vomiting; conscious, but complains of a sensation as if a veil were hanging over eyes; urine very scanty; legs and scrotum greatly swollen; skin cool, pulse little accelerated and pretty full; next day recurrence of convulsions with more or less unconsciousness and complete blindness; deafness.

❙Scarlatina; sequela retarding convalescence; croupy inflammation of nasal mucous membrane; swelling of parotid and submaxillary glands; early decrease of urinary secretion, with traces of albumen and cylindrical tubuli; fully developed dropsy from Bright's disease.

❙After scarlet fever, anasarca and convulsions.

❙Measles, characterized by croupy cough < in morning, without expectoration and rattling in chest.

" Attacks, Periodicity. Attacks: last ten minutes then end in hoarseness; of debility last two or three hours.

After scarlet fever: anasarca and ascites, urine suppressed, tongue clean; next day convulsions and vomiting; next day recurrence of convulsions.

One hour before chill: thirst.

For three hours: chill followed by heat.

Twice a day: fever and bitter taste.

Every morning: boring headache; dull headache; vomiting; violent chill at six or seven o'clock.

Daily attacks: of sudden indescribable debility.

Every night: pain in skull bones; chill.

Four weeks after slight paralysis another attack of complete paralysis of arms and legs.

Every four months: scabby eruptions on head.

Every Winter: whitlows.

Spring and Autumn: bilious attacks.

For three months: l. cornea so hazy that iris could hardly be seen.

Repeated attacks: tonsillitis.

⁴² Locality and Direction. Right: painful throbbing in temple; headache in temple; pressive pain in occiput; cornea involved from periphery toward centre; violent pain over eyebrow; pain in eye <; scurvy formation in half of nose; acute inflammation of parotid gland; sensation in shoulder as of something creeping; large bubo, stony hard in groin; stitching pain in chest; lies immovable on side; lies on hip-joint; side of chest arched like a barrel from axilla downward; side of chest dull percussion sound; side of thorax considerably hollowed; pain in occipital protuberance; ulcer on last rib; red tubercle on buttock; swelling of hand; inside of thumb swollen, livid; whitlow on middle finger; suppuration of middle joint of index finger; carbuncle on thigh; chilly creeping sensation in leg; numbness of arm and hand.

Left: cornea so hazy that iris could hardly be seen; severe inflammation in cornea and iris; small ulcer on cornea; excessive lachrymation of eye; pupil much dilated; unpleasant sensation in side of nose; discharge of bone as large as pea from nostril; severe neuralgic pain in region of orbit; bubo in groin; upper part of side of throat tickling causing cough; as of drops of hot water in chest, side of thorax abnormally bulging; moist râles in lung; upper part of side of thorax dilated backwards; fine stitches in half of chest; carbuncle on side of back; hip pains as if sprained; raised, flat, purplish swelling on thigh; cramp in hand ; mouth drawn to side; paralysis of side; pain in hypochondrium and arm.

From below upwards: internal shivering.

⁴³ Sensations. ▮Bruised sore feeling of body, < from any motion.

▮Burning, throbbing pain, with chilliness.

▮Fainting with the pains.

▮Painful throbbing in different parts.

As if he could murder some one; forehead as if bruised; as if an abscess was forming in head; as if forehead would be torn out; as if eyes would be drawn back into

head; as if skull would burst; as from a plug in head;
wabbling as from water in brain; sense of swashing in
head; as if a nail was driven into occiput; as of sand
in eye; eyelids as if corroded; as of a burn in eyelids;
as if eyes projected; as if eyeballs were bruised; nose as
if bruised; as if blood was entering tooth; tooth as if
too long; pain in throat as from an intense swelling; as
of a plug in throat; sensation of water rising in œsophagus; as if she had eaten sour things; as of a hard body
in epigastrium; as if stomach hung loose; abdomen as
if bruised; as if bladder could not be emptied thoroughly; as if something were running or creeping in r.
shoulder-blade; pain as if in bones of arms and thighs;
as if there was a fishbone in throat; as of dust in lungs;
nose as if bruised; as from a splinter in throat; as if hot
water was floating in chest; as of drops of hot water in
l. chest; as if bruised in small of back and thighs; as if
a weight was resting on it; pain as if bruised in os
humeri; fingers as if dead; left hip pains as if sprained;
knee pains as if bruised; pain in foot as after taking a
misstep; as if something was sticking in throat; as if
he would suffocate; throat as if raw; as if a veil was
hanging over eyes.

Pain: in skull bones; in tumors on head; in pimples; in
eyes and head; on inside of nose; malar bones; in
tooth; in tip of tongue; in throat; in abdomen; in kidneys; in one spot of larynx; in upper part of throat;
extending from ear to ear; in top of chest; in r. occipital protuberance; in neck; in small of back and lumbar
vertebra; in shoulder; in bottom of back; around waist
and shoulders; in abdomen; in l. hypochondrium and
arm; in limbs; in bones.

Intense pain: in throat; in carbuncle on back.

Violent pain in head; over r. eyebrow; in bony part of
nose; in thumb.

Sharp pain: in head.

Severe pain: in r. tonsil; in lower extremities.

Tearing: in arms extending toward suppuration in breast;
in limbs and joints.

Cutting pain: in outer canthus; in abdomen; in thumb.

Lancinating pain: in head; in tumors.

Violent stitch: extending into great toe.

Stitches: in head; in eyes; in region of liver; in region
of spleen; in urethra; extending from ear to ear; in
larynx; in throat; in lungs; in heart; in back; in
joints.

Pulse-like stitches: in lower portion of occiput.

Burning stinging pains: on toes.

Stinging pain: in lids.

Stinging: of ulcers on breast; of blister on thumb.

Stitching: in head; in throat; in hepatic region; in larynx; in r. side of chest.

Severe neuralgic pains: in region of l. orbit; of face, extending in streaks into temple, ear, alæ nasi, upper lip.

Darting pain: in ears.

Ulcerative pain: in nostril; in throat.

Drawing pain: in nose; in tooth; from region of stomach to back; between scapulæ; in limbs.

Throbbing pain: in r. temple; in eyes; in ears; in tooth; in scrotum; in thumb; in last joint of middle finger, r. hand; in abscess.

Clawing: in umbilical region.

Gnawing: in stomach.

Cramp: in calves; in soles and toes; in l. hand.

Pinching: in abdomen.

Burrowing: headache.

Boring: headache; at root of nose; in r. temple.

Burning, bruised pain: in eye.

Burning pain: in eyes; in bones above orbits; in nose; in thumb.

Burning itching: on scalp.

Burning: of body; in throat; in stomach; in rectum; prepuce and pudenda; in urethra; on edges of ulcers; in throat; from pit of stomach to throat and ears; in ulcers.

Smarting pain: in eyelids; in pimple on upper lip; in throat; of vulva.

Pressive pain: in eyes; in lids.

Aching: in forehead; in vertex; in eyes.

Constriction: of chest.

Contractive sensation: in abdomen.

Tensive aching pain: above nose.

Dull aching pain: in stomach.

Rheumatic pains: in limbs and joints; in back.

Acute bruised pain: in eyeballs.

Bruised pain: in anterior muscles of thighs; in limbs.

Oversensitiveness to pain.

Sore pain: on dorsum of nose; in anus; in rectum.

Soreness: of urethra; on genitals; of scrotum; of folds between scrotum and thigh; in chest; in thighs; of all limbs.

Hammering: in head.

Throbbing: in ears; in forehead and temples.

Pulsative sensation: in ulcers on female sexual organs.

Violent pressure: in throat.

Anxious feeling: about heart.

Pressure: in head; in eyes; in stomach; beneath larynx; under sternum; sharp in small of back and lumbar vertebræ; on brain during delivery.

Distressing headache.

Dull headache.

Empty, sinking feeling: in stomach.

Scraping: in throat.

Raw feeling: in side of nose.

Scratching: in air tubes.

Acrid feeling: in stomach.

Unpleasant sensation: in l. side of nose.

Heaviness: in stomach.

Sensation of weight: at back of eyeballs.

Numbness: of r. arm and hand.

Stiffness: of nape of neck; in limbs.

Pricking: in both heels; in tumors.

Tickling sensation: in back of throat; in air tubes; in soles of feet; in arm.

Tingling: in toes; in tips of fingers.

Dry heat: of body.

Dryness: of palms of hands.

Creeping: in rectum; in r. leg; from l. hand up arm.

Formication: in arms.

Intensely violent itching: in bend of elbows; on hands, wrists and in palms; in lower extremities.

Itching: on scalp; in ears; in nose; around mouth; on spot beneath lower lip; on penis; of vulva; of nipples; in throat; of ears; violent at bend of elbow; on hands; in palms; of eruption in bends of joints; dull itching of soles of feet and palms of hands.

" **Tissues.** Child looks plump, yet the flesh is flabby, the muscles withered, digestion weak; intolerant of pressure about stomach after eating; food temporarily > the debility; stools green, watery, undigested, or white, sour smelling and painless; < during day; little tendency to cerebral symptoms; glands swollen and child subject to catarrhs from least draught of cold air; eczema, < morning, when it itches, burns and smarts.

∎Chlorosis with flatulent dyspepsia, delayed menses and leucorrhœa.

∎Hard, burning nodosities.

∎Pains in bones; caries.

∎Caries with watery, foul smelling pus.

∎∎Rheumatic swelling, with heat, redness and sensation as if sprained.

∎Useful in promoting suppuration when a former acute pain suddenly ceases after a chilly feeling, and is followed by a beating pain, or throbbing, indicating formation of pus.

❙Strumous patients, where suppurative process has not been arrested by *Mercur.*, or where suppuration seems inevitable; it hastens formation of abscess.

❙For elimination of foreign bodies by process of suppuration.

❙Suppuration of soft parts, of carious bones, of ulcers, of fistulous tracts, of exanthems.

❙Lacerating and pricking pains in tumors; throbbing and beating in abscess; skin over abscess highly inflamed, hard, hot and swelling; pus scanty, bloody, corroding, smelling like old cheese; pains < night, and by exposure to cold.

❙Felons.

❙Tendency to formation of abscesses.

❙Suppurative adenitis of armpit and of groin.

❙Suppurating buboes in inguinal and axillary regions.

❙Open buboes, which do not heal, especially after mercury or iodine.

❙Glandular swellings, particularly when obstinate and after abuse of mercury; suppuration of axillary and inguinal glands; strumous suppuration of joints with profuse sweats day and night.

❙Absorption of old glandular swellings.

❙Anasarca with tendency to formation of boils, on hairy scalp; tonsils and submaxillary glands enlarged; albuminous urine. θAfter scarlet fever.

❙Anasarca from Bright's disease, especially after so-called light cases of scarlatina.

❙Preventive of dropsy after scarlet fever as soon as traces of albumen are discovered in urine.

❙The child has a sour smell, and white, fetid evacuations.

❙Sour smell of the excretions.

❙❙Scrofulosis.

❙Gout with arthritis, without tophus.

❙Secondary syphilis, especially after mercury and iodide of potassium.

⁴⁵ **Touch. Passive Motion. Injuries.** ❙❙Extreme sensitiveness to contact; dread of contact, out of proportion to actual pain.

Touch: scalp sensitive; nodosities sore; boils on head and neck; head and eye; cornea sensitive; slightest touch acute bruised pain; swelling in lids painful; hemorrhage from ear on slightest touch; interior of nose sensitive; nose very sensitive; bones of nose sensitive; pains in malar bones <; bones of face painful; boils very sensitive; ulceration of face, intolerance of touch; great swelling of upper lip; gums and mouth very painful; renal region sensitive to slightest touch; eruption

on male sexual organs sensitive; larynx and trachea
sensitive; skin very sensitive; muscles of nape of neck
sore.

Pressure: < pain in one spot in throat; on corrosive blister causes stinging.

Binding head up tight: > pressure.

Has to loosen clothing.

Riding in a carriage: vertigo.

When shaking head: vertigo.

From concussion: morning headache <.

After injury: to eye violent inflammation; suppuration
of middle joint of r. index finger.

" Skin. Yellowness of the skin.

■■Constant offensive exhalations from body.

■Child smells sour.

■Great sensitiveness of skin to touch and to slightest cold.

■■Unhealthy, suppurating skin; even slight injuries mat-
urate; every cut or hurt suppurates.

■Cracking of skin and smarting of hands and feet.

■Bruised sensation, or as of subcutaneous ulceration, < by
contact.

■Suppression of exanthems, followed by mania; melancholia; ophthalmia; laryngismus stridulus, with epileptiform convulsions.

I I Erysipelatous inflammation on external parts.

■Suppuration of long inflamed boils on body, or on limbs,
commencing with blisters.

■Burning itching on body, with white vesicles, after
scratching.

■Itching rash in bend of knees and elbows.

■■Eczema, spreading by means of new pimples appearing
just beyond the old parts.

■Humid soreness on genitals, scrotum and folds between
scrotum and thighs.

■Herpes zoster, from spine around l. side to median line;
vesicles, bullæ, some containing dark pus; acute neuralgic pains in seat of eruption; vesicles on an inflamed
base, with severe itching and scratching, and nightly
aggravation.

■Dry and slightly cracked condition in both axillæ, especially left; much itching, < when body becomes heated;
rash generally dry; occasionally slight moisture exuded;
similar eruption about mouth; severe headache, pain <
back of eyeballs, which felt as if they would be drawn
back into head.

■■Nettlerash.

■Chronic urticaria, eruption chiefly in hands and fingers.

■Crusta lactea; tetters; rhagades; excoriations.

❙Fat, pustular and crusty itch.
❙Dry, pimply eruptions.
❙Miliary rash in circles.
❙Adenitis; acne punctata; boils; crusta lactea and serpiginosa; herpes; intertrigo; scurvy; encysted tumors; varices.
❙Eruption after mercurialism.
❙Eruptions very sensitive and sore to touch.
❙Skin inclined to ulcerate; the large sore surrounded by small pustules.
❙Ulcers very sensitive to contact, easily bleeding, burning or stinging, with corrosive pains.
❙❙Bleeding of an ulcer, even on slight wiping.
❙Ulcers: discharge bloody pus, smelling like old cheese; edges very sensitive, and have a pulsating sensation; discharge corroding; burning in ulcers; burning in night only; pains resembling recent excoriations; throbbing and shooting; jagged edges, and surrounded with pustules; bluish, bleeding ulcers; pus laudable, acrid or sanguineous; fetid and ichorous.
❙Margins of ulcers elevated and spongy, without granulations in centre.
❙Little pimples or smooth ulcers surrounding principal ulceration.
❙Severe stitching pain in ulcers when laughing; burning and throbbing at night.
❙The ulcer itches very much.
❙Stinging burning of edges of ulcers.
❙❙Mercurial ulcers.
❙Warts become inflamed and stinging, as if ulceration would set in.
❙Scabs easily torn off, leaving a raw and bleeding surface.
⁴⁷ **Stages of Life, Constitution.** Torpid, lymphatic constitutions; persons with light hair and complexion, slow to act, muscles soft and flabby.
❙Slow, torpid constitutions, with lax fibre and light hair; great sensitiveness to slightest contact of ulcers, eruptions and parts affected.
❙Figure lean, complexion bilious; pimply and subject to erysipelatous inflammation; pallor of face when excited by movement, or very red and flushed.
❙Suitable to scrofulous and debilitated subjects.
❙Psoric scrofulous diathesis.
❙Psora of children.
❙Strumous, outrageously cross children.
❙Purulent diathesis, great tendency to suppuration.
Child, æt. 4½ months; crusta lactea.
Girl, æt. ½ year, weak, scrofulous; laryngismus stridulus.

Boy, æt. ¼ year; croup.

Strong boy, æt. 8 months, since birth has had an eczema of face and head, which five weeks ago began to get better of itself, as eruption was nearly healed, epileptiform spasms set in; laryngismus stridulus.

Boy, æt. 21 months; dropsy after scarlet fever.

Boy, æt. 2, had tinea capitis, for which *Sabad.* was given; inflammation of eyes.

Boy, æt. 2¼; croup.

Boy, æt. 2½; croup.

Boy, æt. 3; parotitis.

Boy, æt. 3; scarlet fever.

Child, æt. 3½; parotitis.

Boy, æt. 4; croup.

Girl, æt. 4, lively temperament; croup.

Boy, æt. 4½, light hair, blue eyes, pale face, of mild, mischievous disposition, had pneumonia when an infant; emphysema.

Boy, æt. 5, healthy and strong; pleurisy.

Boy, æt. 5; croup.

Boy, æt. 5, weak, excitable, after a catarrh which had lasted eight days; croup.

Boy, æt. 6, delicate, weak, muscles flabby, face puffed, upper lip swollen, eyes sunken, frequent swelling of glands of neck; abnormal passages from bowels.   θOphthalmia.

Boy, æt. 6, twenty weeks after pneumonia, treated allopathically; pleuro-pneumonia of r. side, with absorption of pleuritic exudation, but continued presence of pneumonic infiltration in a state of purulent dissolution.

Boy, æt. 7, scrofulous constitution; ulceration of cornea.

Boy, æt. 8; anasarca and convulsions.

Boy, æt. 12; anasarca and convulsions.

Boy, æt. 13, suffering one year; ozæna.

Boy, æt. 16, robust, blonde, exposed to chills and must frequently strain his sight; inflammation of glands of eyelids.

Girl; whitlow.

Young girl, three months after puberty; mind affection.

Mr. K., æt. 18, fast-living, German; affection of cheek.

Girl, æt. 18, strong, healthy, very excitable and has been suffering three months; affection of throat.

Girl, æt. 18, after catching cold; laryngitis.

Miss M., æt. 18; chest troubles succeeding repelled itch.

Needle-woman, æt. 19; whitlows.

Young man, while fencing, received small, scarcely visible fragment of steel in eye, which stuck into cornea; traumatic ophthalmia.

Housemaid, æt. 22; whitlow.

Miss S., æt. 24, dark hair and eyes, pale face; angina pectoris.

Woman, single, æt. 25, menstruation scanty, suffering for three years; skin eruption.

Tenor singer, three years ago had an herpetic eruption in epigastric region which returned after the asthma had been cured; asthma.

Stonecutter, gonorrhœa one year ago, had taken much mercury, struck in eye by small piece of stone; hypopyon.

Waiter, after catching cold when going into cellar; pains in foot.

Mr. R., had been suffering for two weeks, *Arsen.* and *Laches.* without benefit; carbuncle.

Man, after drinking iced milk while in a heated condition; sensation as if a splinter or fishbone were sticking in throat.

Woman, psoric constitution; catarrhal inflammation of eyes.

Woman, suffering for years; indigestion.

Professional man, afflicted for twenty years, has frequently taken mercury; bilious attacks.

Sculptor, suffering for twenty-five years, has been overdosed with mercury; chronic tonsillitis.

Man, æt. 30; kidney disease.

Man, æt. 30; syphilitic bubo.

Man, æt. 30; bubo.

Woman, æt. 33, suffered severely from rheumatic pains, no history of syphilis; keratitis parenchymatosa.

Man, æt. 34, married, tall, slender, dark complexion, lymphatic, torpid temperament, has epilepsy and heart disease, also a recurring eruption which he treated with binoxide of mercury; attacks of debility.

Man, æt. 36, phlegmatic temperament, healthy, strong constitution, for half a year had itch, after bodily exhaustion slept upon ground; affection of brain.

Unmarried woman, æt. 36, has had repeated attacks since eighteenth year; father affected same way; tonsillitis.

Man, æt. 36, another æt. 45; chronic tracheitis.

Miss H., æt. 37, supposed she was bitten by some insect on forearm; carbuncle.

Man, æt. 37, big, strong, after suppressed syphilitic eruption; paralysis.

Woman, æt. 38, weak and flabby, scrofulous during youth, corneitis; hypopyon.

Mrs. P., æt. 40; affection of nose.

Scrofulous woman, æt. 40, subject to suppurating sore throat; tonsillitis.

Mr. W., æt. 40; carbuncle.

Woman, æt. 44, has suffered for many years, has taken large doses of quinine and mercury; hepatic and uterine disease.

Man, æt. 45; ill effects of *Merc. sol.*

Man, æt. 47, carbuncle.

Widow, æt. 52, suffering six years; spinal irritation.

Mrs. H., æt. about 60, large, fleshy woman with frequent attacks of jaundice; carbuncle.

Patient, æt. 63, sick since five years; bronchial catarrh.

Man, æt. 67, has spent much of his life in foreign stations, mercurial history; hepatogenous jaundice.

⁴⁸**Relations.** Antidoted by: *Acet. ac., Bellad., Chamom., Silic.*

It antidotes: mercurial and other metallic preparations; iodine, and especially the iodide of potash; cod-liver oil.

Removes weakening effects of ether.

Compatible: *Acon., Arnic., Bellad., Laches., Mercur., Nitr. ac., Silic., Spongia, Zincum.*

Compare: *Alumina* (constipation); *Calc. ost., Jodum, Kali bich., Mercur., Rheum, Sulphur.*

Complementary: to *Calend.*, in injuries.

HIPPOMANES.

A normally white, usually dark olive green, soft, glutinous, mucous substance, of a urinous odor, which floats in the allantois fluid, or is attached to the allantois membrane of the mare or cow chiefly during the last months of pregnancy.

Triturations were made from the dried substance obtained from Rev. John Helfrich (one of the provers and an associate of the Allentown Academy) who took it from the tongue of a newly born filly.

The provings are by Hering, Helfrich, Floto, Reichhelm, Husman and Neidhard. See Allen's Encyclopedia, vol. 4, p. 589.

As the remedy has not, thus far, had frequent clinical application, we give but a condensed extract from the provings.

¹ **Mind.** ‖Melancholy; a young man sits in the corner and does not want to have anything to do with the world.

Restlessness; must move from place to place.

² **Sensorium.** Sensation of lightness in head.

³ **Inner Head.** Pressive pain in temples.

Headache, with giddiness, heat in head, sleepiness, yawning, thirst.

Violent headache; heaviness on vertex; when walking it feels as if head would fall forward.

Headache > when lying on painful side; < when walking in sun.

4 Outer Head. The head feels so heavy that it falls forward
if he raises himself.

The hair becomes nearly dry; falling off of hair.

5 Sight and Eyes. The light of the candle looks blue.

Stitches in eyes (with headache).

Painfulness of eyes when moving them, with headache.

7 Smell and Nose. Sensation of coldness, when drawing t!
air in.

Bleeding of nose in morning.

9 Lower Face. Involuntary twitching of under lip.

11 Taste and Tongue. Bitter taste in mouth.

Tongue coated white, with redness of tip.

12 Inner Mouth. Increased secretion of saliva, with headache
or sore throat.

13 Throat. Painfulness of l. tonsil.

Sensation of plug in throat (l. side).

14 Appetite, Thirst. Desires, Aversions. Desire for acids,
and aversion to sweet things.

16 Hiccough, Belching, Nausea and Vomiting. Nausea,
especially in a draft of air, with headache.

17 Scrobiculum and Stomach. ●Icy coldness in stomach.

Sensation of emptiness in stomach (and head).

20 Stool and Rectum. Soft stool, with vomiting; discharge
of prostatic fluid after micturition.

Hard stool, in balls.

Spasmodic contraction of sphincter ani.

21 Urinary Organs. Frequent discharge of watery urine.

Urine discharged in a small stream, with straining—it
feels as if a swelling retarded it; prostatitis.

Drawing pain from anus through urethra.

22 Male Sexual Organs. Sexual desire increased.

Prostatitis.

Drawing pain in testicles.

23 Female Sexual Organs. Menstruation too early.

25 Voice and Larynx. Trachea and Bronchia. Larynx
feels raw, as if air were too cold.

26 Respiration. Tickling in throat when breathing.

27 Cough. Cough, barking, during sleep.

28 Inner Chest and Lungs. Stitches in l. side of chest.

32 Upper Limbs. Left arm feels as if paralyzed.

⫯⫯Violent pain in wrists. θChorea.

ǀǀParalysis of wrist, every morning in bed.

Sensation in wrist as if sprained, especially left.

Great weakness of hands and fingers, so that he cannot
hold anything.

Formication on r. hand.

³³ Lower Limbs. Weakness, and as if sprained, in knees.
Weakness and sensation of dryness in foot joints and soles
of feet.
Cramps in soles of feet, in evening.
Cold feet.

³⁴ Limbs in General. Heaviness in limbs.

³⁵ Rest. Position. Motion. Lying: on painful side, head-
ache >.
Desire to lie down, with no relief in doing so.
If he raises himself: head feels heavy.
Must move from place to place.
Walking: head feels as if it would fall forward; in sun
headache <.

³⁶ Nerves. ❙Great weakness of body and mind.
Great weakness and debility, with pale face.
Desire to lie down, with no relief on doing so.
❙Chorea.

³⁸ Time. Morning: bleeding of nose.
Evening: cramps in soles of feet; heat, with dull headache.

³⁹ Temperature and Weather. Sun: < headache.
Draft of air: nausea.
Chill: > being warmly covered in bed.

⁴⁰ Fever. Chill, beginning in back.
Chill, > being warmly covered in bed.
Heat in evening, with dull headache.

⁴¹ Attacks, Periodicity. Every morning in bed: paralysis
of wrists.

⁴² Locality and Direction. Right: formication on hand.
Left: painfulness of tonsil; sensation of plug in throat;
stitches in side of chest; arm feels paralyzed.

⁴³ Sensations. As if head would fall forward when walking;
as of a plug in throat; as if a swelling retarded urine;
as if air was too cold for larynx; left arm feels as if
paralyzed; left wrist as if sprained.
Violent pain: in head; in wrists.
Stitches: in eyes; in l. side of chest.
Drawing pain: in testicles; from anus through urethra.
Cramps: in soles of feet.
Dull headache.
Painfulness: of eyes; of l. tonsil.
Heat: in head.
Heaviness: on vertex; in limbs.
Raw feeling: in larynx.
Sensation of dryness: in foot joints and soles of feet.
Sensation of emptiness: in stomach.
Great weakness: of hands and fingers; of foot joints and
soles of feet; of body and mind.
Lightness: in head.

Tickling: in throat.

Formication: on r. hand.

Itching: on skin, especially on chest, between shoulders.

Coldness: in nose when drawing air in; in stomach.

⁴⁶ Skin. ||Itching as from flannel on skin, especially on chest and between shoulders.

⁴⁷ Stages of Life, Constitution. ‖After growing too fast. θChorea.

⁴⁸ Relations. Antidoted by coffee.

Caustic. relieved paralysis of wrist.

HIPPOZÆNIN.

Glanderine and Farcine.   *A Nosode.*

Introduced by Drysdale.

The extracts (made by Hering) are from Wilkinson, Spinola, Bollinger (Ziemssen) and Virchow. They are the effects observed on horses and men affected with this disease.

Gl. = Glanderine. F. = Farcine. Symptoms so marked are suggested for clinical use by Wilkinson.

CLINICAL AUTHORITIES.—*Ozæna*, Wilkinson, B. J. H., vol. 15, p. 627; Morgan, Raue's Rec., 1873, p. 79; *Chronic ozæna*, Hiller, Organon, vol. 2, p. 381; *Diphtheria*, Wilkinson, B. J. H., vol. 15, p. 627; *Bronchitis*, Wilkinson, B. J. H., vol. 15, p. 625; *Putrid fever*, Wilkinson, B. J. H., vol. 15, p. 627; *Glanderoid influenza*, Baer, Raue's Rec., 1873, p. 108; *Scrofulous swelling of parotid gland*, Nichols, Organon, vol. 3, p. 345.

Cases by Berridge not found.

² Sensorium. Fainting turns with headache.

³ Inner Head. Inflammation of membranes of brain.

Purulent collections between bones of skull and dura mater.

Scattered abscesses in brain substance.

Tubercles may appear in periosteum of skull, in dura mater, in plexus choroides.

A diffused myelitis malleosa, attributable to infiltration.

⁴ Outer Head. Bones of skull and face, most frontal, necrosed.

Hair loses its glisten. Gl.

⁵ Sight and Eyes. Eyes full of tears or slime.

Pupils dilated, with collapse.

Papules on choroid coat of eye.

⁶ Hearing and Ears. Tinkling sounds in ears.

Hoarse and deaf, before fatal termination.

Inflammation of parotid gland.

[7] **Smell and Nose.** Swelling and redness of nose and adjacent parts, with severe pain.

Diffused redness of nose spreading over forehead and face.

Upper portion of nose specially sensitive to touch, exhibiting a diffuse, erysipelatous swelling.

Erysipelas especially upon nose and face.

Gangrenous erysipelas of external integuments of nose, discharge of pus and viscid mucus down one or both nostrils. Gl.

Discharge of a thin, viscid, light colored mucus from nose.

Offensive muco-purulent discharge from nose.

Nasal secretions have a foul appearance, before fatal termination.

Nasal discharge often from one side only.

Discharge from nose becomes later of a thicker consistency, more purulent, often of a brownish-yellow color, sanguineous and offensive.

▮Catarrh: nose inflamed with thick and tinged defluxion; tonsils swollen, fauces gorged. Gl.

▮Obstinate catarrh. Gl.

Ozæna; ulcers inside of nose.

Discharge: often one-sided, albuminous, tough, viscous, discolored, gray, greenish, even bloody and offensive; acrid, corroding.

One nostril appears smaller from swelling.

Little yellow pustules size of a hemp seed on nose.

Ulcers deep, lard-like fundus; edges pectinated, elevated, viscous secretion, no scurfs, most in groups at first size of a lentil, running together.

Ulcerations progress from below upwards.

▮Chronic ozæna.

Small papules of yellowish color are seated upon mucous membrane of nose.

Distinct tubercles situated mostly upon alæ nasi.

Pustules and ulcers on mucous membrane of nose, terminating in erosion of perichondrium and perforation of septum and vomer.

Nostrils covered with foul, crustaceous deposits.

Nostrils covered with a viscous phlegm. Gl.

▮Nose and mouth ulcerated. θCatarrh. Gl.

||Malignant ozæna.

Gangrene of swollen root of nose.

Cartilages of nose become exposed and necrosed, septum, vomer and palatebone disorganized.

Cartilages of the nose are destroyed. Gl.

: Caries of nasal bones.

Catarrhal, inflammatory, ulcerative processes in other mucous membranes than of nose, conjunctiva of eyes, mucous membranes of mouth, gums, fauces and entire respiratory canal.

▮Checks the liability to catarrhal affection. Gl.

⁹ **Lower Face.** Maxillary gland swollen, like a distinct ball or sausage, firmly attached to the maxilla, uneven, rugged, tuberculated; mostly painless, burning only at times.

Submaxillary and sublingual glands swollen and painful at times; abscesses are formed which open externally.

¹⁰ **Teeth and Gums.** Gums show a tendency to bleed.

Gums covered with a black, sooty deposit.

¹¹ **Taste and Tongue.** Act of speaking difficult.

Tongue dry, thickly covered with a black, sooty deposit.

¹² **Inner Mouth.** Dryness of mucous membranes of mouth and pharynx, before fatal termination.

Stomatitis.

Ulcers appear in mouth.

: Buccal passages filled with tenacious lymph and mucus. θScarlatina. Gl.

Croupous exudation upon mucous membrane of mouth and throat.

▮Apparently suffocating from diphtheritis in mouth and nose, agonized with buccal ulcerations. θDiphtheria. Gl.

: Odor of breath putrid. θScarlatina. Gl.

▮Scrofulous swelling of l. parotid gland in a child.

¹³ **Throat.** Ulcerations upon velum of palate.

: Swollen tonsils closing posterior channels. θScarlatina.

Increased difficulty in swallowing, before fatal termination.

Mucous membrane of fauces ulcerated, yellow, like bacon.

Upon mucous membrane of pharynx ecchymoses, redness, swelling, eruptions and foul ulcers.

Inflamed condition of pharynx makes swallowing difficult.

▮Patient apparently suffocating from diphtheritis in mouth and nose; buccal ulceration present.

¹⁴ **Appetite, Thirst. Desires, Aversions.** Appetite failing; loss of appetite. Gl.

Thirst excessive, especially with diarrhœa.

¹⁷ **Scrobiculum and Stomach.** Gastro-intestinal catarrh; loss of appetite, indigestion, constipation, in later stage diarrhœa.

Large ecchymoses on mucous lining of stomach.

Papula shaped formations in substance of lining membrane of stomach.

¹⁸ **Hypochondria.** Liver greatly enlarged, often showing signs of fatty degeneration.

Hepatitis with gangrenous and ulcerative inflammation of gall ducts.

Enlargement of spleen.

Spleen enlarged, filled with blood; softened and liquified, of a grayish-red or dark color; wedge-shaped abscesses in spleen.

[19] **Abdomen.** Inguinal glands swollen.

[20] **Stool and Rectum.** Colliquative diarrhœa with a general cachexia and exhaustion precede the fatal termination.
Involuntary evacuations with collapse.
Constipation.

[21] **Urinary Organs.** Tubercles and abscesses in kidneys.
Suppuration in one kidney.   Gl.
Albumen in urine, also leucine and tyrosine.

[22] **Male Sexual Organs.** Tubercles and abscesses: of glans penis; of testicles; in kidneys.
Sarcocele malleosa.
Swelling and inflammation of testicles.   Gl.
: Syphilis.

[23] **Female Sexual Organs.** Slimy discharge from vagina.
: Uterine phlebitis.   F.

[24] **Pregnancy. Parturition. Lactation.** Abortion.

[25] **Voice and Larynx. Trachea and Bronchia.** Papules and ulcerations in frontal sinuses, pharynx, larynx and trachea.
Extensive lesions in larynx, subsequent œdema of glottis.
Hoarseness from the altered condition of larynx.
❚Neglected cases of bronchitis.
❚❚Bronchitis: in the worst forms; especially in elderly persons; where suffocation from excessive secretion is imminent.   Gl.

[26] **Respiration.** Noisy breathing; loud snoring respiration before fatal termination; breath fetid.
Respiration short and irregular, with collapse.
Slight difficulty in breathing.
❙❙Cough and obstructed respiration, resulting from cicatricial contraction of mucous membrane of nose and larynx; had lasted eleven years; patient presented picture of decided cachexia.
Respiration at first partially impeded, later absolute dyspnœa.
Actual dyspnœa from affection of larynx or lungs.
❚❚Suffocation from excessive secretions.   θBronchitis. Gl.
❚Bronchial asthma.   Gl.

[27] **Cough.** Irritative cough.
Slight cough and hoarseness, sputa often bloody.
❚Cough comenced at Christmas and lasted till June.   Gl.
❚Whooping cough.   Gl.
Patients cough severely and expectorate profusely, sputa usually bearing a strong resemblance to the discharge from the nostrils.

[28] **Inner Chest and Lungs.** Extensive rhonchi are heard over walls of chest.

Large sections of lungs in a state of gray hepatization and purulent infiltration, while other portions are in a state of collateral hyperæmia.

Pneumonia with rusty sputa. Gl.

Pneumonia malleosa; nodules larger, forming isolated hepatizations and abscesses.

One or two infarctions in lungs, size of a bean developed in one lobe, distinctly circumscribed dark red color, in and around which lie small abscesses.

Nodules in lung size of a pea, of a gray whitish appearance and a firm, lardaceous consistence.

Tubercles in lungs.

Tubercles, size of millet seed to a pea, of a firm texture and of a gray, yellowish or reddish color.

Tubercles in lungs are never missed in glanders, rarely in farcy.

Tubercles in lungs, nodules and specific inflammatory processes.

Small tubercles upon pleura; subpleural ecchymoses.

Pulmonary abscesses with pleuritis.

: Given in phthisis, it diminishes expectoration, abates constantly recurring aggravations of inflammation, and checks liability to catarrhal affections.

Suppuration of lungs. Gl.

: Lung diseases of cattle. F.

[29] **Heart, Pulse and Circulation.** Pulse very frequent and small in volume, 110 to 120; in some cases retarded.

[32] **Upper Limbs.** With sore finger, swelling of arm, phlegmonous and erysipelatous with pustules and ulcers.

[33] **Lower Limbs.** : Hip disease.

: Psoas and lumbar abscesses. F.

: Old bad legs (ulcers). Gl.

Suppuration in each knee-joint; a large quantity of pus in bursa of knee-joint. Gl.

∎ Anasarca of lower limbs. F.

[34] **Limbs in General.** Obscure pain in limbs, most in muscles and joints.

[36] **Nerves.** Weakness, fatigue, general discomfort; they give up their business (not in carbuncle).

Malaise, fatigue, prostration, accompanied by headache and chills.

General prostration with considerable emaciation.

[37] **Sleep.** Insomnia and great restlessness.

Nocturnal delirium.

[40] **Fever.** Frequent chilliness. Gl.

Chills and fever in cases of abscesses or ulcers.

Skin becomes cool with collapse.

Symptoms like the early stage of typhoid fever.

Fever exacerbations irregular or of a regular intermittent character.

Febrile disturbances constantly increasing.

As the pains become more severe, regular fever turns often supervene or a continued fever prevails.

Fever when a series of abscesses follow in rapid succession.

Temperature reaches 104° F. and over.

Fever raging without intermission, even in morning, temperature 106° F.

Fever increases, pulse grows weaker, delirium sets in, stupor.

▮Putrid fever. Gl.

: Plague. Gl.

: May be tried in scarlatina, where odor of breath is putrid, buccal passages filled with tenacious lymph and mucus, tonsils greatly swollen.

[41] **Attacks, Periodicity.** At times: burning in maxillary glands; pain in submaxillary and sublingual glands.

Cough commenced at Christmas and lasted till June.

Lasted eleven years: cough and obstructed respiration.

[42] **Locality and Direction.** Left: scrofulous swelling of parotid gland.

[43] **Sensations.** Pain is excessive in acute articular rheumatism.

Attacks of muscular cramps before fatal termination.

Violent pains: in joints and muscles.

Severe pain: in nose and adjacent parts.

Obscure pain: in limbs; in muscles and joints.

Painfulness: of tumors and abscesses; of submaxillary and sublingual glands.

Painful swelling: of joints.

Burning: in maxillary glands.

Dryness: of mucous membranes of mouth and pharynx.

[44] **Tissues.** Greatly debilitated and emaciated, presenting a very similar appearance to that seen in chronic tuberculosis with hectic fever.

Extrusion of contents overbalances supply of nutrition.

Numerous ecchymoses in internal organs.

Inflammation of lymphatic vessels and swelling of glands.

: Lymphatic swellings and inflammation.

On legs, head, sides, chest, near genitals, in long strings, hard swellings from size of a pea to that of a hazel or walnut; after enlarging they break open and discharge a viscous, yellow brownish ichor.

: Phlegmasia dolens.

Entire process presents a strong resemblance to certain forms of pyæmia.

■Pyæmia and inflammation of veins and lymphatics, particularly when pus is formed.

The mucous membranes (first of all that of the nose) manifest symptoms of inflammatory and ulcerative disease.

Inflammatory affection of mucous membrane of mouth followed by swelling of tongue, salivation, ulcers upon gums and throat, finally angina.

Purulent inflammation in serous membranes, especially lining membrane of joints, particularly of knee, hips and hand.

Painful swelling of joints.

Pain in joints and muscles become violent.

: Enlarged joints.

Periarticular nonfluctuating tumefactions.

Large projecting tumors and abscesses becoming extremely painful and hard, then gradually changing to a doughy consistence; fluctuating; after opening, appear as extensive ulcers with irregular edges covered with a white deposit.

The specific nodules mostly in biceps, flexors of forearm, rectus, pectoralis and at point of insertion of deltoid.

Beneath larger blebs well defined sloughs of a dull gray color.

I I Putrescence, destructive, quasi malignant ulcerative tendency to decomposition of tissues. Gl.

■Malignant erysipelas, particularly if attended with large formation of pus, destruction of parts. Gl.

: Dropsy.

All the attacked parts swell, get œdematous.

Beneath œdema are small nodules, varying in size and filled with reddish pus.

Skin cracks in bend of joints, a brownish fluid oozes out, and gets ulcerous.

Purulent infiltrations of skin and cellular tissues, especially upon forehead and eyelids and in vicinity of joints.

Abscesses in various parts of body in course of absorbents.

■Carbuncle.

■Plague.

: Cancer.

: Elephantiasis.

: Obstinate syphilitic sores, with great fetor.

: Scrofula.

■Abates recurring aggravation of inflammation.

: Murrain of cattle.

⁴⁵ **Touch. Passive Motion. Injuries.** Touch: upper portion of nose sensitive.

: Putrid bedsores. Gl.

⁴⁶ Skin. Erythema, erysipelatous or phlegmonous processes, abscesses, pustules and ulcers are spread so extensively over surface of body that hardly any part remains free.

ı Malignant erysipelas, particularly if attended by· large formations of pus, and destruction of parts. Gl.

: Scarlatina. Gl.

Sensation of pain on part of inoculation followed by a redness and inflammation, fever, finally swollen, inflamed lymphatic vessels.

On different parts of skin red spots, changing into pustules like those of small-pox, less often into pemphigus blebs.

Pustules of size of pea often arise in large ·numbers, bursting by discharging a thick, mucous, sanguineous pus, often emitting an offensive odor.

Surrounding subfascial abscesses the numerous layers are pale, discolored and readily torn.

Large abscesses upon different regions of the body, with inflamed lymphatic vessels and glands.

New abscesses are constantly forming in vicinity of the ulcers, especially about joints.

Contents of abscesses often tinged with blood, have a more viscous consistence, while connective tissue or muscular substance is softened.

: Malignant pustule. GL

: Carbuncle. Gl.

Boils and ulcers.

: Confluent small-pox. Gl.

: Malignant external ulcerations; putrid bedsores; obstinate syphilitic sores attended with great fetor.

Ulcers often penetrate so deep as to lay bare the tendons and bone.

Ulcers deep, lard-like fundus, elevated, pectinated edges, slow healing, leaving a star-shaped white scar. ·

: Putrescence, destructive or quasi malignant ulceration, and tendency to decomposition of tissues.

ı Malignant external ulcerations. Gl.

Ulcers have no disposition to heal, livid appearance.

Ulcers assume a corroded, chancroid character and a dirty white hue.

Ulcers enlarge, edges and base acquire an unhealthy aspect, pus offensive.

Sinuous and fistulous ulcers, secreting an offensive, watery pus, showing no tendency to throw out granulations.

Pustules appear gradually on every part of body.

Pustules contain caseous purulent contents.

: Malignant, phagedenic skin diseases. Gl.
: Pustular ringworm. Gl.
; Lupus exedens.
Circumscribed or diffused lesions on skin.
Fluctuating tumors in muscular tissue.
Frequently upon the limbs nodular tumors discharging,
   on being opened, thick, purulent masses mixed with
   blood and serum.
Icterus appears before fatal termination.
Here and there healing by forming cicatricial tissue.

HYDRASTIS CANADENSIS.

Golden Seal; Orange Root.   *Ranunculaceæ.*

Grows in most parts of the United States, in rich woodlands, most abundantly
in the states of Ohio, Indiana, Kentucky and West Virginia.

The tincture is prepared from the fresh root.

This plant was first mentioned by Linnæus, in 1753. The first provings were
made under Hale, by Nichols, Burt and others. (See Hale's New Rem.) About
the year 1866, provings were made by Whitesides, Weaver and others (see Am.
Hom. Obs.), and a year or two later Hydrastis was proved under Lippe by a class
of students of the Hahnemann College of Philadelphia, with different dilutions,
mostly the 30th.

A monograph on Hydrastis, by Chas. Mohr, was printed in the Hah. Mo.,
November, 1886.

CLINICAL AUTHORITIES.—*Ophthalmia*, A. H. O., vol. 3, p. 467; *Nasal catarrh*,
Palmer, Raue's Rec., 1871, p. 65; Webster, Raue's Rec., 1871, p. 84; Moore, Times
Retros., 1877, p. 26; *Diphtheritic deposit in nose and vagina*, Smith, A. H. O., vol. 3,
p. 469; *Epithelial cancer of lip*, Blake, Hom. Rev., vol. 18, p. 491; *Cancerous tumor
of hard palate*, Nankivell, Raue's Rec., 1873, p. 248; *Sore mouth*, Morgan, Hom.
Clinics, vol. 3, p. 131; Williamson, Raue's Rec., 1874, p. 106; *Mercurial salivation*,
Lodge, Hale's Therap., p. 320; *Affection of mouth and throat*, Hale, Hale's Therap.,
p. 319; *Use in diphtheria*, Oehme, Therapeutics, p. 38; *Epigastric tumor with marasmus*, La Brunne, Hale's Therap., p. 322; *Weakness of digestion*, Smedley, A. H. O.,
vol. 4, p. 29; *Dyspepsia*, McClatchey, Raue's Rec., 1875, p. 141; Bradshaw, B. J. H.,
vol. 19, p. 592; *Cancer of stomach*, Hendricks, Raue's Rec., 1872, p. 137; *Subacute inflammation of liver*, Bradshaw, B. J. H., vol. 19, p. 591; *Jaundice*, Albertson,
A. H. O., vol. 3, p. 462; *Constipation* (3 cases), Rogerson, B. J. H., vol. 18, p. 526;
Hughes, B. J. H., vol. 23, p. 257; Hibbard, Raue's Rec., 1874, p. 201; Hale,
Hale's Therap., p. 325; Brown, A. H. O., vol. 3, p. 466; Martin, Trans. Hom.
Med. Soc. Pa., 1882, p. 204; *Constipation of infants*, Hibbard, A. H. O., vol. 10, p.
254; *Constipation and hemorrhoids*, Clark, A. H. O., vol. 3, p. 465; Brown, A. H. O.,
vol. 3, p. 464; *Hemorrhoids*, Hunt, Raue's Rec., 1874, p. 202; Brown, Bernhard

and Strong; Bradshaw, B. J. H., vol. 19, p. 595; *Ulceration of rectum*, Mitchell, U. S. M. and S. J , July, 1871; *Fistula ani*, Morgan, Raue's Rec., 1870, p. 219; *Gonorrhœa*, Brown, A. H. O., vol. 3, p. 467; *Prolapsus uteri*, Boyce, Raue's Rec., 1870, p. 248; *Uterine affection*, Wigand, A. H. O., vol. 2, p. 232; *Uterine hemorrhage*, Hale, Times Retros., 1877, p. 26; *Menstrual disturbances, affections of uterus*, Schatz, Allg. Hom. Ztg., vol. 109, p. 24; *Tumor in breast*, Freeman, B. J. H., vol. 20, p. 8; *Scirrhous of breast*, Maclimont and Marston, B. J. H., vol. 21, p. 639; Marston, Hughes Pharm., p. 409; *Mammary cancer*, Bayes, B. J. H., vol. 19, p. 150; B. J. H., vol. 20, p. 4; *Cough*, Small, Hale's Therap., p. 329; *Disease of heart*, Smedley, A. H. O., vol. 4, p. 21; *Ulcers on leg*, Gilchrist, A. II. O., vol. 3, p. 465, *Scrofulous ulcers on leg*, Eadon, A. H. O., vol. 3, p. 469; *Typhoid fever*, Mohr, Organon, vol. 3, p. 374; *General marasmus*, Rebsher, Raue's Rec., 1870, p. 312; *Scrofulous inflammation of glands*, Bradshaw, B. J. H., vol. 19, p. 596; *Cuts, burns, intertrigo*, Saxton, Hale's Therap., p. 315; *Cancer*, Bradshaw, B. J. H., vol. 19, p. 588; *Epithelioma*, Blake, Raue's Rec., 1875, p. 299; *Erysipelas*, Woodvine, N. E. M. G., 1874, p. 28; *Smallpox* (3 cases), Cleveland, A. H. O., vol. 3, p. 264; *Eczema*, Cooper, Raue's Rec., 1872, p. 256; *Ulcers* (3 cases), Hastings, N. A. J. H., vol. 13, p. 450.

[1] **Mind.** ❙Forgetful; cannot remember what he is reading or talking about.

❙Irritable; disposed to be spiteful.

❙Moaning, with occasional outcries from pain.

❙Despondency.

❙Depression of spirits, sure of death and desires it.

[2] **Sensorium.** ❙Feeling as if intoxicated; headache; weakness.

[3] **Inner Head.** ❙Dull, heavy frontal headache over eyes; catarrhal.

❙Dull frontal headache, with dull pain in hypogastrium and small of back.

❙❙Severe frontal headache.

❙Sharp cutting in temples and over eyes; < over left; > from pressing with hand.

❙❙Dull, pressing pain on top of head, pressing outward from ears, at 10.30 A.M.

❙❙Vertex headache in paroxysms, every other day, commencing about 11 A.M., with excessive nausea, retching and anguish.

❙Headache of a nervous gastric character, almost constant.

❙Frontal headaches; headaches arising from catarrh, gastric difficulties, indigestion, dyspepsia, acidity of stomach, as well as from bilious disorder, constipation, piles, uterine disorder, etc.

[4] **Outer Head.** ❙Myalgic headache, in integuments of scalp and muscles of neck.

❙Weeping eruption on forehead along margin of hair, after taking cold; < from warmth of room after having been in cold air; itching when warm; < washing. θEczema.

‖Scalp and face covered with thick crusts, which upon removal, expose red, raw and infiltrated patches. θEczema.

‖Scalp caked over with a thick, sebaceous secretion; hair dry and lustreless; debility and insufficient nourishment after typhoid fever. θSeborrhœa sicca.

‖Laceration of scalp above l. temple, several inches in length, crescentic in shape; wound suppurated and became a troublesome sore.

⁵ Sight and Eyes. ‖Dark greenish yellow colored conjunctiva.

‖Jaundiced eyes.

‖Lack of accommodative power of eyes and asthenopia.

‖Opacity of cornea; scrofulous ophthalmia, with or without ulceration; thick mucous discharge.

‖Profuse secretion of tears; smarting of eyes; burning of eyes and lids.

‖Pain and burning in eyes.

‖Inflammation and ulceration of conjunctiva.

‖Acute catarrhal ophthalmia, the result of daily exposure to harsh dry winds; inflammation nearly extended to border of iris; lids greatly swollen and excoriated; profuse catarrhal secretion.

‖‖Ophthalmia: catarrhal; scrofulous; thick mucous discharge.

‖Chronic inflammation of eyes.

‖Mucous membrane of eyelids much congested; profuse, thick, white mucous discharge.

‖Discharge of matter from eyes, resulting from catarrhal inflammation.

‖Conjunctivitis siccus with sensation of dryness and scratching, and feeling of weight and heaviness of upper lids.

‖Blepharitis marginalis.

Large painful stye on l. lid.

⁶ Hearing and Ears. ‖Deafness.

‖Roaring in ears, like from machinery.

‖Tinnitus aurium, from catarrh of inner ear.

‖Membrana tympani purplish and bulging.

‖Perforation of membrani tympani.

‖Mucous membrane of middle ear eroded, granular and exuberant with polypoid growths.

‖Purulent inflammation of middle ear, with thick, tenacious discharge, more mucus than pus.

‖Bland mucous discharge, associated with dropping in posterior nares.

‖Thick, offensive, irritating catarrhal and purulent discharges from external auditory meatus.

∎Otorrhœa, thick mucous discharge.
∎Ears red, thickened and covered with scales; skin back
   of each pinna red, thickened and fissured at their connection with side of head.
[7] **Smell and Nose.**   ⁞⁞Tickling, like a hair, in r. nostril.
∎The air feels cold in nose.
∎Stuffed up, smarting sensation in posterior nares, with
   discharge of thin, clear mucus.
∎Stuffiness of nares, and discharge of thick, white or yellow
   tenacious and stringy mucus, or frequent dropping
   down of mucus from posterior nares into throat.
∎Sharp, raw, excoriated feeling in both nares, with con-
   stant inclination to blow nose; hoarseness.
∎Posterior nares clogged with mucus.
∎Secretion, more from posterior nares, thick, tenacious.
⁞⁞Sneezing, with fulness over eyes, dull frontal headache,
   pain in r. breast and down arms.
∎Coryza watery, excoriating; burning in nose, more r.
   nostril; discharge scanty in room, profuse out of doors;
   rawness in throat and chest.
∎Coryza, with copious secretion of white mucus and tears.
∎Fluent coryza, followed by thick catarrhal discharge.
∎Bloody purulent discharge from nose.
∎Influenza in cold, weak, debilitated persons.
∎Catarrhal influenza.
∎Secretions so profuse as to be removed in long tenacious
   shreds or pieces.
∎Constant thick white mucous discharge, with frontal
   headache; discharge of yellowish stringy mucus into
   throat.
∎Constant discharge of thick white mucus from nose;
   coryza with frontal headache. θNasal catarrh.
∎Discharge of thick white mucus from nose; lachryma-
   tion; thickening of membrane of posterior nares; swell-
   ing of turbinated bones; large crusts forming in nasal
   fossæ; occasional thin mucous discharge; raw, smarting sensation in nostrils; pains in ears. θNasal catarrh.
∎Profuse discharge of thick, yellowish, stringy mucus from
   nasal passages.
⁞⁞Discharge of thick yellow matter from nose.
∎Chronic nasal catarrh.
∎Ozæna, with bloody, purulent discharge.
∎Obstruction of nasal passages.
∎Soreness of cartilaginous septum, bleeding when touched;
   inner edge of r. ala sore and thickened.
∎Nosebleed, l. nostril, with burning rawness; followed by
   itching.
∎After apparent recovery from diphtheria, formation of a

diphtheritic membrane in l. nostril and in vagina, the
former being completely plugged up.
- Diphtheritic affections of nose.
⁸ Upper Face. ▪Expression weary, dull, skin pale, or yellow-
white.
- Pale face, worn, weary expression.
- Yellow complexion.
- Erysipelatous eruption following flushes of heat.
- Chills passing down back, followed by burning fever;
pulse 120; headache in supraorbital region, excruciating pain in lumbar region; face red, l. side of nose
swollen; great tenderness of cervical glands, urine high
colored; inflammation passed from l. side of nose to r.
ear, eye, scalp and whole face, r. eye being closed; extreme restlessness, disturbed by least noise; urine suppressed for twenty-four hours; delirium. *θ*Erysipelas
erratica.
- Left cheek swollen; l. eye closed; pain and burning,
chills, flushes; pulse 100. *θ*Erysipelas.
- Forehead, cheeks and nose slightly red and very greasy;
follicles plugged with comedones; skin dirty in patches.
*θ*Seborrhœa oleosa.
- Forehead, cheeks and chin covered with small red elevations with black points—acne punctata—and papulo-
pustules; digestion feeble, bowels torpid.
- Ulcer on nose and eyelid; base of ulcer of a dingy, red-
dish-yellow color, dry, glazed and free from granulations, and discharge but slight.
- Itching, tingling and swelling of face. *θ*Smallpox.
⁹ Lower Face. ▪Aphthæ on lips; tongue swollen.
- ¦¦Pimples about mouth and chin.
- Epithelial cancer of lip.
- Tenacious mucus hangs in shreds from mouth.
¹⁰ Teeth and Gums. ▪Gums dark red and swollen.
¹¹ Taste and Tongue. Taste: flat; peppery; bitter or saltish.
- Tongue and lips parched, red and dry.
- Dryness of tongue, with sensation as if it had been
burned.
- Tongue as if burned or scalded, later a vesicle on tip.
- Tongue coated yellowish-white.
- Tongue foul and coated with thick white fur.
- Large, flabby, slimy looking tongue.
- Tongue large and flabby, showing imprint of teeth.
*θ*Stomatitis.
- Tongue: swollen, showing marks of teeth; coated white,
or with a yellow stripe.
- Tongue raw, dark red, with raised papillæ.
- Cancerous affections of tongue.

[12] **Inner Mouth.** ❙ Excessive secretion of thick, tenacious mucus.

❙ Gums and mucous membrane of mouth dark red and swollen; uvula relaxed and sore; hawking of large quantities of yellow tenacious mucus from throat, leaving a sensation of rawness.

❙ Mucous membrane of fauces studded with round, protuberant spots of a red color, as if injected with blood, < from least exposure to cold.

❙ Soreness and rawness of mouth, with raised papillæ and dark red appearance of mucous membranes.

❙ Follicular and catarrhal ulcers with exceedingly tenacious mucus in mouth.

❙❙ Stomatitis: after mercury or chlorate of potash; in nursing women or weakly children; with peppery taste; tongue as if burned, or raw, with dark red appearance and raised papillæ; during course of eruptive fevers.

❙ Aphthous sore mouth.

❙ Jaws set; liquids swallowed with difficulty; power of articulation lost; ulceration of mouth. θMercurial salivation.

❙ Gangrenous sore mouth after abuse of mercury and chlorate of potash.

❙ Syphilitic affections of mouth, throat and nares.

❙ Syphilitic angina.

❙ Dense, irregular tumor in hard palate, painful to touch, and somewhat elastic, disposed to bleed and to discharge offensive matter; climacteric. θCancer.

[13] **Throat.** ❙ Uvula sore and relaxed.

❙ Hawking of yellow tenacious mucus from posterior nares and fauces; rawness of fauces; ulcers in throat; after mercury and chlorate of potash.

❙❙ Pain on swallowing as from excoriation.

❙ Sensation of rawness in throat, after hawking up large quantities of tenacious mucus.

❙❙ Tingling and smarting in throat.

❙ Soreness of neck and throat, with relaxation of palate.

❙❙ Great swelling, redness and itching, and great soreness of throat.

❙ Sore throat arising from irritation of stomach and lower portion of œsophagus.

❙ Sore throat from gastric derangement.

❙ Ulcerated sore throat: with putrid odor; from salivation by mercury or after chlorate of potash.

❙ Angina with ulceration, accompanying scarlatina.

❙ Chronic angina, with round, protuberant red spots in throat, with sensation of roughness and stiffness when swallowing.

ı ıChilliness although well covered; headache of a beating or darting character, and not confined to any one locality; stools consist entirely of blood; epistaxis. *θ*Diphtheria.

∎Pseudo-membranes, or tenacious mucous secretions, resembling dipthheria, with or without ulceration.

∎Diphtheritic sore throat.

ı ıSyphilitic angina.

∎Syphilitic sore throat.

∎Results of mercurial salivation.

∎Chronic catarrhal affections of throat.

∎Follicular pharyngitis.

¹⁴ **Appetite, Thirst. Desires, Aversions.** ∎Anorexia.

∎Poor appetite, with constipation of seven or eight weeks' standing.

∎Little thirst, with loathing of food.

¹⁵ **Eating and Drinking.** ∎Indigestion from atony of stomach.

∎Bread, or vegetables cause acidity, weakness, indigestion.

¹⁶ **Hiccough, Belching, Nausea and Vomiting.** ∎Eructations putrid, or more commonly sour.

∎Vomits all she eats, except milk and water.

¹⁷ **Scrobiculum and Stomach.** ı ıSinking at epigastrium and palpitation of heart.

∎Violent pulsations in epigastrium, and palpitation of heart, with heavy, dull, hard thumping, fulness of chest and dyspnœa.

∎Even slight pressure of hand reveals strong pulsations in pit of stomach.

∎Feeling of weight in stomach and epigastrium.

∎Anorexia with dyspeptic feeling in epigastrium.

ı ıPain at pit of stomach and extreme emaciation, with vomiting of all food save milk and water. *θ*Cancer of stomach.

∎Pains in stomach five or six years, then loss of strength, great sensitiveness of epigastric region, in which pulsations isochronous with pulse were perceived, and a flattened, resistant tumor of some two inches in diameter; in a few months pains became insufferable, loss of appetite and sleep alarming, frequent vomiting and great anguish about heart almost permanent; tumor pronounced scirrhous. *θ*Epigastric tumor with marasmus.

∎Flat, resistant tumor, two inches in diameter in epigastrium, sensitive to pressure, pulsations synchronous with pulse, insufferable pains, frequent vomiting, loss of appetite, anguish about heart, sleeplessness, loss of strength. *θ*Cancer.

❙Faintness at stomach; sinking, gone feeling, with continued violent palpitation of heart.

❙Dull, aching pain in stomach, which causes a very weak faintish feeling, goneness in epigastric region; acidity; constipation.

❙Stomach actually sunken; weak, faint. θMarasmus.

❙Weight and fulness in stomach, or an empty, aching, "gone" feeling, more or less constant, < by a meal.

❙Food seems to lie heavy in stomach.

❙Pain in pit of stomach.

❙Acute, distressing, cutting pains in stomach.

❙Weakness of digestion, with heavy, dull, hard, thumping fulness of chest and dyspnœa.

❙Weakness of digestion, pale tongue, fulness and uneasiness in stomach after eating, weakness of body and limbs, with depression of spirits.

❙Weakness of digestion with debility, particularly in diseases from exhaustion, and in latter stages of nervous fevers.

❙❙Indigestion from an atonic state of stomach, with debility.

❙Indigestion, with acidity and general weakness.

❙Constant acid mucous vomitings; obstinate constipation; wretched nights; tongue coated; looks ill and pale; is thin and hysterical; pulse quiet; faintings every day from exhaustion; appetite good, but nearly all food returning intensely acid; no actual disease could be detected about her; has taken great quantities of acid and alkaline mixtures and has habitually used purgatives. θMucous irritation et morbus medicinalis.

❙Sympathetic affections of digestive organs arising from uterine disease.

❙Gastric disorders of intemperate people.

❙Flatulency, distension and painful digestion of dyspeptics.

❙Chronic gastric catarrh; chronic dyspepsia.

❙Gastro-duodenal catarrh; sense of sinking and prostration at epigastrium, with violent and continued palpitation of heart.

❙Chronic ulceration of mucous membrane of stomach.

❙Chronic affections of stomach, especially of mucous membrane.

❙Chronic inflammation of stomach.

❙❙Carcinoma, with emaciation; goneness.

[14] **Hypochondria.** ❙❙Fulness and dull aching in r. hypochondrium.

❙Torpor of liver, with pale, scanty stools.

❙Jaundice, with catarrh of stomach and duodenum.

❙Skin very yellow; stools white and frequent; urine very

dark; skin hot; tongue coated; great weariness and
depression; legs anasarcous; bad nights; no appetite;
slight difficulty of breathing; much fulness and tenderness over hepatic region; great aching in shoulder-
blades. θSubacute inflammation of liver.

∎Severe pain in stomach and bowels; skin and eyes dark,
greenish-yellow; urine very dark; feces light colored;
great debility. θJaundice.

∎Jaundice from structural disease of liver.

∎Catarrhal inflammation of mucous lining of gall bladder
and biliary ducts.

∎Functional disorders of liver in connection with intermittent fever.

∎Chronic derangement of liver.

ⅠⅠLiver enlarged, indurated, nodulated, and sensitive
to pressure; tumor in epigastrium as large as a hen's
egg, doughy in consistency, and in centre a small spot
as if filled with fluid; after eating, vomiting of food in-
corporated with sour, putrid mucus; thirst, loss of appetite, diarrhœa, weakness, emaciation, sleeplessness.

∎Liver atrophied. θMarasmus.

∎Sharp pain in region of spleen, with constant dull pain
in stomach and bowels, with hot, burning sensation.

∎Severe cutting pains in splenic and cæcal regions, and in
hypogastrium.

¹⁹ **Abdomen.** Burning in region of navel, with goneness
and faintness in epigastrium.

∎Severe cutting pain in hypogastric region, extending into
testicle, occurring after stool, with faint feeling.

∎Sense of constriction in hypogastric region.

ⅠⅠLoud rumbling, with dull aching in hypogastrium and
small of back; < moving.

∎Flatulent colic, accompanied by faintness.

∎Flatulent colic; sensation of a lump of the size of a hen's
egg, rising and falling in r. iliac and lumbar regions;
sharp pains around umbilicus extending to l. ovarian
and splenic regions; moaning with occasional outcries;
very restless, no sleep; abdominal walls painful on
pressure; discharge of flatulency, sounding like the
report of a pistol; tongue and lips parched and dry;
little thirst and loathing of food; constipation of bowels;
·offensive pus-like discharge from vagina; great tenderness of os uteri; countenance pale and haggard; hiccough; hectic fever; cold sweats and bedsores.

∎Cutting, colicky pains, with heat and faintness; constipation; > after passing flatus.

∎Colicky pains, with fainting turns and heat in bowels,
following constipation.

∎Griping, with profuse light colored diarrhœa.
∎Griping, with light acrid stools.
∎Sharp pain in region of spleen, with dull pain and burn-
  ing in stomach and bowels.
Pain in large intestines and rectum.
∎Sharp pain in cæcal region.
∎Sensation of great fulness in l. iliac region.
∎Dull dragging in groins, cutting pains extending into
  testicles.
∎Pains in groin, as if he had strained himself; clothing
  uncomfortable.
∎Intestinal catarrh, followed by ulceration.
∣∣Blenorrhœa of the intestines.
∎Chronic intestinal catarrh. ·
∎Chronic catarrhal or croupous enteritis.

²⁰ Stool and Rectum. ∣∣Urging to urinate, and sensation as
  if bowels would move, but only wind passes.
∎Discharge of flatus with great noise.
∎Fetid flatus.
∎Stools loose, soft, light colored, with flatus.
∎Soft stool, followed by severe cutting pain in hypogas-
  trium, with dull aching in testicles and faintness.
∎Slimy, tenacious discharges with tenesmus; or when
  feces are in form of hard balls coated over with yel-
  lowish, tough mucus. θChronic enteritis
∎Stool: light colored, soft; acrid; greenish; lumpy, cov-
  ered with mucus; hard, knotty.
∎Stools hard and nodulated, of a gray or brown color.
∎Constipation; feces like bullets.
∎One or two stools a week, very hard but of natural color.
∎Scanty stools occasionally, alternating with discharge of
  membranous casts.
∎Torpidity and want of desire for stool.
∎Constipation more from sluggish state of bowels than
  from diseased condition of system.
∎Obstinate constipation where catarrhal indigestion is coincident.
∎Obstinate constipation and its attendant dull headache
  in forehead; weak feeling in epigastric region; sour
  eructations and "dyspeptic cough," with copious expectoration of thick mucus.
∎Constipation of long standing, aggravated by cathartic
  medicines; patients weak and feeble; complexion sallow; tongue foul; pain in lower bowels and rectum;
  indigestion; stools hard and nodulated.
∎Constipation, one or two stools a week for eight years,
  and then only after use of purgatives; continual pain
  in head, especially in morning; bad taste in mouth with

coated tongue; pain in back and shoulders; sensation
of constriction in hypogastric region, > only by purga-
tion; yellow or rather bilious tint of face, skin smooth
and dry; severe pain after each stool, which is hard and
knotty, and of a brown color.

Constipation: headache and piles; after stools, for hours
severe pain in rectum and anus; colic pains with fainting turns and heat in bowels; anæmia; remittent fever;
after purgative medicines.

Three weeks after confinement was seized, while at stool,
with severe burning, stinging pains in rectum and anus,
lasting six to eight hours after each evacuation; and accompanied with a sensation of heat in intestines, colic
pains and fainting;. every week one or two very hard,
but natural colored stools.

Sore neck, sore throat which is much relaxed and inflamed; headache; cough and expectoration; pain in
side while stooping and rising from recumbent position;
foul breath; tongue foul and coated with a thick white
fur; appetite poor; constipated; after purgatives.

Constipation and hemorrhoids during pregnancy, with
severe pain during stool, no hemorrhage.

Constipated habit since birth, after failure of cathartics
and enemas.

Constipation: with piles; of hepatic origin; following
rheumatic fever; the cause of other ailments.

After stool: long lasting pain in rectum; hemorrhoids
and fainting; exhaustion.

Smarting, burning pains in rectum, during and after
each stool.

Proctitis.

Ulceration of rectum, after bad cases of dysentery.

Prolapsus of rectum; simple prolapsus in children, with
congestion and swelling of mucous membrane, and
marked constipation.

Fistula ani with constipation, piles and ulceration.

Fissures and excoriations of anus.

Hemorrhoids, when a small loss of blood is followed by
excessive weakness.

Painful hemorrhoids, with paroxysms of headache and
constipation; severe burning, smarting pains in rectum,
before and after each stool; colic pains, with attacks of
faintness and heat in intestines, often follow evacuations,
after a constipation of several days.

Hemorrhoidal swellings which bleed profusely at times;
much prolapsus recti; offensive, dirty-looking, hemorrhoidal discharge from anus, obliging him to wear a
bandage.

▮Piles and headache with constipation.

[21] **Urinary Organs.** ▮Dull aching in region of kidneys.

▮Catarrh of bladder, with thick, ropy, mucous sediment in urine.

▮Chronic cystitis; diabetes; gravel.

▮Symptoms of ulceration of bladder.

▮Difficulty in making water.

▮Suppression of urine.

▮Incontinence of urine.

Urine increased and of neutral reaction.

High colored urine which deposits a cloudy sediment while standing.

▮Urine smells as if decomposed.

[22] **Male Sexual Organs.** ▮Debility, after spermatorrhœa.

▮Spermatorrhœa, incipient stricture, chronic gonorrhœa, gleet, inflammation and ulceration of whole internal coat of bladder.

▮Gonorrhœa, second stage, thick, yellow discharge.

▮Long lasting gonorrhœa, accompanied by great moral and physical depression.

▮Acute or chronic gonorrhœa; feeling of debility and faintness after each passage from bowels.

▮Catarrh of urethra; after acute gonorrhœa, a gleety discharge remains; copious, painless, urethral discharge; spurious gonorrhœa; relaxation of urethral mucous membrane, and a consequent weeping, the discharge being almost watery in character.

▮Gleet with debility; copious, painless, sometimes thick discharge.

▮Dragging in r. groin to testicle, thence to l. testicle, thence to l. groin.

[23] **Female Sexual Organs.** ▮Aching pains in small of back at change of life; uterine affections, accompanied by debility and disorder of digestive functions.

▮Offensive, pus-like discharges from vagina.

▮Great tenderness of os uteri.

▮Discharge of tough, stringy mucus from os uteri.

▮Mucous leucorrhœa; uterine and vaginal catarrh.

▮Epithelial abrasion of os and cervix uteri and vagina, with superficial ulceration of parts.

▮Cervix uteri swollen, indurated and eroded.

▮Ulceration of os, cervix and vagina; leucorrhœa; debility; prolapsus uteri.

▮Hot, watery discharge from uterus.

▮Uterine diseases with sympathetic affections of digestive organs.

▮Uterine hemorrhage, menorrhagic form; bleeding excessive for ten days during each period, attended with pain and anæmia; hemorrhage from fibroid tumor; congestive dysmenorrhœa; subinvolution of uterus; metritis; endometritis; menopause.

▮Metrorrhagia: consequent upon fibroid tumors; in girls fifteen to eighteen years of age; puerperal hemorrhages; endometritis.

▮Profuse menses for a year, flowing ten days or more; dysmenorrhœa; great prostration and anæmia.

▮After catching cold by getting feet wet during menstruation, severe pains in bowels and uterine region, "it felt like wind;" a lump, size of a hen's egg, rises and falls in r. iliac and lumbar regions; sharp pains around umbilicus, extending to l. ovarian and splenic region; continual moaning and distressing outcries; very restless; sleepless; abdominal walls painful to pressure; discharge of flatus which sounds like report of pistol.

Tongue and lips parched and dry; little thirst; loathing of food; constipation; injections per anum followed by bullet-shaped feces; offensive, pus-like discharge from vagina; great tenderness of os uteri; pale and haggard; hiccough; hectic fever; cold sweats; bedsores. θUterine affections.

▮Regurgitation of food by mouthful, without nausea, which, however, affords relief; despondent and gloomy; when food is retained suffers from headache, palpitation of heart and nervousness, or restlessness; bad taste in throat from breath; mouth very dry in morning, and tongue thickly coated; sour risings from stomach; great quantities of wind in stomach causing distress until discharged; after eating must keep quiet or she becomes feverish and distressed; pain in bowels three or four hours after eating with inclination to stool; pain and soreness of liver; after dinner nervous and irritable, cannot bear to be spoken to; becomes so nervous that to hear any one speak is unbearable and head aches intensely; on closing eyes sees sparks and light spots; pain in and over eyeballs; pain on opening eyes; cannot sleep until after midnight; epigastric region very tender to touch; sensation as of a tight band around waist, < at night; constant coldness of hands, feet and limbs while head is hot; constipation, feces at first dry and lumpy, afterwards like white of egg; great straining at stool; nosebleed before menses; menses delayed, preceded and accompanied by severe pains in back and headache; constant, acrid, corroding leucorrhœa < ten days after menses cease; when standing feels as if everything would fall out; very tender about vulva; discharge like white of egg, coming on immediately after

menses cease, lasting ten days or longer, profuse and debilitating; severe pain in small of back and in back
part of legs; pain in inside of legs above knees; coition
very painful, with almost constant desire, especially during the time she has "white of egg" discharge, amounting to furor uterinus; after coition prostration and distress in stomach; commences at once to spit up the last
meal, or has taste of it in mouth; the "white of egg"
discharge usually becomes red, bloody fluid, and soon
as it ceases she becomes irritable and angry with every
one, and cannot endure idea of coition, any reference to
it making her angry; constant desire to pass water, and
when a little is passed she is relieved, and it seems to
her that if she could pass a great quantity of water she
would feel still better; in morning this desire is less; at
times, discharges of hot water from womb, which is so
profuse as to wet bed and all her clothes; uterus prolapsed; os indurated and congested; all symptoms >
by lifting womb into place and holding it there; > in
recumbent posture.

‖Tenacious, viscid leucorrhœa, uterine or vaginal.

❙Mucous leucorrhœa, discharge hanging from os in long
viscid strings.

❙Yellow, tenacious leucorrhœa, long threads or pieces in
it; sometimes offensive.

‖Leucorrhœa tenacious, ropy, thick, yellow.

❙Leucorrhœa complicated with hepatic derangement and
constipation.

❙Pruritus vulvæ, with profuse leucorrhœa; sexual excitement.

❙Lancinating pain in breast, extending up to shoulder and
down arms.

❙Pain in l. breast, so bad as to prevent all rest at night.

❙Pain in breast, almost unbearable, causing a worn and
haggard appearance of countenance.

❙Pains accompanying cancer in breast.

❙Scirrhous tumor of l. breast; hard, heavy and adherent
to skin, which is dark, mottled and very much puckered, the nipple being retracted; pains like knives
thrust into the part; cachectic appearance of face.

❙Stony hard, nodulated tumor in l. breast, unattached to
skin, perfectly movable and as large as a filbert; lancinating pains.

❙Cancer of l. breast as large as a small egg, with retraction
of nipple.

❙Hard, irregular enlargement of l. breast; nipple retracted,
and glands of l. axilla enlarged and painful; mother
had died of cancer of tongue.   θCancer.

▮Irregular nodule of scirrhus of mamma, with retraction of nipple; enlargement of axillary glands; health poor; sallow complexion.

▮Epithelioma of mamma.

In a case of open cancer of l. breast, which had been ulcerated for four or five years, it diminished the ulcerated surface, which was as large as half crown, to a size not as large as a pea.

▮In open cancer of r. mamma, relieved the constant burning pain and favored healing, healthy granulations making their appearance.

²¹ **Pregnancy. Parturition. Lactation.** ▮Sore mouth of nursing women; tongue large, and retains the impression made by teeth.

▮Abraded, cracked and sore nipples of nursing women.

²⁵ **Voice and Larynx. Trachea and Bronchia.** ▮Scraping in larynx.

▮Cough, with rawness of larynx; tingling and smarting in throat; hawks up tenacious, yellow or white mucus; pain on swallowing as if throat were excoriated; cough rough, harsh and rattling, and continued day and night; abdominal congestion. θLaryngo-tracheitis. θBronchitis.

▮Bronchial catarrh of old people, with debility, loss of appetite, and a general cachectic condition.

▮Catarrhal cough of long standing, with febrile symptoms in evening and night, with debility in children.

▮Rough, harsh and rattling cough, day and night.

²⁷ **Cough.** ▮Dry, harsh cough, from tickling in larynx.

▮Chronic catarrhal cough, with febrile paroxysms in evening and night, with debility; cough rough, harsh and rattling, continued day and night.

▮Chronic cough, accompanied by febrile paroxysms evenings and night, and excessive prostration; sputa thick, yellowish, very tenacious, stringy and profuse.

▮Old man's cough; senile catarrh.

²⁸ **Inner Chest and Lungs.** ▮Rawness, soreness and burning in chest.

▮Bronchitis of old, exhausted people; thick, yellow, tenacious, stringy sputa.

▮Phthisis, to relieve goneness in stomach, emaciation, loss of appetite.

▮▮Cancer of r. lung, with nodules in external walls of chest (relieved).

²⁹ **Heart, Pulse and Circulation.** ▮Palpitation, with faintness.

▮Dyspnœa, with heavy beating of heart.

▮Intermittent pulsation of heart.

▮Palpitation of heart, with heavy, dull, hard, thumping

fulness of chest and dyspnœa, in connection with dyspepsia.

▌Palpitation, pain shooting from chest to l. shoulder, with numbness of arm; irregular, and at times labored action of heart; cannot lie on either side; feeling of immediate suffocation on attempting to lie on l. side; unable from weakness and dizziness to sit in erect posture; sounds of chest dull on percussion; heart has a muffled sound, as if laboring in a sac of water; a blowing and rushing sound in under portion, and peculiar noise at each stroke, like striking knuckle against a hard substance; swelling of abdomen, particularly upper portion; œdema of legs; urine scanty and turbid; constipation; tongue yellowish-white; no appetite; food causes nauséa; frequent sinking spells. θHeart disease.

▌Pulse slow, during the chill.

⁰⁰ Outer Chest. ⅠⅠPain in r. breast and down arm.

▌Thoracic or intercostal myalgia.

³¹ Neck and Back. ▌Ulcers under r. and l. inferior maxilla from broken down lymphatic glands.

▌Chronic suppuration and swelling of cervical glands; great weakness. θScrofula.

ⅠⅠExcoriations in folds of skin of neck. θIntertrigo.

▌Muscles of neck feel sore.

▌Pain in back and shoulders.

▌Aching pain in small of back in women, at change of life.

▌Debility and weakness in back and lower limbs, > by walking about.

▌Tired aching across small of back and in limbs; knees ache.

▌Stiffness in muscles of lumbar region while bending over for a short time, causing great difficulty when assuming an erect posture; dull, heavy, dragging pain and stiffness of back, especially across lumbar region, necessitating use of arms to rise from a seat; must walk about some time before being able to straighten up.

³² Upper Limbs. ▌Pain from head to shoulders, with aching in both, more the left.

▌Rheumatic pains in elbow, forearms, right shoulder and first finger of l. hand.

▌Right arm, from tips of fingers to shoulder, greatly swollen, and one mass of sores, discharging fetid pus; glands in axilla tender and swollen; elbow enlarged and full of sores; exceedingly weak and nervous, owing to severe pain and constant loss of sleep; emaciation.

Small boils, two or three inches apart on hands, arms and shoulders, some papular with inflamed area, others pustular.

❚Ulcer from a burn, on back of hand, greatly inflamed and very painful; could hardly move wrist.

ᴴ Lower Limbs. ❚Pain from r. hip to knee, while walking; cannot stand or bear one's weight.

❚Legs feel weak; knees weak; aching.

❚Outer part of l. knee aches while sitting, < when walking.

❚Erysipelas of lower extremities.

❚Bright efflorescence from patella to bend of foot; scaly skin slightly broken here and there, having in some places a jagged and cracked appearance; slight serous moisture; intolerable itching.

❚Irritable and indolent ulcers on legs.

❚Atonic old ulcers on legs.

❚Scrofulous ulcers on leg and foot.

❚Ulcers on both legs resulting from injuries.

❚Dry, superficial, angry looking ulcers on legs; covered by a yellow scab; stinging burning pain; areola inflamed, and covered by pimples, which frequently degenerate into ulcers; faint fetid odor; circular shape with flat edges; one of ulcers had high and thick edges; no pus; < at night also from warmth of bed, on motion, or on touching them; l. side. .

❚Three large ulcers each one of which seems to belong to a separate class, around r. ankle; one in front is circular with high elevated edges slightly rounded, surrounded by inflamed skin; irregular base, bleeds readily and discharges a thin corrosive ichor; one on outside is circular, with clean, sharp cut edges, deep, smooth, shining base, but with ichorous discharge; inside one is largest, ragged, irregular and deep; rough base; high, rounded and swollen edges at upper part, well defined at the lower; discharge of grayish, putrid, thick pus and has one or two patches of large, flabby, pale granulations; pain from motion and from warmth of bed; on stepping on ground pricking sensation in sores, and on sitting down to rest after motion, shooting or lancinating ain in ulcers.

❚Extensive œdema of foot and ankle.

❚Aching in sole of l. foot; no > from change of position.

❚Dorsal surface of feet red, infiltrated, especially about toes, between which are deep fissures; aggravations from ointments; poor digestion; constipation alternating with diarrhœa.

❚Hard, nodulated tumor as large as a walnut on dorsum of foot; occasionally painful.

❚Scrofulous ulcers in hollow of sole of foot, and over tarsal and metatarsal bones, discharging pus and sanious matter; loss of appetite; pale face; melancholia.

** Limbs in General.** ❚Limbs tired and aching. θCoryza.
❚Shifting pains in r. arm and leg, then l. leg.

** Rest. Position. Motion.** Lying: on l. side causes feeling
of immediate suffocation; cannot lie on either side.

Recumbent position: > womb complaints.

Sitting: outer part of l. knee aches after motion; shooting
pains in ulcers; in erect posture, dizziness.

Standing: feels as if everything would fall out.

Dull, heavy, dragging pain and stiffness of back especially
across lumbar region, necessitating use of arms to rise
from a seat; must walk about some time before being
able to straighten up.

Rising from recumbent position: pain in side.

Stooping: pain in side; causes stiffness of muscles in lumbar region.

Walking: weakness in back and lower limbs; pain in r.
hip and knee; outer part of l. knee aches.

Moving: < rumbling in abdomen with dull aching in
hypogastrium and small of back; can hardly move
wrist on account of ulcers; ulcers on legs <.

** Nerves.** ❚Frequent sudden attacks of fainty spells, with
profuse cold sweat all over. θCancerous ulcers on l.
side of throat, inside.

❚Cachectic condition with loss of appetite and fainting.

❚After measles, great emaciation, depression of spirits;
easily excited to anger; liver reduced in size; urine
scanty and high colored. θMarasmus.

❚General debility.

❚Debility from gastric, bilious and typhoid fevers.

❚Faintness, goneness, great weakness and physical prostration.

** Sleep.** ❚Awakened by backache and dull pains in navel
and hypogastric region.

❚Dreams worrisome; restless sleep.

❚❚Difficulty in awaking.

** Time.** Morning: continual pain in head; mouth very dry;
desire to pass water >; chill.

10.30 A.M.: dull, piercing pain on top of head, outward
from ears.

Day: cough.

Evening: febrile symptoms; chill; dull, burning pain.

10 P.M.: great heat of whole body.

Night: feeling of tight band around waist <; cannot
sleep on account of pain in l. breast; cough; febrile symptoms; ulcers on legs <; chilliness; delirium; erysipelatous rash; pains <.

Before midnight: cannot sleep.

** Temperature and Weather.** Warmth: < weeping erup-

tion on forehead after having been in cold air; causes
itching; ulcers on legs.

In room: discharge scanty from nose.

Washing: < eruption on forehead.

Getting feet wet during menses: severe pain in bowels.

Harsh, dry winds: cause acute catarrhal ophthalmia.

Out of doors: discharge from nose profuse.

⁴⁰ **Fever.** ❙Chill morning or evening; chilliness, especially in
back or thighs, with aching, or around shoulders and
.chest; pulse slow.

❙Chilliness at night.

❙Heat, in flushes, over face, neck and hands.

❙Great heat of whole body, dull, burning pain all evening.

❙Great heat of whole body, at 10 P.M., followed by great
debility.

❙Profuse, offensive sweat of genitals.

❙Gastric, bilious or typhoid forms of fever, with gastric
disturbances, jaundice and great debility following.

❙Fevers which do not reach a high grade of inflammatory
action, but which are attended with gastric and bilious
disturbances, or complicated with jaundice, and the del-
eterious effects of mercury or quinine.

❙Intermittent fever: cachectic subjects; gastric and hepatic symptoms, showing atony and torpor; vertex
headache in paroxysms every other day, commencing
at 11 A.M., with excessive nausea, retching and anguish.

❙Quotidian fevers, with gastric disturbance; jaundice.

❙Catarrhal symptoms which frequently precede measles;
also favors development of eruption.

❙Typhoid fever with characteristic temperature; for days
before attack feeling of entire goneness in pit of stomach,
with no desire for food; abdominal tenderness, gurgling
in ileo-cæcal region, with bloated abdomen; delirium
at night; a feeling that he could not recover.

❙Typhoid fever; retarded convalescence; will eat nothing;
tongue large, flabby, thickly coated, and shows imprint
of teeth; bowels constipated; urine scanty; copious
sweats; sleeplessness.

❙Hectic fever.

⁴¹ **Attacks, Periodicity.** Every day: faintings.

For hours: after stool, severe pain in rectum.

Three or four hours after eating: pains in bowels.

Twenty-four hours: urine suppressed.

Every other day: vertex headache at 11 A.M.

For days before attack of typhoid fever: feeling of entire
goneness in pit of stomach.

For ten days: excessive bleeding, uterine hemorrhage;
after menses leucorrhœa <.

Three weeks after confinement: seized after stool with
severe burning, stinging pains in rectum and anus,
lasting six or eight hours after each evacuation.

For a year: profuse menses flowing for ten days.

For four or five years: open cancer of l. breast.

For eight years: one or two stools a week.

" Locality and Direction. Right: tickling like a hair in
nostril; pain in breast; burning in nostril; inner edge of
ala nasi sore and thickened; inflammation in ear; eye
closed from inflammation; dragging in groin to testicle;
lump rising and falling in iliac and lumbar region;
fulness and dull aching in hypochondrium; open cancer of mamma; cancer of lung; pain in breast and
down arms; ulcer under inferior maxilla; rheumatic
pains in shoulder; arm greatly swollen; pain from hip
to knee; three large ulcers around ankle; shifting pains
in leg and arm.

Left: sharp cutting over eyes <; laceration of scalp above
temple; stye on lid; nosebleed l. nostril; formation of
diphtheritic membrane in nostril; side of nose swollen;
inflammation from nostril to r. ear; dragging in testicle
to groin; sharp pain extending to ovarian region; fulness in iliac region; scirrhous tumor of breast; stony
hard nodulated tumor in breast; cancer of breast; hard,
irregular enlargement of breast; glands of axilla enlarged and painful; open cancer of breast; pain shooting from chest to shoulder; ulcer under inferior maxilla;
aching in shoulder; rheumatic pains in first finger of
hand; outer part of knee aches; ulcers on legs; aching
in sole of foot; cancerous ulcer on side of throat.

Shifting pains from r. leg to left.

" Sensations. As if intoxicated; tickling like a hair in r. nostril; as if tongue had been burned; pain on swallowing
as from excoriation; food seems to lie heavy on stomach;
small spot in epigastric tumor as if filled with fluid; as
if a lump of size of a hen's egg rising and falling on r.
iliac and lumbar regions; pains in groins as if he had
strained himself; pain in uterine region felt like wind;
as of a tight band around waist; as if everything would
fall out when standing; as if knives were thrust into
breast; as if throat was excoriated.

Pain: in eyes; over eyeballs; in r. breast and down arms;
in ears; at pit of stomach; in large intestines; in rectum; in groin; in back; in shoulders; in bowels; in
liver; on opening eyes; in l. breast; from head to
shoulders; from r. hip to knee.

Insupportable pains: in epigastric region.

Excruciating pain: in lumbar region.

Intense pain: in head.

Severe pain: in forehead; in stomach and bowels; in abdomen after stool; in rectum and anus; in uterine region; in back; in small of back; in back part of legs.

Lancinating pain: in breast extending up to shoulder and down arms; in ulcers.

Cutting pains: from groins into testicles.

Acute, distressing, cutting pains: in stomach.

Sharp cutting: in temples; in splenic and cæcal regions; in hypogastric. region, extending into testicle; in lower bowels and rectum; on inside of legs above knees.

Cutting, colicky pains: in abdomen.

Sharp pains: in region of spleen; around umbilicus; extending to l. ovarian and splenic regions; in cæcal region; around umbilicus.

Great anguish: about heart.

Shooting pains: from chest to l. shoulder; in ulcers.

Darting pain: in head.

Griping: in abdomen.

Beating pain: in head.

Stinging pains: in rectum and anus; in ulcers on legs.

Severe burning pain: in rectum.

Pricking pains: in ulcers.

Rheumatic pains: in elbow, forearm, r. shoulder and first finger of l. hand.

Shifting pains: in r. arm and leg, then l. leg.

Continual pain: in head.

Tired aching: across small of back; in limbs.

Aching: in shoulder-blades; in small of back; in knees; in head and shoulders; in outer part of l. knee; in soles of l. foot.

Dull dragging: in groins; from groin to r. then to l. testicles across lumbar region.

Dull, aching pains: at stomach; in r. hypogastrium; in hypogastrium and small of back; in region of kidneys.

Dull, burning pains: all over body.

Dull, heavy frontal headache.

Dull pain in hypogastrium; in small of back; on top of head; in stomach and bowels; in navel.

Fulness: over eyes; of chest; of stomach; of r. hypogastrium; in hepatic region; in l. iliac region.

Great sensitiveness: of epigastric region.

Tenderness: of cervical glands; over hepatic region; of os uteri; of abdomen.

Soreness: of cartilaginous septum; of inner edge of r. ala; of uvula; of mouth; of neck and throat; of liver; of nipple; in chest.

Pricking sensation: in ears.

Burning heat: of skin.

Burning: of eyes and lids; in nose; in r. nostril; l. nostril;
in stomach; in bowels; in region of navel; in rectum
and anus; in chest; in ulcers; on legs.

Heat: in intestines; of whole body.

Smarting: of eyes: in posterior nares; in nostrils; in
throat; in rectum.

Sharp, raw, excoriated feeling: in both nares.

Sensation of roughness and stiffness: on swallowing.

Scraping: in larynx.

Rawness: in nares; in throat and chest; of l. nostril; of
mouth; of fauces; of larynx; in chest.

Tickling: in r. nostril.

Tingling: of throat.

Dryness: of upper lids; of tongue.

Constriction: in hypogastric region.

Stuffed up sensation: in posterior nares.

Heaviness: of upper lids.

Weight: in stomach and epigastrium.

Roaring: in ears.

Stiffness: in muscles of lumbar region.

Numbness: of arm.

Faintness: at stomach; in hypogastrium.

Goneness: at epigastrium; in pit of stomach.

Debility: in back and lower limbs.

Weakness: of body and limbs.

Itching: of l. nostril; of face; of throat; of foot; of skin.

" Tissues. ▮Great emaciation; weight reduced 70 pounds;
very moody and depressed in mind; averse to conversing;
at times so excited as to curse his mother for the least
thing, and throwing food or medicine across room; liver
atrophied, not more than two-thirds the natural size;
kidneys affected, urine scanty and high colored. θGen-
eral marasmus.

▮Small wounds bleed much.

▮General anasarca; great difficulty in passing water, which
is high colored and deposits a cloudy sediment on standing; constipation.

Mucous membranes: secretions increased, tenacious, ropy;
erosions.

▮Catarrhal affections: in patients of a cachectic habit.

▮▮Muscles greatly weakened; atony.

▮Marasmus; scrofula; cancer cachexia.

▮Cancers: hard, adherent, skin mottled, puckered; cutting
like knives; in mammæ.

In cancer it removes the pain, modifies the discharge, depriving it of its offensiveness, and improves the general
health in a marked degree.

In early stage of scirrhus, and chiefly when its situation
is in a gland or in the immediate vicinity of a gland.

Stage of degenerative softening in scirrhus.

Touch. Passive Motion. Injuries. Touch: causes bleeding of cartilaginous septum which is sore; epigastric region very tender; ulcers on legs <.

Pressure: cutting over eyes >; abdominal walls painful; liver sensitive; of hand > head; clothing feels uncomfortable about groins.

Skin. Skin jaundiced, of a dark greenish-yellow color.

Skin of a dark purplish hue, with heat and tingling, < from motion.

Hot, dry skin, with fever.

Burning heat and itching of skin.

Itching in small-pox.

Yellowish looking vesicles, filled with a limpid fluid.

Hyperidrosis; excessive sweat of axillæ or about genitals; offensive.

Obstinate excoriations of skin, intertrigo, in children.

Nettlerash from head to foot, next day face affected, and through scratching became much swollen; lids puffed; itching, burning and stinging, < at night; rash resembled scarlatina, both in color and in disappearing a long time on pressure.

Erysipelatoid rash on face, neck, palms, joints of fingers and wrist, with maddening, burning heat, later skin exfoliates; pains < at night.

Fissures around mucous outlets, as on lips, about anus, or on flexor surfaces, and between fingers and toes of syphilitic subjects, who have used too much mercury or iodide of potash; debilitated subjects, broken down by excessive use of alcohol.

Margins around anus thickened and fissured, fissures extending into mucous membrane.

Ulcers with indolent granulations; unhealthy and scanty pus; scrofulous or cachectic persons.

Chronic ulcers arising from contusions, incised and lacerated wounds, burns, scalds, or some disease of skin.

Ulcers following removal of tumors, pricking pain on motion of part.

Bedsores.

Small-pox; itching; tingling of skin; great redness, swelling and aching of skin; very sore throat; intense aching in small of back and legs; pustules dark; ulcers in mouth and fauces; sleeplessness.

Variola, itching tingling of eruption: face swollen; throat raw; pustules dark; great prostration.

Face greatly swollen, eyes closed, nose enormously large and entirely stopped up; throat very sore; pustules dark; almost unconscious, having no hope of recovery θSmall-pox.

∎Face covered with a fine rash which subsequently proved
to be confluent small-pox; face greatly swollen, eyes
closed; throat sore.

In small-pox it relieves the irritation almost instantly,
removes the swelling, diminishes the odor, obviates secondary fever, prevents pitting to very great degree, and
destroys the contagious character of the disease.

∎Lupus; lupus exedens and ulcerative stage of leprosy.

" Stages of Life, Constitution. Weakened, debilitated subjects, with mucous discharges.

Cachectic persons, with marked disturbance of gastric and
hepatic functions.

∎Scrofulous diathesis.

∎Old people.

Child, æt. 1; constipation.

Boy, æt. 6, light complexion, light curly hair, had not
been vaccinated; small-pox.

Girl, æt. 8, after a fall; lacerated wound of scalp.

Little girl, after burn; ulcer on back of hand.

Girl, æt. 14, as she was about recovering from an attack
of diphtheria; diphtheritic deposit in nose and vagina.

Man, æt. 18, cachectic, consumptive appearance; scrofulous ulcers on leg.

Woman, æt. 20, brunette, black eyes, delicate features, but
strong and energetic, two months pregnant with third
child; constipation and hemorrhoids.

Woman, æt. 21, mother of one child, nervous temperament, blue eyes, light hair, has prolapsus uteri and
leucorrhœa of several years standing; uterine affection.

Unmarried woman, æt. 22; cancer of breast.

Man, æt. 22, after measles two and one-half years ago;
marasmus.

Miss ——, æt. 25, a teacher, was given up by the old
school; cancer of stomach.

Married woman, æt. 26, light hair, pale complexion, feeble
constitution, tea drinker, has suffered for twelve years;
headache and constipation.

Young unmarried woman, for two years under allopathic
treatment; cancer of breast.

Sanguine young lady, after confinement; sore mouth.

Unmarried woman; erysipelas.

Man, suffering from itch, for which corrosive sublimate
was used; salivation.

Man, æt. 28, blue eyes, light hair, unmarried, of dissipated
habits, has had three epileptic seizures, has had gonorrhœa three times; gonorrhœa.

Man, æt. 29, after habitual use of purgatives; constipation.

Woman, æt. 29, mother of two children, habitually takes
castor oil and senna; constipation.

Colored woman, æt. 30, next day after confinement; small-pox.

Woman, æt. 32, blue eyes, light hair, delicate skin, mother of two children, has used tea and coffee for fifteen years; suffering for three years; hemorrhoids.

Man, æt. 32, mason, three years ago fell from a scaffold and injured r. arm; ulceration of arm.

Man, æt. 35, mill operator, habits moderately temperate; ulcers on leg.

Mrs. J., æt. 37, laundress, health good; tumor in l. breast.

Woman, æt 38, bilous temperament, dark hair, suffering eight years, has taken much purgative medicine· constipation.

Man, æt. 40; jaundice.

Man, æt. 40, railroad engineer; small-pox.

Woman, æt. 45; cancerous tumor.

Man, æt. 46, during Crimean campaign was attacked with rheumatic fever, consequent upon exposure; anasarca and constipation.

Woman, æt 50, has suffered many years; cancer (improved).

Woman, single, æt. 52, of phthisical family, ill fourteen years, but always delicate; dyspepsia.

Mrs. D., æt. 55, suffering two years; tumor on foot.

· Woman, æt 60, widow, seven children, previously stout and healthy, after getting wet one year ago, affection of liver for which she was leeched, blistered and salivated, since which she has not been well; subacute inflammation of liver.

Woman, æt. 70; sore leg.

Man, æt. 70; epigastric tumor.

" Relations. Antidoted by: *Sulphur* (head symptoms and sciatic pains).

It antidotes: *Mercur.* and chlorate of potash.

Compare: *Amm. mur., Ant. crud., Kali bich., Pulsat.* (action on mucous membranes); *Aloes., Collin., Sepia, Sulphur* (action on lower bowels); *Berber., Digit., Gelsem.* (gastro-duodenal catarrh involving bile ducts); *Nux vom.* (gastric catarrh of alcoholism); *Amm. mur., Graphit., Nux vom.* (constipation); *Ant. crud.* (indigestion); *Kali bich.* (otorrhœa); *Arsen., Merc. corr., Euphras.* (ophthalmia); *Arg.· nitr., Kali bich.* (nasal catarrh); *Hepar* (syphilitic ozæna after abuse of mercury or iodide of potash); *Aloes, Sulphur* (cough with abdominal congestion); *Arsen., Aurum mur., Hydrocotyle, Kali bich.* (lupus); *Ant. tart., Baptis, Thuja* (variola); *Thuja* (epithelioma); *Arsen., Baptis., Conium, Condur., Kreos., Phytol., Trifol. prat.* (cancer of mammary glands); *Cinchon.* (intermittents); *Strychnia* (action on spinal cord).

HYDROCOTYLE ASIATICA.

Indian Pennywort.   *Umbelliferæ.*

A small plant long known as an Indian remedy, growing in India and Southern Africa. First employed by Boileau in the treatment of leprosy.
Experiments by Andouit; see Allen's Encyclopedia, vol. 4, p. 625.

CLINICAL AUTHORITIES.—*Lupus exedens of nose*, Andouit, B. J. H., vol. 16, p. 585; *Lupus, tuberculous, erythematic*, Martin, Hom. Rec., vol. 2, p. 177; *Ulceration cervix uteri*, Andouit, B. J. H., vol. 16, p. 588; *Pruritus vaginæ*, Andouit, B. J. H., vol. 16, p. 588; *Eczema*, Andouit, B. J. H., vol. 16, pp. 586–87; *Lepra tuberculosa*, Andouit, B. J. H., vol. 16, p. 584; *Gangrene after operation*, Andouit, B. J. H., vol. 16, p. 589; *Lepra*, Boilieu, Sinnasamy, B. J. H., vol. 16, p. 462; *Syphilitic lesions*, Martin, Hom. Rec., vol. 2, p. 177

1 **Mind.** Gayety or gloomy thoughts.
2 **Sensorium.** ∎Vertigo.
4 **Outer Head.** Intense pain with some tumefaction in posterior portion of skull; occiput acutely sensitive, especially to touch.
 Tinea favosa; painful constriction of posterior and superior integuments of skull; general lassitude and prostration.
5 **Sight and Eyes.** ∎∎Tumors of lid, especially in epithelioma.
9 **Upper Face.** ∎Copper colored eruption on face; large tubercle on r. alæ nasi, as large as sixpence, and covered with a thick crust, under which yellowish matter mixed with blood; edges of ulcer irregular and livid; five other tubercles, as large as lentils, near root of nose at both sides, and painless. *θ*Lupus exedens.
 ∎Papular eruption on face.
 ∎Neuralgic affections of supra and infraorbital nerves.
12 **Inner Mouth.** ∎∎Stomatitis aphthosa.
 ∎∎Syphilitic patches in mouth.
14 **Appetite, Thirst. Desires, Aversions.** ∎∎Loathing of food.
18 **Hypochondria.** ∎Cirrhosis of liver; hypertrophy and induration of connective tissue; obstruction in whole hepatic region; slight pain in upper portion of liver; crampy pains in stomach, without nausea.
19 **Abdomen.** ∎Flatulent colic.
20 **Stool and Rectum.** ∎Constipation.
22 **Male Sexual Organs.** ∎Acute and secondary gonorrhœa.
 ∎Gonorrhœa, which had been suppressed for fifteen years.
23 **Female Sexual Organs.** Dull pain in region of ovary.

Pains in uterus, especially of l. side.

Violent pains in uterus and neighborhood, like labor pains.

ı ıUterus feels heavy.

ı ıRedness of os uteri and cervix.

ıPartly fungous, partly granular ulcer on upper lip of neck of uterus, with profuse leucorrhœa.

ıGranular ulceration of entire neck of uterus, which is very red; prolapsus of uterus; profuse leucorrhœa.

Menses too early.

ıDeep seated heat in vagina; shooting and itching in orifice.

ıInsupportable itching of vagina.

ı ıHeat and redness of vagina and vulva.

ıProfuse leucorrhœa.

²⁹ **Heart, Pulse and Circulation.** ı ıAlleviated the sufferings in stenosis of aorta.

³⁰ **Outer Chest.** ıTwo small pustules on chest.

³¹ **Neck and Back.** ı ıSwelling of lymphatic vessels of neck.

ıOn lower third of inner surface of l. loin a large oval patch, about four and three-fourths inches in length, covered with a powder resembling pulverized chalk; the edges of a yellowish color; small eruption having the appearance of millet.

³³ **Lower Limbs.** ıYellowish spots on legs.

ıInsupportable itching of soles of feet.

ıBack of r. foot, over a space of two inches in diameter, was covered with small indurations, having a large thick crust, some grayish-white, others light yellow, the whole resting on a purple base. θTuberculous, erythematic lupus.

³⁴ **Nerves.** ıGeneral weariness.

ıDepression, heaviness and dull feeling.

ıBruised feeling in all the muscles.

Hyperæmia of nervous centres.

Acts especially upon nervus trigeminus.

⁴² **Locality and Direction.** Right: large tubercle on alæ nasi; back of foot covered with small indurations.

Left: pains in side of uterus.

⁴³ **Sensations.** Pains: in uterus.

Intense pain: in posterior portion of skull.

· Violent pains: in uterus and neighborhood.

Shooting: in orifice of vagina.

Crampy pains: in stomach.

Neuralgic affections: of supra and infraorbital nerves.

Gout: with very severe paroxysms.

Dull pain: in region of ovary.

Slight pain: in upper part of liver.

Painful constriction: of posterior and superior integuments of skull.

Acute sensitiveness: of occiput.

Bruised feeling: in all muscles.

Deep seated heat: in vagina.

Heavy feeling: of uterus.

Insupportable itching: in orifice of vagina; of vagina; of soles of feet.

" Tissues. ❙Rheumatic disorders.

❙❙Gout with very severe paroxysms.

❙Gangrene in newly formed flap on little finger.

❙Syphilitic affections of skin and mucous membranes.

" Touch. Passive Motion. Injuries. Touch: occiput acutely sensitive.

" Skin. ❙Intolerable itching in several places.

❙Pricking on different parts.

❙Erysipelatous redness.

❙Eczema.

❙Three spots, almost completely circular, with slightly raised, scaly edges.

❙Pemphigus benignus.

❙Lepra tuberculosa, especially in face, abdomen, thighs and genitals; in latter there was a large tubercle, secreting a reddish pus.

❙Arabian elephantiasis.

" Stages of Life, Constitution. It had a beneficial effect in fifty-seven cases of leprosy treated by Boileau.

Boy, æt. 15; lupus, tuberculous and erythematic, on r. foot and l. loin.

Man, æt. 16, has never suffered either from syphilis or scrofula, has lived for a long time in a damp dwelling, suffering about six·months; lepra tuberculosa.

Young woman, æt 20, delicate, weakly, during childhood suffered frequently from swelling of glands, mother has a copper colored eruption on face; suffered for eight years; lupus exedens of nose.

Man, æt 22, after an operation; gangrene of flap.

Lady, æt. 30, suffering for two months; pruritus vaginæ.

Woman, æt. 34, childless, tolerably robust constitution, melancholic, skin yellow, has suffered much from grief; ulceration of cervix uteri.

Woman, æt. 40, melancholic temperament, mother of three children; affection of uterus.

Married woman, æt. 46, delicate, has had nine children, and much anxiety; ulcer on neck of uterus.

" Relations. Compare *Hydrast.* (in lupus exedens).

HYDROCYANIC ACID.

Prussic Acid. *HCy.*

Provings by Jœrg and pupils, see Allen's Encyclopedia, vol. 5, p. 1.
Most of the symptoms are toxicological, clinically verified.

CLINICAL AUTHORITIES.—*Catarrh of stomach and small intestines*, Moore, Allg.
Hom. Ztg., vol. 105, p. 46; *Chronic dyspepsia*, Hendricks, Allg. Hom. Ztg., vol.
105, p. 144; *Asthma* (3 cases), Frank, N. A. J. H., vol. 8, p. 89; *Varicose ulcers on
legs*, Schüssler, Raue's Rec., 1870, p. 330; *Nervous exhaustion*, Chapman, B. J. H.,
vol. 7, p. 387; *Hysteria*, Payne, N. E. M. G., vol. 6, p. 432; *Convulsions*, Gallagher,
N. E. M. G., vol. 4, p. 447; *Epileptiform seizures*, Cooper, B. J. H., vol. 29, p. 783;
Hemiplegia (benefited), Swan, Hah. Mo., vol. 10, p. 322; *Traumatic tetanus*, Moore,
B. J. H., vol. 24, p. 506.

[1] **Mind.** Inability to think.
Vexed mood, despondency, oppression.
Could not remain in middle of road when he saw a vehicle
approaching him even at a considerable distance, but
was forced, as it were against his will, to stand aside
without waiting for it to come nearer. (After recovering from poisoning.)
:Insanity, when there is much excitement present, as
shown in gesture or speech.
◧Hysteria. See Chap. 36.
[2] **Sensorium.** ◧Loss of consciousness.
Dizziness with feeling of intoxication.
Sudden feeling as though everything about him moved
slowly; dizzy without reeling; slight pressure l. side of
occiput over l. half of head to frontal region.
Vertigo with reeling; with headache.
Insufficiency of arterial contraction, with frequent headaches, stupefaction and falling down; cloudiness of
senses, objects seem to move; he sees through a gauze;
is scarcely able to keep on his feet after raising head
when stooping, or rising from one's seat, < in open air.
[3] **Inner Head.** Pressure from vertex towards forehead on
both sides and to orbits where it became fixed, while
from occiput it extended down nape of neck; it caused
confusion of head.
Violent pressure in occiput and forehead, < r. side; pressure soon leaves, but confusion lasts.
◧Headache with giddiness.
Stupefying headache.
Pricking in various parts of head.

∎Sudden and desperate cases of cerebro-spinal meningitis; insensibility, with protruded, half open eyes; dilated, immovable pupils, with blindness; roaring and deafness in ears; distorted, bloated and bluish face; tongue paralyzed and protruded; loss of speech; retention of or involuntary urine and stool; rattling, slow respiration; irregular, feeble beating of heart; general coldness with heat in head.

Sudden cerebral congestion, with profound coma; preceded by vertigo, weight and great pain in back of head.

⁵ Sight and Eyes.   ⵊⵊOpen eyes, with fixed eyeballs.

∎Distorted, half open eyes.

ⵊⵊDimness of sight; gauze before eyes.

Pupils dilated, immovable, insensible to light; paralysis of lids; protrusion of eyes.

⁶ Hearing and Ears.   Roaring and buzzing in ears; hardness of hearing.

⁷ Smell and Nose.   Dryness of nose.

Stinging high up in nose, discharge of disorganized, greenish brown looking fetid pieces of hardened mucus.

Enlarged, bluish wings of nose.

⁸ Upper Face.   Sallow and gray complexion.

∎Pale, bluish face, looks old.

Face bloated; distorted.

Sudden supraorbital neuralgia, with much flushing of same side of face.

⁹ Lower Face.   ⵊⵊPale, bluish lips.

Distortion of corners of mouth.

∎Jaws firmly clenched in rigid spasm.

ⵊⵊFroth at mouth.

¹¹ Taste and Tongue.   Taste acrid, sweet or fetid.

Tongue coated white.

Lameness and stiffness of tongue.

Cold feeling of tongue.

Burning on tip of tongue.

¹² Inner Mouth.   Increased secretion of saliva.

¹³ Throat.   Scraping sensation in throat, followed by secretion of mucus in bronchia.

Heat and inflammation of throat.

ⵊⵊDrink which is swallowed rolls audibly down throat, as though it were poured into an empty barrel.

∎Spasm in pharynx and œsophagus.

∎Paralysis of œsophagus.

¹⁴ Appetite, Thirst. Desires, Aversions.   Absence of thirst, with heat of whole body, or violent thirst.

¹⁵ Eating and Drinking.   ∎Gurgling noise on drinking, like fluid running into a barrel.

¹⁶ Hiccough, Belching, Nausea and Vomiting.   Vomiting of a black fluid.

Acidity and heartburn.

[17] **Scrobiculum and Stomach.** Anguish in pit of stomach.
 ▮Great sinking sensation at epigastrium and stomach.
 Spasmodic contraction of stomach.
 ▮▮Fluids enter stomach with gurgling noise.
 ▮Gastrodynia.
 ▮Attacks of indisposition coming on particularly in evening, about two hours after a delayed dinner; during
  attack refuses all food; intense sourness, sometimes preceded by waterbrash; loss of flesh and depression of
  spirits. θCatarrh of stomach and small intestines.
 ▮Burning pain in region of navel, extending to œsophagus
  and throat, two or three hours after eating; loss of appetite; white coated tongue; pyrosis; bitter eructations;
  flatulency and constipation; region of navel sensitive to
  touch, and upon deep pressure there is a sensation as of
  a resistant body; this condition frequently alternates
  with hepatic disturbance, which manifests itself by attacks of colic; there is also present vomiting of food, or
  of a slimy, bilious matter, < evening and night; emaciation. θChronic dyspepsia.
 ▮Intense gastrodynia and enterodynia, with much flatulence, especially when heart sympathizes with the dyspeptic symptoms.
 ▮Dyspepsia dependent upon chronic inflammation of stomach and bowels.
 ▮Inflammation of stomach and bowels.

[19] **Abdomen.** Coldness of abdomen alternating with burning.
 Cold feeling in abdomen with stitches.
 ▮Enteralgia, with distension of abdomen.
 Yellow or brownish spots on abdomen.

[20] **Stool and Rectum.** ▮Involuntary stools, hiccough and
  great prostration.
 ▮Involuntary stool in bed.
 ▮Sudden prostration; long lasting fainting spells resembling apoplectic attacks. θCholera Asiatica.
 ▮Sudden cessation of all discharges. θCholera.
 ▮Rapid progress towards asphyxia; marble coldness of
  whole body; pulselessness; cessation of vomiting and
  diarrhœa; hiccough; paralysis of œsophagus; when
  drinking, fluid runs gurgling down the œsophagus;
  long fainting spells; trismus; tetanus. θCholera.
 ▮Last stage of Asiatic cholera, when diarrhœa has ceased
  and the vomiting has decreased, when there is anguish
  with pressure on chest, and the patient becomes cold,
  with gradual extinction of pulse.
 ▮Dry cholera.

[21] **Urinary Organs.** ▮Uræmia, action of heart diminished;
  pulse accelerated, soft; stagnation of circulation in heart

and lungs; palpitation, with indescribable anguish and
dyspnœa; depression of sensibility; first convulsions
and afterwards paralysis; extreme apathy; slow moaning breathing; rattling in trachea; paralysis of larynx
or sudden paralysis of heart. θ Asphyctic form of uræmia.
Retention of urine.
Copious emission of watery urine.
Involuntary urination.
" Female Sexual Organs. Gone or sinking sensation in
epigastrium, with frequent hot flashes, at climacteric
period.
" Voice and Larynx. Trachea and Bronchia. Loss of
speech.
Tickling and scraping in larynx and bronchial tubes, with
expectoration of yellowish or whitish mucus.
ǀScraping and burning in larynx.
ǀSensation as if larynx were swollen.
" Respiration. ǀǀNoisy and agitated breathing.
ǀRattling, moaning, slow breathing.
Arrest of breathing caused by stitches in larynx.
Tightness in chest, sensation of suffocation.
Feeling of suffocation with torturing pains in chest.
Asthma, especially when the minute bronchial tubes are
chiefly involved, with puffy face and feeble action of
heart; or heart's action may be violent.
ǀPeriodical asthma, and violent attacks of suffocative,
spasmodic cough.
ǀSpasmodic asthma; asthma Millari.
" Cough. Violent paroxysms of cough, or frequent cough excited by a pricking sensation, which begins in larynx
and extends down into trachea, followed by dryness of
mouth and larynx; slow, enfeebled and anxious respiration, with much rattling of mucus.
ǀDry, tickling cough in consumptives, especially if reflex
from heart disease.
Nervous cough with dyspnœa.
ǀWhooping cough; dry, spasmodic, suffocating cough.
" Inner Chest and Lungs. Threatened pulmonary apoplexy.
" Heart, Pulse and Circulation. ǀHeart's action very weak.
ǀIrregular feeble beating of heart.
ǀHeart's action irregular, pulse hardly to be felt.
: Palpitation and other functional irregularities of organ,
of no very energetic character, whether purely nervous
or associated with organic disease.
ǀSudden outcry; spasmodic sensations; long fainting
spells; heart disease with violent palpitations; feeling of
suffocation with torturing pains in chest; irregularity
of motions of heart; feeble beating of heart. θ Angina.
ǀPulse sometimes ceases.

■Pulselessness; cold, clammy sweat; involuntary stools; staring, fixed look, with dilated pupils; breathing slow, deep, gasping, difficult and spasmodic, at long intervals; apparently dead.

30 Outer Chest. Brownish spots on chest and abdomen.

31 Neck and Back. ■Muscles of back and face are principally affected.

33 Lower Limbs. ■Varicose ulcers on legs.

34 Limbs in General. Languor and weakness of limbs.

35 Rest. Position. Motion. Lies on bed: with head fixed and thrown backwards, and legs fixed and rigid; no distinct bend backwards or sideways of trunk and leg.

Lies in an apparently unconscious state, limbs and jaws rigid, forearms flexed on arms, which are firmly pressed on side.

Lies like one dead.

Frequently rises in bed, gazes vacantly about for a minute, then throws herself forcibly upon pillow, or flings herself from one side to the other.

Can scarcely stand: after raising head from stooping; on rising from one's seat.

Falls down with vertigo.

36 Nerves. ■General weakness; loss of power; great exhaustion.

Languor and weakness of limbs, especially of thighs.

■Long lasting fainting spells.

■Nervous exhaustion, the result of overwork and anxiety; loss of appetite; circulation languid; at times is forced to scream out suddenly, she knows not why; this scream is followed by faintness, sometimes even swooning; at such times either before or subsequent to faintness, tightness of chest and acute pain as of spasm of heart; at times is wakened out of sleep by this scream and the overpowering sensations. *θ*Nervous dyspepsia.

■Lies in an apparently unconscious state, limbs and jaws rigid, forearms flexed on arms, which are firmly pressed to sides; eyes fixed and drawn somewhat to the right; eyeballs slightly sensitive to touch; constant succession of tears roll down cheeks; beat of heart very irregular and feeble; occasionally utters a groan or a sigh, and presses hand forcibly over region of heart, as if suffering pain there; at these times limbs become more relaxed, and she frequently rises in bed and gazes vacantly about for a minute, then throws herself forcibly upon pillow, or flings herself from one side of bed to the other; at times great force has to be exercised to prevent her from injuring herself; if any means are used to extend the contracted arms, or open clenched teeth, she exerts greater power to prevent it; after twenty-four hours this form of attack ceased, and she became very busy packing and folding bedclothes, and placing them carefully under head, or elsewhere about bed, at same time guarding them with watchful eyes, allowing no one to touch or take them; if this is attempted, she strikes with her full strength; seems to notice no person in room, unless they interfere with her plans, but if any one enters, she seizes a pillow or anything within reach, and throws it forcibly at the intruder: at other times fixes eyes on a particular spot on wall, or on a picture, or follows an imaginary figure or object with her eyes, as if watching its motions; frequently talking, laughing loudly, or scolding vehemently; imagines herself surrounded by many friends, shaking hands with them, and calling them by name as they appear before her; she asks no questions and returns no answers; during this time, which lasted four days, she took no nourishment voluntarily. *θ*Hysteria.

- Anxious feeling and fretfulness; uneasy confusion of head; hysterical spasms; semi-consciousness; limbs and jaws rigid; eyes fixed.

▪Convulsions when muscles of back, face and jaws are principally affected, and the body assumes a bluish tint.

▪Convulsions complicated with whooping cough.

▪Infantile convulsions.

Tonic spasms; catalepsy.

▪Affects upper spine, especially medulla oblongata; blueness of surface; marked trismus, face blue, threatened suffocation; paralytic weakness quickly developed; water runs down œsophagus like through a pipe.

▪Sudden complete loss of consciousness and sensation; extreme coma for several hours, only interrupted by occasional sudden convulsive movements; confusion of head and vertigo; jaws clenched, teeth firmly set, froth at mouth, forming large bubbles; unable to swallow; involuntary discharge of urine and feces; upper extremities contracted and hands clenched; unusual stiffness of legs; spasms commencing in toes, followed by distortion of eyes, towards right and upwards, afterwards general spasms; distortion of limbs and frightful distortion of face; trunk spasmodically bent forward; great exhaustion, prostration and aversion to all work, mental or physical.

▪Sudden epileptiform seizures coming on about every three months, lasting for two or three weeks and leaving him completely prostrated; falls down with vertigo accompanied by vomiting of food; lies like one dead; in some attacks the patient remains about for several days, in which case he vomits quantities of green fetid fluid, accompanied by green motions from bowels; during attacks can drink, but cannot eat; lies in a drowsy, semi-comatose state, at times being plunged into convulsions, during which he grinds his teeth.

∎Epileptic form of hysteria.

∎Tetanic grin; jaws firmly fixed; masseters hard; lies on bed with head fixed and thrown backwards, and legs fixed and rigid; no distinct bend backwards or sideways of trunk and legs; abdominal muscles firmly contracted and hard as a board, severe spasms of all muscles, during which breathing becomes hurried and labored, < at night, when dropping off to sleep; feels on verge of suffocation; can hardly be kept in bed; paroxysms come on without any apparent provocation and leave him prostrate with exhaustion and apprehension; dreads their approach, and cannot sleep for fear of these attacks seizing him just as he closes his eyes; has not slept for several days; fluids can be swallowed when poured into mouth, but the act is painful and difficult; pulse 80; constipated. θTraumatic tetanus.

∎Cyanotic appearance; cold; heart beats slower and slower, until it almost ceases, then suddenly rises in frequency, with each return of spasms. θTetanus.

∎Traumatic tetanus.

∎Tetanic convulsions during course of diarrhœa and dysentery.

∎General coldness, long lasting syncope; anguish and pressure on chest; hiccough; rattling, moaning, slow breathing; distorted features; pupils dilated; eyelids paralyzed; filiform pulse. θShock.

∎Darting pains; inability to think; feeling of approaching paralysis; unsteadiness of gait.

Loss of sensation in limbs, with stiffness of same.

Staggering and trembling; immobility; insensibility; stiffness of body.

Paralysis first of lower, then of upper limbs.

❙❙Paralysis of l. side; could recognize persons, but was unable to speak; intermittent pulse and heartbeat; fingers cold; nose pinched, eyes turned up. θHemiplegia.

∎Diseases of cerebro-spinal system that come on with great suddenness and severity; mind depressed and very irritable.

³⁷ **Sleep.** Irresistible, constant drowsiness.

Prolonged sleeplessness, or very heavy sleep; fear and great anxiety.

³⁸ **Time.** For several hours: extreme coma.

Two or three hours after eating: burning pain in region of navel, extending to œsophagus and throat.

For several days: in some attacks the sickness remains; has not slept.

Evening: attacks of indisposition; two hours after delayed
    dinner; vomiting of food or slimy, bilious matter <.
.Night: vomiting of food or slimy, bilious matter; severe
    spasms of all muscles, during which breathing becomes
    hurried and labored <.

³⁹ Temperature and Weather. Open air: vertigo <.

⁴⁰ Fever. ❙Coldness within and without, like marble.
    ❙❙Cold extremities.
    ❙Heat in head with coldness of extremities.
    Heat and perspiration over whole body.
    ❙❙Body covered with sweat.
    ❙Scarlatina, when the eruption in its early appearance is
        dark colored and soon becomes livid, only slowly regain-
        ing its color when this is expelled by pressure of finger;
        rapid, feeble pulse; coma and great prostration.
    ❙❙Bad cases of small-pox.

⁴¹ Attacks, Periodicity. Attacks last four days.
    At times: is forced to scream out suddenly, she knows not
        why; tightness of chest; acute pain at heart; is awakened
        out of sleep by this scream; plunges in convulsions.
    About every month: sudden epileptiform seizures lasting
        for two or three weeks.

⁴² Locality and Direction. Right: side of head violent pres-
    sure.
    Left: slight pressure of occiput over l. half of head to
        frontal region, paralysis of side.
    Towards right and upwards: distortion of eyes.

⁴³ Sensations. As though everything about him moved slowly;
        as if drink was poured down throat like an empty
        barrel; as if a resistant body in region of navel; as if
        larynx was swollen.
    Torturing pains: in chest.
    Acute pain: of heart.
    Great pain: in back of head.
    Darting pains: general.
    Stitches: in abdomen; in larynx.
    Anguish: in pit of stomach; in chest.
    Stupefying headache.
    Supraorbital neuralgia.
    Stinging: high up in nose.
    Burning pain: in region of navel.
    Burning: on tip of tongue; on larynx.
    Scraping sensation: in throat; in larynx; in bronchial
        tubes.
    Pricking sensation: from larynx to trachea.
    Pricking: in various parts of head.
    Tickling: in larynx.
    Violent pressure: in occiput and forehead.
    Slight pressure: l. side of occiput over l. half of head to

frontal region; from vertex towards forehead on both
sides and to orbits, where it became fixed, while from
occiput it extended down nape of neck.

Heat: in head; in throat.

Confusion: of head.

Gone sensation: in epigastrium.

Weight: in back of head.

Tightness: in chest.

Stiffness: of tongue; of legs.

Lameness: of tongue.

Weakness: of limbs.

Dryness: of nose; of mouth; of larynx.

Roaring and deafness: in ears.

Buzzing: in ears.

Coldness: in body.

Cold feeling: of tongue; of abdomen.

⁴⁴ Tissues. Acts upon cerebral veins, producing congestion;
secondarily upon heart, nerves, etc.

⁴⁵ Touch. Passive Motion. Injuries. Touch: region of
navel sensitive; eyeballs slightly sensitive.

Pressure of finger: scarlatina, when eruption, in its early
appearance, is dark colored and soon becomes livid,
only slowly regaining its color when this is expelled by
pressure of finger.

⁴⁶ Skin. Paleness with a blue tinge.

Dryness of skin.

Itching; formication; erythema.

⁴⁷ Stages of Life, Constitution. Boy, æt. 3; epileptiform
seizure.

Joiner, æt. 20, after scalding legs; traumatic tetanus.

Married woman, æt. 23, after undergoing the most heroic
treatment, even to trephining, two months after abortion;
hysteria.

Woman, æt. 30, drawing teacher; nervous exhaustion.

Man, æt. 39, bilious temperament, dark complexioned,
married; catarrh of stomach and small intestines.

Woman, æt. 80; hemiplegia (benefited).

⁴⁸ Relations. Antidoted by: *Ammonia, Camphor., Coffea, Ipec.,
Nux vom., Opium, Verat. vir.*

Compare: *Camphor.* (first stage of cholera); *Acon., Cicuta*
(action on spinal cord); *Œnanthe crocata* (in epilepsy).

HYDROPHOBINUM. (See Lyssin.)

HYOSCYAMUS NIGER:

Henbane. *Solonaceæ.*

Provings by Hahnemann and his provers. See Allen's Encyclopedia, vol. 5, p. 25.

CLINICAL AUTHORITIES.—*Affections of mind,* Gauwerky, Woost, Bathmann, Rück. Kl. Erf., vol. 5, p. 4; (2 cases) von Störk, N. A. J. H., vol. 3, p. 547; *Effects of jealousy,* Stapf, Analytic Therap., vol. 1, p. 86; *Melancholia,* Bethmann, Analytic. Therap., vol. 1, p. 192; *Hallucinations,* Moore, Organon, vol. 1, p. 358; *Hallucinations,* Moore, Organon, vol. 1, p. 358; *Delirium,* Bœnninghausen, Analytic. Therap., vol. 1, p. 109; *Mania,* Guernsey, Dunham's Lectures; *Mania from jealousy,* Stapf, Analytic. Therap., vol. 1, p. 109; *Maniacal fury,* Chapman, B. J. H., vol. 8, p. 229; *Madness,* von Störk, N. A. J. H., vol. 3, p. 546; *Mania,* Grissel, Martini and Spohr, Szotar, Hahnemann, Thorer, Hanstein, Weber, Rück. Kl. Erf., vol. 4, pp. 26–29; *Insanity,* Sstaraveszki, Hom. Clinics, vol. 1, p. 55; Haywood, B. J. H., vol. 35, p. 162; *Delirium tremens,* Müller, Rück. Kl. Erf., vol. 1, p. 143; Moore, B. J. H., vol. 8, p. 497; *Hydrophobia,* Rück. Kl. Erf., vol. 4, p. 623; *Affection of brain,* Gross, Rück. Kl. Erf., vol. 1, p. 125; *Inflammation of brain,* Mossbauer, Rück. Kl. Erf., vol. 1, p. 125; *Apoplexy,* Elwert, Rück. Kl. Erf., vol. 1, p. 92; *Hemeralopia,* Hauptmann, Rück. Kl. Erf., vol. 1, p. 340; Martin, Norton's Ophth. Therap., p. 95; *Photophobia,* Garay, Rück. Kl. Erf., vol. 5, p. 125; *Strabismus,* Gallavardin, Rück. Kl. Erf., vol. 5, p. 141; *Toothache,* Kreuss, Hering, Bœnninghausen, Knorre, Altschul, Rück. Kl. Erf., vol. 1, p. 462; *Loss of speech,* Rück. Kl. Erf., vol. 5, p. 18; Hahnemann, Rück. Kl. Erf., vol. 1, p. 70; Rampel, Rück. Kl. Erf., vol. 1, p. 69; *Affection of throat,* Altschul, Rück. Kl. Erf., vol. 5, p. 240; *Vomiting,* Löw, Rück. Kl. Erf, vol. 5, p. 260; *Flatulent colic,* Hartman, Rück. Kl. Erf., vol. 1, p. 753; *Diarrhœa,* Miller, Cin. Med. Adv., vol. 3, p. 381; *Paralysis of sphincter ani,* Gross, Rück. Kl. Erf., vol. 1, p. 1010; *Frequent micturition,* Chapman, B. J. H., vol. 8, p. 230; *Uterine hemorrhage,* Hirsch, Rück. Kl. Erf., vol. 5, p. 625; Hahnemann, Hering, Hartmann, Rück. Kl. Erf., vol. 2, p. 311; *Metrorrhagia,* Z. S. Hahnemann, B. J. H., vol. 12, p. 271; *Affections during pregnancy,* Gaspar, Rück. Kl. Erf., vol. 2, p. 382; *Diarrhœa in lying-in woman,* Martin, T H M S Pa., 1886, p. 95; *Convulsions during labor,* Rückert, Rück. Kl. Erf., vol. 2, p. 407; *Cramps in calves of legs during labor,* Wielobicky, Rück. Kl. Erf., vol. 2, p. 408; *Child-bed fever,* Hartmann, Rück. Kl. Erf., vol. 2, p. 448; *Bronchitis,* Miller, Raue's Rec., 1875, p. 115; *Cough,* Caspar, Trinks, Hartmann, Elwert, Rück. Kl. Erf., vol. 3, p. 15; Eidherr, Löw, Müller, Rück. Kl. Erf., vol. 5, pp. 683, 720; *Chest affection,* von Störk, N. A. J. H., vol. 3, p. 546; *Inflammation of lungs,* Watzke, Buchner, Müller, Rück. Kl. Erf., vol. 3, p. 298; *Catarrhal pneumonia,* Gross, Raue's Rec., 1871, p. 100; *Spasms of chest,* von Störk, N. A. J. H., vol. 3, p. 550; *Cramps of diaphragm,* Adler, Rück. Kl. Erf., vol. 1, p. 944; *Hæmoptysis,* von Störk, N. A. J. H., vol. 3, p. 547; *Palpitation of heart,* von Störk, N. A. J. H., vol. 3, p. 546; *Rheumatic endocarditis,* Marchal de Calvi, Hom. Clinics, vol. 3, p. 25; *Hysteria,* von Störk, N. A. J. H., vol. 3, p. 550;

Convulsive tremors and convulsions, von Störk, N. A. J. H., vol. 3, p. 545; *Chorea,*
Rückert, Shellhammer, Rück. Kl. Erf., vol. 4, p. 510; *Spasms and epilepsy,* von
Störk, N. A. J. H., vol. 3, p. 548; Hartmann, Jahr, Tietzer, Müller, Rückert,
Hoffendahl, Schubert, Caspari, Knorre, Kleinert, Rück. Kl. Erf., vol. 4, p. 562;
Sleeplessness, Schrön, Rück. Kl. Erf., vol. 3, p. 517; *Remittent fever,* Morrison, Hah.
Mo., vol. 10, p. 222; *Typhoid fever,* Knorre, Diez, Elwert, Rück. Kl. Erf., vol. 4,
pp. 735-740; McGeorge, Hah. Mo., vol. 15, p. 540; *Typhus,* Smith, Raue's Rec.,
1874, p. 284.

[1] **Mind.** Stupor, unconsciousness; does not reply to questions;
does not recognize any one; answers properly, but immediately stupor returns.

Stupefaction: depressing mental influences; hypochon-
driacal; from smell of flowers, gas, etheric oils, etc.

Imbecility, or illusions of imagination and senses.

Inability to think; cannot direct or control thoughts.

Loss of memory.

Quiet, reflective mood; no complaints; no wants.

Answers no questions; cannot bear to be talked to.

Makes irrelevant answers.

While reading, interpolates improper words and sentences.

Raises head from pillow and gazes about.

Thinks he is in the wrong place.

Sees persons who are not and have not been present.

Does not know whether or not to take what is offered.

Dread of drinks; of water.

Anxious apprehension; chronic fearfulness.

Fears: being left alone; poison, or being bitten; being
poisoned or sold; being betrayed, or injured; wishes to
run away.

Complains of having been poisoned.

Horrid anguish, fits of anxiety.

Very suspicious.

Reproaches others, complains of supposed injury done him.

Quarrelsomeness; indomitable rage.

Impatience, precipitate liveliness, talkativeness, tells
everything.

Picking at bedclothes; mutters and prattles.

Mutters absurd things to himself.

Makes abrupt, short answers to imaginary questions.

Cries out suddenly.

While awake talks irrationally, as if a man were present.

Talks more than usual, and more animatedly and hur-
riedly.

Constant unintelligible chattering.

Lies naked in bed and prattles.

Delirium: talks of business · of imaginary wrongs.

Loves smutty talk.

Frequently breaks out into a loud laugh.

Scolds; raves; abuses those about him.

Cries and laughs alternately, gesticulations lively.

Whines, but knows not why.

Silly, smiling, laughs at everything, silly expression.

Foolish laughter.

Talks in an absurd way.

Does foolish things, behaves like one mad.

Comical alienation of mind; ludicrous actions like monkeys; makes ridiculous gestures like a dancing clown; like one intoxicated.

Plays with his fingers (not picking bedclothes).

Catches at air, or at some imaginary appearance, and pulls bedclothes about.

Carphologia and muttering.

Sings constantly and talks hastily, but indistinctly.

Sings amorous and obscene songs.

Excessive animation, restless hurry.

Insulting, shouting, brawling, ungovernable rage, with exhibition of unusual strength.

Insane passion for work.

Tendency to action; wants to kill somebody or himself.

Is violent, and beats people.

Bite, scratch and nip everyone interfering with them.

Child makes violent exertions to get out of bed, tries to bite, and raves.

Tries to injure those around him; convulsions after trying to swallow.

Working and clutching of hands, strikes his attendants; movements very quick, with difficulty held upon lap; wants to fight, attempts to bite; at intervals would sing and at times burst out laughing; when anything is offered him clinches hold of it with both hands greedily.

Delirium: with physical restlessness; would not stay in bed; moves from one place to another; complete: lively; wild; busy, with constant muttering or talking, and meddling with hands; about usual employments; wants to get up and attend to business or go home; without apparent heat; face pale, limbs cold, though temperature is high; with jerking of limbs, and diarrhœa, red face, wild, staring look, and throbbing of carotids; comes back to consciousness when spoken to; continued while awake; from jealousy or vexation; murmurings; incoherent talk; from pain.

Delirium tremens: with clonic spasms; averse to light and company; visions, as if persecuted; preceded by an epileptic attack; constant talking at night; seeks to escape from men by whom he imagines himself surrounded and who are trying to capture him; does not recognize his wife who is standing by his side, but imagines he sees her under a distant bed.

∎Insanity brought on by drinking; will neither eat nor drink; face flushed, expression wild; tears clothes; wanders up and down room during night; strikes at keepers, and can scarcely be restrained.

∎Trembling all over, looking very wild, and constantly pointing to serpents which she saw creeping up towards her, and fancied they were in bed approaching her; had to be held to be kept quiet; metrorrhagia. θDelirium tremens.

∎Epileptiform fit precedes the attack; continuous talking at night; wants to run away for fear of being persecuted by police; tremor of limbs. θDelirium tremens.

∎Loquacious and quarrelsome mania, especially inclined to unseemly and immodest acts, gestures and expressions.

∎∎Jealousy: with rage and delirium; with attempt to murder.

∎Erotic mania accompanied by jealousy.

∎Serious illness from jealousy and grief about a faithless lover; fever <after midnight; high redness of face, with constant delirium and desire to run away; continual throbbing toothache.

∎Violent and threatening nervous symptoms, even spasms; hectic fever; sleepless nights; mind nearly deranged; disturbed by unfounded jealousy.

∎A gentle, lovable woman became extremely jealous of her husband, and although fully realizing that she did him injustice, she was so filled with grief that she found no rest day nor night, and could neither eat nor drink.

∎Amativeness; nymphomania; erotomania.

∎Onanism since childhood; has always been greatly attracted by opposite sex and prematurely busied himself with thoughts of marriage; for last half year has been very ill humored and irritable; memory impaired; reserved; secretly wrote his love affairs; speech incoherent; restlessness and sleeplessness; attacks of mania with profuse sweating, hasty and vehement talking, one idea rapidly following another, all in some way concerning love; masturbates at every opportunity, and is full of obscene talk; constant walking about; strikes at and destroys everything; spits in face of attendant and raves; face pale and sunken; eyes wild, piercing, shining; severe pain in nape of neck and small of back.

∎∎Lascivious mania, uncovers body, especially sexual parts; sings amorous songs.

∎Goes about nearly naked; will not be covered.

∎Constantly throwing off bedcovers or clothes; entire loss
of modesty.

∎He lies in bed nude and chatters; walks about insane,
naked, wrapped in a skin during summer heat.

∎Desires to be naked (hyperæsthesia of cutaneous nerves).

∎Disappointed love followed by: epilepsy; melancholy; rage
or inclination to laugh at everything; despair and pro-
pensity to drown himself.

Morose dejection, despair.

∎After a fit of passion, melancholia, gradually developing
into true madness; appetite gone; nights restless; continual delirium attended with timorousness; loss of
strength; complains of frequent shudderings and rigors
in spine going up into head during lucid intervals;
hard, constipated stool.

∎After fit of passion and sudden fear, became so melancholy and timorous as to hide himself in every corner,
and even to dread and run away from flies; speechless,
could not get a word out of him; no appetite; sleepless;
loss of strength; seemed as one out of his senses:

∎Groundless suspicion of being watched by members of
family with whom he had some slight misunderstand-
ing; to avoid being recognized by them, clothed himself
differently every day, and seldom left his house; this
monomania gradually developed into insanity; recognized his physician but at once went off again into
delusions; uncovered and exposed himself; continually
counting, at one time in French, at another in English,
and at another in both; continually fixing himself to
correspond with the points of the compass and looking
through his fingers; tracing the pattern of carpet with
his feet and twisting his legs till he nearly fell down;
grasping at imaginary objects; watching his relations
suspiciously and imagining he might be poisoned; talking to himself. θInsanity.

∎After being harshly accused of theft, continual delirium;
fancies herself surrounded by objects of a terrifying
nature; not a moment quiet, continual calling out that
she saw the devil; denies herself guilty of theft, or that
she has any concern with witches; tremor all over
body; struggles with such violence to escape, that she
must be tied to bed; pulse and respiration shift according to the various phantoms which offer themselves to
her imagination; tongue extremely moist; eyes stern,
grim, wrathful; involuntary stool and urine in bed.

∎Mania during lactation; extreme irritability; raving;
when thwarted in anything scolds and strikes indiscrim-
inately at persons; talkative, irrational speech; crying,

alternating with a merry humor; anxiety with trembling in limbs; very profuse secretion of milk.

∎Great restlessness, piercing, staring look; jerking motion of head with rapid glances here and there; face pale; pulse slow and soft; attempts to escape from room; frightful hallucinations of figures coming to seize him, hens bound with chains, numbers of large crabs being driven into room; general epileptic convulsions; θInsanity.

∎Raving, scolding, singing; chatters day and night; will not eat, drink or sleep; seeks to escape; breaks the window; use of straight-jacket necessary. θMania.

∎Restless, talking delirium, yet when spoken to answering rationally; imagining that her deceased sister was sitting by her bedside, and talking to this imaginary person; pulse 80, full; head ached, but not hot; hearing decreased; loquacious. θHallucinations.

∎Face earthy pale; wild, strange expression; constant talking, particularly on religious subjects; believes himself poisoned, or that there is a stinking odor from his mouth; occasionally scolds and cries, and declares that he hears loud noises. θInsanity.

∎Could not bear the light, nor to be spoken to; repelled with rage and seeming disgust his mother, of whom, in his natural state, he was doatingly fond, did not know her, said she was not his mamma; talked wildly and could with difficulty be kept covered. θManiacal fury.

∎Face red and hot; wild expression of eye; respiration quick and impeded; constant scolding and cursing; tears her clothes; walks about room at night; strikes viciously at those about her and can scarcely be restrained; will neither eat nor drink. θMania.

∎Refused to rise from bed and dress herself; assigned no reason; after a few hours insisted on rising, but would not wear a single garment of any kind; received her physician without any apparent consciousness of her singular condition, conversed intelligently, but would not admit that she needed any advice to clothe herself; refused medicine, and cunningly evaded all stratagems to give it; escaped from room, went through house, and sought to escape into street. θMania.

∎Frequent looking at hands because they seem too large.

∣∣Considers the stove a tree and wants to climb it.

∣∣Looks at men as hogs.

∎Does not know her relatives.

∎Puerperal mania, with desire to be uncovered and nude.

∎Nervous irritability without hyperæmia.

∎Consequences of fright.

▮Syphilophobia.

² Sensorium. ▮▮Complete loss of consciousness.

▮Unconsciousness, from congestion of blood to head, with delirium; answering all questions properly; pupils dilated.

Stupor, loss of consciousness, delirium, patient talking of his domestic affairs.

Stupor, with incoherent speech; patient is unconscious of severity of his case.

▮Sopor with loud snoring, from which she can only be partially aroused by hard shaking or loud calling; does not answer any questions; unable to swallow; involuntary stool and urine; face red; bloodvessels of body swollen; pulse quick and full; this condition lasted several days and was accompanied by numbnes of hands. θApoplexy.

▮Sudden falling, with a shriek, sopor.

▮Apoplexy, snoring; involuntary stool and urine.

▮Rolls head, stertor, hiccough. θConcussion of brain.

▮Repeated attacks of fainting.

▮▮Stupefaction.

▮Confusion of head.

▮▮Vertigo; giddiness.

▮Vertigo, with drunkenness.

▮Vertigo from smell of flowers, gas, etc.

³ Inner Head. Constrictive, stupefying headache in upper part of forehead, and general malaise, alternating with absence of all pain.

Pressing, stupefying pain in forehead.

Aching, stupefying pains over eyes.

Pressure in vertex and drawing in nape of neck, when turning head.

Heaviness of head and violent pains, alternating with pains in nape of neck.

▮Heaviness, vacant feeling, confusion, severe pain; pains in meninges; pressure in l. side of forehead, changing to shooting.

▮▮Brain feels as if loose.

▮Sensation as if water was swashing in head.

▮Shakes head to and fro; swashing sensation in brain.

Undulating sensation in brain, as if from throbbing in arteries.

▮Heat and tingling in head: violent pulsations, like waves, head shakes; < becoming cold, after eating; > bending head forward, and from heat.

▮Congestion of blood to head; red, sparkling eyes; face purple red; < in evening.

▮Cerebral hyperæmia, unconscious, blue red face; red, sparkling eyes.

Nervous headaches.

▮Pain and heat in head, after a meal.

▮Headache, better walking.

▮Inflammation of brain, with unconsciousness; heat and tingling in head; violent pulsations in head, like waves; head shakes; < from becoming cold and after eating; > bending head forward (stooping) and from heat.

▮Hydrocephalus, with stupor; head is shaken to and fro; twitching motions.

' **Outer Head.** ||Catches cold in head, especially from dry, cold air.

▮Rolling the head.

||Head sinks on one or other side.

' **Sight and Eyes.** ▮Farsighted, clearsighted; pupils dilated.

▮Illusions; objects look red as fire.

||Illusions of vision; small objects seem very large.

▮Deceptive vision; flame of one light seems smaller, that of another larger, though both were of equal size.

▮Double sight.

▮When reading the letters move about, from mydriasis.

▮Dimness of vision, as though a veil were before eyes; could scarcely see three steps.

▮Obscuration of vision; objects seem indistinct; is near-sighted and obliged to hold book nearer when reading.

||Momentary loss of sight.

▮Amblyopia. θEpilepsy.

▮Night blindness.

▮Hemeralopia in a myopic eye, with shooting pains from eyes into nose and head; headache > closing eyes.

||Eyes become shortsighted; distorted, stare and protrude.

▮Eyes open; distorted; rolling about in orbits; squinting.

▮Spasmodic action of internal rectus.

▮Eyes red, wild, sparkling.

||Constant staring at surrounding objects, self-forgetful.

▮Stupid staring, distorted eyes.

|▮Brilliant lustre to eyes.

||Pupils dilated; insensible.

||Albugineæ red, and pupils so widely dilated that irides seemed like a narrow circle; they were also insensible to light.

▮Pupils altered, dilated or contracted; slow respiration.

▮Conjunctiva red.

▮Excesssive photophobia of scrofulous ophthalmia.

▮Tearing, beating in r. eye, which waters and seems projected.

Twitching in eyes; dim vision, as if a veil before eyes.

▮Quivering of eyeball.

⁶ Hearing and Ears. ▮Buzzing, singing, rushing in ears.
▮Hard hearing, as if stupefied, especially after apoplexy.
▮Hardness of hearing from paralyzed auditory nerves.
▮▮Deafness.

⁷ Smell and Nose. ▮▮Sense of smell weak, or lost.
▮Sudden jerking from above downwards in root of nose.
▮Pressing pinching in root of nose and in zygomata.
▮Cramp pressure at root of nose and malar bones.
▮Nostrils sooty, smoky.
▮Nosebleed bright red, with salivation.
▮▮Dryness of nose.
Liability to catch cold in head, principally from dry,
cold air.

⁸ Upper Face. ▮Heat and redness of face.
▮Flushed and excited countenance.
▮Face: flushed; dark red, bloated; cold and pale; dis-
torted; stupid expression; muscles twitch, makes grim-
aces.
▮Distorted, bluish face, with wide open mouth; approach-
ing cerebral paralysis. θTyphoid.
▮Twitching of muscles of face.

⁹ Lower Face. ▮▮Foam at the mouth.
▮Lips, dry.
Large pustules on chin.
▮Lockjaw; fully conscious.

¹⁰ Teeth and Gums. ▮Closes the teeth tightly together.
▮Toothache, driving to despair; tearing, throbbing, ex-
tending to cheeks and along lower jaw.
▮Violent attacks of toothache with sense of strangulation
and difficult deglutition; cramps; sense of mental fatigue.
▮Violent tearing and pulsating pain, causing spasmodic
jerks of fingers, hands, arms and facial muscles.
▮Toothache, driving to despair, in sensitive, nervous, excitable persons.
▮Tearing in teeth as if blood was forced into them, flushes
of heat, congestion to head; < from cold air, morning.
▮Toothache, jerking, throbbing, tearing, drawing, extending into forehead.
▮Throbbing toothache, appearing generally in morning,
usually due to a cold; throbbing in tooth, tearing sensation in gums, and in masticating the tooth seems
loose as if it would fall out; congestion to head, with
great heat all over body.
▮Teeth feel loose when chewing; also, too long.
Tearing raging pain in gums, with buzzing sensation in
tooth.
▮▮Intense pain in gums after extraction of a tooth.
▮▮Presssing of gums together, putting hands to jaws,
fingers into mouth; during dentition.

❙❙Sordes on teeth and in mouth.

❙❙Grating the teeth.

¹¹ **Taste and Tongue.** ❙Putrid or salt taste.

❙Parching dryness of tongue.

❙❙Tongue: red or brown, dry, cracked, hard; looks like burnt leather; clean, parched; white; tremulous.

❙❙Tongue shaken to and fro, with a trembling movement.

❙Tongue does not obey, difficult mobility.

❙Tongue protruded with difficulty, can hardly draw it in.

❙Biting the tongue when talking.

❙Paralysis of tongue.

❙After fright complete loss of speech; motions of tongue much impaired with sensation of numbness and lameness; chewing and swallowing unaffected; frequent stitching headaches.

❙Loss of speech; utters inarticulate sounds.

❙❙Speech impaired, difficult and unintelligible, from arrest of secretion.

❙Speech embarrassed.

❙Very talkative.

¹² **Inner Mouth.** ❙Soft and hard palate dry and glazed.

❙Dryness of mouth, lips and fauces.

Soreness of soft parts between gums and cheeks.

❙Salivation.

❙Foaming, bloody saliva, tasting salty.

❙Cadaverous smell from mouth, < morning and evening.

¹³ **Throat.** ❙Elongated palate.

❙Throat and mouth dry, parched and red, inability to swallow.

❙Throat dry, burning; shooting, pricking pains, difficult swallowing, as from constriction; dread of liquors.

❙Constriction of throat, with inability to swallow fluids.

❙Spasms of throat; an attempt to swallow renews spasm.

❙Spasmodic contraction of œsophagus after injury; solid and warm food swallowed best; fluids cause spasm; hiccough, nausea, stiff neck.

¹⁴ **Appetite, Thirst. Desires, Aversions.** ❙❙Unusually great appetite; hungry gnawing.

❙Voracious appetite and thirst, with inability to swallow.

❙Unquenchable thirst.

❙❙Much thirst with tenderness of stomach.

❙❙Thirst, drinks but little at a time.

❙❙Dread of water.

¹⁵ **Eating and Drinking.** Solid and warm food are swallowed best; fluids cause spasm.

¹⁶ **Hiccough, Belching, Nausea and Vomiting.** ❙❙Hiccough: with spasms and rumbling; after eating and at night; with inflammation of intestinal organs.

Eructations: empty; incomplete; bitter.

Nausea: with vertigo and vomiting; with stiff neck.

❚Vomiting and retching: with colic, extorting cries; after coughing.

❚Vomiting: of food and drink; of blood, with convulsions; of bloody mucus, with dark red blood.

¹⁷ **Scrobiculum and Stomach.** ❚Pit of stomach tender to touch.

❚Violent pain in stomach with vomiting and hiccough.

❚Cramps in stomach, with loud shrieks, vomiting, convulsions; cramps > after vomiting.

❙❙Burning and inflammation of stomach.

❚❚Inflammation of stomach, or peritonitis, with hiccough.

❚Hæmatemesis, pit of stomach sensitive; dull aching about liver; abdomen bloated.

¹⁸ **Hypochondria.** ❚Stitches or dull pain in region of liver.

¹⁹ **Abdomen.** ❚Abdomen distended, sore to touch, tympanitic.

❙❙Pinching in abdomen.

❚Colic, as if abdomen would burst; presses fists into sides; cutting, vomiting, belching, hiccough, screaming.

❚Colic > by vomiting.

❚Hysterical colic.

❙❙Abdominal muscles sore.

❚Pain, as from soreness in abdominal walls, when coughing.

❚Pains in abdominal muscles: as if he had fallen upon them; while sitting; as after excessive exertion or a strain.

❚Sticking in umbilical region, during inspiration.

❙❙Umbilicus open, urine oozing through.

❚❚Cutting low down in abdomen.

❚Distension of hypogastrium, which is painful to touch.

❚Enteritis or peritonitis, with typhoid symptoms.

❚Roseola on abdomen.

²⁰ **Stool and Rectum.** ❙❙Frequent desire for stool; with small discharges.

❚Watery diarrhœa.

❚Stools: painless; watery; mucous; nearly odorless; yellow, watery, involuntary during sleep, in old men.

❚Stools involuntary, unconscious, painless, yellowish, watery; attack coming on suddenly and without apparent cause. θDiarrhœa in lying-in women.

❚Hysterical females and young girls whose bowels are apt to bloat, and who are subject to attacks of diarrhœa, with colicky pains and frequent urging to stool, or where sphincters are weak, causing great difficulty in retaining the feces, and where excitement or mental trouble produces the attack.

❚Relaxed state of bowels dependent on or connected with irritation of uterine system.

▮Involuntary stool while urinating.

▮Diarrhœa: during pregnancy; in childbed; at night; during typhoid fever.

▮Bright, staring eyes; muttering delirium; flushed face; dry tongue; teeth incrusted with brown mucus; scanty urine; rolling of head; dilated pupils; difficulty in swallowing liquids; involuntary stools; night cough. θCholera infantum.

▮Typhoid symptoms after the vomiting diarrhœa and coldness have ceased, with dulness of sense, wandering looks; red and hot face; spasms and rumbling in abdomen; hiccough, with involuntary micturition and foaming at mouth. θCholera.

▯▯Stool small in size.

▮Constipation, with epilepsy.

▯▯Paralysis of rectum, or sphincter ani.

▮Paralysis of sphincter ani and vesicæ; involuntary stool and urine.

▮Piles bleed profusely; fulness of veins, full pulse, skin and muscles lax.

²¹ Urinary Organs. ▮Paralysis of bladder; after labor, and in children with affections of head.

▮Retention of urine with constant pressure in bladder; atony or apparent paralysis of bladder.

Urination: frequent, scanty; difficult, from spasmodic or inflammatory condition of neck of bladder; involuntary; has no will to urinate, difficult, with pressing.

Urine: scanty; retained or suppressed; turbid, with mucopurulent deposit; with red, sandy sediment.

▮Frequent emission of urine as clear as water.

▮Frequent urination at night, so that his rest was broken to such a degree as to make him miserable; prostate slightly enlarged.

²² Male Sexual Organs. ▮Sexual desire excessive; lascivious, exposes his person.

▯▯Impotence.

²³ Female Sexual Organs. ▯▯Lascivious, uncovers sexual parts.

▮Lascivious furor without modesty.

▮Excited sexual desire without excitement of fancy.

▮Metritis, especially if inflammation is developed by emotional disturbances; typhoid state.

▮Uterine cramps, with pulling in loins and small of back; irritable uterus.

▮Metrorrhagia, accompanied by cramps of whole body, interrupted by jerks and starts of entire frame, or of single parts, succeeded by general stiffness of limbs.

▮Metrorrhagia in patients who have been subject to

cramps during pregnancy; blood bright red, and issues
more and more freely at every jerk of body, while action
of pulse diminishes.

▮Continuous bright red flow, with spasmodic jerkings,
great vascular excitement. *θ*Metrorrhagia.

▮Metrorrhagia, blood pale, with convulsions.

▮Labor-like pains, previous to menstruation, with draw-
ings in loins and small of back.

▮Menses preceded by hysterical or epileptic spasms;
loud, uninterrupted laughing; profuse sweat and nausea.

▮During menses: convulsive trembling of hands and feet,
headache, profuse sweat; lockjaw; enuresis.

▮Profuse menses, with delirium; convulsive trembling of
hands and feet; silly manners, rage.

▮Menstruation appears with profuse perspiration, headache
and nausea.

▮▮Irregular menses.

▮Suppressed menstruation; suppressed lochia.

Pregnancy. Parturition. Lactation. ▮Twitching in
cheeks; cramp-like pains in abdomen; violent pain in
pit of stomach. *θ*Pregnancy.

▮Cold perspiration; pale face; suffocating spells and convulsions; facial muscles greatly agitated. *θ*During parturition.

▮Spasms during parturition with much nervous irritability.

▮Every ten or fifteen minutes an attack of twitching of
limbs and muscles of face; unconsciousness. *θ*Parturition.

▮▮Puerperal spasms, shrieks, anguish; chest oppressed,
unconscious.

▮After miscarriage or labor, hemorrhage of bright red
blood, flowing steadily; commences with spasms, single
shocks, twitchings and startings, with every start more
blood comes.

▮Puerperal fever.

▮▮No will to make water, in child-bed.

▮Watery, painless diarrhœa of lying-in women.

▮Total suppression of milk or lochia.

▮Children at breast have singultus.

Voice and Larynx. Trachea and Bronchia. ▮Loss of
speech with aphonia, although she makes great efforts
to speak cannot produce a sound or syllable.

▮Hysterical aphonia.

▮Speech impaired; confused; difficult and irrational.

▮Hoarseness, with dry and inflamed throat; hysteria.

▮Voice husky, as from mucus.

▮Constriction of larynx.

▮▮Much mucus in larynx and air passages, which makes
speech and voice rough.

²⁶ Respiration. Spasms of chest with arrest of breathing, compelling one to lean forward.

❙Loss of breath, as from rapid running.

❙Oppression of chest, with internal stinging, < during inspiration.

❙Slow rattling breathing.

❙Mucous râles during stupor or furious delirium.

²⁷ Cough. Tickling sensation in throat causing an incessant cough, < when lying down, > when sitting up.

❙Dry, tickling, hacking cough, which seems to come from air passages.

❙Violent spasmodic cough; short consecutive coughs, caused by tickling in throat, as if palate was too long, or as if some mucus was lodged there.

❙Shattering spasmodic cough, with frequent, rapidly succeeding coughs, excited by tickling, as from adherent mucus, at night without, in daytime with expectoration of saltish mucus, or of bright red blood mixed with coagula.

❙Tickling cough, with anxiety at night and expectoration of blood streaked mucus. *θ*Chest affection.

❙❙Dry, hacking or spasmodic cough, < lying down, > sitting up; < at night, also after eating, drinking, talking or singing; velum palati elongated.

❙Dry, spasmodic, persistent cough. *θ*Bronchitis.

❙❙Frequent cough at night, which always wakes him, after which he again falls asleep.

❙Paroxysms of dry cough come on more frequently at night; during cough face reddens and respiration may be arrested; vomiting of white mucus; after cough, exhaustion. *θ*Pertussis.

❙Paroxysmal cough, severely shaking chest, abdomen, whole body, and causing a sense of excoriation in abdominal muscles.

❙During cough: spasms of larynx; painful epigastrium and hypochondria.

❙Cough < after midnight, when at rest, during sleep, in cold air, and from eating and drinking.

❙Cough in incurable cases of pulmonary and laryngeal phthisis.

❙Cough after measles.

❙Expectoration of saltish mucus, or bright red blood, mixed with coagula.

²⁸ Inner Chest and Lungs. ❙Tight feeling across chest, as from overexertion, running.

❙Spasms of chest, arrest of breathing, must lean forward.

❙Alternate difficult breathing with anxiety or oppression; continual strong convulsive twitchings of abdomen;

diaphragm apparently affected in same manner, for
breast seemed suddenly to become strongly dilated and
ribs to rise and sink suddenly; at intervals violent hiccough and risus sardonicus; loss of voice; difficult deglutition; pulse full, strong and quick; restless at night;
feels as if heart and breast were torn to pieces; after
paroxysms great weakness. θSpasms of chest.

∎Exhausted from long talking, body, and especially chest,
weak; green sputum, weak pulse.

∎Stitches in sides of chest.

∎Restless, delirious; tongue and lips dry, brownish; great
heat and great thirst; watery, yellowish diarrhœa; intense spasmodic cough, causing him to jump up; dull
percussion sound from lower edge of scapula downwards on l. side; bronchial breathing; bronchophony.
θCatarrhal pneumonia.

∎Pneumonia: cerebral symptoms, delirium, sopor; dry,
fatiguing night cough, or rattling in chest; senilis, with
acute œdema of lungs; of drunkards; complicated with
typhus; hypostatic, in course of chronic affections.

∎Atelectasis pulmonum; bluish color of face; great difficulty in inspiring; must be raised up.

∎Hæmoptysis, bright red, with spasms, also in drunkards.

²⁹ Heart, Pulse and Circulation. ∎Chronic palpitation of
heart so that she could not move body without greatest
anxiety, or apprehension of suffocation or swooning;
unquenchable thirst in morning; frequent, copious discharge of limpid urine; appetite impaired.

Pulse: accelerated, full, hard and strong; rapid, intermitting; slow and small; weak and irregular; small, weak,
scarcely perceptible.

∎Parotids beat violently.

Ⅰ Ⅰ Inflammation of bloodvessels.

³⁰ Outer Chest. ∎Muscles of chest sore.

∎Roseola on chest.

∎Spasms of muscles of chest.

³¹ Neck and Back. Ⅰ Ⅰ Stiffness of cervical muscles, with tension as if too short, on bending neck.

∎Contraction of muscles on one side of neck, twisting neck
to one side; neck turned obliquely.

Ⅰ Ⅰ Herpetic spots on nape of neck.

Ⅰ Ⅰ Abscesses on l. side of neck.

∎Spinal meningitis, with convulsions, jerks of muscles;
after injury.

³² Upper Limbs. ∎Trembling of arms and hands.

∎Arms tremble, especially in evening and after exercise.

Two pimples at elbow.

Ⅰ Ⅰ Painful numbness of hands.

I I Rigor of hands.

I Fingers look and feel too thick.

⁸³ Lower Limbs. Weakness of legs; staggering gait.

I Cramps in thigh.

I I Gangrenous spots and vesicles here and there on lower limbs.

I Convulsive tremor in r. foot, can neither lie, sit, nor walk; constipation, stool hard and discharged with much straining; urine limpid, watery and inodorous.

I Coldness and swelling of feet.

I I Toes spasmodically contracted, in walking or going up stairs.

⁸⁴ Limbs in General. I Trembling of limbs.

I I Frequent twitching of hands and feet.

I Cramps and spasms of extremities.

I Lancinating pains in joints, especially on motion.

I I Cold hands and feet.

⁸⁵ Rest. Position. Motion. When at rest: cough <.

Lying down: cough <.

Lying on back: suddenly sits up, then lies down again.

Lies on back: eyes wide open, staring and immovable.

Bending head forward; > violent pulsation.

Spasm of chest compels one to lean forward.

Pressing gums together, hands to jaws, fingers into mouth, during dentition; presses fists into sides with colic.

Must be raised up: great difficulty in inspiring.

While sitting: pain in abdominal muscles; cough >.

Motion: lancinating pains in joints; bruised feeling.

Movements quick.

Moves from place to place.

Turns from one place to another.

Turning head: pressure in vertex and drawing in nape of neck.

Walking: headache >; toes spasmodically contracted.

Attempts to jump out of bed and run away.

Jump up: cough causes patient to.

Could not move body without greatest anxiety.

Can neither lie, sit, nor walk on account of convulsive tremor in r. foot.

Going up stairs: toes spasmodically contracted.

⁸⁶ Nerves. I Blunted sensibility.

I Loss of smell and taste.

I Weakness; uncommon sinking of strength.

I Long talking exhausts patient.

I I Wants to get away, but cannot stand alone.

I Repeated attacks of fainting.

I Restless, turns from one place to another.

I Contraction of stomach with difficult breathing; can

hardly swallow anything, even a few spoonfuls of broth cause great fatigue; pulse unequal; urine limpid; restless day and night; perpetually watchful. *θ*Hysteria.

■About 10 A.M., chilliness in extremities, followed by heat, first in head, then descending to extremities; sings; bawls out aloud; covers face with handkerchief; stands in awe of those about her; this continued for two hours and was followed by sleep which lasted three hours, during which body was very hot, with much sweat, and short, quick respiration; on awakening does not remember. *θ*Hysteria.

■Constant state of erethism; not a single part of whole body nor a solitary muscle in a quiet state for a moment; general uninterrupted, irregular motion full of impetuosity; eyelids opened and closed with a sudden force, features fairly grinned, made grimaces, rubbed head steadily on pillow, and whole body twisted and turned continually; unceasing spitting, but without saliva; answers no questions, as if it was impossible for him to collect his senses. *θ*Endocarditis rheumatica.

■Hysteric and asthenic delirium, with attempts to run away, prompted by fear.

■Concussive startings, alternating with tremblings and convulsions.

■■Angular motions; jerks of single muscles or sets of muscles.

■Convulsive jerks; long lasting spasms.

■■Subsultus tendinum.

■Violent tearing and pulsating pains causing spasmodic jerks of fingers, hands, arms, and facial muscles.

■Convulsions, beginning with twitchings of muscles of face, especially about eyes; dark colored, bloated appearance of face and deep sleep after spasm goes off.

■Violent convulsions, not all over body but wandering, at one time affecting breast, belly, feet, arms, etc.; great pain; strength and appetite impaired; sleepless; vomiting of large quantities of bile; while convulsions seized abdomen, strong contraction of sphincter ani followed by strangury with continual and very painful tenesmus.

■Falls suddenly to ground, with cries and convulsions.

■Every muscle in body convulsed; frothing at mouth.

■Eyes staring and distorted, with spasmodic closure of lids, bluish face, clenching of teeth, foaming at mouth, constriction of throat.

■Alternate convulsions of upper and lower extremities.

■■Convulsions: of children, especially from fright; after meals; child sickens after eating, vomits or shows distress at stomach, sudden shriek, and then insensible; from intestinal worms; puerperal.

∎Convulsion during deep, heavy sleep.

∎∎Suffocating spells and convulsions during labor.

∎Rigid all over, as in tetanus.

∎The forces sink quickly; patient gets easily fatigued; syncope is readily produced; limbs become cold and tremble; these symptoms, with those of sleep, paralysis of sphincters, point to its use in some conditions occurring in course of continued fevers.

ı ıFell down unconscious with whole body cold and stiff like a piece of wood.

∎The spasms flex the limbs, and the bent body is tossed upward.

∎Toes becomes spasmodically flexed, as from cramps, when walking or carrying foot forward, and ascending.

ı ıStiffness of arms and legs, jerking of hands and feet.

After attack : sopor, snoring, dark colored, bloated appearance of countenance.

∎Chorea, the result or consequence of long and debilitating diseases; every muscle of body from eyes to toes twitches; great agitation and loquacity; tendency to laugh at everything.

∎Throws arms about, misses what is reached for, gait tottering. θChorea.

∎Epileptiform spasms, hyperæsthesia of skin.

∎∎Epilepsy ; before the attack, vertigo, sparks before eyes, ringing in ears, hungry gnawing; during attack, face purple, eyes projecting, shrieks, grinding teeth, urination.

∎Epileptic fits, almost daily ; convulsions so violent that it seemed as if joints or spine would be broken.

∎∎Epileptoid spasms.

∎Epilepsy : from grief, after emotion ; in consequence of drinking.

∎Nervous apoplexy with somnolency; paralysis of œsophagus and numb feeling; paralysis of sphincter muscles.

∎Paralysis after spasms, or after diphtheria.

∎Paralysis agitans.

∎Lockjaw.

Hydrophobia.

[37] **Sleep.** Sleepiness; falls asleep while answering.

ı ıVery deep slumber.

∎Constant slumber, with picking.

∎Deep sleep, with convulsions.

∎Deep sleep which continued without interruption at least three days; only by hard shaking and loud calling she could be awakened sufficiently to take hold of breast, but before she had drawn a few swallows she went off again. θLethargy.

∎Stupid and drowsy, or excitable and sleepless.

❚Drowsy or sleepless; wild expression; delirious; after chloroform.
❚❚Laughing expression during sleep.
❚Child sobs and cries in sleep.
❚Sleep, with outcries.
❚Drowsy, jerks in sleep, cries out, grates his teeth.
❚❚Starts up from sleep in affright, or after a fright.
❚Awakening with screams.
❚Restless sleep.
❚Frequent micturition at night, preventing sleep.
❚❚Lying on back, suddenly sits up, then lies down again.
❚Unable to sleep whole night; tried lying upon one side then the other, yet he was unable to get quiet; only shortly before daybreak sleeps a little from time to time; during short naps perspiration all over, especially about neck.
❚Sleeplessness from nervous irritation.
❚❚Intense sleeplessness of irritable, excitable persons, from business embarrassments, often imaginary.
❚❚Sleepless, on account of a quiet mental activity.
❚Sleeplessness or dozing, with brain full of ideas, figures and bewildering images.
❚Excessive wakefulness, alternating with drowsiness.
❚❚Sleepless, or constant sleep, with muttering.
❚Sleeplessness, after violent disease.
❚Sleeplessness from renal affections; very excitable.
❚❚Long continued sleeplessness.
❚Dreams: anxious; lascivious.

³⁶ **Time.** Morning: toothache <; cadaverous smell from mouth; unquenchable thirst.
10 A.M.: chilliness in extremities.
Afternoon: fever.
Day: chatters; cough; restless.
Evening: congestion of blood to head <; cadaverous smell from mouth <; arms tremble; external heat, coldness ceases, thirst commences; inflamed ulcers <.
Night: constant talking; tears clothes; sleepless; chatters; walks about room; hiccough; frequent urination; cough without expectoration; anxiety; cough <; dry fatiguing cough; restless; cold; burning heat, with tearing cough.
After midnight: fever <; cough <.

³⁷ **Temperature and Weather.** Cannot get warm in bed.
Cold: < violent pulsations in head.
Cold air: toothache <; cough <.
Cold dry air: catches cold in head.
Will not be covered; throws off bed clothes.
Getting warm: inflamed ulcers >.
Heat: pressure in vertex >.

Bad effects from cold air.

⁴⁰ Fever. ▮Cold at night, up back from small of back; cannot get warm in bed.

▮Chill commencing in feet and running up spine to nape of neck.

▮Sudden chilliness; coldness of spine; body cold and stiff, cannot get warm in bed.

▮Chill from feet upward; shivering, heat of face.

▮▮Cannot bear to be talked to, or least noise during chill.

Chill without thirst; alternate days, 11 A.M.

▮Congestive chill with cold extremities.

▮▮Chill, alternating with heat.

▮Whole body cold, with burning redness of face.

Afternoon fever, coldness predominates; pain in back.

▮Heat of head and face, with general coldness of body, without thirst, followed in evening by external heat, coldness ceases, thirst commences.

▮▮Heat of head and face, with coldness and loss of sensibility of external surface of body.

▮Burning heat all over, every evening congestion to head; putrid taste.

▮Burning heat of body every evening, always with thirst.

▮▮Skin burning hot to examining hand, which leaves a burning in place touched.

▮Burning heat, no external redness; blood burns in veins.

▮▮Burning heat all over, skin hot and dry to touch, with distended veins.

▮▮Burning heat all through night, with tearing cough.

Heat: over whole body, much thirst, or no desire to drink; lips sticky; along whole spine; runs up back; ascending from feet to face.

During heat: pain in region of liver; epileptiform convulsions; sleeplessness.

▮They throw the bedclothes entirely off, not because they are too warm, but they will not remain covered. *θ*Fever.

Sweat: cold; sour; weakening; during sleep; on back and pit of stomach; mostly on legs.

Violent sweat after thirst.

▮Dry nocturnal cough, disturbs sleep; extreme nervous excitement, epileptic attacks, or other spasmodic affections; hot stage without much sweat; after each paroxysm pressure in head, vertigo, apyrexia, extreme weakness, luminous spots before eyes, dryness in mouth and frequent hiccough; pulse small. *θ*Intermittent.

▮Intermittent fever, quartan, with short, dry, hacking cough at night.

▮Pulse 100; temperature 104° F.; tongue red and cracked; heavy, sour sweats; troublesome dreams; bronchial complications, with difficult, frothy, hemorrhagic expectoration. θRemittent fever.

■Entire loss of consciousness and of functions of organs of sense; does not recognize relatives or friends; illusions of imagination and senses; delirium continued while awake; sees persons who are not and have not been present; indistinct and muttering loquacity; muttering with picking of bedclothes; inability to think, thoughts cannot be directed or controlled; constant staring at surrounding objects, with apparent entire self-forgetfulness. θTyphoid fever.

■Great agitation; restlessness; jumping out of bed; attempts to run away; eyes red and sparkling, staring, rolling about in orbits; squinting; deafness; distorted face, stupid expression; tongue red or brown, dry and cracked, paralyzed; loss of speech, or indistinct speech; cadaverous smell from mouth; involuntary or unnoticed stools in bed; suppressed secretion or retention of urine; involuntary discharge of urine, leaving streaks of red sand on sheet; paralysis of spincter ani and vesicæ; convulsive motions; grating of teeth; jerkings; subsultus tendinum; trembling; sleeplessness, or constant sleep with muttering; coma vigil; roseola spots on chest and abdomen; cold extremities. θTyphoid fever.

■Delirium, with attempt to jump out of bed and run away, sometimes with fear, sometimes without; when spoken to answers correctly in whole or in part, and then is gone again, muttering to himself; loquacity; talks nonsense continually with his eyes open, but does not pay attention to any one; thinks he is in the wrong place but does not want to go home; picking at bedclothes and playing with hands; throws off bedclothes so as to leave the genitals uncovered; plays with the genitals. θTyphoid fever.

■Staring or squinting, either with one or both eyes; involuntary stools in bed and involuntary urination; paralysis of sphincter ani and vesicœ; marked subsultus tendinum. θTyphoid fever.

■In typhoid and typhus fevers, especially typhus, when brain is active but wandering, patient laboring under hallucination of various kinds, but all centering in a desire to escape from room or from those around.

■Lies on back, eyes wide open, staring and immovable; unconscious; face red, lips black, tongue dry and black; lower jaw hangs down; urine involuntary, it leaves large streaks of red sand on sheet; skin dry; pulse over 200; ill nine days. θTyphus.

∎Fever cases in which torpor of entire organism predominates; dull, fixed expression of face, delirium is
lacking, or if present it consists of a confused farrago
of complex images; the perceptive faculty is almost
suspended.

∎Convulsions, mania, delirium, cough, and sleeplessness,
all occur almost absolutely without any manifestations
of fever.

⁴¹ **Attacks, Periodicity.** Chill and heat: last two hours,
followed by sleep which lasts three.

Every ten or fifteen minutes: an attack of twitching of
limbs and muscles of face.

Every evening: congestion to head; burning heat of body.

Alternate days, 11 A.M.: chill without thirst.

Almost daily epileptic fits.

Three days: sleeps without interruption.

⁴² **Locality and Direction.** Right: beating in eye; convulsive tremor in foot.

Left: pressure in side of forehead changing to shooting;
dull percussion sound from lower edge of scapula downwards on side; abscesses on side of neck; inflamed ulcers.

From above downwards: sudden jerking in root of nose.

From within outward: pricking stitches.

⁴³ **Sensations.** Brain as if loose; as if water was swashing in
head; undulating sensation in brain, as if from throbbing in arteries; as though a veil was before eyes;
hands as if too large; hard hearing, as if stupefied; as
if strangling; as if blood was forced into teeth; as if
tooth would fall out; teeth feel loose and too long; as if
abdomen would burst; as if he had fallen on abdominal
muscles; as if heart and breast were torn to pieces; as
if cervical muscles were too short; fingers feel too thick;
as if palate was too long; as if mucus was lodged in
throat.

Pain: in nape of neck; in meninges; in head; in teeth;
in back; in region of liver.

Intense pain: in gums.

Severe pain: in head; in nape of neck.

Violent pains: in head; in teeth; in stomach; in pit of
stomach.

Tearing raging pain: in teeth; toothache driving to despair.

Violent tearing and pulsating pains.

Great pain: during convulsion.

Very painful tenesmus.

Tearing: in r. eye; in teeth, extending to cheeks and
lower jaw.

Beating: in r. eye.

Cutting: low down in abdomen.

Lancinating pain: in joints.
Stitches: in sides of chest.
Stitching pain: in head; in region of liver.
Shooting: in l. side of forehead; from eyes into nose and head; in throat.
Stinging: in internal chest.
Sticking: in umbilical region.
Pricking pains: in throat.
Pinching: in root of nose; in zygomata; in abdomen.
Throbbing pain: in teeth.
Jerking: in teeth.
Labor-like pains: previous to menstruation.
Cramp pressure: at root of nose and malar bone.
Cramps: in stomach; of whole body; in thigh; of extremities.
Cramp-like pain: in abdomen.
Hysterical colic.
Pulsating pain: in teeth.
Painful epigastrium and hypochondria.
Burning heat: all over.
Burning: in throat; in stomach.
Heat: in head; over whole body.
Painful warmth: after applying hands to parts.
Soreness: of soft parts between gums and cheeks; of abdominal muscles; of muscles of chest; of throat.
Constrictive, stupefying pain: in upper part of forehead.
Pressing, stupefying pain: in forehead.
Aching, stupefying pain: over eyes.
Dull pain: in region of liver.
Dull aching: about liver.
Bruised feeling: on moving parts.
Pulling: in loins; in small of back.
Drawing: in nape of neck; in teeth; in loins; in small of back.
Contraction: of stomach; of sphincter ani.
Painful numbness: of hands.
Vacant feeling: in head.
Tickling: in throat.
Pressure: in vertex; in l. side of forehead; in root of nose and zygomata; in bladder; in head.
Heaviness: of head.
Oppression: of chest.
Constriction: of throat.
Tight feeling: across chest.
Stiffness: of cervical muscles; of arms and legs.
Numbness: of hands; of tongue; of œsophagus.
Weakness: after paroxysms; of legs.
Tingling: in head.

Buzzing sensation: in teeth.
Buzzing, singing, rushing: in ears.
Parching dryness: of tongue.
Dryness: of mouth; of throat.
Violent pulsation, like waves: in head.
Tremor: of limbs; all through body.
Quivering: in eyes.
Twitching: in eyes; of muscles of face; in cheeks; of limbs; convulsive, of abdomen.
Shudderings and rigors: in spine going up into head.
Trembling: of arms and hands; of limbs.
Convulsive trembling: of hands and feet; in r. foot.
Itching: around part.
Coldness: of hands and feet; of spine.

" **Tissues.** ▮Convulsions, spasms, cramps, epilepsy, chorea and other spasmodic affections; in women and children.
▮Expanded and puffed up veins; full pulse.
▮Hemorrhages usually light red.
A constant flow of bright red blood, with bluish face.
Obesity.
Skin and muscles lax.
Obstinate dropsy.

" **Touch. Passive Motion. Injuries.** Touch: pit of stomach tender; abdomen sore; hypogastrium painful; inflamed ulcers <.
After applying hand to parts: painful warmth.

" **Skin.** ▮Great sensitiveness of skin.
▮Hot, dry, brittle skin, want of sensation.
▮Painful warmth after applying hand to parts.
▮Skin often pale, with delirium; body hot.
▮Skin red, or with red rash.
▮Skin of bright red hue, resembling scarlet fever, with dry, sore throat and much nervousness.
▮Scarlatina, with marked mental symptoms.
▮Stupid drowsiness, or else great nervous excitability and sleeplessness; utter stupidity, or else illusions of imagination and senses; vacant staring at things, or else sparkling red, prominent eyes; embarrassed, indistinct speech; answers no questions, or else indistinct muttering loquacity; mouth and throat dry and red; inability to swallow; abdomen distended, tympanitic; watery, involuntary and unnoticed stools in bed. *θ*Scarlatina.
▮Scarlatina with acute inflammatory affections of brain, or when there is a condition between erethism and torpor.
▮Miliary eruption especially after abuse of *Bellad.*
▮Varicella; vesicles in crops, sleepless; nervous, dry cough, must sit up.
▮Large pustules, clustering from hips to knees.

| | Eruption of dry pimples like confluent small-pox.
| Repelled eruptions, with tendency to diarrhœa.
| Frequent large blood boils.
| | Ulcers painful, bleeding; bruised feeling on moving part.
| Inflamed ulcers, surrounding skin being of a bright vermilion redness; large pustules around ulcers; < evening, during menses, from touch; > when getting warm; l. side.
| Anthrax in nervous and hysterical persons; coma vigil; great restlessness caused by excessive nervous excitement, shaking of head in all directions; constriction of pharynx; itching around part.
| Gangrene, with nervous restlessness.
| Brown or gangrenous spots.

Stages of Life, Constitution. | | Nervous, irritable, excitable, sanguine temperaments.

Light haired people.

| Hysterical women and young girls; old men; drunkards.

Child, æt. 6 weeks, without any premonitory symptoms; lethargy.

Boy, æt. 2, sudden attack; maniacal fury.

Boy, æt. 6; catarrhal pneumonia.

Boy, æt. 13; rheumatic endocarditis.

Boy, æt. 14; insanity.

Girl, æt. 15; chronic palpitation of heart.

Girl, æt. 18; epilepsy.

Girl, æt. 20; spasms of chest.

Woman, æt. 21, strong and healthy, after fright; loss of speech.

Man, æt. 23, previous good health, sudden insanity.

Woman, æt. 24, suffering five weeks; convulsive tremor in foot.

Woman, æt. 25, quiet and peaceable disposition, after some mental shock, epileptic attacks, which, five days after childbirth, were followed by mania.

Woman, æt. 27, suffering four weeks; hysteria.

Young woman, apparently well, except recently had irregular menses; mania.

Very irritable lady; effects of jealousy.

Mrs. R., weak, nervous temperament, three weeks after confinement; diarrhœa.

Woman, after having been cured of a previous fit of insanity, after drinking; insanity.

Brandy drinker, within six years has had attacks; delirium tremens.

Woman, æt. 30, after being accused of theft; affection of mind.

Man, æt. 30, after fit of passion; melancholia followed by
madness.

Man, æt. 33, suffering several weeks; chest affection.

Woman, æt. 36, tradesman's wife, lymphatic temperament;
delirium tremens.

Woman, æt. 37, drunkard; mania.

Woman, æt. 37, suffering from daily paroxysms for more
than a year; convulsions.

Man, æt. 38; frequent micturition.

Man, æt. 48; insanity.

Man, æt. 50, for some years monomania; insanity.

Woman, æt. 59, unmarried; apoplexy.

Old man; diarrhœa.

Man, æt. 70, suffering a year; frequent micturition.

Mrs. P., æt. 85, health has been failing for several weeks,
less activity of mind and body, restless at night, fearing
to be alone in the dark; hallucinations.

⁴⁸ Relations. Antidoted by: Vinegar, *Bellad.*, *Citric acid*, *Cinchon.*, *Stramon.*

It antidotes: *Bellad.*, effects of ether, *Plumbum*, *Stramon.*

Compatible: *Bellad.*, *Pulsat.*, *Stramon.*, *Veratr.*, all follow
well when indicated; *Phosphor.* often cures lasciviousness
when *Hyosc.* fails; *Hyosc.* follows *Bellad.* well in deafness
after apoplexy; *Nux vom.* or *Opium* in hæmoptysis of
drunkards; *Bellad.* and *Opium* in congestive chills.

HYPERICUM PERFORATUM.

Hypericaceæ.   *St. John's Wort.*

Provings by Mueller, Thorer, Stokes, Bruckner and Schelling. See Allen's
Encyclopedia, vol. 5, p. 53.

CLINICAL AUTHORITIES.—*Affection of mind,* Müller, Analyt. Therap., vol. 1, p.
134; *Headache,* C. Hering, Analyt. Therap., vol. 1, p. 332; *Bone pains in head,* Lyford,
Organon, vol. 3, p. 361; *Pain and irritation of eye,* Moffat, Norton's Oph. Therap.,
p. 95; *Spasmodic asthma,* Ludlam, Rück. Kl. Erf., vol. 5, p. 871; *Spinal irritation,*
Dornberg, Raue's P., p. 798; *Traumatic meningitis,* Winterburn, Trans. Hom. Med.
Soc. N. Y., 1884, p. 149; *Injury to spine; concussion of spine,* Winterburn, Trans.
Hom. Med. Soc. N. Y., 1884; *Affection of spine,* Ludlam, B. J. H., vol. 17, p. 524;
Crushing of foot, Winterburn, Trans. Hom. Med. Soc. N. Y., 1884, p. 148; *Injury to
foot,* Farrington, Organon, vol. 3, p. 91; *Shock,* Winterburn, Trans. Hom. Med. Soc.
N. Y., 1884, p. 148; *Tetanic symptoms,* Hocking, Raue's Rec., 1874, p. 264;
Wounds, Franklin, B. J. H., vol. 27, p. 325; *Gunshot wounds,* Franklin, Trans.
W. H. Con., 1876, p. 794; *Compound fractures and dislocations,* Franklin, T. W. H. C.,
1876, p. 194; *Pain after operation,* Gilchrist, Organon, vol. 2, p. 241, vol. 3, p. 366.

¹ **Mind.**   ı ıMakes mistakes in writing; omits letters; forgets
  what she wanted to say; confused.
  Increase of intellectual power.
  ı ı Erotic ideas; brain excited, as after tea.
  Sees spirits; spectres; delirium.
  ıTalking nonsense in her sleep at 4 o'clock in morning;
    disturbed look, stares at people; head hot, carotids
    throbbing; flushed and bloated face; eyes fixed, pupils
    dilated; frequent pulse; hair moist, rest of body burning
    hot; great anxiety; singing, followed by weeping and
    loud screaming, with gasping for breath; beating head-
    ache, especially in vertex; tearing stitches in brain;
    crawling in hands and feet, as if they were numb; great
    thirst; white coated tongue.
  ı ıGreat anxiety.   θMeningitis.
  Melancholy.
  Irritable, inclined to speak sharply; slept badly, languid
    on waking.
  ıConsequences of fright; effects of shock.
² **Sensorium.**   Heaviness and dizziness in head.
  ıVertigo: at night, with urging to urinate; with loathing
    on waking; with pain in temples; in afternoon, with
    feeling of weakness and trembling of limbs; sensation
    as if head became suddenly elongated.

∎Sensation as if being lifted up high into air; tormented by anxiety that the slightest touch or motion would make her fall down from this height; with headache after a fall on occiput.

∎Confused sensation in vertex with buzzing sensation at night, as if something living were in brain.

∎Asphyxia after a fall; when jerkings or shooting pains appear.

³ **Inner Head.** ∎Tearing stitches in brain; beating, mostly on vertex. θMeningitis.

∎Burning in vertex, pulsation and heat.

∎Dull headache, only on vertex, gradually increasing as if whole brain would be pressed asunder, with inability to perform any kind of labor; loathing; tingling, drawing pains in cheeks and chin.

∎Violent headache after puerperal rash; throbbing in vertex, moves to cheeks and chin, where it changes to tingling, drawing pains; brain feels compressed, becomes stupefied.

∎Throbbing in vertex, and heat in head in afternoon.

∎Headache as if brain would be torn to pieces.

∎Sensation as if head became elongated.

∎Dull headache, head heavy; morning.

∎∎Headache after breakfast.

∎Headache, with sore eyes, after a fall.

∎Headache, extending into zygoma or cheeks.

∎Pressive pain in occiput on motion; also with drawing stitches; tearing; back of head feels "bothered;" severe scalp headache l. side of occiput, after breakfast, at other times dull; shoot of dull pain up l. occipital nerve.

∎Headache after a fall upon occiput, combined with a sensation as if being lifted up high into air; she was tormented by the greatest anxiety that the slightest touch or motion would make her fall down from this height.

⁴ **Outer Head.** Sensation in forehead as if touched by an icy cold hand, in afternoon, after which a spasmodic contraction is felt in r. eye.

∎Pressure in l. temple, after breakfast.

∎Curling sensation on vertex.

∎Head hot, carotids throbbing.

∎Hair moist, rest of body burning hot.

∎∎Heat and pressure on vertex.

∎Severe bone pains in cranium.

∎Fractured skull; bone splintered.

∎∎Humid eruption on scalp with children.

⁵ **Sight and Eyes.** ∎Disturbed look, stares at people, eyes fixed; pupils dilated.

∎Pain and irritation of eye, from an anterior synechia resulting from an injury several years previously; healthy eye also irritable.

▮Stitches in r. eye.

▮Stye on lower left lid.

⁶ Hearing and Ears. ▮Sensitiveness of hearing; during catamenia.

ı ıShooting through the ear.

ı ıEars hot; scurf on ear.

⁷ Smell and Nose. ▮Exceedingly fine sense of smell.

ı ıNose dry, very annoying.

ı ıSneezing, leaving a raw sore feeling in throat.

▮Sores inside nose, itching; all the time picking nose.

ı ıDryness of nostrils; crusts in it.

⁸ Upper Face. Suffering expression.

▮Face hot, bloated. *θ*Meningitis.

ı ıCheeks red·; erysipelatous redness.

ı ıDull faceache, aching in brows; afternoon, evening; < at night, disturbing sleep.

▮Headache extending into zygoma or cheek.

▮Red eruption on both cheeks, chin and nose; sometimes dry, with thin crusts; sometimes fiery red, oozing yellow drops.

⁹ Lower Face. Tension in the cheek.

ı ıLips dry, feel hot.

▮Eruption around mouth and on r. ear.

▮Yellow-greenish scabs, with cracking and moisture.

¹⁰ Teeth and Gums. ▮Severe aching in decayed tooth at night; restless, wakeful; > lying on affected side, and keeping quiet.

Injuries to dental nerves.

¹¹ Taste and Tongue. Taste: insipid; of blood.

▮Tongue coated white or yellow; great thirst. *θ*Meningitis.

▮Great soreness of tongue, from lacerated wounds, with inability to speak, not from stiffness or swelling, but extreme soreness.

¹² Inner Mouth. ▮Dry, burning heat in mouth and on lips.

¹³ Throat. Expansion of throat and abdomen.

ı ıSensation as if a worm was moving in throat.

ı ıHot rising in œsophagus after a fright, or with anxious feelings.

ı ıWith hemming, some bright, red blood comes up.

¹⁴ Appetite, Thirst. Desires, Aversions. ▮Desire for warm drinks. *θ*Meningitis.

ı ıGreat thirst, white tongue; in morning after heat and delirium.

▮Thirst with feeling of heat in mouth; violent thirst.

ı ıDesire for wine; for pickles.

ı ıAppetite increased morning and evening.

¹⁵ **Eating and Drinking.** Tastelessness.
I I Belching, when drinking water.
I I Smoking tobacco does not taste well.
After breakfast: headache, eructations, gastric symptoms,
pressure in stomach toward back; pains in limbs.
After supper; flatulence and diarrhœa.

¹⁶ **Hiccough, Belching, Nausea and Vomiting.** Eructations:
tasteless; bitter; preventing sleep at night; < after
drinking water.
I Nausea: weakness every morning; abdomen distended,
pains in bowels, awaking in night; with headache on
vertex.
I Vomiting.

¹⁷ **Scrobiculum and Stomach.** Pressure at stomach on eating
but little.
Sticking in stomach.
Pain in stomach, nausea, diarrhœa and chill after eating.

¹⁸ **Hypochondria.** Sticking or dragging pain in r. hypochon-
drium.

¹⁹ **Abdomen.** I Tympanitic distension of abdomen; relieved
by a stool.
I I Cutting in belly, in region of navel.
I I Pinching pains; diarrhœa; catamenia.
I Colic.
I Pain after operation for incarcerated hernia.

²⁰ **Stool and Rectum.** Awakes with distended abdomen, re-
lieved by stool.
I I Diarrhœa driving out of bed in morning.
I I Loose, bilious, yellow stools evening or morning.
I Summer diarrhœa, with eruptions on skin.
I Cholera morbus, slimy stools; afterward constipation; .
flesh sore all over; feet swollen, urine lessened.
I Constipation; violent tenesmus, with discharge of a hard
little ball; with nausea.
I Rectum feels dry, morning.
: Hemorrhoids.

²¹ **Urinary Organs.** Vesical tenesmus.
I Swelling and hardness of female urethra, with burning,
soreness and sensitiveness; especially if caused by
instruments for uterine prolapsus.
I Nightly urging to urinate, with vertigo.
Retention of urine.
Urine: much diminished; bloody; turbid; of peculiar
odor.

²² **Male Sexual Organs.** Sexual functions excited.
Tearing in genital organs, with desire to urinate.

²³ **Female Sexual Organs.** Inflammatory conditions of
mucous membranes of uterus and vagina.

Menses: delay a fortnight; too late, with tension in
uterine region, as from a tight bandage; increased in
quantity; three days before their appearance, pinching
in abdomen, diarrhœa, cold feet; headache, wrenching
pain over eyes, > in motion ; severe headache; attended
by sickening pain in belly and sensitiveness of hearing.

Leucorrhœa: with delayed menses, palpitation, pressure
in small of back; with heaviness in lower bowels; in a
child, milky, but corroding.
: Chlorosis of marriageable girls.
: Scirrhus of breast caused by injury.

²⁴ **Pregnancy. Parturition. Lactation.** Labor pains tardy.
❙Afterpains violent, in sacrum and hips, with severe headache; after instrumental delivery.

²⁵ **Voice and Larynx. Trachea and Bronchia.** Hoarseness, with scraping and roughness in larynx, upper part
of pharynx and nares, in a foggy atmosphere.

²⁶ **Respiration.** ❙Spasmodic asthmatic attacks: with changes
of weather from clear to damp, or before storms; cannot
lie for any length of time upon back; attacks > by
copious expectoration from bronchial tubes ; after lesion
of spinal cord, by a fall, years before.

²⁷ **Cough.** ❙Spells of short, barking cough. θMeningitis.
❙Frequent dry, hacking cough.
❙❙Hacking cough, from irritation in throat, < by heat
· and cold air.
Dry cough and prostration in morning.
❙Whooping cough, worse from 6 to 10 P.M.; great nervous
prostration.

²⁸ **Inner Chest and Lungs.** Anxiety in chest, in forenoon,
with short breath, dizziness and bitter belching.
❙Tightness in chest.
Pressure and burning in chest.
Stitches in chest between breasts.
Stinging in left chest, < when moving.
Cutting in upper right chest, then in lower left.
: Consumption with hæmoptysis.

²⁹ **Heart, Pulse and Circulation.** . Violent beating of heart. ˍ
Pulse: quick and hard; frequent.
Local congestions, and capillary erethism, with or without
hemorrhages and great nervous depression, following
wounds.

³⁰ **Outer Chest.** Stitches under mammæ.
Continual stitches from within outward, through l. breast
and sternum, < from motion.
Stinging burning pain on one edge of l. pectoral muscles.
Dull pressure, r. chest, from seventh rib downwards, after
breakfast.

[31] **Neck and Back.** ▮Cervical vertebræ very sensitive to touch.
▮Stinging near edge of right scapula near spine; morning.
▮Cutting between scapulæ.
▮Back lame and painful.
▮Stitches in small of back.
▮Aching pain and sensation of lameness in small of back.
▮Backache after confinement.
▮After falling out of hammock, great pain in spine, growing daily more severe; she could not sit except upon an
air cushion.
▮Every four weeks attack of illness lasting 4 to 8 days,
beginning with chill, followed by long continued fever,
with dry, parched skin, headache, especially towards
evening, restlessness, jactitation, supersensibility of surface of neck and of superior extremities, great dread of
motion, would not walk and screamed outright if any
one proposed to lift her from one place to another, in-
sisting all the while that she should be held in lap;
face pale and anxious, white around mouth, and expression of suffering and uneasiness; anorexia; slight thirst
for warm drinks; dry, hacking cough from irritation in
throat, < from least exposure to cold air; tongue white,
taste insipid; cervical vertebræ very sensitive to touch.
θAfter a fall.
▮After a fall: slightest motion of arms or of neck extorts
cries; cervical vertebræ very sensitive to touch; headache; desire for warm drinks; asthmatic spells, or spells
of short, hacking cough.
▮An ice-man struck back violently against curbstone by
being thrown from wagon; he felt a momentary intense
pain shoot down both legs, but was afterwards able to
get up, and serve out the rest of his route; in afternoon
was unable to hold urine, which dribbled away without
his being aware of it; next morning on attempting to
rise legs seemed "as if drunk;" pulse feeble; temperature normal; breathing slightly labored, no pain
along spine, nor any spasmodic movement; sphincter
muscles partially paralyzed; walks with a rolling
motion; legs felt "as if dead." θConcussion of spine.
▮Boy fell from shed, but did not seem much hurt; next
night, however, began vomiting; in morning was slightly
delirious, but could easily be aroused to answer questions; severe pain in head and down spine, greatly
intensified by attempting to move arms or legs; pupils
dilated; face puffed and hot; tongue coated yellowish;
mouth dry, but did not wish to drink water, desired
warm milk; pulse 140, full and hard, temperature
104½ F.; constipated, stools consisting of small, hard

lumps; urine thick and muddy, and had the appearance of beer. θTraumatic meningitis.

▮Boy, æt. 14, fair, of lively temperament, was attacked
while husking corn with numbness of limbs, and pain in
upper part of spinal cord; spinal column from cervical
vertebræ to region of kidneys, tender to touch; paroxysms
of pain with symptoms of mania, pains principally in
joints and changing about; almost constant dull
headache; least touch on spine between cervical and
lumbar regions made him shrink.

▮Violent pains and inability to walk, or to stoop after a fall
on coccyx; feet feel pithy, as if pricked with needles.

▮Lies on back jerking head backward.

▮▮Consequences of spinal concussion.

²² Upper Limbs.   Flying pains in r. shoulder.
Cutting under left scapula.
Pressure at insertion of right deltoid.
Stitches on top of shoulder at every inspiration.
Hard pain running down left median nerve.
Numbness in l. arm; > from rubbing.
Dry herpetic eruption on outer side of arms, < on right.
▮Excruciating pain after amputation of arm; fainting.
Tension in both arms and in hands.
Cutting in fleshy ends of fingers.
▮Compound dislocation of two fingers, with severe lacera-
tion and tearing of external structure, the members
being severed except by a narrow bridge of skin uniting
them to the body (applied locally).
Pain in last phalanges of fingers, < in thumb, fore and
little fingers.
▮Panaritium.

²³ Lower Limbs.   ▮After severe injury to sciatic nerve, sharp,
cutting pains, darting along course of nerve and termi-
nating in a twisting or wrenching sensation in foot.
▮▮Sciatica, rheumatism.
▮▮Coxalgia after confinement.
▮Left leg numb, cold while sitting.
Weakening drawing, over front of legs; shoots of pain, as
if in periosteum.
Fearful pains in knees, sharp, could hardly touch them.
▮▮Articular rheumatism in knee; effusion around joint;
muddy urine, looking like settlings of beer; pains sharp,
< least touch; tearing pains.
▮The feet feel pithy, as if pricked with needles.
▮Lying in bed the feet tingle.
Sensation as if l. foot was strained or dislocated.
▮Same evening, after running pin into foot, intense pain
at seat of injury; toes became rigid, ankle stiffened,

chills chased each other down back, followed by nausea and vomiting; she fainted, and on coming to, still complained of the agonizing pain; strange expression of face, eyes set, lips drawn tightly across teeth.

∎After running pins in r. foot pain runs up limb through spine to neck and face; muscles of neck and jaw become rigid, < r. side, and also muscles of abdomen and thorax. θTetanic symptoms.

∎Toes of r. foot crushed by heavy iron shutter, and almost severed from foot, the bones protruding in several places; considerable hemorrhage; excruciating pain; depressed and cold.

: Gout.

∎Bunions excruciatingly painful (locally).

∎Cannot walk, spine affected.

³⁴ **Limbs in General.** Feeling of weakness and trembling of all the limbs.

Bruised sensation in all the joints.

Rheumatoid inflammation of joints.

∎Crawling in hands and feet, as if they were numb.

Sensation of lameness of l. arm and right foot.

∎Crawling in hands and feet, they felt fuzzy.

∎Compound fractures of hands and feet, with great laceration of soft parts.

∎∎Affections of joints.

³⁵ **Rest. Position. Motion.** Keeping quiet: toothache >.

Lying in bed: feet tingle.

Lying on affected side: toothache >.

Lies on back: jerking head backwards.

Sitting: l. leg cold.

On rising: languor.

Cannot lie for any length of time upon back.

Could not sit except on air cushion; screamed when it was proposed to lift her to another place.

Motion: pressive pain in occiput; wrenching pain over eyes >; continual stitches through l. breast and sternum.

Slightest motions of arms or neck extorts cries, after a fall.

Great dread of motion.

Physical effort causes fainting.

Would not walk.

Cannot walk or stoop: after a fall on coccyx.

³⁶ **Nerves.** ∎∎Effects of nervous shock.

∎Great weakness.

Weariness on awaking; goes off by noon.

∎Great nervous depression following wounds.

∎After being frightened by a practical joke, became very pale and hysterical; pulse 54, very weak and compressible; respiration 15 and sighing; temperature 96°; skin cold and clammy; slight vomiting. θShock.

Jerks in limbs.

∎Convulsions from blows upon head or concussion; dull headache, on vertex, or severe headache, with throbbing on top of head.

∎Spasms after slight injuries, in children.

∎Epileptiform spasms after hard knocks.

∎∎Tetanus after traumatic injuries.

∥Opisthotonos.

∎Prevents lockjaw from wounds in soles of feet, fingers, or palms of hands.

∎Removes ill effects of local shock, prevents in a great measure sympathetic irritation of system from local derangement and modifies subsequent inflammation and sloughing. θGunshot wounds.

∎∎Injuries to nerves, attended by great pain.

∎Especially adapted to mechanical injuries of spinal cord, and nerves at their peripheral extremities.

∎Nervous disorders arising from falls and hurts.

∎Lacerated nerves, causing excruciating pain.

[57] **Sleep.** Constant drowsiness.

Spasmodic jerks of arms or legs on going to sleep; twitchings.

On awaking: weary, > by noon; feels refreshed; bowels distended.

Dreams: with activity, traveling; vivid; distressing.

[58] **Time.** 4 A.M.: talking nonsense in sleep.

Morning: dull headache, head heavy; great thirst, white tongue; appetite increased; diarrhœa drives out of bed; loose, bilious, yellow stools; rectum feels dry; dry cough and prostration; stinging near scapula; after a fall slightly delirious.

After breakfast: headache; severe scalp headache; pressure in l. temple; eructations; gastric symptoms; pressure in stomach; pains in limbs; dull pressure in r. chest.

Noon: weariness >.

Afternoon: feeling of weakness and trembling of limbs; throbbing in vertex; sensation as if forehead was touched by an icy cold hand, after which contraction of r. eye; dull faceache; brows ache; unable to hold urine.

4 P.M.: eruption like nettlerash on both hands.

Evening: dull faceache, brows ache; appetite increased; loose, bilious, yellow stools; dry, parched skin, headache; intense pain at seat of injury; eruption on both hands.

After supper: flatulence and diarrhœa.

Night: vertigo; urging to urinate; dull faceache <; severe aching in decayed tooth; eructations preventing sleep; awakening at night from pain in bowels; vomiting, after a fall.

³⁹ Temperature and Weather. Sensitiveness to cold.

Attacks return with changes of weather from clear to damp, or before storms; after lesion of spine by a fall, spasmodic asthma.

Foggy atmosphere: hoarseness, with scraping and roughness of larynx, upper part of pharynx and nares.

Heat: hacking cough <.

Cold air: hacking cough <; least exposure < symptoms.

⁴⁰ Fever. Shuddering over whole body, with desire to urinate.

Heat, with delirium, wild staring look, hot head, throbbing of carotids, bright red bloated face, moist hair on head, burning heat of skin, great oppression and anguish.

Chill followed by heat, with sweat on hands and feet.

⁴¹ Attacks, Periodicity. Every morning: nausea, weakness.

From 6 to 10 P.M.: whooping cough <.

Three days before menses: pinching in abdomen.

Every four weeks: attacks of illness, lasting 4 to 8 days.

Summer: diarrhœa.

⁴² Locality and Direction. Right: spasmodic contraction of eye; stitches in eye; dull depression in chest; stinging near edge of scapula near spine; flying pains in shoulder; pressure at insertion of deltoid; dry, herpetic eruption on outer side of arm; pains through limb, spine, neck and face; excruciating pain in crushed toes; lameness of foot.

Left: severe scalp headache in side of occiput; shoot of dull pain up cervical nerve; pressure in temple; stye on lower lid; continual stitches through breast and sternum; stinging burning pain on one edge of pectoral muscles; cutting under scapula; hard pain running down median nerve; numbness in arm; leg numb; leg cold while sitting; sensation as if foot was strained or dislocated.

Before backward: pressure in stomach.

Upper r. to lower l.: cutting in chest.

Left upper and r. lower: sensation of lameness of arm and foot.

Above downward: pain down l. median nerve; pain down from vertex to face.

⁴³ Sensations. Brain excited as after tea; as if hands and feet were numb; as if head became suddenly elongated; as if being lifted up high into air; as if something alive was in brain; as if whole brain would be pressed asunder; brain feels compressed; as if brain would be torn to pieces; as if forehead was touched by icy cold hand; as if a worm was moving in throat; as from a tight bandage in uterine region; legs as if dead; feet feel pithy as if pricked with needles, as if l. foot was strained and dislocated; hands and feet as if numb; skin as if full of knots.

Pain: in temples; in head; in head extending to zygoma or cheeks; in eye; in limbs; in bowels; in stomach; after operation for incarcerated hernia; in back; in upper part of spinal cord; in joints; in last phalanges of fingers; in old cicatrices.

Intense pain: in momentary shoots down both legs.

Excruciating pain: after amputating arm; in r. foot, after crushing toes with heavy iron shutter; in bunions.

Fearful pains: in knees.

Agonizing pain: in foot after running in a pin.

Sickening pain: in belly.

Violent pain: in head.

Great pain: in spine.

Severe pain: in head; in spine; in cranial bones.

Severe headache: in scalp; l. side of occiput.

Sharp pain: in knees.

Sharp, cutting pain, darting along course of sciatic nerve terminating in a wrenching, twisting sensation in foot.

Cutting: in belly and in region of navel; between scapula; under l. scapula; in fleshy ends of fingers.

Beating: headache; in vertex.

Tearing: in male genitals.

Tearing stitches: in brain.

Wrenching pain: over eyes ; in foot.

Pinching pain: in abdomen.

Stitches: in r. eye; under mammæ; through l. breast and sternum; in small of back; on top of shoulder at every inspiration

Drawing stitches: in occiput.

Shooting: through ear.

Flying pains: in r. shoulder.

Tingling, drawing pain: in cheeks and chin.

Dragging pain: in hypochondrium.

Sticking: in stomach; in hypochondrium.

Stinging: near edge of r. scapula.

Throbbing: in vertex, moves to cheeks and chin.

Severe aching: in decayed tooth.

Aching pain: in small of back.

Pressive pain: in occiput.

Hard pain: running down l. median nerve.

Stinging, burning pain: on one edge of l. pectoral muscle.

Burning soreness: of female urethra.

Burning heat: in whole body; in mouth; in lips.

Burning in vertex.

Dull pressure: in r. chest.

Shoot of dull pain: up l. occipital nerve; in legs.

Dull pain: in head; in face; in brows.

Soreness: of eyes; of inside of nose; of tongue; all over.

Bruised sensation: in all joints.

Sensitiveness: of female urethra.

Raw, sore feeling: in throat after sneezing.

Heat: in vertex; in ears; in lips.

Weakening drawing: over front of legs.

"Bothered" sensation back of head.

Confused sensation: in vertex.

Spasmodic contraction in r. eye.

Pressure: in l.temple; on vertex; in stomach toward back; in small of back; at insertion of r. deltoid.

Tension: in cheek; in both arms and both hands.

Lame feeling: in back.

Weakness: of limbs.

Heaviness: in head; in lower bowels.

Pulsation: in vertex.

Shuddering: over whole body.

Hot rising: in œsophagus.

Scraping and roughness: in larynx; upper part of pharynx; of nares.

Dryness: of nostrils; of rectum.

Fuzzy feeling: in hands and feet.

Buzzing sensation: in head.

Curling sensation: on vertex.

Tingling: in carotids; in feet.

Trembling: of limb.

Crawling: in hands and feet.

Numbness: of limbs; in l. arm.

Violent itching: of skin; of tetter.

Itching: of nose; in sacral region.

" **Tissues.** ▮Local congestions; nervous erethism, with or without hemorrhage; great nervous depression following wounds.

Congestion to head, lungs or heart.

▮Next to nervous tissues, the joints are affected; all articulations feel bruised.

▮Injuries of parts rich in sentient nerves, particularly fingers and toes, and matrices of nails; open, painful wounds, with general prostration from loss of blood, and great nervous depression; lacerated wounds.

▮Mashed, punctured and torn wounds, when nervous tissues are mainly concerned; lacerations of skin; injuries of vertebral region, of tissues of animal life, as hands and feet.

▮Lacerated wounds, or other injuries to nerves, in which there is much soreness, with jerking in the muscles.

▮Violent, excruciating pains from laceration of nerves.

▮Excessive painfulness of affected parts, showing nerves to
be attacked.

▮Preserves vitality of torn and lacerated members when
almost entirely separated from the body.

▮Lacerations when intolerable pain shows nerves are severely involved.

▮In slighter forms of lacerated wounds, if applied early,
will sometimes arrest, and always modify the occurrence
of ulceration and sloughing.

▮Gunshot wounds when the parts have been extensively
lacerated and torn, with engorgement of the capillaries,
attended with more or less discharge of bloody serum.

▮Piercing wounds from pointed instruments.

▮▮Punctured, incised, contused or lacerated wounds, when
pains are extremely severe, and particularly if they are
of long duration; pains like those of a severe toothache;
pains spread to neighboring parts and extend up limb.

▮Open, painful wounds, with general prostration from loss
of blood, feeling of weakness and trembling in all the
limbs; languor on rising, fainting from physical effort,
thirst and heaviness of head.

▮Mechanical injuries, wounds by nails or splinters in feet;
needles under nails; squeezing or hammering of toes
and fingers; when the nerves have been lacerated,
wounded, or torn, with excruciating pains. It prevents
lockjaw from wounds in soles of feet, or of fingers and
palms of hands.

Always modifies and sometimes arrests ulceration and
sloughing.

▮▮Hard, yellow crusts form on the healing wound.

▮Pain in old cicatrices.

▮▮Stings of insects and bug bites; burns.

"**Touch. Passive Motion. Injuries.** ▮▮Punctured wounds
feel very sore: from treading on nails, needles, pins,
splinters, rat bites, etc.; prevents lockjaw.

▮Wounds from crushing, as mashed fingers, especially
tips.

▮Nerves lacerated, pains excruciating.

▮▮Painful wounds before suppuration.

▮Rheumatism, bunions, corns, etc., when pains are so dis-
proportionately severe as to show nerves are attacked.

After a knock or blow on head: spasms.

▮▮Consequences of spinal concussion. See chaps. 31 and 44.

Touch: cervical vertebræ sensitive; on spine between cervical and lumbar region made him shrink; < sharp
pains in knees.

Rubbing: > numbness of arm.

After using instruments for uterine prolapsus: burning soreness of female urethra.

After a fall: asphyxia; headache with sore eyes; lesion of spinal cord; asthmatic attacks; great pain in spine; unable to hold urine; sphincter muscles partially paralyzed; vomiting at night; slightly delirious in morning; severe pain in head and down spine.

After a fall upon occiput: headache with sensation as if she was being lifted high up into air.

After a fall on coccyx: violent pains and inability to walk or stoop.

After hard knock: epileptiform spasms.

Blows upon head: convulsions.

Following wounds: great nervous depression.

❙Gunshot wounds.

❙❙Piercing wounds: from sharp instruments.

Compound fracture of hands and feet.

After severe injury to sciatic nerve: sharp cutting pains darting along course of nerve.

❙Slight injuries in children: cause spasms.

❙Injuries to dental nerves.

Injury several years ago: pain and irritation of eye from anterior synechia.

❙After running pins into foot: intense pain; toes rigid, ankle stiffened, chills in back; pains run up limb, ·through spine to neck and face; muscles of neck and jaw become rigid.

⁴⁶ **Skin.**   Great itching when undressing, most in sacral region.

Violent itching; smarting.

Skin rough, as if full of small knots.

Pimples on forehead, throat, back, hips.

Eruption like nettlerash on both hands, at 4 P.M. and in evening.

Smarting eruption, like nettlerash, on hands.

❙Tetters, beginning with sore places, and forming hard, yellow crusts, with violent itching.

❙❙Eruptions accompanying diarrhœa in Summer time.

❙Hard, dry, yellow crusts form on wounds or open sores.

❙Foul, torpid and phagedenic ulcers.

⁴⁷ **Stages of Life, Constitution.**   Girl, æt. 6, three years ago fell down steps, since which time she has been in poor health; affection of·spine.

Boy, æt. 7, after falling from roof of shed; traumatic men-ingitis.

Girl, æt. 14, timid and impressionable, after being greatly frightened by a practical joke; shock.

Robust young lady, after fall upon occiput; headache.

Mason, æt. 29; crushing of r. foot.

Mrs. E. M. C., æt. 32, after falling from hammock; pain in spine.

Ice-man, æt. 32, after being thrown from wagon; concussion of spine.

Woman, æt. 40, stepped upon a paper of pins, a number of which penetrated sole of r. foot quite deeply; tetanic symptoms.

Strong woman, æt. 45, mother of five children, in fifteenth year fell down steps and injured spine, has suffered with chest affection for ten years; spasmodic asthma.

[48] **Relations.** Antidoted by: *Arsen.* (weakness or sickness in the morning); *Chamom.* (pains in face).

Antidotes: Effects of mesmerism (*Sulphur*).

Compare: *Acon., Agar.,* **I I** *Arnic., Arsen.,* **I I** *Callend., Chamom., Coccul., Ruta, Staphis., Sulphur.*

IBERIS AMARA.

Bitter Candy Tuft.   *Cruciferæ.*

Provings by Sabin and Dodge, under supervision of Hale. See Allen's Encyclopedia, vol. 5, p. 60.

CLINICAL AUTHORITIES.—*Heart affections,* Williams and Sylvester. See Note, Allen's Encyclopedia, vol. 5, p. 61.

[1] **Mind.** Sad, downhearted, oppressed, with desire to sigh.

I I Very irritable, with dulness of mind and lack of memory.

Nervous and irritable on rising in morning.

Feels as if frightened; an indefinable dread with trembling.

An excited, frightened feeling, with cold sweat on face.

Peculiar inability to fix mind on any one thing.

[2] **Sensorium.** Vertigo: with dull pain and chilliness; when rising, morning, had to lie down; when making any exertion, with nausea; when standing, < on stooping; in back part of head, as if occiput was turning around.

Entering the house after walking felt faint.

Heat and fulness in neck and head, with flushed face and cold feet and hands.

Heaviness of head, with roaring in ears.

[3] **Inner Head.** Pain in r. side of head.

I I Frontal headache: on rising in morning; with nausea and loss of appetite.

Heat in head and neck and flushed face.

Dull pain in head, with vertigo and feverish chilliness.

⁵ Sight and Eyes. Red eyes with flushed face.

ı ı Feeling in eyes as if being forced outward.

Flashes before eyes, with dull headache and palpitation of heart.

⁷ Hearing and Ears. Dulness of hearing and comprehension.

Dull hearing and labored breathing.

Roaring in ears, with heaviness of head, slight nausea and palpitation of heart.

⁸ Upper Face. Looks as if he had been ill a long while.

Flushed hot face and red eyes, with palpitation.

Cold sweat on face, with fearfulness.

¹³ Throat. Throat dry as if filled with dust.

Throat feels as if both tonsils were enlarged.

ı ı Constant hawking up of thick, viscid, stringy mucus > after a meal.

Choking sensation: in throat, with fulness and heat; just above cricoid cartilage.

Constrictive sensation in throat, with stabbing pains in heart, dyspnœa and palpitation.

¹⁴ Appetite, Thirst. Desires, Aversions. Loss of appetite, with feeling of indigestion.

Desire for stimulants.

¹⁵ Eating and Drinking. After eating: sour belching; hawking of stringy mucus >.

¹⁶ Hiccough, Belching, Nausea and Vomiting. Nausea, with cold, chilly feelings over body.

¹⁸ Hypochondria. Fulness and oppression in r. hypochondriac region.

Pain in region of liver with clay colored stool.

¹⁹ Abdomen. Fulness and distension of bowels.

Tenderness of bowels, with thin, whitish stool.

²⁰ Stool and Rectum. Stool: clay colored; thin, whitish; large, white.

²¹ Urinary Organs. Frequent but scanty urination.

Excessive evacuation of urine.

²⁵ Voice and Larynx. Trachea and Bronchia. Choking sensation just above cricoid cartilage.

Dryness in larynx and throat, with hawking up of thin, stringy mucus, for many hours; > after eating.

Tickling in throat, with expectoration of stringy mucus.

Tightness and constrictive feeling in larynx.

²⁶ Respiration. ı ı Dyspnœa and palpitation on going up stairs.

Constant desire to draw a long breath, without relief.

Respiration more frequent and labored.

²⁸ Inner Chest and Lungs. Slight pain under sternum, at articulation of third rib.

Fulness and constriction under sternum, with lancinating pain through chest.

Continued feeling of weight and anxiety in chest.

Fulness in chest, with fulness and heat in head and neck, and flushed face.

⁎Heart, Pulse and Circulation. Increased action of heart, full feeling in neck and head.

Palpitation: with flushed hot face and red eyes; with dull headache and flashes before eyes; with heaviness of head, roaring, slight nausea; on going up stairs.

Stabbing pains in heart with constriction in throat.

❘❘Palpitation, with vertigo and choking in throat after walking, and on entering house felt faint; tingling and numbness commencing in fingers of l. hand, gradually extending up arm, with irregular, tremulous and not well defined pulse; dull, heavy aching in l. arm.

Increase of heart's action from 72 to 88, after fifteen minutes.

A wavy, tremulous sensation in radial artery, felt by finger, pulse intermitting every third beat, easily compressible.

Pulse has peculiar double beats, which seem to run into each other, full, soft and easily compressed.

❘❘Palpitation of heart on slight exertion (pulling down a window).

❘Palpitation plainly visible over whole chest, < by walking, > sitting still, but renewed by slightest exertion.

Much pain over base of heart with dull, heavy pain in l. arm, and tingling and numbness in tips of fingers.

❘❘Sensation of weight and pressure in region of heart, with occasional sharp, stinging pains, passing from before backwards; heart's action from 70 to 96.

❘Hypertrophy of heart.

Pulse rises from 60 to 94 after fifteen minutes, with slight pains in region of heart.

Pains darting through heart at night, in bed ; < lying on l. side.

Dull, dragging pain in heart not > by any position nor by pressing with hand.

❘❘Sharp, sticking pain in heart, with constriction in throat, red eyes, flushed face.

❘❘Pain as if needle were crosswise in ventricles, and pricked at each contraction.

❘❘Palpitation with marked increase of force of apex beat, with irregular, jerking pulse, and a peculiar thrill under finger.

Strong palpitation, with forcible impulse; hand placed on heart was visibly moved.

Palpitation when going up stairs, obliged to lie down, with dyspnœa and weak feeling.

Constant dull pain in heart < lying down.

Distressing palpitation with increase of dull pain, caused by coughing, laughing or slight exertion.

With the full, intermittently irregular pulse auscultation revealed great excitement of heart.

Contractions at intervals of three or four beats, after which there was a much longer interval.

Near end of proving sounds of heart increased in intensity, especially region of semilunar valves.

Force of apex beat visibly increased, heart impulse raised the touching hand; pulse hard, jerking, intermitting every third beat; rising from 70–90.

Heart's action apparently weakened for the first few moments, in ten minutes pulse rose to 100, full, strong, somewhat irregular.

Heart's action weak and fluttering, with small weak pulse.

[31] **Neck and Back.** I I Sensation of fulness in neck and head.

[32] **Upper Limbs.** Tingling and numbness commencing in fingers of l. hand, gradually extending up l. arm, with irregular, tremulous pulse, not well defined.

Dull, heavy aching in l. arm.

Tingling and numbness in finger tips, < lying on l. side.

Dull aching in l. arm, as if he had slept on it all night.

Rheumatic pains in r. shoulder.

[33] **Lower Limbs.** Trembling of lower limbs after exercise.

[34] **Limbs in General.** Cold feet and hands.

[35] **Rest. Position. Motion.** Any position: does not > pain in heart.

Lying down: dull pain at heart <.

Lying on l. side: darting pains through heart <; tingling and numbness in finger tips <.

Had to lie down: on rising in morning.

Desire to lie down.

Sitting still: palpitation passes off.

When stooping or standing : vertigo.

When making any exertion: vertigo with nausea; palpitation; trembling of lower limbs.

Walking causes indescribable sensation under the sternum.

After walking: faint feeling; choking sensation in throat; palpitation <.

On going up stairs: dyspnœa and palpitation.

Feeling of inability to move even a finger.

[36] **Nerves.** Feels weary, with desire to lie down.

Feeling of general nervous excitement.

Feeling of inability to move even a finger; great weakness and debility.

Nervous and irritable on rising in morning.

Feeling of lameness and soreness through whole body, as from a cold.

Looks as if he had been ill a long while.

Trembling sensation all over, had to lie down.

Desire for stimulants.

37 Sleep.   At night in bed darting through heart.

ι ιSleep at night disturbed by all sorts of dreams.

Restless, turning in bed, with ludicrous dreams.

ι ι Restless nights with horrid dreams.

38 Time.   Morning: on rising nervous and irritable; dull pain, chilliness, vertigo; frontal headache.

Night: darting pain through heart; sleep disturbed by all sorts of dreams; restless with horrid dreams.

40 Fever.   Heat and fulness in neck and head with flushed face and cold feet and hands.

Feverish chilliness.

Cold, chilly feeling with nausea.

Quickly passing febrile paroxysms.

41 Attacks, Periodicity.   Quickly passing febrile attacks.

After ten minutes: pulse rose from weak to 100.

After fifteen minutes: a wavy, tremulous sensation in radial artery, with pulse intermitting every third beat; pulse rises from 60 to 94.

For many hours: dryness of larynx and throat, with hawking up of thin, stringy mucus.

42 Locality and Direction.   Right: pain in side of head; fulness and oppression in hypochondriac region; rheumatic pain in shoulder.

Left: tingling and numbness commencing in fingers, extending up arm; dull, heavy aching in arm.

From before backward: sharp, stinging pains in heart.

43 Sensations.   As if frightened; as if occiput was turning around; as if eyes were being forced out; as if throat was filled with dust; as if both tonsils were enlarged; as if needles were crosswise in ventricles; as if he had been asleep on l. arm all night.

Pain: in r. side of head; in region of liver.

Much pain: over base of heart.

Stabbing pains: in heart.

Lancinating pain: through chest.

Darting pains: through heart.

Sharp, sticking pain: in heart.

Sharp, stinging pain: passing from before heart backwards.

Pricking pain: at each contraction of heart.

Dull, dragging pain: in heart.

Dull, heavy aching: in l. arm.

Dull pain: in head; in heart.

Rheumatic pains: in r. shoulder.

Slight pain: under sternum at articulation of third rib; in region of heart.

Feeling of lameness and soreness: all over body.

Heat and fulness: in neck and head; in throat.

Fulness and distension: of bowels.

Fulness and constriction: under sternum.

Fulness and oppression: in r. hypochondriac region.

Fulness: in chest.

Tenderness ot bowels.

Great weakness and debility.

Faint feeling: after walking.

Weary feeling.

Choking sensation: in throat.

Constrictive sensation: in throat; in larynx.

Tightness: in larynx.

Tickling: in throat.

Dryness: in larynx and throat.

Sensation of weight and pressure: in region of heart.

Continued feeling of weight and anxiety: in chest.

Heaviness: of head.

Roaring: in ears.

Tingling and numbness: commencing in fingers of l. hand, extending up arm.

Wavy, tremulous sensation: in radial artery.

Trembling: of lower limbs; all over.

Chilly feelings: over body.

" **Tissues.** Cardiac affections; bronchitis; asthma; dropsy.

" **Touch. Passive Motion. Injuries.** Pressure: by hand does not > pain in heart.

" **Relations.** Compare: *Amyg. amara, Bellad., Cact. grand., Digit.*

ICTODES FŒTIDA.

Skunk Cabbage.   *Aracex.*

Experiment by Bigelow, Amer. Med. Botany, vol. 2, p. 48. Symptoms in
Jahr's Symptomatology are from provings by C. Hering and others.

[1] **Mind.** Cross; impetuous; inclined to contradict.
Absence of mind and inattention; enters sick-room without knocking, does not listen to patient.

[2] **Sensorium.** Vertigo and dimness of sight.

[3] **Inner Head.** Headache on single places, lasting a short while, then changing place; dulness; pressing in temples now more in one, then more in the other, with violent pulsation of arteries.
Drawing in forehead in two lines from protuberances to glabella, where it draws outward as from a magnet.

[5] **Sight and Eyes.** Dimness of sight, with vertigo.

[7] **Smell and Nose.** The nose is swollen as far as the nasal bones extend, red like a saddle, sore to touch, < l. side.
Cartilage cold and bloodless, with red spots on cheeks and small pimples on l. side of face.
Violent sneezing, with pains in palate, fauces and œsophagus to stomach, hurting for a while after in cardiac end of stomach.

[9] **Lower Face.** Swollen submaxillary glands.

[10] **Teeth and Gums.** Scurvy.

[11] **Taste and Tongue.** Numbness of tongue, cannot touch teeth with it.
Papillæ elevated.
Tongue red and sore on tip and edges.

[13] **Throat.** Burning from fauces downwards through chest.
Œsophagus painful on sneezing.

[14] **Appetite, Thirst. Desires, Aversions.** Inclined so smoke, but it does not taste good.

[16] **Hiccough, Belching, Nausea and Vomiting.** Nausea and vomiting.

[17] **Scrobiculum and Stomach.** With every firm step, pain in pit of stomach as from something breaking loose.

[19] **Abdomen.** Expansion and tension in abdomen.
Pain in abdomen here and there, in single spots.
When walking sensation as if the entrails were hanging loose and flabby, without any pain.

²¹ Urinary Organs. Great urging; urine darker.
²² Male Sexual Organs. ❙Titillation voluptuous, but painful, around corona glandis.
²³ Female Sexual Organs. Amenorrhœa.
²⁶ Respiration. ❙Spasmodic asthma.

❙Sudden anxiety, with dyspnœa and sweat, followed by stool and relief of that and other complaints.

Inclined to take a deep breath; with hollowness of chest; with constriction in fauces and chest.

❙❙Asthma, aggravated or caused by dust. θHeaves in horses from dusty hay.

²⁷ Cough. ❙Spasmodic cough.

❙❙Senile catarrh.

²⁸ Inner Chest and Lungs. Pain in chest and in axillæ; seems to have a connection with burning in œsophagus.
³⁰ Outer Chest. Pressing pain on sternum.
³¹ Neck and Back. Glands on throat swollen.
³⁴ Lower Limbs. Aching along r. cresta tibiæ.
³⁵ Rest. Position. Motion. With every firm step: pain in pit of stomach as from something breaking loose.

When walking: sensation as if entrails were hanging loose and flabby.

On sneezing: Painfulness in œsophagus.

³⁶ Nerves. ❙Hysterics.

: Epilepsy.

³⁷ Sleep. Sleepiness early in evening.
³⁹ Temperature and Weather. All complaints disappear in open air.
⁴² Locality and Direction. Right: aching along cresta tibiæ.

Left: small pimples on side of face.

Outward: drawing in forehead.

⁴³ Sensations. Erratic and spasmodic pains.

Drawing as if from a magnet in forehead; pain in pit of stomach as from something breaking loose; as if entrails were hanging loose and flabby, without pain.

Pain: in palate; in fauces; in œsophagus to stomach; in pit of stomach; in abdomen here and there in single spots; in chest and in axillæ.

Painful titillation: around corona glandis.

Pressing pain: in sternum.

Drawing: in forehead, in two lines from protuberances to glabella, where it draws outward as from a magnet.

Pressing: in temples, now in one, then in the other.

Aching: along r. cresta tibiæ.

Burning: extends from fauces downwards through chest.

Soreness: of tip and edges of tongue.

Violent pulsation: of arteries of temples.

Expansion and tension: of abdomen.

Constriction: of fauces and chest.

Dulness: in head.

Numbness: of tongue.

" **Tissues.** ❙Spasmodic asthma; senile catarrh.

❙Dropsy.

❙Chronic rheumatism.

" **Touch. Passive Motion. Injuries.** Touch: nose sore; tongue numb, cannot touch teeth with it.

" **Skin.** ❙Herpes and cutaneous affections.

" **Stages of Life, Constitution.** Catarrh of aged persons.

" **Relations.** Compare: *Arum triph., Asaf., Mephit.*

IGNATIA.

Loganiaceæ.   *Bean of St. Ignatius.*

A species of strychos native to the Phillipine Islands. The tree bears a pear-shaped fruit, containing intensely bitter seed, from which is obtained the alcoholic tincture.

Introduced and proved by Hahnemann and his provers. See Allen's Ency-clopedia, vol. 5, p. 66.

CLINICAL AUTHORITIES.—*Melancholy,* Gross, Analyt. Therap., vol. 1, p. 178; *Effects of mortification,* Attomyr, Analyt. Therap., vol. 1, p. 91; *Insanity,* Gross, Analyt. Therap., vol. 1, p. 223; *Affection of mind,* Schmid, B. J. H., vol. 5, p. 269; Rück. Kl. Erf., vol. 1, p. 31; Griess, Rück. Kl. Erf., vol. 1, p. 31; Hermel, Rück. Kl. Erf., vol. 5, p. 6; (6 cases), Goeze, Allg. Hom. Ztg., vol. 103, p. 10; *Vertigo,* Goullon, Raue's Rec., 1872, p. 57; *Headache,* Shuldham, Raue's Rec., 1872, p. 213; Hom. Rev., vol. 15, p. 285–7; Stow, Raue's Rec., 1870, p. 286; Schwarze, Hrg., Black, Rück. Kl. Erf., vol. 1, p. 177; *Nervous periodical headache,* Bender, Raue's Rec., 1873, p. 197; *Hydrocephaloid,* Butman, Raue's Rec., 1871, p. 53; *As a prophy-lactic in apoplexy,* Pommerais, Rück. Kl. Erf., vol. 5, p. 29; *Hyperæsthesia of retina,* Fowler, Norton's Oph. Therap., p. 97; *Ophthalmia,* Tülff, Rück. Kl. Erf., vol. 5, p. 137; *Traumatic ophthalmia,* Dessaix, B. J. H., vol. 6, p. 367; Norton, T. W. H. C., 1876, p. 601; *Catarrhal conjunctivitis,* Lewis, Norton's Oph. Therap., p. 96; *Ulcers on cornea,* Buffum, Norton's Oph. Therap., p. 96; *Herpes cornea,* Payr, Raue's Rec., 1872, p. 71; *Affection of eye,* Billig, Allg. Hom. Ztg., vol. 101, p. 98; *Ciliary neural-gia,* Norton's Oph. Therap., p. 97; *Exophthalmus,* Wanstall, Norton's Oph. Therap., p. 96; *Coryza,* Rummell, Rück. Kl. Erf., vol. 1, p. 388; *Prosopalgia,* Gerson, B. J. H., vol. 20, p. 417; *Neuralgia of face,* Käsemann, Rück. Kl. Erf., vol. 5, p. 186; *Toothache,* Hrg., Altschul, Rück. Kl. Erf., vol. 1, p. 463; *Ptyalism,* Meyer, Rück. Kl. Erf., vol. 5, p. 256; *Sensation of lump in throat,* Hofrichter, Rück. Kl. Erf., vol. 5, p. 240; *Angina of throat,* Tietze, Rück. Kl. Erf., vol. 1, p. 530; *Diph-theria,* Boskowitz; (20 cases cured) Slough, Raue's P., p. 303; Guernsey, T. H. M. S. Pa., 1876, p. 304; Raue, MSS.; Knerr, MSS.; *Singultus,* Hilberger, N. A. J. H., vol. 8, p. 278; *Affection of stomach*, Kreuss, Rück. Kl. Erf., vol. 1, p. 636; *Affection of stomach*, Schlosser, Huber, Montgomery, Hofrichter, Rück. Kl. Erf., vol. 5, p. 310; *Colic*, Hartmann, Rück. Kl. Erf., vol. 1, p. 753; *Diarrhœa*, Gross, Analyt. Therap., vol. 1, p. 246; *Constipation*, Hirsch, B. J. H., vol. 26, p. 223; *Hemorrhoids*, Rafinesque, Raue's Rec., 1870, p. 218, and 1874, p. 202; Diez, Rück. Kl. Erf., vol. 1, p. 999; *Ascarides*, Pierson, Raue's Rec., 1872, p. 154; *Worms*, Hirsch, B. J. H., vol. 26, p. 223; *Tænia*, Eidherr, B. J. H., vol. 19, p. 116; Wurmb, Rück. Kl. Erf., vol. 5, p. 388; *Menorrhagia*, Weber, Rück. Kl. Erf., vol. 2, p. 312; Knorr, Rück. Kl. Erf., vol. 2, p. 234; *Amenorrhœa*, Kallenbach, Rück. Kl. Erf., vol. 2, p. 234; *Dysmenorrhœa*, Hilberger, Rück. Kl. Erf., vol. 5, p. 590; N. A. J. H., vol. 8, p. 277; *Vaginismus*, Skinner, Organon, vol. 1, p. 78; *Threatened abortion*, McNeil, Organon, vol. 2, p. 125; *Puerperal convulsions*, Johnson, Raue's Rec., 1872, p. 192; *Sciatica*, Nankivell, Raue's Rec., 1872, p. 219; *Tumor on thigh*, Willard, T. H. M. S. Pa. 1869, p. 43; *Spasms after fright*, Rückert, B. J. H., vol. 30, p. 581; Raue's Rec., 1873, p. 205; *Convulsions*, Hirsch, B. J. H., vol. 26, p. 221; *Hysteria*, Lobeth, Rau, Diez, Rück. Kl. Erf., vol. 2, p. 285; Bartlett, T. H. M. S. Pa., 1885, p. 193; *Chorea*, Hirsch, B. J. H., vol. 26, p. 221; Goullon, Müller, Wurmb., Rück. Kl. Erf., vol. 4, p. 511; *Epilepsy*, Hilberger, N. A. J. H., vol. 8, p. 278; Herzberger, B. J. H., vol. 36, p. 376; *Hysterical paraplegia*, Kapper, Rück. Kl. Erf., vol. 4, p. 471; *Nervous affections; epilepsy; spasms; tetanus; convulsions;* Lobeth, Gross, Tietzer, Werber, Segin, Rothanel, Sturm, Bigel, Tietze, Biez, Bethmann, Hromada, Hoffendal, Haustein, Rück. Kl. Erf., vol. 4, p. 566–73; *Intermittent fever*, Hahnemann, Hering, Rummel, Tripi, Nagel, Neumann, Vehsem, Seidel, Käsemann, Baertl, Rück. Kl. Erf., vol. 4, p. 922–6; Miller, Raue's Rec., 1872, p. 237; (6 cases), Brigham, Allen, Allen's Int. Fever, p. 145; Gosewisch, MSS.; *Ague*, Brigham, Organon, vol. 2, p. 133; *Typhoid fever* (report of 200 cases), Wohlfart, Rück. Kl. Erf., vol. 4, p. 743; *Chlorosis*, Müller, Rück. Kl. Erf., vol. 5, p. 603; *Rheumatism*, Haustein, Rück. Kl. Erf. vol. 5, p. 899; *Tobacco poisoning*, Sanborn, Organon, vol. 3, p. 365.

[1] **Mind.** ▮Memory weak and untrustworthy.
▮Heaviness of head; very great weakness of memory; forgets everything except dreams; hardness of hearing; sees everything as if through a fog; sits quietly, with a vacant gaze, always thinking of the mortification endured, and knowing nothing of what passes around him; prefers to be alone; thinking of the past mortification prevents him from going to sleep as early as usual; restless sleep, starts during sleep, much dreaming; pain in l. hypochondrium < by pressure and continuous walking; loses hair; face colorless, hollow; voice low, trembling, with distortion of muscles of face; does not like to talk; no desire to eat or drink; appetite is soon satisfied; feels cold, especially in evening; very weak; staggering walk; walks carefully; increased stool and urine. θMelancholy after mortification.
▮▮Absent-mindedness.
▮▮Difficult comprehension; mental dulness; mental effort is irksome.

ı ı Incapacity for thought in evening.

ı ı Brooding over imaginary or real troubles; is wrapt in thought.

ı ▌Hurry of mind, after exerting brain, especially in morning; is unable to talk, write or do anything else as rapidly as he wishes, whereupon there occur anxious behavior, mistakes in talking and writing and awkward actions requiring constant corrections.

▌A torrent of words pours out of mind, and confusion of writing is caused by profusion of thought.

▌Fancies; delirium; insanity.

▌Spasms and insanity after fright; imagines her soul cannot be saved and cries very much; at times rages and tears clothes, can scarcely be restrained by four strong persons.

▌After catamenia, which came at night time, symptoms of insanity; believes herself married and pregnant; is tormented by remorse for imagined crimes; seeks constantly to escape to drown herself; terrible anxiety from rush of blood to head and heart; is only quiet when lying undisturbed and brooding over her troubles, which she rehearses in a doleful tone; if disturbed, screams, strikes and tears things, crying all the while "I am neglecting my duty, breaking my vow;" face pale and distorted; desire for sour things; difficulty to get her to eat; conscientious scruples after eating; menses suppressed.

ı ı Desire to be alone.

▌Sighs and sobs; will not be comforted.

ı Inclined to be very secretive and passive.

▌Changeable disposition, laughing and crying almost in same breath.

ı ▌Looks about bed as if to find something.

▌Taciturn, with continuous sad thoughts; still, serious melancholy, with moaning.

ı ı Aversion to being alone.

ı ı Incredible changes of mood; at one time jokes and makes merry, at another is lachrymose, alternating every three or four hours.

ı ı Apprehensive feeling.

ı ı Sadness and sighing, empty feeling in pit of stomach.

ı Melancholia from suppressed mental sufferings, with much sighing; desire to be alone so as to give way to her real or imaginary grief; weeps bitterly.

▌Silent melancholy; twitching of one muscle at a time.

ı ı Melancholy after disappointed love, always combined with spinal symptoms.

▌Fright is followed by grief.

¶¶Great grief after losing persons or objects very dear.

¶¶Unhappy love with silent grief.

¶Senseless staring at one object, with sighing and moaning; remorse about imaginary crimes, intolerance to noise; great inclination to have fixed ideas.

¶Appetite and digestion left him .   θMorbid grief.

¶Became bilious, nervous, depressed, and would scarce move from the fire, for days together. θMorbid grief.

¶A peculiar trembling of hands disturbs her very much in writing, most when she has to write in any one's presence, gets worse as soon as she fancies any one might notice it.

¶¶Unusual tendency to be frightened.

¶Dread of every trifle, especially of things coming near him.

¶Fear of thieves, on waking after midnight.

¶Fearfulness; does not like to talk; prefers to be alone.

¶Anxiety as though something terrible had happened; cannot speak because of it; hurry, fearfulness, terror, alternating with irresolution and inertness.

¶Tears wept inwardly, the pain and penalty of unrequited love; desires solitude so that one may nourish inward grief; great anxiousness at night or when awaking in morning, with taciturnity; aversion to every amusement.

¶Anxiety, as if he had committed some crime.

¶Anxiety and disquiet as if she had done something wrong, or as if some great misfortune were about to happen, this so overpowers her, that she can with difficulty refrain from weeping; has oppression of breathing, but feels distinctly that oppression begins at stomach and spreads up into throat; becomes very weak, incapable of work, and disinclined to company; no appetite; bowels torpid and insufficiently moved; paroxysms about twice a day, one lasting often for hours.

¶Anxiety, sleeplessness, despair; severe palpitation; loss of appetite; constipation.

Altered appearance; made an unsuccessful attempt to end his almost unendurable sufferings, by eating the phosphorus from matches; after business embarrassments.

¶A state of anguish in which she shrieks for help, with suffocating constriction of throat, difficult deglutition; comes out of spasms with deep sighing. θParturition.

¶Indifferent to everything; seemed to live without his usual good humor.

¶Suppressed menstruation with melancholy; indifference to things she loved best; sits alone and weeps, imagines things, especially that she might go crazy; in all parts crawling sensation as if gone to sleep, as if she had no

feeling in epigastrium; sleep unrefreshing and disturbed by dreams.
■ ■Sensitive disposition and hyperacute feeling.
ι ιTender mood, with very clear consciousness.
■ ■Finely sensitive mood, delicate conscientiousness.
■Amiable disposition if feeling well; every little emotion disturbs her.
■Mild disposition; bears suffering, even outrage, without complaining. θLeucorrhœa.
ι ιJealousy, disappointed love.
■ ■Inconstant, impatient, irresolute, quarrelsome.
■The slightest contradiction irritates.
■ ■Slight blame or contradiction excites him to anger, and this makes him angry with himself.
Peevish, capricious and quarrelsome; impatient.
■Anger, followed by quiet grief or sorrow.
■Fright; inclination to start.
Headache < from reading and writing.
■Palpitation while engaged in deep thought.
■Spasmodic affections of children, consequent on being put to sleep soon after punishment.
■After fright: disturbed, introspective, taciturn; insomnia and great restlessness; anorexia.
■Melancholia after great grief and much domestic trouble; complete sleeplessness; suicidal thoughts and desire to escape.
■Ill effects from hearing bad news; from vexation with reserved displeasure; from grief, or suppressed mental sufferings; of shame and disappointed love.

² Sensorium.   ι ιVertigo.
■Periodical fits of vertigo, with intolerable pain in back following; slightest motion of head, especially stooping, increases vertigo; gastric symptoms; gaping; coated tongue; anæmia; tingling as of ants; jerkings; heaviness of r. arm, which had been paralyzed.
ι ιEpileptic vertigo.
ι ιHeaviness of head.

³ Inner Head.   ■Pressive pain in frontal region; above root of nose, must bend head forward, followed by qualmishness.
■Pressive headache in r. side of forehead, extending down into r. eye; it seems as though eyeball would be pressed out; burning in eyes and increased lachrymation, with much mucus.
■Pressive, drawing headache above r. orbit at root of nose, renewed by stooping low down.
■Pressure in r. frontal region, above eyebrow.
■Intense pain over r. eye and seemingly through supra-

orbital foramen; pains as though needle were pushed
through into brain, pressure from without inward;
appetite disordered; sometimes mad delirium; nausea
and vomiting; eyes red, swollen and protruding; pains
come on about 9 A.M, generally stopping at 2 P.M.;
< from noise, washing hands in cold water, dropping
head forward, stepping heavily; > from soft pressure,
lying on back, and heat.

∎Throbbing pains in r. side of forehead beginning at inner
end of r. eyebrow and running around eye, at 8 A.M.
every morning, gradually < until 10.30 when gradually
>, and entirely disappear about 1 P.M.; when attack is
at its height, must lie down; lachrymation and redness of eye.

∎Pain beginning in forehead, drawing, extending down
one-half of nose; pain extends to middle of vertex,
where there is a pressure as of a weight, with nausea
and tendency to vomit; < morning till afternoon, then
gradually getting better until evening; sensitive to least
noise or loud talking; pale face; suffering expression;
great lassitude of limbs.

∎Pressing pain over nose, > leaning forward; pressure
from within outward; twitching, throbbing, tearing
pain in forehead, or as if a nail was being driven in;
lancinating, boring, deep in brain, with nausea, darkness before eyes, photophobia, pale face, copious, watery
urine; pains often > by change of position, come again
after eating, in evening after lying down, or early in
morning while rising; patient anxious, fickle, or silent
and depressed.

∎Periodical headache, weekly, fortnightly or monthly;
gradual increase with sudden abatement; unilateral
headache, which affects chiefly the eye, eyebrow or side
of head, with general chilliness; crisis with secretion of
copious limpid urine; momentary disappearance of pain
by change of position.

∎Anxious suffering expression of face, eyes almost fear
the light, frown across brow, from frequent closure of
eyes in pain; extreme pain in both temples, with pain
in back and nape of neck; great mental and physical
prostration; bowels relaxed; tongue covered with white
fur; skin cold; pain > from pressure and rest; < from
light, sound and thinking; pulse thin and weak.

∎Dull headache, confined to r. half of forehead and involving r. eye, which was very sensitive.

∎Pain extending from head into l. eye; burning in eyes
and lachrymation.

Pressing, stinging pain from within to without, in forehead and root of nose.

Pressure in temples sometimes with deep sleep.

Headache as if temples would be pressed out.

When lying in bed on the side, furious headache as if pressing through temples, > by lying on back.

❚❚Pain as if a nail was driven out through side of head, > by lying on it.

Aching in one half of head, when walking in open air, < by talking and reflecting.

❚Headache in morning on awaking, as if brain was beaten and bruised; on rising it disappears and a toothache takes its place, as if nerve of tooth was shattered and crushed, changes to a similar pain in small of back; headache always renewed on thinking.

❚Jerking headache; on ascending steps; < by raising eyes.

❚Headache like a pressure with something hard on upper surface of brain; in paroxysms.

❚Sudden pressure in head, now in one place, now in another, in evening.

Throbbing headache; pain with every throb of arteries.

❚Congestion to head, from being spoken to harshly.

❘❘Heat in head.

❘❘Talking aloud excites a headache, as if head would burst, going off entirely when reading to himself or writing.

❚Deep sighing and sobbing with a strange compressed feeling in brain.

Headache with heaviness and heat in head.

❚Head feels sore, bruised.

❚Headache in highly nervous and sensitive temperaments, or in those whose nervous system has given way to anxiety, grief, or mental work.

❚Periodical headache increases gradually in severity, and then suddenly abates.

❚Headache passes off with a flow of pale, limpid urine.

❚Nervous headaches in hysterical women, suddenly appearing and disappearing.

❚Headache: from abuse of coffee; from smoking, or abuse of snuff; from inhaling smoke; from being where others smoke; from tobacco or alcohol; from close attention.

❚Headache > by warmth, rest, and sometimes by stimulants; < by cold winds, turning head suddenly, at stool, stooping, change of position, running, looking up long, from moving eyes; noise and light.

❚Throbbing pain in occiput, < when pressing at stool.

❚Pain in occiput; < from cold, snuffing or smelling tobacco; > from external heat; good appetite, even keener than usual; headache > whilst eating, but < soon after.

∎Weight at back of head; tendency of head to incline backward.

∎Stabbing pain, deep seated, in eyes, going to occiput and nape of neck, and finally to vertex; pain very acute, driving him almost frantic; pain generally begins on rising in morning, is at its height at 4 P.M., and passes off with a night's rest; > from warmth, < from sound; irritability of disposition day before headache; scalp tender to touch, and dull, uncomfortable feeling as if headache might return, day after; headaches occur every month.

∎Nervous headaches coming at same hour and day, weekly lasting forty-eight hours; come and go at 11 A.M.; their coming is preceded by a sense of vacuity in stomach and chest, stiffness of nuchæ and muscles (trapezius) on each side of this ligament; at end of twelve hours from attack, pain extends to vertex and remains there several hours, being of a compressive and burning character; after some time they continue their course towards sinciput and eyes, latter feeling hot and heavy; nausea and salivation, but without vomiting; first night of attack cannot sleep, though with eyes closed perceives figures and objects moving about; in acute stage cannot lie down, but must, with closed eyes, remain in a dark room; sleeplessness, profuse diuresis of pale urine, melancholia, and much sighing succeed each attack.

∎Sudden metastasis from bowels to brain during dentition, with sudden pale face; rolling, tossing of head; difficult swallowing; delirium, with convulsive motions of eyes and lids. θHydrocephaloid.

Cerebro-spinal meningitis; hysterical symptoms or complications, or rapid alternation of symptoms.

Threatenings of apoplexy; head feels empty, face is pale. Nervous apoplexy.

⁴ **Outer Head.** ∎Trembling and shaking of head.

∎Pain in a spot in r. parietal bone, < by stooping, with pain in r. breast.

∎Pain in outer part of head, which is painful on feeling it.

∎Weight in back of head, tendency of head to incline backward against back of chair, probably from congestion to cerebellum.

∎Head bent backward, during spasms.

∎∎Inclines head forward; lays head forward upon table.

⁵ **Sight and Eyes.** ∎Hyperæsthesia of retina with hysteria; intense photophobia; ciliary neuralgia; general nervous symptoms.

∎Cannot bear glare of light; sunlight causes headache.

∎Zigzag and serpentine white flickering at one side of field of vision.

∎Dim-sighted.

∎Asthenopia and amblyopia in females, due to onanism or ciliary neuralgia; hysterical subjects.

∎Dimness before one eye while reading, as if tears were in it, which is not the case.

∎Two "chipping ulcers" at upper margin of r. cornea, with periorbital pains, sharp sticking generally in one spot in superciliary ridge, temple or side of head; sleep disturbed; digestion poor.

∎In commencement before pimples have formed, where there is only slight injection, pain, dacryorrhœa, and photophobia. θHerpes cornea.

∎Intense but fitful photophobia.

∎Sensation as of sand in eyes.

∎Excessively nervous, starts at slightest noise; after working late at night, feeling as of sand under eyelid, with great dryness. θConjunctivitis.

∎Catarrhal inflammation of eyes when subjective symptoms are particularly marked, rather than objective; pressive pain in eyes; photophobia; lachrymation; coryza.

Upper part of eyeball, as far as covered by lid, inflamed.

∎Traumatic ophthalmia, with violent pains and sensation as if sand was rolling around beneath lids.

∎Catarrhal ophthalmia, with sensation of sand in eye and great dryness, lachrymation only in sunlight.

∎Ophthalmia of newborn infants.

∎Convulsive movements of eyes and lids.

∎Pain under upper lid, as if it was too dry.

∎Swelling of upper lid.

∎Nightly agglutination of lids.

∎Morbid nictation, with spasmodic action of various muscles of face.

Eyelid turned upward.

∎Occasionally l. eye appears smaller than r. in consequence marked ptosis of upper lid; lachrymation, < when exerting eye in open air; vision impaired; occasional twitching pain and sensation of pressure and heaviness as if eye would fall out, < reading, sewing, etc.; loss of sense of smell; diminished sense of taste; foul odors seem to be perceived in mouth.

∎Very nervous and restless at night, walking and talking in her sleep; "swelling of eyes," lachrymation and pain in eyes, with headache for six months, after having had tooth drawn; moderate amount of exophthalmus present, together with palpitation of heart; pulse 120; congestive headaches; no enlargement of thyroid gland; menses regular.

∎∎Sensation as if a particle were in l. external canthus.

❙Acrid tears in eyes, during day.

❙Ciliary neuralgia; severe pains extending from eye to top of head, producing nausea, and often alternating with swelling in throat (globus hystericus); pains begin very slightly, increase gradually until they become very severe, and only cease when she became exhausted.

❙Pain from head into l. eye; latter burns and waters.

⁷ **Smell and Nose.** ❙❙Stoppage of one nostril; dry coryza.
❙Fluent coryza.

❙Coryza in nervous persons; general hysterical irritability; dull pain in forehead.

❙Soreness and sensitiveness of inner nose, with swelling.

❙Nostrils ulcerated.

❙❙Itching of nose.

⁸ **Upper Face.** ❙Convulsive twitchings of muscles of face.
❙❙Face distorted, deathly pale and sunken.

❙Face clay colored and sunken, blue rings around eyes.

❙Redness and heat of one cheek and ear.

❙Alternate redness and paleness of face.

Sweat on face while eating.

❙Prosopalgia coming on suddenly without any warning, or preceded by slight premonitory symptoms, such as bruised feeling, tension, twitching in face; duration of paroxysm, and time of occurrence very various; exciting causes chiefly mental emotions; but sometimes they were excesses in mental work, in musical performances, in venere and in baccho; also suppressed perspiration, blenorrhœa and hemorrhoidal fluxes, were frequently remote causes; seat of pain usually in smaller twigs of facial nerves, and having no tendency to radiation; the attacks by day are preceded by uneasy sleep, waking with a bruised feeling, pandiculations and ill humor; pains boring, dart-like shoots, giving quite a shock, dull drawing, twisting, formication, being borne in dull resignation; partial convulsions of facial muscles; trismus; paleness and coolness of face; lachrymation and photophobia; spasms in cheek; yawning; shuddering; diuresis; urinary tenesmus; pulse quickened, small; cutaneous temperature cool; quiet weeping; pusillanimity.

❙Prosopalgia: in women of the upper ranks, delicate, soft fibred, anæmic, nervous, of melancholic or melancholic-sanguine temperament; in those suffering from special irritation due to sexual excesses or to inordinate mechanical irritation of spinal nerves, as in case of some musical virtuosi; due to presence of ascarides; arthritic form; in course of typhoid and miliary fevers; in roués during prolonged course of gonorrhœa; due to prolonged nursing, pollutions, musical excesses, etc.; during pregnancy; after diuresis; after lancinating uterine pains; after attacks of proctalgia.

⁹ Lower Face. ▮Twitching of corners of mouth.

▮Spasmodic closing of jaws.

▮Every evening, about half an hour after going to bed, pains in r. lower jaw, which continue until she falls asleep; pains last one to one and a half hours, with exacerbations, and are followed by quiet sleep and sweating.

▮Lips dry, cracked, bleeding.

ı ıUlceration of one of corners of mouth.

▮Inside of lower lip painful, as if raw and sore.

▮Eruption on lips and corners of mouth. θIntermittent.

▮Pain in submaxillary glands, when moving neck.

¹⁰ Teeth and Gums. ▮Jaws feel as if crushed.

▮Soreness and tenderness in teeth, felt more between meals than when eating.

▮Boring pain in front teeth.

ı ıOdontalgia as if teeth were crushed into fragments.

▮Toothache from cold in molars, as if they were crushed.

▮Toothache: < after drinking coffee, after smoking tobacco; after dinner; in evening; after lying down; in morning on awaking; < in intervals between meals.

ı ıDifficult dentition, with convulsions.

¹¹ Taste and Tongue. ▮▮Sour taste in mouth; with sour eructations; saliva tastes sour.

Taste: flat, like chalk.

▮Food has a bitter, repulsive taste, or no taste.

ı ıTongue white, flabby, shows marks of teeth, trembles protruded.

▮▮When talking or chewing, bites cheek or tongue.

¹² Inner Mouth. ı ıSticking in palate extending to inner ear.

▮Putrid odor from mouth.

▮Inner mouth inflamed and sore.

▮Copious secretion of saliva.

ı ıAccumulation of acid saliva.

▮Sudden attack of ptyalism without any apparent cause; < from every motion of tongue, as in talking, chewing, etc.; after eating, sensation as if food lodged over orifice of stomach and could not get down; fluids taste bitter; bitter belching and regurgitation of food; loss of strength; pulse small, quick; slight fever in evening; papillæ of tongue enlarged and turgescent; mucous membrane of mouth very red and in several places corroded, with raw pain; orifices of salivary glands swollen; constant flow of saliva prevents sleep; inner surface of lower lip pain as if raw and sore; anterior half of tongue as if numb; when eating tongue feels as if burnt or raw; painful swelling of orifice of salivary duct; sensation as if whole mucous membrane of mouth was about to become raw; difficult deglutition; mouth constantly full of mucus; constant discharge of white, frothy mucus; increased secretion of saliva with constant spitting of frothy saliva; everything eaten, and especially beer, tastes bitter or putrid; loss of appetite, could not swallow bread, as if it was too dry; pain in epigastrium on pressure, as if it was raw inside.

¹³ **Throat.** ▮Stitches in soft palate, extending to ear.
▮▮Crawling in pharynx.
▮Hysterical spasm of throat and gullet, result of suppressed grief; cannot swallow either liquids or solids.
▮Retching (constrictive) sensation in middle of throat, as if a large morsel of food or plug was sticking there; felt more when not swallowing; disappears on continuing to swallow but returns.
▮▮Choking sensation from stomach up into throat.
▮▮Sensation as from a lump in throat, when not swallowing.
▮Stinging in throat between acts of deglutition; sensation when swallowing as if swallowing over a bone, with a rolling around.
▮Stitches in throat, only between acts of swallowing.
▮▮Sore throat; sticking in it when not swallowing, and even somewhat while swallowing; the more he swallows, however, the more it disappears; if he swallows anything solid, like bread, it seems as though the sticking entirely disappeared.
▮Unable to swallow bread, it seems too dry.
▮Both tonsils greatly swollen and inflamed; several small openings filled with pus on tonsils; pharynx red, inflamed; stitching pains in throat < swallowing; stitches extend to ear when swallowing; r. parotid, swollen, hard to touch, but painless; stitches in parotid; tongue covered with tenacious white mucus; foul taste in mouth; offensive odor from same; chilliness, in afternoon fever with red cheeks, and at same time chilliness and coldness of feet; despondent, depressed, tearful. *θ*Angina.
▮Inflamed, hard, swollen tonsils, with small ulcers.
▮Acute paroxysms in chronic tonsillitis, with feeling of swelling in throat; painful soreness during deglutition.
▮▮Follicular tonsillitis.
▮Whitish tough mucus in spots on tonsils, simulating diphtheria.
▮Green vomiting, substance scum-like or membranous; putrid throat, seldom painful (the painful cases were less likely to prove fatal); greenish-yellow patches; de-

lirium; headache; pain in limbs; nosebleed; dilated
pupils; diarrhœa; green stools; suppression of urine;
chilliness; high fever. θDiphtheria.

❚Commences on r. side; high fever; delirium characterized
by fearfulness or dread; soreness of throat greatest between acts of deglutition; pains in back of head, nuchæ
and sometimes in ears. θDiphtheria.

❚Throat < when not swallowing, and when swallowing
liquids; > when swallowing food.

" **Appetite, Thirst. Desires, Aversions.** ❚Hunger and nausea
at same time.

❚Feeling of hunger in evening, prevents sleep.

❚❚Good appetite: headache > while eating, < soon after.

❚Appetite for: sour things; bread, particularly rye bread.

❚❚Thirst, with a chill.

❚Desire for various things, but when offered appetite fails.

❚❚Fanciful aversion to special articles of food, or craving
for a particular article, and after a small portion has
been enjoyed, sudden and great aversion to it.

❚❚Extreme aversion to tobacco smoke.

❚Aversion to: tobacco; warm food; meat; spirituous liquors.

" **Eating and Drinking.** ❚It is difficult to persuade her to
eat; after doing so she is tormented with conscientious
scruples.

Sweat on face while eating.

Symptoms renewed after dinner.

Headache < from coffee, tobacco and alcohol.

Better from partaking of sour things.

Worse from drinking coffee.

" **Hiccough, Belching, Nausea and Vomiting.** ❚Hiccough:
after emotions; after eating and drinking; from smoking; especially in children.

❚❚Eructations: of food into mouth; of bitter fluid; with
pressure in cardia.

❚Spasmodic ructus and singultus, occurring periodically
every afternoon, and lasting for hours; after violent
mental excitement.

❚Qualmishness from smoking.

❚❚Nausea, without vomiting.

❚Empty retching, better by eating.

❚❚Vomit: bitter; of food.

" **Scrobiculum and Stomach.** ❚❚Weak, empty feeling at pit
of stomach, not > by eating; involuntary sighing; must
take a long breath.

❚Sensation of weakness, sinking, or "goneness" in pit of
stomach, with qualmishness and flat taste.

❚Feeling of weakness in epigastrium, and pain as if
sprained, with great depression.

❚Fulness, heaviness or pressure in pit of stomach.
❚Fulness and swelling in epigastrium.
❚Burning, darting in epigastrium.
❚Anxious feeling in præcordia.
❚Feeling in stomach as from fasting, with physical exhaustion.
❚❚Feeling of flabbiness in stomach; stomach and intestines seem to hang down relaxed.
❚Feeling of emptiness or goneness in stomach, with sensation as if a number of pins were sticking in it; not > by eating.
Sensation as if stomach was shortened.
❚Painful pressure as from a stone, especially after eating or at night, in region of pylorus; sensitiveness to contact, and burning in stomach.
❚Bloated stomach.
❚Stitches in region of stomach.
❚Burning in stomach, especially after brandy.
❚Gnawing, cutting pain in stomach.
❚Spasmodic pains in stomach; > when eating.
❚Gastralgia, with sticking pains, brought on by starvation.
❚Gnawing sensation in stomach in morning, > by eating; swelling in region of stomach, cannot button, or is frequently obliged to unloosen clothing; frequent sensation of rawness in throat, a little below larynx, and on l. side of throat when swallowing; ptyalism and accumulation of saliva in throat; constipation.
❚Pressure in stomach after eating, < at night, with nausea and sensation of rawness in stomach; on moving pain becomes cutting in character; trembling in stomach.
·❚Twitching in pit of stomach, with periodical attacks of weakness and qualmishness, so severe that she becomes pale and almost faints, accompanied by a sensation of hunger.
❚Attacks of extremely severe pains in stomach 7 to 8 P.M., but more frequently about midnight, lasting two to three hours; vomiting of slime; can only eat broths or other fluid food with any comfort; digestion greatly impaired; stools regular; urine pale, watery, profuse; nausea with great restlessness and anxiety; pressing pains; sensation in region of stomach as if he would like to vomit, with oppression and spasmodic constriction of chest; < from pressure over stomach; frequent vomiting of food with great restlessness and anxiety; hemorrhoidal pains in anus and pressure in sacrum.
❚Periodical attacks of cramps in stomach, coming on usually at night, or after eating; < by slightest contact, mitigated by change of position. θGastralgia.

∎Catarrh of stomach from grief and worriment.

∎∎Dyspepsia with great nervous prostration, caused by mental depression.

[18] **Hypochondria.** ∣∣Great distension of hypochondria, pit of stomach and small of back; unable to breathe on account of fulness and tension under ribs.

∎Jaundice, with silent melancholy, twitching of one muscle at a time.

∎Swelling and induration of spleen.

∎Painful pressure in region of spleen and pit of stomach.

∎Pain in l. hypochondrium; < from pressure.

[19] **Abdomen.** ∎∎Peculiar sensation of weakness in upper abdomen and pit of stomach.

An anxious feeling mounts up from abdomen, after breakfast.

∎Pulsation (throbbing) in abdomen.

∣∣Drawing and pinching in umbilical region.

∣∣Sensation of protrusion in umbilical region.

∎Stitching and lancinating in sides of abdomen.

∣∣Sharp sticking, above and to left of umbilicus.

∎Colic pains, first griping, then stitching, in one or other side of abdomen.

∎Drawing and griping in abdomen; in rectum it occurred like a pressure, with qualmishness and weakness in pit of stomach, and paleness of face.

∎Periodical abdominal spasms, colic particularly at night, waking out of sleep, with stitches running up into chest and to sides; pains > passing wind, which, however, is difficult.

∎Spasmodic pains, cutting stinging, like labor pains; spasmodic colic.

The colic pains are < by brandy, coffee and sweet things.

∎Flatulent colic; flatus incarcerated, rumbling and rolling about, making a loud noise; rumbling as from hunger.

∣∣Wind presses on bladder.

∎Excessive flatulence; hysterical females.

∎Protrusions on various parts of abdomen.

∎Unsatisfactory, short and abrupt emissions of flatus, of offensive odor, not without exertion of abdominal muscles.

[20] **Stool and Rectum.** ∣∣Bowels inclined to be loose; with stabbing pains in rectum.

Diarrhœa: painless, with rumbling of wind; < at night and from fright, with great timidity; with smarting in rectum; stools frequent; but scanty.

∎Copious diarrhœa, < at night, painless, with much wind; emaciated; great nervousness; in a little girl, after a great fright which almost produced convulsions.

∎Great nervous erethism and tenesmus, occurring only after stool. θDysentery.

▮Pale, cold, fixed, staring look, occasional screams, vomiting food. θCholera infantum.

▮Stools large and soft, but passed with difficulty.

▮Excessive desire for stool, more in upper intestines and upper abdomen; it causes great urging, nevertheless stool is insufficient, though soft.

▮▮Great urgency and desire for stool, in evening, felt mostly in middle of abdomen, but no stool follows, only rectum protrudes.

▮Constant urging to stool, which causes smarting pain.

ΙΙIneffectual urging to stool with erections.

▮Difficult stool, causing prolapse of rectum.

▮Hard stools, tries often, but in vain.

Constipation: from taking cold; of a paralytic origin.

▮Alternate diarrhœa and constipation following inflammation of bowels; tenesmus only after a discharge.

Stools: whitish, yellowish white, slimy; thin; pasty; mucous; bloody mucus; acrid; mucous, with colic.

Before stool: rumbling; urging, felt mostly in middle and upper abdomen.

▮▮Sharp, pressive pain in rectum.

▮Frequent cutting deep in rectum.

▮Sudden sharp stitches in rectum, extending upwards into body; < from excessive grief.

Spasmodic tension in rectum.

▮▮Contractive sore pain in rectum, like from blind hemorrhoids, one or two hours after stool.

▮Sensation of excoriation and contraction in rectum.

▮Neuralgia of rectum; pains in anus, returning regularly every day; < walking or standing; > sitting.

ΙΙDull pain in rectum as if distended with gas, after stool.

▮Unpleasant crawling low down in rectum, near anus, as from thread worms.

▮Violent itching in rectum, in evening, in bed.

▮Passive hemorrhage from rectum, after stool (of long standing); flow bright red; stools regular; bowels flatulent; faintness when hemorrhage is profuse; must lie down after stool.

▮Bleeding during and after stool; hemorrhage and pain are < when stool is loose.

▮Ennervation of longitudinal and circular muscles of rectum, causing a semi-paralyzed state of bowel and allowing feces to accumulate.

▮Anxious desire for stool, with inactivity of rectum; is unable to evacuate feces without danger of eversion and prolapsus of rectum.

▮▮Prolapsus of rectum from moderate straining at stool.

▮Tenesmus; prolapsus recti after stool.

▮Prolapsus of rectum, with a male child, æt. 4; parents
have to return the bowel after each stool, sometimes
twice a day and with great difficulty.

▮Severe, constant, stitching and sore, burning pains in rectum, completely robbing her of sleep; prolapsus of rectum; hard, bloody stools greatly aggravating the pains;
ulcerated hemorrhoids in rectum.

▮Hemorrhoids: after confinement, with sharp, painful
pressure in rectum after stool, even a soft stool; also
sharp stitches from anus to rectum; bleeding slightly
and protruding at stool, followed by severe contractive
pain in anus and stitches up rectum, lasting until exactly 5 P.M. each day, when pain suddenly ceases; with
sensation of excoriation or contraction of anus; tumors
prolapse with every stool, and have to be replaced; they
are sore as if excoriated; hemorrhage and pain <
when stool is loose; dragging pains around pelvis.

▮Blind piles, pressure and soreness in anus and rectum;
painful while sitting and standing, less while walking,
though renewed and < after taking fresh air.

▮Stitches in hemorrhoidal tumors during cough.

▮Pain in anus as from blind piles, sore pain after soft stool.

▮▮Sore pain in anus, without reference to stool.

▮▮A coarse stitch extending from anus deep into rectum.

▯▯Pain in anus returning at same hour each day, <
walking and still < standing, > on sitting down.

▮Constriction of anus after stool, < while standing.

▮Painless contraction of anus for many days.

▮Itching and tingling in anus.   θPruritus.

▮Itching of anus: at night; child is nervous and spasmodic; from seat worms.

Fissures of anus.

Blotches at anus.

▮Stitches, itching and a creeping sensation in lower part
of rectum.   θAscarides.

▮Ascarides causing itching in rectum and anus.

▮Thread worms in rectum, especially when there are traces
of blood in stools.

▮Convulsions; suddenly fell prostrate and remained unconscious for half an hour; after which she was unable
to speak for several minutes; after *Ignat.* passed tapeworm, and convulsions did not recur.

Increased accumulation of flatus and increased discharge
of it.

²**Urinary Organs.**   ▮Sudden, irresistible desire to urinate.

▯▯Painful pressure, with a scraping sensation in neck of
bladder, especially when walking; turbid urine.

▮Pressure to urinate, from drinking coffee.

¹¹Frequent discharge of much watery urine. *θ*Hysteria.
Urine: nervous, watery; clear, lemon colored; scanty,
  dark and acrid.
¹¹Involuntary discharge of urine.
¹Burning, smarting or soreness during urination.
¹¹Itching in forepart of urethra.
²² Male Sexual Organs. Lasciviousness without erections.
¹Sexual desire weak, or sexual desire with impotence.
¹Erections during stool; emission of prostatic fluid.
¹Hysterical-spasmodic stricture.
¹¹Contraction of penis, it becomes quite small.
¹Itching around genitals and on penis, in evening after
  lying down; passes off after scratching.
¹¹Soreness and ulcerative pain, combined with itching, at
  margin of prepuce.
¹¹Sweat on scrotum.
²³ Female Sexual Organs. **¹**Cramp pains in uterus, with
  lancinations, < from touching parts.
¹Uterine spasms with lancinations or labor-like pains.
¹Metrorrhagia from chamomile tea.
¹Menses: too soon and profuse; scanty, delayed.
¹Menses too early and profuse, appearing every 10–14
  days; before and during menses heat and heaviness in
  head, severe pressing pain in forehead, eyes sensitive
  to light, ringing in ears, loss of appetite, sensation of
  emptiness in stomach, cramping pains in abdomen,
  chilliness alternating with heat, anxiety, palpitation,
  extreme prostration of whole body and especially of
  extremities.
¹Menstruation profuse and irregular; leucorrhoea, with
  bearing-down pain.
¹Menorrhagia with sighing and sobbing, faint feeling at
  pit of stomach; great despondency, seems full of suppressed grief.
¹Brought on a flow in a lady, æt. 62, who had suffered
  from grief; also in a lady, æt. 30, whose menses had
  been suppressed for three months.
¹Menstrual blood black, of putrid odor, in clots.
¹Irregular menstruation, especially dysmenorrhœa, originating in irritation of nervous system, and not in
  uterine congestion.
¹Menses scanty, attended by violent spasms and pains,
  lasting several days, and resembling pains of parturition;
  nervous system in very excitable state. *θ*Dysmenorrhœa.
¹¹Amenorrhœa; ulcers on feet; anæmic; region of liver
  and spleen swollen.
¹Suppression of menses caused by suppressed grief; much

involuntary sighing and sobbing; præcordial anguish; weak and empty feeling in pit of stomach.

▮During menstruation uterine spasms, with crampy pressing, > by pressure and in a recumbent posture.

▮During menses: photophobia; contractive colic; anguish; palpitation of heart; backache; lassitude approaching faintness.

▮Pain from sacral region through to front, followed by leucorrhœa and a numb and stupid feeling in brain; difficulty in answering questions.

▮Violent labor-like pain; purulent, corrosive leucorrhœa..

▮Chronic leucorrhœa, with excited sexual desire.

▮Menses scanty, stringy, with dark clots; great dysmenia both before and after; fearful griping and cutting uterine colic; milky whites; constant burning heat in vagina, < before menses; very acute darting pains in vulva, only during day; intensely sore pain at entrance of vagina during coitus, almost driving her frantic; heavy and sleepy after meals, must lie down after dinner; pain and sickness at stomach while standing, > sitting down; sinking and emptiness at epigastrium; total loss of appetite except at supper time; stitches in breasts; feet burning hot, or cold; feels as if stockings were cold and damp; one cheek generally hot, the other not so; hysteria; constipation with great pain, dreads to go to closet; deep sighing inspiration; inflammation of vagina and vulva. θVaginismus.

▮Pruritus of young girls, with leucorrhœa and associated with ascaris vermicularis.

" **Pregnancy. Parturition. Lactation.** ▮Emptiness, qualmishness and weakness in region of stomach, with flat taste; distension of abdomen after eating; hiccough; sour eructations; frequent regurgitation of food, and of bitter liquid; vomiting at night of food taken in evening; empty retching, > by eating. θMorning sickness.

▮After great fright, during seventh month of pregnancy, severe pain in epigastrium; undefined anxiety; restlessness; falls asleep late at night; also pain low down in l. side of abdomen.

▮After fright during pregnancy, trembling, followed next day by labor pains and hemorrhage, > lying on back without pillow and with lower end of mattress elevated.

▮Deep sighing and sobbing with strange, compressed feeling in brain; groaning and stretching of limbs at termination of each spasm. θSpasms during labor.

▮Spasms with twitching of muscles of mouth and eyes; wild expression; eyes upturned; constant attempt to tear her hair; laughing and crying; nervous and excitable. θPuerperal convulsions.

▮Puerperal convulsions commence and terminate with groaning and stretching of limbs; vomiting.

▮The labor does not progress.

▮Afterpains with much sighing, sadness and despondency.

▮Infantile colic after taking breast of mother or nurse, who suffers from grief.

▮Milk diminished.

²⁵ Voice and Larynx. Trachea and Bronchia. Voice: low; trembling; hoarseness from cold.

▮Subdued, low voice; is unable to talk loud.

▮Hysterical aphonia, mental anxiety, spinal symptoms.

▮Sensation of soreness in larynx.

▮Constrictive sensation in trachea and larynx.

▮Uninterrupted provocation to a hacking cough in larynx (not tickling) in evening after lying down; it does not disappear on coughing, only on suppressing cough.

²⁶ Respiration. ▮Frequent sighing.

▮Sighing and sobbing continue long after crying.

▮Snoring inspiration during sleep.

▮▮Desire to take a deep breath. *θ*Hysteria. *θ*Dyspepsia.

▮Frequently obliged to take a deep breath, which momentarily relieves pressure upon chest.

▮Impeded inspiration, like from a weight on chest.

▮Oppressed breathing, alternating with convulsions.

▮Oppression of chest at night, < after midnight.

▮▮Slow breathing.

▮Inspiration slow; expiration quick.

▮Loses breath when running.

²⁷ Cough. ▮Tickling cough which may be suppressed by an effort of will.

▮Constant, dry cough, excited by tickling in suprasternal fossa; as from inspired feathery dust, not < by coughing, but more excited the more he allows himself to cough; especially < towards evening.

▮Cough caused by constrictive sensation above throat pit.

▮Constant hacking cough in evening in bed.

▮Dry, spasmodic cough.

▮Hollow, spasmodic cough, caused, in evening, by a sensation like from fumes of sulphur, or from dust in pit of throat; in morning, from a tickling above pit of stomach.

▮Hollow, spasmodic cough, < evening, with but little expectoration, leaving pain in trachea.

▮▮Cough dry and rough, with fluent coryza, headache and weak voice.

▮Nervous cough and oppression frequently accompanying catarrhal affections in young people and women.

Spasmodic cough in nervous, sensitive persons.

▮▮Cough every time he stands still during a walk.

ⅠⅠCough after warm drink.

❚The longer the cough, the more irritation to cough.

❚Sleepy after each coughing spell.

During cough: nauseous feeling in epigastrium; concussions in hypogastrium; pain in penis; convulsions.

❚Expectoration: in evening, rarely in morning; difficult, in evening; tasting and smelling like old catarrh.

²⁸ **Inner Chest and Lungs.** ❚Stitches: in chest, from flatulent colic; in l. side of chest.

❚❚Spasmodic constriction of chest.

❚Chest feels as if too small; spasmodic yawning.

²⁹ **Heart, Pulse and Circulation.** ❚❚Anxious feeling in præcordia.

❚After excessive anxiety followed by sudden joy; uncertain, weak, weary sensation in chest; sinking sensation and emptiness in pit of stomach; heart's impulse feeble; pulse small, soft and 100 to 110 per minute. *θ*Cardiac hyperæsthesia.

❚Constriction at heart, with anxiety and disposition to cry; loss of appetite; pressure in stomach; palpitation; menses more profuse than usual; sleepiness; weakness of eyes; after grief.

❚Palpitation: at night, and in morning, in bed; at night, with stitches in heart; during deep meditation.

❚Pulse: generally hard, full and frequent, with throbbing in bloodvessels; less frequently small and slow; variable, very changeable; frequent in morning, slower during day and evening.

³⁰ **Outer Chest.** ⅠⅠStitches in nipple on deep inspiration.

³¹ **Neck and Back.** ❚❚Stiffness of nape of neck. *θ*Diphtheria.

ⅠⅠStitch in nape of neck.

ⅠⅠPressive pain in cervical glands.

❚Painless glandular swellings on neck.

Tensive pains in back on standing erect.

Simple pains which are apt to become excessive when touched; jerks through whole body.

Pains in back during chill.

ⅠⅠStitches in small of back.

❚Lancinating stitches as from a sharp knife, in back through loins, extending to legs.

Pain in sacrum, also when lying on back, morning in bed.

❚Spine disease, with gressus gallinaceus.

ⅠⅠThe back is bent forward.

³² **Upper Limbs.** ❚Quivering jerks in deltoid muscle.

❚After anxiety sudden stroke as if r. shoulder had been paralyzed by a stroke of lightning, which extended through whole arm, extending to tips of thumb, index and middle fingers; use of arm completely lost, can

hardly raise it; sensation as if arm did not belong to
her; on touching objects it seems as if they were covered
with fine felt. *θ*Hysterical paraplegia.

▮Pain in shoulder-joint as if dislocated, on moving arm.

▮Lancinating, cutting pain in shoulder-joint when bending arm forward.

▮Numb feeling of arms at night, in bed, with it a sensation
as if something living were running in arm.

▮Pains in joints of arms, when bending them backwards,
like from overexertion, or as if bruised.

▮Warm sweat in palms and on fingers.

²³ Lower Limbs. ▮Lancinating, cutting pains in hip-joint.

▮Pains, incisive, throbbing, intermittent; at first every
other day, then daily; chilliness; mild, melancholic
temperament; fever, but no thirst; returns every winter.
*θ*Sciatica.

▮Paroxysms of excruciating neuralgia of sciatic nerve and
its perineal branches preceded by intense coldness
and shivering, < at night, obliging her to get up and
walk about room; pain acute, of a tearing, digging,
boring character, and lasts sixty to ninety minutes, when
it slowly departs.

▮Ischias: intermitting, chronic; > in summer, < in winter; beating as though it would burst hip-joint, accompanied by chilliness, with thirst, flushes of heat,
particularly in face, without thirst.

Boil on inner side of thigh.

▮Tumor large as an egg, a short distance above knee, quite
movable, hard upon pressure; great nervousness, continually sighing, afraid she would die; great fear of
coming sorrow or trouble; very despondent; slight
twitching of muscles; drawing limbs to body.

▮Knees are involuntarily drawn upwards when walking;
gressus gallinaceus.

▮Heat of knees, with coldness of nose.

Cracking of knees.

▮Tearing pains in back of legs.

▮Tearing pain in tendo achillis and calf, as though parts
would be cut off; < standing, walking, or exerting
muscles.

Numbness of feet, legs, and sometimes of lower limbs.

▮▮Coldness of feet and legs, extending above knee.

▮Heaviness of feet.

▮Burning in heels, at night; when they come in contact,
however, they feel cold.

▮Bruised or stinging sensation in soles of feet.

▮▮Corns painful as if sore.

▮Convulsive jerking of lower limbs.

∎Staggering walk.
³¹ Limbs in General. ∎Trembling of limbs; languor.
∎Single jerks of limbs, when falling asleep.
∎Sudden spasmodic action of a muscle; limbs jerk;
∎Crawling, asleep sensation in limbs.
∎Tingling in limbs.
∎Pain as if sprained or dislocated, in shoulder, hip and
    knee-joints.
∎Neuralgic pain in r. shoulder when raising arm or when
    turning it towards chest; loss of sensation in r. knee
    and tension in same when stretching leg.
∎∎Painfulness of limbs on going to sleep.
∎Cold hands, and cold feet up to knees.
³⁵ Rest. Position. Motion. Rest: pains >: headache >.
∎Change of position > pain.
Lying: pains in head >; vertigo.
Lying down: pains come again; toothache; itching around
    genitals; uterine pains >; hacking cough; jerking in
    forearm.
Lying on back: > headache; labor pains and trembling
    >; pains in sacrum; chorea >.
Lying on side: headache <; pain as if nail was driven
    in head >.
Must lie down: when pain in head is bad; after hemor-
    rhage from rectum; after dinner.
Must bend head forward; lays it upon table.
Inclines head backward, or is drawn powerfully back.
Leaning forward: pain over nose >.
Bends himself backward, so that he rests on head and feet.
Sitting: pain in anus >; blind piles painful; pain and
    sickness at stomach >; tremor of legs <.
Sitting and standing very difficult: on account of chorea.
Drawing limbs to body.
Lower jaw thrust forward.
When fingers are extended: trembling of hands.
Change of position: often > pains; headache <; cramps
    in stomach >; frequent at night in bed.
Moving: pressure in stomach becomes cutting; pain in
    shoulder-joint on moving arm.
Slightest motion: of head < vertigo; of tongue < ptyalism.
Slight motion: knees give way.
Exerting muscles: < tearing in tendo achilles and calf.
Bending arm forward: lancinating pain in shoulder-joint.
Bending arms backward: pains in joints.
Turning arm to chest: neuralgic pain in r. shoulder.
Raising arm: neuralgic pain in r. shoulder.
Stretching leg: tension in it.
Dropping head forward: < headache.

Turning head suddenly : headache <.
Tossing head : during dentition.
Trembling and shaking : of head.
Stooping : < vertigo; renews pain at root of nose; head-
ache >; pain in a spot in r. parietal bone <.
Walking : pain in anus <; blind piles less painful; pain-
ful pressure in neck of bladder <; knees involuntarily
drawn upwards; tearing pain in tendo achilles and calf
<; as though breath would fail, becomes qualmish.
Standing : pain in anus <; blind piles painful; pain and
sickness at stomach; tensive pain in back; tearing pain
in tendo achilles and calf <; goes to sleep.
Obliging her to get up and walk about rooms : pain in
sciatic nerve.
On ascending steps : jerking headache.
Stepping heavily : headache <.
Stands still during walk : on account of cough.
Running : headache <.
Throws himself wildly about in bed.
³⁶ **Nerves.** **Persons mentally and physically exhausted by
long concentrated grief.
**Oversensitive to pain.
*Trembling and languor of limbs.
*Trembling of hands when writing, most in anyone's pres-
ence, and getting < as soon as she fancies any one
might notice it; appears also when fingers are extended..
*Her trembling does not make much difference to her
writing, but shows itself when she extends her fingers,
more marked on r. side.
**Great languor or deep sleep, with stertorous breathing
after or during fever.
||Sensation as if she had been fasting a long time with
flat taste and languor in limbs.
*Faint feeling; false hunger; nausea and vomiting of mu-
cus; habitual smoking.
*Great weakness of whole body; on walking seems as
though breath would fail, becomes qualmish in pit of
stomach, and then coughs.
*Great weakness and exhaustion of whole body; lassitude
in evening.
*Debility after arrest of hemorrhage, with disposition to
be vehement or vexed.
*A simple violent pain here and there in a small spot, as
for example, on ribs, only noticed on touch.
||Emotional hyperæsthesia ending in depression and tor-
por; sexual desire with impotence.
*Hysterical debility and fainting fits.
*Mind very irritable; easily becomes sad; frequent attacks

of pressing, cramping pain in forehead and occiput, face
red, lachrymation; spasmodic constriction of throat,
with difficult deglutition; much belching, hiccough;
constriction of chest, respiration impeded, trembling of
head, twitching of arms and legs with semi-consciousness, finally a deep sigh followed by profound sleep.
*θ*Hysteria.
▮After a quarrel with her husband, awoke next morning
with a rhythmical tremor of entire l. leg which gradually
involved both legs; < sitting, did not interfere with
walking; on following day was accompanied by choreic
jerking of head from l. to r., and slightly from above
downwards. *θ*Hysteria.
▮Anguish, shrieks for help, with suffocating constriction
of throat; difficult deglutition; comes out of spasm with
deep sighing. *θ*Hysteria.
▮Hysteria characterized by a mental character which is
mild, gentle, yielding though whimsical and introverted.
▮Hemicrania, globus hystericus, or sudden toothache
attacking a healthy tooth, in hysterical subjects.
▮Great tendency to start.
▮Jerkings and twitchings in various parts of muscles.
▮Jerking, as if a mouse was crawling under skin, in one
part of muscles of forearm, in evening after lying down.
▮Convulsive twitchings, especially after fright or grief.
▮Screaming with violent trembling all over; single parts
seem to be convulsed.
▮▮Children are convulsed in sleep after punishment.
▮Convulsions in children in first period of dentition, with
pale complexion, or in consequence of irregular inner-
vation of capillaries, with remarkable redness of one
cheek and cold nose; increased temperature of body
transient; skin cool to touch.
▮▮Spasms in children: from fright or from worms; child
pale, cold; fixed, staring look; occasional screams; vomits food; preceded by hasty drinking.
▮Spasms with cries or involuntary laughter.
▮Convulsions alternating with oppressed breathing.
▮Convulsions, with loss of consciousness, and temporary
inability to speak.
▮Convulsions: during dentition, with frothing at mouth,
kicking with legs; during commencement of exanthe-
matic fevers; of children, after punishment; after fear
or fright; return at same hour, daily.
▮Suddenly feels sleepy and lies down, or goes to sleep standing and falls; lies quietly and unconsciously for half an
hour, or several hours; eyes closed; makes fists; hides
under bedcover, and peeps timidly from under it; ex-

tremities jerking upwards; body thrown upward and lower jaw thrust forward; suddenly wakes up gasping, and complains of hunger. ϑSpasms after fright.

■Loss of consciousness, sudden or preceded by headache, especially at night; bends himself backward so that he rests on head and feet, throws himself wildly about and tumbles out of bed if not prevented; violent shocks affect the body and particularly chest; froth mixed with blood escapes from mouth; after ten or fifteen minutes spasms pass off but unconsciousness lasts for five or six hours; confused speech of which later he remembers nothing; passes stool or urine in every corner of room if not prevented; severe chill, during which body is cold as ice, ends the attack, which is followed by great mental and physical prostration.

■Children during dentition, or even at an earlier or later period, are suddenly seized with spasms resembling epilepsy; they often occur without apparent cause or come on after child has been reprimanded for a fault and then put to bed; twitchings begin at corners of mouth so that child appears to smile, then spasms rapidly affect muscles of face, forehead, eyes, and often eyeballs, or eyes may be open, fixed and staring, with dilated pupils; frothing at mouth, biting of tongue or cheeks, teeth firmly clenched and immovable, trismus, twitching of arms, less often of feet, attacks last from five minutes to half an hour, after which child is covered with sweat and presents all the symptoms of congestion of brain, followed by soporous sleep, from which they are awakened by renewed spasms, or spasms return after a complete intermission; pulse frequent, often delirium and involuntary urination.

■Clonic convulsions, in hysterical, fitful women.

■Violent convulsions; often tonic spasms predominate.

■Tetanic convulsions, with frequent inclination to yawn.

■Tetanus after fright.

■Spasms and tetanic convulsions in hysterical women and children; especially when falling asleep.

‖Catalepsy with bending backwards.

■After fright, cataleptic attacks, lasting several hours and returning regularly every two months; gradually attacks became epileptiform in character, with violent convulsions and loss of consciousness; attacks also became more frequent, occurring every month, just before or after menstruation, and finally occurring after any accidental excitement; spasms and pain during menstruation.

■Emotional trismus or opisthotonos; head drawn powerfully back, countenance livid, pupils dilated, respiration and deglutition of fluids difficult.

▮Children with pale complexion and blue rings around eyes; there gradually ensues a great degree of timidity and tendency to start, followed by involuntary movements of facial muscles, and of upper and lower extremities, gradually attaining the intensity of chorea.

▮Chorea: after fright or grief; < after eating; > lying on back.

▮Emotional chorea, especially after fright, grief, or other mental excitement, with sighing and sobbing; vacillating gait; liability to stumble and fall over small objects; trembling and twitching of various muscles; precipitancy of volition; patient expresses anxiety in his movements; < after eating, especially after dinner; after deep grief; > while lying on back.

▮Chorea in girls who have been frightened by threats or punishment; constant and involuntary twitching and throwing about of arms; objects are dropped from hands; twitching of eyes and shaking of head.

▮Sudden and severe chorea after being frightened by mouse running up arm; twitching in facial muscles and active movements in upper extremities, so that hands seemed always to be engaged in some sort of voluntary work; at one time put her hand to hair, at another to ear, now quickly extended arm as if to smooth dress, and so on the whole day; voluntary movements of hands so far lost that she could neither eat nor drink unassisted.

▮All sorts of motions and contortions of extremities, head also being affected; cannot walk nor use hands even to eat. θChorea after fright.

▮Cries out when any one approaches bed, and at intervals repeats her crying, but is not capable of speaking a single word; hands and feet thrown violently about; convulsive distortion of muscles of face; head one moment bent backward, at another to side, and whole body is thrown violently about, tophi on hands and feet. θChorea.

▮Chorea in such aggravated form that sitting and standing is extremely difficult; previous bright and active mind degenerated almost to a condition of idiocy.

▮Chorea; convulsions are greatest in mouth, producing much distortion of face; globus hystericus.

▮Nervous condition in influenza, with general convulsions and frothing at mouth; attacks resembling epilepsy.

▮Emotional epilepsy; caused by fright and suppressed grief; especially suitable for children; recent cases.

∎Convulsive movements in limbs with spasmodic closure of jaws; attacks lasted about half an hour, and recurred every four to seven days; they came on at all hours of day and night, and were occasioned by any mental excitement; finally attacks became more violent; fell down, became unconscious, thumbs turned into palms, convulsions and foaming at mouth, terminating in sleep; the longer the attacks were delayed the more violent they were; expression of face one of extreme melancholy. *θ*Epilepsy after fright.

∎Face red; pulse full, 100; loss of consciousness; eyes fixed; convulsions of extremities with frothing at mouth; thumbs clenched; great thirst after consciousness is restored.

∎Silent, stupid state, with jerking of body, partial spasms of extremities, one limb or only certain muscles at a time; lassitude after a fit. *θ*Epilepsy.

∎Chorea-like and epileptiform convulsions; paresis; anæsthesia combined often with hyperæsthesia of legs; subsultus tendinum; jerking of limbs; trembling of tongue; delirium tremens.

∎∎Paralysis after great mental emotion and night watching in sick chamber.

∎Hysterical paraplegia.

∎Perversion of co-ordinations of function; clavus hystericus.

∎Great mobility in nervous phenomena.

Sleep. Sleeplessness: from grief, care, sadness; anxious thoughts and depressing emotions; after overstraining mind by racking business cares; before midnight; from ebullition of blood; with starting when falling asleep; inward restlessness, thirst, fever with anxiety from 2 to 5 A.M.

∎Sleep very light, hears everything, even distant sounds.

∎Restless sleep.

∎Spasmodic yawning: with pain in lower jaw, as if dislocated; so that water runs from eyes.

∎Hiccough in children; restlessness at night, and screaming during sleep.

∎When going to sleep jerks through whole body, or in a single limb, or a single muscle.

∎Very restless at night in bed; hysterical subjects.

∎Frequently changes his position at night in bed.

∎Snoring inspiration during sleep.

∎During sleep of children: chewing motion of mouth and startings (flexors); stamping feet and grinding teeth.

∎Child awakens from sleep: with piercing cries and trembles all over; in spasms after being punished and sent to bed.

■Somnambulism; describes¹ clearly the interior of brain;
again sees everything that passes in street, but recollects
nothing of it when awake. θEffects of wounded honor.
■In his dream is occupied thinking of the same object
throughout whole night; a fixed idea, which does not
leave him on waking.
■Dreams with reflections and deliberations.
** **Time.**   The morning is the best time to give this remedy. H.
Aggravation at 4 A.M. and 4 P.M., lasting till evening.
Morning: pains come on at 9 o'clock and last till 2 P.M.;
pain < till afternoon; when rising pains <; on awakening, headache which disappears on rising; headache <;
stabbing pain in head begins on rising; toothache;
gnawing pain in stomach; hurry of brain; great anxiousness, hollow, spasmodic cough; palpitation; pulse frequent; pains in sacrum, lying in bed; general heat.
From 2 to 5 A.M., inward restlessness, thirst, fever with
anxiety.
11 A.M.: hungry.
During day: acrid tears; darting pains in vulva; pulse slow.
Afternoon: pain gradually > till evening; fever; heat of
whole body; severe shaking chill.
4 P.M.: stabbing pain in head at its height.
At sunset: chilly.
Evening: incapacity for thought; hacking cough; hollow,
spasmodic cough <; expectoration difficult; pulse
slower; lassitude; jerking as if a mouse was crawling
under skin in forearm; shaking chill, with redness of
face; warm sweat in hands; when lying down, pains
come on again; sudden pressure in head now in one
place, now in another; toothache; slight fever; feeling
of hunger; desire for stool; violent itching in rectum;
itching around genitals; chilliness.
Night: agglutination of lids; nervous and restless painful
pressure in region of pylorus; pressure in stomach <;
cramps in stomach; colic; rumbling of wind <; diarrhœa <; itching of anus; anxiousness; vomiting; falls
asleep late; oppression of chest; palpitation with stitches
in breast; numb feeling in arms; sciatica; burning of
heels; loss of consciousness; restlessness; frequently
changes position in bed; fever.
After midnight: fear of thieves on waking; oppression of
chest <.
** **Temperature and Weather.**   Open air: walking in, aching in one-half of head; lachrymation < when exerting
eye; itching > when getting heated, out doors.
Fresh air: blind piles <.
Warmth: headache >; stabbing pains in head; chills <.

Warm room: > chilliness.
Warm drink: cough.
Warm food: aversion to.
External warmth is intolerable; must be uncovered as .
   soon as heat begins.
Heat: > headache.
Lying on a hot bed: > chill.
As soon as back is the least uncovered: chill begins.
Cold: pain in occiput <; pain in teeth.
Cold air: causes chilliness.
Cold winds: headache <.
Cold water: washing hands < pain.

ᴷ **Fever.** ▮Chill and chilliness, with increased pains.
   ⁞⁞Chilliness in face and on arms, with chattering of teeth
      and gooseflesh.
   ⁞⁞Chill commences in upper arms, spreads to back and
      chest, with heat of ears.
   ▮Coldness and chilliness of whole body, or only of poste-
      rior portions, > in warm room, or by a warm stove.
   ▮Chill proceeding from abdomen.
   ▮Chilliness about knees, which are not cold externally.
   ▮Chill of single parts only.
   ▮▮Shaking chill, with redness of face, in evening.
   ▮▮Chill: with great thirst for large quantities of water;
      > from external warmth.
   ▮Chilly at sunset or in cool air; very cold all over, with
      one-sided headache.
   During chill: ill humor; violent thirst; colic; nausea;
      vomiting of food, bile or mucus; great paleness of face;
      pain in back; lameness of lower limbs; urticaria.
   ▮Chill > after eating.
   ▮Internal chill, with external heat.
   ▮External coldness, with internal heat.
   ▮Continuous quick alternations from heat to cold.
   ▮Hot knees, with cold nose.
   ▮One ear and one cheek red and burning; the other cold
      and pale.
   ▮Heat with cold feet.
   ▮Heat or coldness of single parts.
   ▮One-sided burning heat of face.
   ▮External warmth is intolerable, must be uncovered as
      soon as heat begins.
   ▮▮External heat and redness, without internal heat;
      flushes.
   ▮▮Heat of whole body, in afternoon, without thirst, with
      sensation of dryness of skin, though with some perspira-
      tion on face.
   ⁞⁞General heat in morning in bed, with thirst, does not
      wish to be uncovered.

Ι Ι Frequent flushes of heat with sweat.

Ι Fainting during the heat or sweat.

Ι Sudden attack of continued fever, consequence of reverse of fortune.

During heat: deep snoring sleep; frequent sighing; beating headache; vertigo; delirium; pain in stomach and bowels; no thirst; vomiting of ingesta, with coldness of feet and spasmodic twitching of extremities; nettlerash over whole body, with violent itching, easily relieved by scratching, disappears with sweat.

Ι Ι Hunger after fever.

Ι Sweat slight, or only on face.

Ι Sensation as if sweat would break out, which, however, does not follow.

Ι Ι Warm perspiration of extremities.

Ι Warm sweat on hands, or on inner surface of hands and fingers, in evening.

Ι Sweat: at times cold, but generally warm and somewhat sour smelling; without thirst; during a meal; when eating, only on small spot on face; often confined to upper part of body; in hands.

Ι Paroxysm preceded by much yawning and stretching; in afternoon severe shaking chill, particularly on back and arms, with thirst, lasting about an hour, followed by heat of whole body, with cold feet; internal shuddering with red cheeks and warm skin which is only > by onset of sweat, which usually lasts several hours; during heat and sweat no thirst; short periodical attacks of pressing pains in head from within out; accompanied by tearing in forehead, both > lying; dull, pressing pain in epigastrium; oppression of chest; appetite increased; ineffectual urging to stool followed by hard stool; heaviness in limbs with pain in joints; during apyrexia great lassitude; knees give way on slight motion; sound sleep with snoring respiration; taciturn, indifferent, startled when spoken to; tongue white and moist; lips cracked and dry; face pale; pulse small, and somewhat increased during fever. θTertian ague.

Ι Slight chilliness gradually extending over whole body, and finally becoming a shaking chill with chattering teeth; stretching, yawning, tearing in limbs, and great thirst; nausea with vomiting; vomits the water she drinks, mixed with slime; oppression of chest; vomiting at end of chill, followed by heat without thirst; headache; sweat without thirst; chilliness of long duration, heat and sweat being much shorter. θTertian ague.

Ι Paroxysm assuming all types—quotidian, tertian, quartan, anticipating or postponing, and coming on at all hours of day or night; chill severe and pronounced, lasting usually about an hour, with intense thirst only during chill; chill > by external warmth; as soon as chill began, although temperature was .over 90, would go at once to stove, and "over a hot fire drink the hydrant dry;" fever well developed, with much headache and vertigo, but no thirst; rarely any perspiration, and with exception of some vertigo felt well during apyrexia.

▮Slight chill lasting about half an hour, and accompanied by violent thirst and vomiting; after chill pains in breast, followed by heat with headache; no sweat.

▮During paroxysm: vertigo on lying; palpitation of heart; chilliness with thirst; chilliness > by external warmth; heat and sweat without thirst; chill > by lying in a hot bed; great weakness during fever.

▮Severe chill followed by dry heat, sweating stage absent; thirst before, during and after chill, with pains and lassitude in lower limbs and diarrhœa. *θ*Quartan ague.

▮Chill > by wrapping up warm; begins as soon as back is least uncovered; jerking of limbs; jactitation.

▮Ague recurring each Spring for several years and annually suppressed by Quinine; thirst during chill.

▮Quotidian fever with violent thirst at commencement of violent and continuous chills; is quiet and taciturn.

▮Return of chill in one month, in a boy, æt. 7, of mild, quiet disposition, very laconic in speech; headache between paroxysms, chill with thirst > from external warmth; fever with heavy sleep, perspiration light.

▮Strumming sensation in body. *θ*Intermittent.

Apyrexia: heaviness in head; throbbing in temples; sensation as if head was smaller; burning in head with cold hands and feet; face pale; eruption on lips and in corners of mouth; lips dry and chapped; pappy taste in mouth; hungry about 11 A.M, but little or no appetite at time of meals; aching pain in pit of stomach; colic, with hard stools and ineffectual urging; pain in back and limbs; irritation to cough in larynx, sensation as ●f a foreign body lying over it; languor, apathy, giving away of knees, starting in sleep, or sound sleep with snoring; sleep usually continues from heat through sweating stage into apyrexia.

Type: quotidian; tertian; quartan; irregular; continually changing, especially after abuse of quinine; paroxysms accompanied by spasmodic symptoms.

Time: irregularity of hour; paroxysm at sunset, late in afternoon or evening, then fever heat all night; anteponing paroxysms, usually postponing.

Attacks irregular both in periodicity and evolution of their stages.

∎Typhoid fever in women or in young men; for some time
before attack patient does not feel well, then suddenly
and without any gradual exacerbations the paroxysm
sets in and is usually very severe; fever begins in afternoon and continues through whole night; patient although suffering greatly cannot clearly describe his
symptoms, and does not know where he is ailing or what
is the matter with him; almost beside himself with impatience and despair, and cries out for help to those
standing about; easily frightened, fears this or that may
hurt him; sensation as if swung to and fro in a swing
or cradle; least noise or jar aggravates the complaints;
during first five days paroxysms begin with slight chilliness and coldness, with or without thirst, followed by
heat with chilly creepings and thirstlessnness; as the
disease progresses chilliness precedes fever; yawning
and stretching; severe throbbing headache in forehead
and over eyes, < from light; pain in nape of neck,
neck as if stiff; bitter taste and dryness in mouth, without thirst, latter being only present during chill; choking sensation from stomach up into throat with oppression of chest, > from belching; pressure as from a stone
in pit of stomach; indescribable sensation in pit of
stomach over which there is a feeling of constriction accompanied by shortness of breath, as if lower part was
tightly laced; severe palpitation of heart, patient often
losing consciousness, eyes are closed and respiration
seems suspended; trembling and shaking of single parts;
attacks begin and end with stretching and yawning;
pressure, or weak and empty feeling in stomach, which
is somewhat painful to touch; constipation; severe, indescribable pains in back and limbs; strumming
through limbs; jerking of tendons ; at no time sweat,
skin generally dry; great sleeplessness; on falling into
a doze starts up, affrighted by various visions; troublesome dreams.

" **Attacks, Periodicity.** ∎Complaints return at precisely
the same hour.

Acute paroxysms: chronic tonsillitis.

Momentary disappearance of pain by change of position.

Periodical: fits of vertigo ; headache weekly, fortnightly
or monthly; headache gradually increases, suddenly
abates; attacks of weakness; attacks of cramps in stomach; abdominal spasms; attacks of pressing pain in
head; convulsions.

Irregularity of hour: paroxysm at sunset, late in afternoon
or evening.

Every 3 to 4 hours: merry and lachrymose moods alternate.

Twice a day: bowel must be returned after stool; paroxysms of anxiety lasting for hours.

Every morning at 8 A.M.: < until 10.30, when gradually
> and entirely disappears at about 1 P.M.

Every day: pain in anus; pains in lower limbs; at same
hour, convulsions.

Periodically every afternoon: spasmodic ructus and singultus.

7 to 8 P.M. attacks of extremely severe pains in stomach,
more frequently at midnight, lasting 2 to 3 hours.

Every evening: half hour after going to bed, pain in r.
lower jaw lasting from one to one and a half hours.

Every other day: incisive pains in lower limbs.

Day before headache: irritable disposition.

Day after headache: feels as though it might return.

Every four to seven days: attacks of convulsive movements in limbs.

Weekly: same hour (11 A.M.) and day, nervous headache.

Every ten to fourteen days: nausea.

Every month: headache; just before or after menstruation,
cataleptic attacks.

Every two months: cataleptic attacks.

Every Spring: ague recurs.

Every Winter: pains in lower limbs.

During dentition: metastasis from bowels to brain; spasms.

During menstruation: spasms and pain.

Five minutes to half an hour: duration of spasms.

Lasting sixty to ninety minutes: pain in sciatic nerve.

Chill lasts one hour, sweat lasts several hours.

Lasting till 5 P.M. every day: contractive pain in anus and
stitches up rectum.

Lasting several hours: cataleptic attacks.

Lasts from five to six hours: spasms.

For many days: painless contraction of anus.

For six months: lachrymation; pain in eyes with headache.

" Locality and Direction. Right: heaviness of arm; pressive headache in side of forehead extending to eye;
headache above orbit at root of nose; pressure in frontal
region; intense pain over eye; throbbing pains on side
of forehead from eyebrow around eye; pain in a spot
in parietal bone; pain in breast; two chipping ulcers
at upper margin of cornea; pain in lower jaw; parotid
swollen; diphtheria commences r. side; shoulder as if
paralyzed; neuralgic pain in shoulder; loss of sensation in knee; trembling of hands < r. side.

Left: pains from head into eye; eye smaller; as if a particle was in external canthus; pain in eye; burning

and watering of eye; rawness on side of throat; pain in
hypochondrium; sharp sticking left of umbilicus; pain
low down side of abdomen; stitches side of chest; rhythmical tremor of entire leg.

From l. to r.: choreic jerking of head.

From above downward: jerking of head.

From within outward: pain over nose in forehead; pressing pain in head.

From without inward: in brain.

" Sensations.   ‖ Oversensitiveness to pain.

❚ Pressing pain from in out, like from a hard, pointed body.

‖ Tension in internal parts.

‖ Pain in small, circumscribed spots.

Pain as from dislocations in joints; cutting as from a
knife; tingling as of ants; as though eyeball would be
pressed out; as though needles were pushed through
into brain; pressure as of a weight on vertex; as if a
nail was being driven out through side of head; as if
temples would be pressed out; as if brain was beaten
and bruised; as if nerve of tooth was shattered and
crushed; as if head would burst; as if headache might
return; as if tears were in one eye; as of sand in eyes;
as if upper lid was too dry; as if eye would fall out;
as if a foreign particle was in l. external canthus; as
if inside of under lip was raw and sore; jaws feel as if
crushed; as if teeth were crushed into fragments; as if
food lodged over orifice of stomach and could not get
down; anterior half of tongue as if numb; tongue as if
burnt or raw; bread feels as if too dry; as if epigastrium
was raw inside; as if large morsel of food or plug was
sticking in middle of throat; as from a lump in throat;
as if swallowing over a bone; feeling in stomach as
from fasting; as if stomach and intestines were hanging down relaxed; as if a number of pins were sticking
in stomach; as if stomach was shortened; as if a stone
was pressing in region of pylorus; as if he would like
to vomit; as if rectum was distended with gas; hemor-
rhoidals as if excoriated; sees everything as through a
fog; as if all parts were asleep; as if she had no feeling
in epigastrium; as if stockings were cold and damp;
chest as if too small; pains as from a sharp cutting
knife through back; as if r. shoulder had been paralyzed;
as if arm did not belong to her; as if objects touched
were covered with fine felt; looks around bed as if to
find something; as if he had committed some crime;
as if she had done something wrong; as if some great
misfortune was about to happen; as if shoulder-joint
was dislocated; as if something living was running

in arm; pain in joints of arms as if bruised; beating as
though hip-joint would burst; as if back of leg would
be cut off; corns as if sore; hip and knee-joints as if
dislocated; as if she had been fasting a long time; as if
a mouse was crawling under skin in forearm ; as if jaw
was dislocated; as if sweat would break out; as if head
was smaller; as of a foreign body lying over larynx; as
if swung to and fro in a swing or cradle; neck as if stiff;
pressure as from a stone in pit of stomach; as if lower
part of stomach was tightly laced; as if flesh was loose
on bones on account of blows.

Pain: from forehead to middle of vertex; in back and nape
of neck; from head to l. eye; in head with every throb of
arteries; in occiput; in a spot in r. parietal bone; in r.
breast; in outer part of head; in periorbital region; in
upper part of lid; in eyes; from head into l. eye; in
smaller twigs of facial nerves; in r. lower jaw; in submaxillary glands; in teeth; in limbs; in back of head,
nuchæ; in ears; in l. hypochondrium; in anus; from
sacral region through to front; at stomach low down l.
side of abdomen; in trachea; in penis; in back; in
sacrum; in shoulder-joint; in joints of arms; in lower
jaw; in back; in stomach and bowels; in joints; in breast;
in lower limbs.

Intolerable pain: in back.

Furious headache.

Intense pain: over r. eye and seemingly through supraorbital foramen.

Extreme pain: in both temples; from eye to top of head;
in epigastrium; in stomach.

Intensely sore pain: at entrance to vagina.

Indescribable pain: in back and limbs.

Excruciating neuralgia: of sciatic nerve and its branches.

Simple violent pain: in small spots.

Pain very acute, driving him almost frantic: through eyes
to head.

Tearing pain: in forehead; in back of legs; in tendo
achilles; in calf; in limbs.

Acute, tearing, digging, boring pain: in sciatic nerve.

Lancinating: in sides of abdomen; in uterus.

Lancinating, cutting pain: in shoulder-joint; in hip-joint.

Lancinating boring: deep in brain.

Lancinating stitches: in back through loins to legs.

Stabbing pain: deep seated in eyes, going to occiput and
nape of neck finally to vertex; in rectum.

Darting: in face; in epigastrium; in vulva.

Cutting: deep in rectum.

Cutting stinging: in abdomen.

Gnawing cutting: in stomach.

Stitches: in soft palate extending to ear; in throat; in parotid; in stomach; from abdomen into chest; in sides of abdomen; up rectum; in hemorrhoidal tumors; in lower part of rectum; in breast; in l. side of chest; in nipple; in nape of neck; in small of back.

Sharp sticking: generally in one spot; in superciliary ridge, temple or side of head; above and to l. of umbilicus.

Sticking: in palate to inner ear; in throat; in stomach.

Stinging pain: in forehead; in throat.

Twisting pain: in face.

Fearful griping and cutting: in uterus.

Drawing and griping: in abdomen.

Pinching: in umbilical region.

Boring pain: in face; in front teeth.

Pressing, cramping pain: in forehead; in occiput.

Cramp pains: in stomach; in abdomen; in uterus.

Twitching pain: in forehead; in eye; in stomach.

Incisive, throbbing pains: in lower limbs.

Throbbing pain: in r. side of forehead; in head; in occiput; in temples.

Labor-like pains: in uterus.

Bearing-down pain: in abdomen.

Neuralgic pain: in head; in eyes; in rectum; in r. shoulder.

Beating: in hip-joint; in head.

Ulcerative pain: on margin of prepuce.

Severe contractive pain: in anus.

Contractive colic.

Contractive sore pain: in rectum.

Dragging pains: about pelvis.

Crampy pressure: in uterus.

Pressing pain: in head; in forehead; in stomach.

Pressive pain: in frontal region; above root of nose; in r. side of forehead, extending down into r. eye; in eyes; in rectum; in cervical glands.

Pressive, drawing pain: above r. orbit at root of nose.

Painful pressure: on upper surface of brain; in region of pylorus; in region of spleen; at pit of stomach; in rectum; with scraping sensation in neck of bladder.

Dull, pressing pain: in epigastrium.

Sudden pressure: in head, now in one place, now in another.

Pressure: in r. frontal region above eyebrow; from without inward in head; as of a weight on vertex; in temples; in eye; in pit of stomach; in stomach; over stomach; in sacrum; in rectum; in anus; on chest.

Drawing pain: beginning at forehead, extending down one-half of nose; in face; in umbilical region.

Spasmodic pains: in stomach; in abdomen.
Jerking: of head; through whole body when going to
  sleep; in a single limb; in a single muscle; of tendons.
Bruised pain: in small of back; in soles of feet.
Dull pain: in head, confined to r. half of forehead and r.
  eye; in forehead; in face; in rectum.
Aching: in one half of head; in pit of stomach.
Raw pain: in mucous membrane of mouth.
Soreness: of inner nose; in teeth; of inner mouth; of
  throat; of anus and rectum; in urethra; on margin of
  prepuce; in larynx.
Sore, burning pain: in rectum.
Burning heat: in vagina; in feet.
Burning: in head; in eyes; in epigastrium; in stomach;
  in urethra; in heels; in one ear and cheek.
Heat: in head; of whole body; of knees.
Stinging: in soles of feet.
Smarting: in rectum; in urethra.
Sore and bruised feeling: of head; of face.
Tenderness: of teeth.
Tensive pain: in back.
Tension: under ribs; in rectum; in r. knee.
Compressive, burning pain: extending through sinciput
  and eyes.
Suffocating constriction: of throat.
Constrictive sensation: in trachea and larynx; above throat
  pit; of chest; of anus; at heart.
Spasmodic constriction: of throat.
Choking sensation: from stomach up into throat, with
  oppression of chest.
Anxious feeling: in præcordia; mounts up to abdomen.
Hemorrhoidal pains: in anus.
Indescribable sensation: in pit of stomach over which
  there is a feeling of constriction.
Fulness: in pit of stomach; in epigastrium; under ribs.
Sensation of protrusion: in umbilical region.
Weight: at back of head.
Heaviness: of head; of r. arm; of eye; in pit of stomach;
  of feet; in limbs.
Oppression: begins at stomach spreads to throat; of chest.
Lameness: of lower limbs.
Weakness: in pit of stomach; of whole body.
Lassitude: of limbs.
Sinking sensation: in pit of stomach.
Peculiar sensation of weakness: in upper abdomen and
  pit of stomach.
Weary sensation: in chest.
Empty feeling: of head; of stomach and chest; at pit of
  stomach; at epigastrium.

Faint feeling: at pit of stomach.
Sinking: in pit of stomach.
Flabby feeling: in stomach.
Stiffness: of nape of neck; of nuchæ and muscles (trape-
zius) on each side of this ligament.
Dryness: of skin; of mouth.
Strumming: through limbs.
Quivering jerks: in deltoid muscle.
Trembling: in stomach.
Ringing: in ears.
Numb feeling: of arms; of feet; of legs.
Numb and stupid feeling: in brain.
Trickling: above pit of stomach.
Tingling: in anus; in limbs.
Crawling, asleep sensation: in limbs.
Crawling: in pharynx; low down in rectum.
Creeping sensation: in lower part of rectum.
Formication: in face.
Itching: of nose; of anus; in lower part of rectum; in
forepart of urethra; on genitals; on margin of prepuce.
Violent itching: over whole body; in rectum.
Chilliness: in face; on anus spreads to back; of whole
body or of posterior portions ; about knees.
Coldness: of nose; of feet and legs ; of hands and feet up
to knees.

" Tissues. Inflammation of external parts.
External parts become black.
Hemorrhages, blood dark.
Anæmia.
Painless swelling of glands.
Sensation as of dislocation in joints.
Chlorosis in sensitive, nervous and hysteric women,
inclined to spasmodic and intermittent complaints;
induced by mental emotions, such as grief, fright, dis-
appointed love.
Chlorosis; stomach very delicate; œdema of lower limbs;
globus hystericus.
Suitable to persons who had been starving either from
want or other causes.
Pains as if contused or sprained, or sensation as if flesh
was loose on bones in consequence of blows.

" Touch. Passive Motion. Injuries. ﹗Generally < from
slight touch ; > from hard pressure; > from scratching.
Worse during passive motion, riding and after it.
Touch: scalp tender; head painful; region of pylorus sensitive; cramp pains in uterus <; heels when they come
in contact feel cold; simple, violent pain in small spot

here and there, only noticed on touch; stomach painful;
ulcers <.

Pressure: soft, > headache; pains >; pain in epigastrium;
pain in stomach <; pain in l. hypochondrium <;
uterine pains >; ulcers > from hard pressure.

Slightest contact < cramps in stomach.

Frequently obliged to loosen clothing.

⁴⁶**Skin.** ▮Great sensitiveness of the skin to a draft of air.

Itching: better from gentle scratching; when getting
heated in open air.

Fine pricking like flea bites.

Eruption on face.

Skin chafed, sore.

Chilblains, excoriation and vesicles.

Ulcers: painless; discharge scanty; burning; generally <
from slight touch, > from hard pressure.

⁴⁷**Stages of Life, Constitution.** ▮▮Especially adapted to
nervous temperament; women of a sensitive, easily excited nature; dark hair and skin, but mild disposition;
quick to perceive, rapid in execution.

▮The patient is sensitive, peevish, excitable, hysterical,
with sanguine, nervous temperament; is delicate; falls
easily in love; is romantic; bears trials meekly; readily
falls into clonic spasms after mental agitation.

Stands in same relation to children and women that *Nux
vom.* does to sanguine, bilious men.*

Healthy child, æt. 9 months; mother suffering from nervous disorders; spasms.

Child, æt. 1½, mother had severe fright during pregnancy;
epileptiform spasms.

Boy, æt. 4, girl, æt. 6; epilepsy.

Boy, æt. 7, mild, quiet disposition, laconic in speech; intermittent.

Girl, æt. 9, after fright; spasms..

Boy, after fright; spasmodic affection.

Girl, æt. 10, blonde, graceful; after fright; epilepsy.

Boy, æt. 10, robust, but pale, had tapeworm after fright;
spasms.

Girl, æt. 10, after catching cold, pain in limbs, followed by
gouty swellings of joints; chorea.

Girl, æt. 11, sick eight days; angina.

Girl, æt. 11; chorea.

Boy, æt. 12, suffering seven months; chorea.

Girl, æt. 12, after being frightened by a fire; spasms.

---

* There are many more *Ignatia* persons in North America than *Nux vom.* persons, at least this side of Mason and Dixon's line.—C. Hg.

Girl, æt. 14; hysterical cramps.

Girl, æt. 17, weak; affection of mind.

Man, æt. 17; tertian ague.

Colored girl, æt. 17; exophthalmus.

Girl, æt. 18, delicate appearance, white skin, somewhat pale face, menses regular, has suffered several years; hysteria.

Italian girl, æt. 18, commenced menstruating at 12; four years ago in consequence of fright, epilepsy.

Girl, when five years old was pushed into a stream, the chill and fright bringing on violent fever; followed a fortnight later by attacks from which she has since suffered; menstruation set in at 14 without bringing relief; epilepsy.

Man, æt. 19; quartan ague.

Girl, æt. 19; amenorrhœa.

Man, æt. 20, sanguine, choleric temperament, strong and well nourished, after deep mortification; melancholy.

Girl, æt. 20, deformed; affection of stomach.

Girl, æt. 20, sanguine temperament, very sensitive to joy or sorrow; melancholy.

Girl, æt. 20; affection of mind.

Man, æt. 21, cheerful disposition, after fright; epilepsy.

Woman, æt. 24, since fifteenth year suffering from attacks of headache, vertigo and vomiting; for last two years after least mental disturbance, convulsions.

Nursing woman, æt. 24, after fright; convulsions.

Woman, æt. 24, has conceived four times within the last seven months; headaches.

Girl, æt. 25; after grief; affection of stomach.

Woman, æt. 25, married eight years, but had never borne children; hysteria.

Woman, æt. 26, very irritable, dark hair, delicate build, well educated, childless, has suffered since first appearance of menses; dysmenorrhœa.

Woman, æt. 26, had ague three years ago, delicate, yellow skin, spleen enlarged, suffering four days; intermittent fever.

Married woman, æt. 27, strumous, leuco-phlegmatic diathesis; vaginismus.

Man, æt. 28, soldier, strong and healthy, coming from a swampy district; tertian ague.

Woman, æt. 28, half year ago was greatly frightened by a cat which tore to pieces her canary bird; affection of mind.

Woman, æt. 29, mother of two children, has suffered for several years; hemorrhoids.

Woman, æt. 30, nervous temperament, irritable, lively and

responsive disposition, after long nursing; hysterical paraplegia.

Strong man, æt. 30, gardener; facial neuralgia.

Delicate lady, has had children in rapid succession; prosopalgia.

Lady artist, dark complexion, excessively nervous; conjunctivitis.

Young widow, tall, slender, dark hair, eyes and skin; affection of stomach.

Woman, after being cured of headache, pains in stomach and fluor albus, by *Pulsat.;* affection of stomach.

Woman, suffering eleven years, since birth of first child; hemorrhoids.

Woman, æt. 33, seven months pregnant with her fifth child; puerperal convulsions.

Man, æt. 33, carpenter, after great mental excitement, eight years previously; epilepsy.

Woman, æt. 34, during lactation; affection of shoulder and knee.

Plethoric lady, æt. 35, mother of eleven children; prosopalgia.

Woman, æt. 35, mother of three children, for three years; tumor above knee.

Man, æt. 36, weak, after quarrelsome life; epilepsy.

Woman, æt. 36, thin, weak, confined three weeks ago; hemorrhoids.

Woman, æt. 37, corpulent, twelve years ago gave birth to child, since which time has been suffering; affection of eyes.

Woman, æt. 39, unmarried, spare habit, bilious temperament; headache.

Woman, æt. 40; affection of mind.

Patient, æt. 40; prosopalgia.

Woman, æt. 40, pregnant, after fright; pain in epigastrium and abdomen.

Woman, æt. 42, from the country; affection of mind.

Woman, æt. 42, subject to attacks of migraine, after typhoid fever; ptyalism.

Woman, æt. 42; after being greatly frightened by seeing grandson carried into house apparently drowned; affection of mind.

Woman, æt. 44, wife of inn keeper, after grief and much trouble; melancholy.

Strong woman, æt. 46; ague.

Strong woman, æt. 46, blonde, after being angered and overheated; spasms.

Strong, healthy woman, æt. 46; neuralgia of face.

Man, æt. 48, married, red hair, blue eyes; headache.

Woman, æt. 50, sedentary habits, suffering for three months; sciatica.

Manufacturer, æt. 54, after business embarrassments; affection of mind.

Mrs. G., æt. 54, blonde; leuco-phlegmatic; rather fleshy; passed climacteric four years ago; till eight years ago healthy, since then subject to nervous periodical headaches.

Man, æt. 68, artist, thin and weak, sanguine and lively temperament; affection of stomach.

Aged women, oversensitive to external impressions; spinal affection (paralysis, fixed pain in spine); habitual constipation; r. half of body weakest; vertigo.

⁴⁸Relations. Antidoted by: *Arnic., Camphor., Chamom., Coccul., Coffea,* **¹¹***Pulsat.*

It antidotes effects of brandy, coffee, chamomile tea, tobacco, *Zincum.*

Compatible: *Arsen., Bellad., Calc. ostr., Cinchon., Lycop., Nux vom., Pulsat., Rhus tox., Sepia, Sulphur.*

Incompatible: *Coffea, Nux vom., Tabac.*

Compare: *Calc. ostr., Chamom., Coffea, Nux vom., Stramon.*

ILLICIUM ANISATUM.

Star Anise.   *Magnoliaceæ.*

Tincture of the seeds.

Provings by Franz and Mure. See Allen's Encyclopedia, vol. 5, p. 91.

CLINICAL AUTHORITIES.—*Infantile colic,* Jeanes, Hom. Clinics, vol. 4, p. 132.

³Inner Head. Pains in head; > evenings, < mornings.

⁶Hearing and Ears. Buzzing in ears.

Ringing in ears, followed by sleep.

Itching over l. ear, going off when touching place.

⁷Smell and Nose. Acute catarrh.

Watery discharge from nostrils.

Warm smarting sensation in nose, succeeded by sneezing.

Sharp stitches in tip of nose.

⁹Lower Face. Stinging sensation in upper lip, as if blood would press out, > from touch.

Dryness of upper lip, which is drawn closer to teeth.

Burning in inner surface of lower lip, with sensation as if it had gone to sleep.

11 Taste and Tongue. Rye bread tastes good, its odor is refreshing.

◼Tongue covered with aphthæ; most on edges.

◼Edges of tongue folded like little bags.

12 Throat. ◼Tough, viscid phlegm from stomach; with old drunkards.

13 Eating and Drinking. Satiety, after eating but little.

All food, except rye bread, tastes too salty or bitter, yet appetite is good.

14 Hiccough, Belching, Nausea and Vomiting. Nausea in stomach, extends to chest, then ceases.

Nausea, with gagging and inclination to vomit.

17 Scrobiculum and Stomach. Bloating of stomach; acidity.

18 Hypochondria. Pain in splenic region.

19 Abdomen. ◼Three months' colic, especially if it recurs at regular hours; bowels disturbed.

◼Violent wind colic.

Rumbling in abdomen.

20 Stool and Rectum. Stools: bilious; compact and dark colored.

21 Urinary Organs. Retention of urine.

22 Respiration. ◼Dyspnœa in old asthmatics.

23 Cough. After coughing, feeling of emptiness.

◼Frequent cough, with pain.

Spitting blood in small quantities and with pus-like phlegm, pain in r. chest.

Whitish expectoration.

24 Inner Chest and Lungs. ◼Tough, viscous phlegm, with old drunkards.

Pain in region of third rib, about one or two inches from sternum, generally on r. side, but occasionally left.

Pain about junction of third r. rib with its cartilage; hemorrhage; cough; congestion; enlarged liver.

28 Heart, Pulse and Circulation. ◼Palpitation, with aphthæ and weakness.

31 Neck and Back. Cramp-like drawing, as from a cold, in l. side of dorsal vertebræ.

33 Lower Limbs. Left thigh feels as if broken at middle, when sitting, ceases on rising.

35 Rest. Position. Motion. Sitting: l. thigh feels as if broken at middle.

Rising: sensation as if l. thigh was broken ceases.

36 Time. Morning: pains in head <.

Evenings: pains in head >.

41 Attacks, Periodicity. Three months' colic, especially if it recurs at regular hours.

42 Locality and Direction. Right: pain in chest; pain in region of third rib; pain about junction of third rib with its cartilage.

Left: itching over ear; occasionally pain in region of third rib; cramps like drawing in side of dorsal vertebræ; l. thigh feels as if broken at middle.

⁴³ Sensations. As if blood would press out of upper lip; as if lower lip had gone to sleep; cramp-like drawing as from a cold in l. side of dorsal vertebræ; l. thigh feels as if broken at middle.

Pain: in head; in splenic region; in r. chest; in region of third rib; generally on r. side, but occasionally left; about junction of third rib.

Sharp stitches: in tip of nose.

Violent wind colic.

Warm smarting sensation: in nose.

Stinging sensation: in upper lip.

Burning: in inner surface of lower lip.

Rumbling: in abdomen.

Dryness: of upper lip.

Itching: over l. ear.

⁴⁴ Touch. Passive Motion. Injuries. Touch: itching ceases when touching place; stinging sensation in upper lip.

⁴⁷ Stages of Life, Constitution. Babies with three months' colic. Old drunkards, catarrh of stomach. Old asthmatics.

⁴⁸ Relations. Compatible: after *Acon.* and *Bryon.* in hæmoptysis.

INDIGO.

Indigo.   *Leguminosæ.*

Proved extensively by German provers. See Allen's Encyclopedia, vol. 5, p. 92.

CLINICAL AUTHORITIES.—*Prolapsus ani*, Schüssler, Raue's Rec., 1871, p. 123; *Sciatica*, Preston, T. H. M. Soc. Pa., 1872, p. 120; *Epilepsy*, four cases, Kenyon, Raue's Rec., 1875, p. 254-255.

¹ Mind. Melancholy, sadness.

‖Sad, discontented, ill humored, introverted.

‖Gloomy; endeavors to hide it, has spent many nights alone crying. *θ*Epileptic convulsions.

² Sensorium. Excessive giddiness with headache.

Vertigo with headache, fulness of abdomen, great discharge of flatus, and nausea, going off in evening after remaining some time in open air.

Undulating sensation through whole head from behind forward.

3 Inner Head. Sensation as if head were tightly bandaged around forehead.

Constant pain in sinciput, attended with an aching pain in r. hypochondrium.

Tearing in vertex.

Heaviness of head, as from a heavy load on vertex, when stooping.

Beating, with painful stinging in occiput.

Beating in whole head.

Feeling as if brain was distending at centre.

Headache with redness and heat of face.

Severe, lacerating pain in head.

❚Sick headache, originating in a state of debility.

❚Migraine.

Pains are characterized by great intensity, are < during rest and when sitting, and can frequently be entirely suppressed by rubbing and pressure, or by motion, or alleviated, so as to reappear with less intensity.

4 Outer Head. Sensation as if a bunch of hair was pulled from vertex.

5 Sight and Eyes. Pressure in ball of eye.

Inflammation of meibomian glands on lower lids.

Violent jerking and twitching in lids.

7 Smell and Nose. ❚Excessive continued sneezing, succeeded by violent bleeding of nose.

Nose bleeding, with dry cough.

Epistaxis.

8 Upper Face. Pricking in r. malar bone.

Small blisters on l. side of face, from forehead to neck.

10 Teeth and Gums. Toothache, of a rheumatic character.

11 Taste and Tongue. ❚❚Metallic taste in tongue, with contracted feeling in pharynx.

Vesicles on tip of tongue.

12 Inner Mouth. Numbness of inner mouth.

Pain in submaxillary glands, extending to teeth.

16 Hiccough, Belching, Nausea and Vomiting. Retching and vomiting of watery fluid.

Vomiting of glue-like mucus.

17 Scrobiculum and Stomach. Tingling pain in pit of stomach.

Bloating of stomach.

Catarrh of stomach and intestines, with colic.

20 Stool and Rectum. Emission of excessive quantity of flatus.

Diarrhœa; stool liquid, with flatulence; creeping over skin, cold hands and colic.

❚Prolapsus ani after each stool.

Pin worms.

21 Urinary Organs. Inflammation of kidneys.

Renal colic.

Catarrh of bladder with pustules and boils on body, menses
often appearing too early.

Chronic catarrh of bladder.

Frequent desire to urinate, burning in fundus of bladder;
painful emissions of small quantities of turbid urine.

Increased emission of turbid urine, containing much
mucus, without thirst, with violent contraction of urethra
and pain in bladder.

22 Male Sexual Organs. Depressed sexual desire.
∎Urethral stricture following gonorrhœa.

Itching of urethra, glans and scrotum.

23 Female Sexual Organs. Menstruation too early.
Burning in mammæ during menses.

Stinging in mammæ, going off momentarily by rubbing.

27 Cough. ∎Dry cough, always attended by nosebleed.
Violent cough; inducing vomiting; bleeding of nose.
Suffocative cough in evening and after going to bed.
∎Cough dry, always accompanied with expectoration.
Spasmodic cough with tough, mucous expectoration.

28 Inner Chest and Lungs. Severe sharp stitch in middle of
sternum, passing through chest, when sitting.

29 Outer Chest. Painful spot, size of hand, in region of r. lower
ribs, with stitch extending to shoulder joint when sitting,
going off by motion.

Stitch in region of lower false ribs, toward small of back.

31 Neck and Back. Drawing, lancinating pains, following
course of l. rhomboideus muscle.

Boils on neck and buttocks.

Stitch between scapulæ.

Stitch in small of back, > after an evacuation.

32 Upper Limbs. Excessive itching (preceded by a dull headache), especially on r. elbow joint.

Blotches on hands.

33 Lower Limbs. ∎Intense aching, stinging and bruised pain
in middle of the posterior of thigh, extending to knee;
boring pain in knee-joint; sharp tearing, stinging or
pricking in calf above ankle; < sitting; > by motion,
though motion also painful; < afternoon and evening;
much pricking in calf just below knee and in popliteal
space; must lie down. θSciatica.

∎Indescribable pain, extending from middle of thigh to
knee, in the bone, > walking, returning during rest, in
afternoon.

∎Tearing pain four fingers' breadth above l. knee joint, extending to a hand's breadth above ankle; in afternoon
while sitting, > rising and walking about.

35 Rest. Position. Motion. Rest: pain <; pain in thigh
bone <.

Must lie down: pain in calf so severe.

Sitting: pain <; stitch in middle of sternum; stitch extending to shoulder joint; sharp tearing, stinging in calf <; tearing above knee joint.

Stooping: heaviness of head.

Motion: pains >.

Rising: tearing above knee-joint >.

Walking: indescribable pain in thigh bone >; tearing above knee-joint >.

⁸⁸ Nerves. Excessive nervous irritation.

Illusory sensations.

Subsultus tendinum.

█Paroxysms come suddenly; falls down or out of chair, becomes convulsed all over; frothing at mouth; convulsive movements followed by a rigid condition of body; before attacks he had a furious disposition, excitable, easily angered, since then had become mild and even timid. θEpilepsy.

█Paroxysms lasting five minutes, clonic and very violent; occur every nine or ten days; very melancholy, exceedingly timid; did not want to live. θEpilepsy.

█Convulsions regularly once a week; gloomy, but endeavors to hide it, has spent many nights alone crying. θEpilepsy.

█Fits every day; exceeding melancholic. θEpilepsy.

█Flushes of heat from abdomen to head, with sensation as if head was tightly bandaged around forehead; fits begin with dizziness. θEpilepsy.

█Epilepsy, originating from plexus solaris, or from abdominal ganglia, or from a cold or fright.

⁸⁸ Time. Afternoon: sharp tearing in calf <; pain in thigh bone returns; tearing above knee joint.

Evening: vertigo with headache >: suffocative cough; sharp tearing in calf <.

⁸⁹ Temperature and Weather. Open air: vertigo with headache.

⁴⁰ Fever. Chilliness, with cold hands and violent headache, with constant desire to urinate; urine turbid.

Flushes of heat from abdomen to head.

Great heat, particularly in face, with increased secretion of urine.

█Worm fevers in children.

⁴¹ Attacks, Periodicity. Paroxysms: come suddenly.

Last five minutes: paroxysms.

Every day: fits.

Once a week: convulsions.

Every nine or ten days: paroxysms.

⁴² Locality and Direction. Right: aching pain in hypochon-

drium; pricking in malar bone; painful spot in region
of lower ribs; excessive itching on elbow joint.

Left: small blisters on side of face, from forehead to neck;
drawing, lancinating pains following course of rhomboideus muscle; tearing pain in knee joint.

From behind forward: undulating sensation through
whole head.

" **Sensations.** As if head was tightly bandaged around forehead; as if a heavy load was on vertex; as if brain
was distending at centre; as if a bunch of hair was
pulled from vertex.

Pain: in submaxillary glands; in bladder.

Pains: characterized by great intensity.

Constant pain: in sinciput.

Painful spot: size of hand in region of r. lower ribs, with
stitch extending to shoulder joint.

Indescribable pain: extending from middle of thigh to knee.

Severe lacerating pain: in head.

Sharp tearing, stinging or pricking: in calf above ankle.

Tearing: in vertex; four fingers' breadth above l. knee-
joint, extending to a hand's breadth above ankle.

Drawing, lancinating pains: following course of l. rhomboideus muscle.

Severe sharp stitch: in middle of sternum.

Stitch: extending from ribs to shoulder-joint; in region of
lower false ribs; between scapulæ; in small of back.

Boring pain: in knee joint.

Intense aching, stinging and bruised pain: in middle of
the posterior of thigh.

Stinging: in mammæ.

Aching pain: in r. hypochondrium.

Beating, with painful stinging: in occiput.

Beating: in whole head.

Tingling pain: in pit of stomach.

Toothache: of rheumatic character.

Painful emissions: of small quantities of turbid urine.

Picking: in calf just below knee and in popliteal space.

Pricking: in r. malar bone.

Burning: in fundus of bladder; in mammæ.

Heat: of face.

Contracted feeling: in pharynx.

Pressure: in ball of eye.

Heaviness: of head.

Fulness: of abdomen.

Undulating sensation: through whole head.

Creeping: over chin.

Numbness: of inner mouth.

Excessive itching: especially on r. elbow joint.

Itching: of urethra, glans and scrotum ; of skin.
" Tissues.   Congestive,condition of head and lungs, with palpitation of heart.
Rheumatic and gouty affections of nerves and joints, ac-
companied by slight fever and great debility.
⁴⁵ Touch.   Passive Motion.   Injuries.   Pressure: pains >.
Rubbing: pains > ; stinging in mammæ, going off mo-
mentarily.
⁴⁶ Skin. ▮Itching of skin with constipation (improved).
Pimples on face and body.
⁴⁷ Stages of Life, Constitution.   Little boy ; prolapsus ani.
Boy, æt. 9, suffering three years; epileptic fits.
Boy, æt. 12, has had fits ever since he could remember.
Boy, æt. 17 ; epileptic fits.
Woman, æt. 33, unmarried ; epilepsy.
Married woman, æt. 35, tall, slender build, phthisical habit,
nervo-bilious temperament ; sciatica.
⁴⁸ Relations.   Compare *Sulphur* in epilepsy, hot flushes, and
worm fever.

INDIUM METALLICUM.

Trituration of the pure metal.   *In.*

"This metal was discovered by Reich and Richter in the zinc-blende of Freiberg.
Its spectrum is characterized by two indigo colored lines, one very bright and more
refrangible than the blue lines of Strontium, the other fainter but still more refrangible, approaching the blue line of Potassium.   It was the production of this
peculiar spectrum that led to the discovery of the metal.   The ore, consisting
chiefly of blende, galena and arsenical pyrites, was roasted to expel sulphur and
arsenic, then treated with hydrochloric acid, and the solution was evaporated to
dryness.   The impure zinc chloride thus obtained, exhibited, when examined by
the spectroscope, the first of the indigo lines above mentioned.   The chloride was
afterwards obtained in a state of greater purity, and from this the hydrate and the
metal itself were prepared.   The first line then came out with much greater bril-
liancy and the second was likewise observed."—*Am. Hom. Pharm.*

The provings, under the direction of Bell (See Allen's Encyclopedia, vol. 5, p.
107), were mostly made with the higher dilutions, as was also the one by C. Mohr.

¹ **Mind.**   Mental depression.
Mind feels tired ; does not care to work.
Feels stupid and careless ; cannot fix thoughts on anything.
Restless, cannot sit still, must walk about.
Sleepy and irritable with headache.

Feels almost crazed when attempting to study, with headache.

² Sensorium. Vertigo: on rising from a seat; after retiring, with nausea; when sitting and stooping slightly; between 3 and 4 A.M., < on turning and on rising, cannot sit up.

³ Inner Head. ▮Dull headache in temples and forehead, with sleepiness and nausea.

Headache beginning at night and continuing all next day; pain mostly on r. side of occiput; occasional pains over l. eye, with a tired, sick feeling.

Very distressing headache in forenoon; pains commence on r. side of occiput and extend over head to l. eye.

Pain at 8 A.M., extending over r. side of head from occiput, leaving a bruised spot on vertex.

Pain in r. occipital region, with occasional dull, aching pain in forehead.

Severe l. sided headache in evening.

Beating, throbbing pain in head, with much heat, and a stupid, cross feeling; > washing in cold water.

Beating, throbbing headache at 3 P.M., lasting till bedtime; head very hot; face red.

Slight throbbing headache, lasting two hours, with hot head and cold, clammy hands; afterwards, bruised feeling of brain in vertex, > in cold air.

Headache, in morning, on rising, > eating; an hour afterwards headache returns and lasts till noon.

⁴ Outer Head. Severe itching of scalp on vertex lasting several days, < in morning.

⁵ Sight and Eyes. People and things look ghastly and pale or saffron colored.

Mist before eyes, in evening.

Sharp pain in eyeball from before backward, on turning or moving eyes.

Irritation in l. eye, as if heavy with sleep, coming and going, not affected by daylight, < from artificial light, and from closing eye, with a desire to close it; in evening r. eye affected in same way.

Spasmodic twitching at outer angle of l. eye.

⁶ Hearing and Ears. Throbbing in ears, in evening.

Bright redness of whole r. ear, with a row of very sore pimples on helix.

⁷ Smell and Nose. ▮Violent attacks of sneezing.

Epistaxis; nose bleeds whenever blown or touched.

Nasal discharge: green; bloody; then watery; thin, yellowish.

⁸ Upper Face. Very painful suppurating pimples on forehead; feel as though pierced with a needle; skin very red far around each pustule.

Sore pustules all over face; burning and stinging.

Face: red during headache; red and hot; complexion sallow.

Fiery red places about an inch long over l. eye.

⁹ Lower Face. Patches of small vesicles on mucous membrane of lower lip; vesicles contain a colorless, limpid fluid.

Corners of mouth cracked and very sore.

¹³ Throat. Uvula greatly enlarged, back part of pharynx covered with thick yellow mucus, very tough and hard to remove.

। ।Destructive ulceration of uvula, soft palate and tonsils, with thick yellow secretion in ulcers.

Left tonsil swollen; pain and difficulty in swallowing.

Throat sore on r. side.

Tickling in throat inducing continual hawking.

Dryness, throbbing, stinging soreness; swallowing painful.

Throat: < in evening; > eating and drinking cold water.

¹⁵ Eating and Drinking. After eating lobster: taste of iodide of potash.

¹⁶ Hiccough, Belching, Nausea and Vomiting. Qualmishness.

▮Nausea: with headache; during breakfast; with faintness at 11 A.M. and on rising; after retiring, with dizziness and pain in liver.

Sick feeling at stomach for two days; felt as if vomiting would relieve.

¹⁷ Scrobiculum and Stomach. Fulness and pressure at stomach with soreness.

¹⁸ Hypochondria. Stitches in region of liver.

¹⁹ Abdomen. Colic: griping; from umbilicus downward; as if diarrhœa would set in.

²⁰ Stool and Rectum. Stool: pasty, brownish-yellow, fetid, with particles of undigested food, preceded by colic; involuntary, slight, when urinating; small and hard, afterwards pappy; hard, with blood.

Diarrhœa: < by drinking beer; with headache on r. side.

Burning tenesmus and pain in anus, after stool.

Violent pain in head when straining at stool.

²¹ Urinary Organs. Painful urination.

When urinating: loss of power over sphincter ani.

▮▮Horribly offensive smell of urine after standing a short time.

²² Male Sexual Organs. Sexual desire and power diminished, emission too soon, thrill deficient.

। ।Increase of sexual desire.

Emissions: twice the same night; four nights in succession; at night without knowledge.

Itching of glans penis.

Severe pain in r. testicle.

⬛Testicles tumefied and very tender·to touch; drawing pains along spermatic cords upwards; l. testicle much <.

²³ **Female Sexual Organs.** Menses two weeks too soon; bearing down pains, with cross temper and weeping mood; face very red.

²⁵ **Voice and Larynx. Trachea and Bronchia.** Hoarseness: on rising; with sore throat.

Habitual bronchial expectoration freer, but a little blood appeared in mucus.

²⁶ **Respiration.** ⬛Frequent desire to take a deep breath, when lying down; < lying on l. side, > lying on back.

²⁸ **Inner Chest and Lungs.** Severe pain behind lower r. portion of sternum.

Sharp pains through upper part of chest.

Burning pain on l. side of chest near sternum, which feels as if drawn towards back.

ǀǀDull pain in l. pectoral region.

³⁰ **Outer Chest.** Dull pain in l. axilla.

³¹ **Neck and Back.** ⬛Stiffness of neck and shoulders.

Drawing through side of head and neck to clavicle, first r. side, next day left.

Pressing pain in upper scapular region, with stiffness on sitting still, pain < on beginning to move.

Severe pain under scapula of l. side.

Dull pain under r. shoulder blade.

Rheumatic drawing across shoulders up to head; < in riding, turning in bed, flexure or rotation of head, and morning and evening.

Dull, aching pain in back and lumbar regions.

³² **Upper Limbs.** Constant pain in l. shoulder, as if bruised.

Intermitting pains in l. shoulder.

Pain in l. shoulder, with soreness extending down arm.

Severe pain in l. shoulder; pain runs down to elbow, at times so severe as to disable arm.

Shooting pains in fingers.

Muscles of l. arm and shoulder feel flabby and soft; no power in arm.

Severe lancinating pains in biceps of l. arm, extending into shoulder; pains < extending arm; paralytic weakness.

Left elbow feels sore.

Slight pains in l. arm.

Palms of hands sweat continually.

Itching in palms.

³³ **Lower Limbs.** ǀǀTired feeling, weariness in legs.

Drawing, strained feeling of muscles of inside of r. thigh, while walking.

Sharp, shooting pains in r. leg.

A narrow streak of severe pressing pain in back of l. thigh,
sudden, when sitting.

Severe pain and lameness in lower r. leg.

Legs from knees downward and feet feel heavy as if loaded.

Peculiar hot tingling in legs.

Dull, boring pain in l. great toe joint, almost unbearable,
must move foot to > it, for three evenings, from 8 to 9.

Burning and intense itching of all the toes the whole day.

Itching of toes in evening.

Feet sweat easily and feel cold.

Profuse foot sweat.

³⁵ Rest. Position. Motion. Walking: causes weak feeling,
particularly in legs.

Restless, cannot sit still, must walk about.

Lying on back: desire to take long breath >; nightmare.

Lying on l. side: desire to take a long breath <.

Sitting: vertigo; stiffness in scapular region; a narrow
streak of severe pain in back of l. thigh.

Rising from a seat: vertigo.

Stooping slightly: vertigo.

Cannot sit up: on account of vertigo.

On rising: vertigo; headache; hoarseness.

Beginning to move: pressing pain in upper scapular
region <.

Moving: high fever with chilliness.

Must move foot to > pain in great toe joint.

Turning: vertigo; rheumatic drawing across shoulders <.

Moving eyes: < pain.

Closing eye: irritation <.

Rotation of head: rheumatic drawing across shoulders <.

Walking: strained feeling in muscles of r. thigh.

³⁶ Nerves. Felt as though he was his natural size, during fever.

Tired feeling, weariness and restlessness in legs; tremor
of thighs.

³⁷ Sleep. Sleepiness: with headache and nausea; with irritability; in morning; from 4 to 6 P.M.; in evening, in a
warm room.

Dreams: lascivious; amorous; of having unsuccessful
intercourse with men; vivid, of what had occupied his
mind during day; of annoying accidents; of being in
foreign countries; chased by mad bulls; lost in
mountains.

Nightmare: from lying on back; very stupid on awaking.

³⁸ Time. 3.30 A.M.: wakes with great restlessness, especially
in legs.

3 to 4 A.M.: awake with vertigo.

Morning: headache on rising; itching of scalp <; rheumatic drawing across shoulders; sleepiness.

8 A.M.: pain in r. side of head.

11 A.M.: faintness.

Forenoon: very distressing headache.

The whole day: burning and itching of toes.

3 P.M.: pain in head lasting till bedtime.

From 4 to 6 P.M.: sleepiness.

Evening: l. sided headache; mist before eyes; irritation in r. eye; throbbing in ears; throat <; rheumatic drawing across shoulders; itching of toes; sleepiness.

Night: headache begins lasts all next day; emission without knowledge.

³⁹ Temperature and Weather. In a warm room: sleepiness.

Out doors: fever >.

Cold air: headache >.

Working in cold water: pain in head >.

Cold water: throat >.

⁴⁰ Fever. Sensitive to cold.

High fever with chilliness on moving, great weakness, sore throat; thirst, stretching, violent headache and backache.

Fever: with nausea, after eating; > out doors.

Easy perspirations.

⁴¹ Attacks, Periodicity. One hour after eating: headache returns and lasts till noon.

For two hours: throbbing headache.

For two days: sick feeling in stomach.

For several days: itching of scalp.

Twice the same night: emissions.

For three evenings from 8 to 9: severe pain in toe joint.

Four nights in succession : emissions.

Two weeks too soon: menses.

⁴² Locality and Direction. Right: pain mostly on side of occiput; from occiput to side of head ; in occipital region; eye as if heavy with sleep; bright redness of whole ear; side of throat sore; headache; severe pain in testicle; severe pain, behind lower portion of sternum; dull pain under shoulder blade; strained feeling of muscles of side of thigh ; sharp shooting pains in leg; severe pain and lameness in leg.

Left: occasional pains over eye ; headache in side; irritation in eye, as if heavy with sleep; spasmodic twitching of outer angle of eye; fiery red place about an inch long over eye; tonsil swollen ; testicle tender to touch ; lying on side desires to take long breath <; burning pain along side of chest; dull pain in pectoral region; dull pain in axilla; severe pain under scapula; constant pain in shoulder; intermitting pains in shoulder; severe pain from shoulder to elbow; severe lancinating pain in biceps of arm; elbow sore; slight pains in arm; a narrow streak of severe pressing pain in back of thigh; dull, boring pain in great toe joint.

Right then left: drawing through side of head and neck to clavicle.

From before backwards: sharp pain in eyeball.

" **Sensations.** Frequent pressing pain here and there, all over.

Soreness of whole l. side of body.

Soreness all over body; severe pain in l. side, making it difficult to move; > after continued motion.

Body feels sore all over; sickish feeling and sensation as though bones would crush through flesh.

Irritation in l. eye as if heavy with sleep; pimples on forehead feel as though pierced with a needle; felt as if vomiting would relieve; as if diarrhœa would set in; sternum feels as if drawn towards back; l. shoulder as if bruised; legs feel as if loaded.

Pain: in liver; in anus; in l. shoulder.

Violent pain: in head.

Severe pain: in r. testicle; behind lower r. portion of sternum; under l. scapula; in l. shoulder down to elbow; in lower r. leg.

Severe lancinating pains: in biceps of l. arm, extending into shoulder.

Sharp pains: through upper part of chest; in eyeballs.

Shooting pains: in fingers; in r. leg.

Stitches: in region of liver.

Beating, throbbing pain: in head.

Griping: from umbilicus downwards.

Pressing pain: in back of l. thigh.

Burning pain: on l. side of chest near sternum.

Burning, stinging: in pustules all over face.

Burning tenesmus.

Drawing pain: along spermatic cords upwards; through side of head and neck to clavicle.

Drawing strained feeling: of muscles of side of r. thigh.

Dull, almost unbearable boring pain: in l. great toe joint.

Bearing down pains: during menses.

Pressing pain: in upper scapular region.

Rheumatic drawing: across shoulders.

Dull aching: in forehead; in back and lumbar region.

Dull pain: in l. pectoral region; in l. axilla; under r. shoulder blade.

Dull headache: in temples and forehead.

Bruised feeling: in vertex after pain in head.

Constant pain: in l. shoulder.

Intermitting pains: in l. shoulder.

Slight throbbing: headache.

Slight pains : in l. arm.

Dryness, throbbing, stinging soreness : in throat.

Sore pimples : on helix of ear.

Soreness : of corners of mouth; of throat; of stomach ; down arm ; of l. elbow.

Burning and intense itching: of toes.

Hot tingling : in legs.

Throbbing : in ears.

Tickling : in throat.

Spasmodic twitching : in outer angle of l. eye.

Fulness : at stomach.

Pressure : at stomach.

Tired feeling : in legs.

Sick feeling : at stomach.

Faintness : on rising.

Stiffness : of neck and shoulders; in scapular region.

Lameness : in lower r. leg.

Itching : of scalp; of glans penis; in palms; of toes.

⁴⁵ Touch. Passive Motion. Injuries. Touch : makes nose bleed; testicle tender.

Riding : rheumatic drawing across shoulders <.

⁴⁶ Skin. Itching of scalp, toes, etc.

Very painful sore pimples on various parts of body.

⁴⁸ Relations. Compare : *Bellad.* (headache, menses); *Asparagus* (offensive urine); *Sanguin.* (headache, rheumatism); *Ferrum* (headache, ebullitions, lameness of shoulder muscles).

INULA.

Elecampane; Scabwort.   *Corymbiferæ.*

An ancient medicine known to Hippocrates, Dioscorides, Eben Sina, etc.

The plant is a native of Europe, Central Asia and Siberia, but grows wild along roadsides in the Northern part of the United States.

The tincture is prepared from the fresh root dug in Autumn of its second year.

Proving with the juice of the root on a female prover, by Fischer. See Allen's Encyclopedia, vol. 5, p. 112.

CLINICAL AUTHORITIES.—*Bronchitis*, Chargé, Hahn. Mo., vol. 10, p. 228; *Laryngitis*, Lingen, MSS.

[1] **Mind.** Excessive anxiety and trembling of whole body, chattering of teeth from cold, during menstruation.

[2] **Sensorium.** Vertigo, on stooping.
Confusion of head with nausea, in evening.
Headache, in r. side, afterward in left.
Sticking headache in r. side.
Jerking, tearing pain in occiput.

[3] **Inner Head.** Rush of blood to head with sleeplessness.
Tearing, throbbing pain in forehead and vertex, after eating.
Burning headache in l. temple, in a spot as large as a silver dollar, in evening.

[5] **Sight and Eyes.** Twitching in upper lids.
Burning in l. eyeball.
Swimming before eyes and pressure in temples and forehead.

[6] **Hearing and Ears.** Dull stitches in l. ear, with transient sticking above r. eyebrow, in evening.

[7] **Smell and Nose.** Stitches in r. side of middle of nose.
Sticking, crawling in root of nose, extending to eyebrows.

[8] **Upper Face.** Left side of face red and hot, a white spot near nose.
Flushes of heat; l. cheek glowing.

[10] **Teeth and Gums.** Pain in decayed teeth, < at night.

[12] **Inner Mouth.** Dryness of mouth with scraping and tickling in throat, swallowing difficult.

[13] **Throat.** Pain in throat on swallowing; tickling causing cough.

[16] **Hiccough, Belching, Nausea and Vomiting.** ‖Nausea in morning coming from stomach.

[17] **Scrobiculum and Stomach.** Twisting as of a ball in epigastric region, above umbilicus.

Sticking pain in epigastric region.

[18] **Hypochondria.** Violent motion beneath r. hypochondrium, as though something living were moving about, during menstruation.

[19] **Abdomen.** Sticking: as with two pins to r. of umbilicus; as from a knife between umbilicus and r. groin.

Stitches in l. side of abdomen, towards l. groin.

[20] **Stool and Rectum.** Pressing dragging towards rectum and genitals, as in labor; as if a substance would come out, occurring repeatedly.

[21] **Urinary Organs.** Urging to urinate ten times in one hour; urine passes by drops.

Urine smells of violets.

[23] **Female Sexual Organs.** Movings about in abdomen, as at appearance of menstruation, followed by yellowish leucorrhœa.

Pain in uterus, with pain in small of back, very violent, with pressure as in labor; urging to stool, which she dreads; is obliged to remain lying.

Dragging in genitals, with more violent backache than she had ever had before.

Stitches in region of uterus and genitals.

Menses too early and painful.

[23] **Voice and Larynx. Trachea and Bronchia.** ❚Violent tickling in larynx, producing dry cough, < lying down, < at night; larynx painful.

❚Cough with abundant thick expectoration; accompanied by weakness of digestive tract, general languor and debility and much leucorrhœa; skin has been the seat of psoric manifestations; engorged glands. *θ*Chronic bronchitis.

[24] **Respiration.** Difficult breathing with dry, tickling cough.

[27] **Cough.** Dry, tickling cough.

[28] **Inner Chest and Lungs.** Stitches behind sternum and beneath l. seventh and eighth ribs.

Throbbing, jerking pain as from suppuration, in middle of chest.

[31] **Neck and Back.** ❚Pain through back and chest, on inspiration.

Transient pain in r. scapula.

Violent backache during menstruation.

[32] **Upper Limbs.** Stitches and tearing pain in r. shoulder and wrist.

Tearing, cramp-like pain in tip of l. shoulder; in scaleni muscles on l. side of neck, as if pulled by pincers.

Tearing, jerking in r. arm.

Upper arms as far as elbow fall asleep.

Tearing in palm of l. hand, unable to double fingers.

Fine stitches in index finger.
Tearing in r. little finger, it seems dead.
[33] Lower Limbs.   Tensive drawing in hips extending to nates.
Sticking in r. hip extending to groin; in middle toes of
r. foot; in r. heel.
Stitches: in thighs; in left ankle, when walking; as if
sprained; in r. heel.
Spasmodic sticking beneath bend of r. knee, hot face and
chilliness.
Cramp in calves at night during sleep.
[36] Rest. Position. Motion.   Lying down: tickling in larynx.
Obliged to remain lying: on account of pain in uterus.
Stooping: vertigo.
[37] Sleep.   Sleep restless, starting and crying out.
Dreams: lascivious; disgusting.
[38] Time.   Morning: nausea.
Evening: confusion in head with nausea; burning in l.
temple; sticking above r. eyebrow.
Night: toothache $<$; tickling in larynx $<$; cramp in calves.
[40] Fever.   Coldness, shaking in bed, cold, blue hands and nails.
[41] Attacks. Periodicity.   Ten times in one hour: urging to
urinate.
[42] Locality and Direction.   Right: sticking headache; transient sticking above eyebrow; stitches in side of middle
of nose; sticking side of umbilicus; cutting between
umbilicus and groin; transient pain in scapula; stitches
and tearing pain in shoulder; tearing, jerking in arm;
tearing in little finger; sticking in hip, in toes, in heel;
spasmodic sticking beneath bend of knee.
Left: burning in temple and eyeball; dull stitches in ear;
side of face red and hot; cheek glowing; stitches between seventh and eighth rib; tearing, cramp-like pain
in tip of shoulder, in muscles of side of neck; tearing in
palm of hand.
Right then left: headache.
[43] Sensations.   As though some one was poking him with
finger, in various parts of body, especially in diaphragm,
so painful he awoke and clenched his teeth; as of a ball
twisting in epigastric region; as though something living was moving about beneath hypochondrium; sticking as with two pins to r. of umbilicus; as from a knife
between umbilicus and r. groin; as if a substance would
come out of rectum and genitals; pain as from suppuration in middle of chest; neck as if pulled with pincers;
itching as from fleas.
Pain: in decayed teeth; in throat; in uterus; in small of
back; through back and chest.
Violent pain: in back.

Tearing pain: in r. shoulder and wrist; in palm of l. hand;
  in r. little finger.
Tearing, throbbing pain: in forehead and vertex.
Tearing, cramp-like pain: in tip of l. shoulder; in scaleni
  muscles on l. side of neck.
Throbbing, jerking pain: in middle of chest.
Sticking pain: on r. side of head; in epigastric region; to
  r. of umbilicus; in r. hip to groin; in middle toes of r.
  foot.
Jerking, tearing pain: in occiput; in r. arm.
Sticking, crawling: in nose, extending to eyebrows; in r.
  heel.
Spasmodic sticking: beneath bend of r. knee.
Stitches: in r. side of middle of nose; in l. side of abdomen;
  in region of uterus and genitals; behind sternum and
  beneath l. seventh and eighth ribs, in r. shoulder and
  wrist, in thighs; in l. ankle; in r. heel.
Fine stitches: in index finger.
Burning pain: in l. temple; in l. eyeball.
Transient stitching: above r. eyebrow.
Transient pain: in r. scapula.
Dull stitches: in l. ear.
Burning: on skin.
Headache: in r. side, then in left.
Cramp: in calves.
Twisting: as of a ball in epigastric region.
Pressing and dragging: towards rectum and genitals.
Tensive drawing: in hips.
Pressure: in temples and forehead.
Violent tickling: in larynx.
Scraping and tickling: in throat.
Dryness: of mouth.
Confusion: of head.
Twitching: in upper lids.
Trembling: of whole body.
Itching: on legs.
" **Skin.** Itching: as from fleas; violent on legs during menses,
  with burning after scratching, in bed.
" **Relations.** Compare: *Crocus* and *Thuja* (movements as of
  something alive in abdomen); *Tereb.* (urinary symp-
  tons); *Ignat.* (cough < lying down and in evening);
  Sulphur (psora).

IODOFORMUM.

Iodoform. *CHI*₃

Provings by Underwood and Haines. See Allen's Encyclopedia, vol. 5, p. 116.
CLINICAL AUTHORITIES.—*Sphacelous chancre*, Windelband, B. J. H., vol. 36, p. 367.

[1] **Mind.** Feels happy and elated.
[2] **Sensorium.** Confusion of head, with slight nausea.
 Head feels as if he had been intoxicated the day previous.
[3] **Inner Head.** Dull pain in forehead, with shooting in r. ear; < coming down stairs.
 Sharp, neuralgic pains in forehead, < stooping.
 Dull, pressing pain in both temples, following the pain in r. maxillary bone; temples felt as if something heavy was pressing on them.
 Sharp, neuralgic pain in temples, < r. side, extending to back of head, behind ears.
 Stitches in temples.
 Stitch pain in r. side of head.
 Heavy feeling in head, and a dull aching in top of head.
 Stitching pains in head.
 Head felt heavy, as if he could not lift it from pillow.
 Headache on awakening.
[4] **Outer Head.** Violent itching of occiput.
[5] **Sight and Eyes.** Eyes sensitive to light.
 Objects appear tesselated, red.
 Pain in eyes; eyes bloodshot.
 Smarting, burning, stinging in eyes.
 Right eye felt sore and as if bruised.
[6] **Hearing and Ears.** Hearing dull; must be spoken to quite loudly.
 Ears feel full, dry and feverish.
 Shooting in r. ear.
 Stitches in r. ear.
 Neuralgic pain in l. ear.
[7] **Smell and Nose.** Sensation as of smelling fumes of Iodine.
 Peculiar smell, like the odor arising from decaying leaves in a swamp.
 Membrane of nose feels full and dry; constant snuffing, yet no discharge.
[8] **Upper Face.** Dull pain in malar bones.

Drawing and pressing in malar bone.

⁹ Lower Face. Feeling of stiffness in zygomatic muscles.

Slight pain in zygomatic muscles, < from motion and bending forward.

Dryness and stinging of lips.

Dull aching, increasing to a heavy pain, like something pressing heavily in r. lower maxillary bone.

¹⁰ Teeth and Gums. Teeth feel sore and as if too long.

Toothache; pain leaving teeth and going quickly to temples.

Sharp pains in upper teeth.

I I Toothache in decayed teeth.

¹¹ Taste and Tongue. Metallic taste in mouth.

¹³ Throat. Dryness of throat and lips.

Dryness of throat, with rawness on swallowing; with bitter taste.

Stitch pain in r. side of throat.

¹⁶ Hiccough, Belching, Nausea and Vomiting. I I Nausea.

¹⁹ Abdomen. Rumbling in bowels.

Flatulent colic.

I I Cutting pain in bowels.

Feeling of warmth in bowels and rectum, with slight nausea and desire for stool.

Sharp cutting in r. inguinal region, with desire for stool.

Sore pain in r. inguinal region.

²⁰ Stool and Rectum. Desire for stool with cutting in r. inguinal region.

Desire as for a liquid stool.

Bowels not moved as usual; anus felt as if drawn up into rectum.

²¹ Urinary Organs. Urine very yellow and smelling like saffron tea.

²⁶ Respiration. Felt as if something heavy was resting on chest, preventing free expansion; after half an hour less intense, and appeared to diffuse itself to extremities.

Felt as though smothering; room felt too close, although freely ventilated.

²⁷ Cough. Cough from dryness of throat.

Cough and wheezing from mucus in throat, going to bed.

²⁸ Inner Chest and Lungs. Chest feels sore when taking a long breath.

Dull sore pain in apex of r. lung; on breathing lung felt as though two ulcerated surfaces were in contact.

Both lungs felt as if a heavy cold had settled there.

Severe pain concentrated in l. breast, a little to right of nipple; at first felt as if a deep ulcer had formed there, then became like a hand grasping base of heart; aching in l. breast at times, < night.

Sharp pain in r. chest.

Stitch in r. chest, through to angle of shoulder blade.

⁹⁰ Heart, Pulse and Circulation. Occasional stitches through heart.

³¹ Neck and Back. Back of neck sore as if bruised.

Sharp pain in angle of shoulder blade.

Pain in back along spine.

Spine feels sore, does not wish it touched.

Pain along r. side of dorsal vertebræ.

Continued pains in lumbar region, with weakness when straining.

³² Upper Limbs. Stitching pain in l. arm and shoulder.

Severe aching in l. humerus; muscles around bone feel as if severely bruised ; < from touch.

Pain in course of median nerve of l. arm.

Sharp pains in nerves of l. arm and back.

Rheumatic pain in r. arm, < when using it.

Pain in l. elbow.

Sharp pain in nerves of l. hand.

³³ Lower Limbs. Rheumatism in flexor muscles of legs.

Pain along course of l. crural nerve.

Weakness of knees when going up stairs.

Weakness and pain in knees, < standing.

Pain in inside of knees.

Neuralgic pain in l. knee.

Rheumatic pain in both gastrocnemii.

Cutting pain in l. ankle, when walking in open air.

Pain in l. foot, < walking.

Stitch pain in r. instep.

³⁴ Limbs in General. Left arm and leg pain as if bruised; as pain increases muscles feel as if ulcerated.

Severe pain in l. arm and leg, < at lower half of tibia and fibula, extending into foot.

³⁵ Rest. Position. Motion. Pain renewed in bed: r. side of head, r. shoulder, r. arm, hand and fingers, thigh, leg, foot and toes.

Stooping: neuralgic pain in forehead <.

Bending forwards: pain in zygomatic muscles.

Standing: weakness and pain in knees <.

Motion: pain in zygomatic muscles <; perspires easily.

When using r. arm: rheumatic pain <.

Coming down stairs: dull pain in forehead and shooting in ear <.

Going up stairs: weakness of knees.

Going to bed: cough and wheezing from mucus.

Walking: cutting pain in l. ankle; pain in l. foot.

³⁶ Nerves. Jerks and shocks in nerves when trying to sleep.

Susceptible to the heat of the weather.

Feeling of faintness.

Pain seems to sharply define course of nerves.

Neuralgic pains in various parts of body.

Neuralgic pains flying all over him at times.

⁷ Sleep. Very drowsy.

Slept soundly until 1.30 A.M., then awakened suddenly; restless and unable to sleep any more till 4.30; then slept about an hour and a half, being partially conscious, and then followed a deep, heavy sleep; on awaking it seemed as though he could not get aroused.

Wakefulness.

Restless sleep, tossing, turning, full of dreams.

Dreams: confused; of accident.

⁸ Time. Night: aching in l. breast <.

1.30 A.M.: awakened suddenly, restless and unable to sleep until 4.30.

⁹ Temperature and Weather. Lays covers off the bed.

Open air: when walking, cutting pains in l. ankle.

Heat of weather: susceptible to.

⁴⁰ Fever. Shuddering after urination.

Heat, lays covers off the bed.

Perspiration on head.

Perspires easily from motion.

⁴¹ Attacks, Periodicity. At times: neuralgic pains flying all over him.

⁴² Locality and Direction. Right: pain in maxillary bone; pain in temple <; stitch pain in side of head; shooting in ear; stitches in ear; heavy pain in maxilla; stitch pain in r. side of throat; sharp cutting in inguinal region; sore pain in inguinal region; cutting in r. inguinal region; dull, sore pain in apex of lung; sharp pain in chest; stitch in chest; pain alongside of dorsal vertebræ; rheumatic pain in arm; stitch pain in instep.

Left: neuralgic pain in ear; severe pain in breast; aching in breast; stitching pain in arm and shoulder; severe aching in humerus; pain in course of median nerve of arm; sharp pain in nerves of arm; pain in elbow; sharp pain in nerves of hand; pain along course of crural nerve; neuralgic pain in knee; cutting pain in ankle; pain in foot; arm and leg pain as if bruised; severe pain in arm and leg.

⁴³ Sensations. Feels strangely.

Thinks he has taken a bad cold.

Fine, sharp pains all over.

Head feels as if he had been intoxicated the day previous; temples feel as if something heavy was pressing on them; head as if he could not lift it from pillow: r. eye felt sore as if bruised; sensation as of smelling fumes of

Iodine; as if something was pressing heavily on r. lower maxillary bone; teeth as if too long; anus felt as if drawn up into rectum; as if something heavy was resting on chest; felt as though smothering; on breathing lung felt as though two ulcerated surfaces were in contact; both lungs felt as if a heavy cold had been taken; breast felt as if a deep ulcer had formed there; as if a hand was grasping base of heart; base of neck sore as if bruised; muscles around 'bone feel as if severely bruised; l. arm and leg as if bruised; muscles of l. arm and leg feel as if ulcerated.

Pain: in r. maxillary bone; in eyes; in teeth extending to temples; in decayed teeth; in back along spine; along r. side of dorsal vertebræ; in lumbar region; in l. elbow; in course of median nerve of l. arm; along course of l. crural nerve; in knees; in inside of knees; in l. foot; in l. arm and leg.

Severe pain: concentrated in l. breast; in l. arm and leg.

Sharp cutting: in r. inguinal region.

Cutting pain: in bowels; in r. inguinal region; in pharynx; in l. ankle.

Sharp pain: in upper teeth; in r. chest; in angle of shoulder blade; in nerves of l. arm and back; in nerves of l. hand.

Shooting: in ear.

Sharp, neuralgic pains: in forehead; in temples, extending to back of head behind ears.

Stitches: in temples; in r. ear; in r. chest through to angle of shoulder blade; through heart.

Stitching pains: in head; in l. arm and shoulder.

Stitch-like pain: in r. side of head; in r. side of throat; in r. instep.

Severe aching in l. humerus.

Neuralgic pain: in l. ear; in l. knee.

Rheumatic pain: in r. arm; in flexor muscles of legs; in both gastrocnemii.

Aching in l. breast.

Drawing and pressing: in malar bones.

Dull, pressing pain: in both temples.

Smarting, burning, stinging: in eyes.

Dull pain: in forehead; in malar bones.

Sore pain: in r. inguinal region.

Heavy pain: in r. lower maxillary bone.

Slight pain: in zygomatic muscles.

Dull, sore pain: in apex of r. lung.

Dull aching: in top of head; in r. lower maxillary bone.

Sore feeling: in teeth; in chest; in base of neck; in spine.

Dryness and stinging: of lips.

Feeling of stiffness: in zygomatic muscles.
Weakness: in knees.
Rawness: of throat.
Dryness: of throat and lips.
Feeling of warmth: in bowels and rectum.
Heavy feeling: in head.
Violent itching: of occiput.

" **Tissues.** ∎Relieves pain of cancerous tumors, (locally).
∎Sphacelous chancre (locally).

" **Touch. Passive Motion. Injuries.** Touch: muscles around
bone feel as if severely bruised.
Pains renewed: when riding in cars.

" **Relations.** Antidoted by: *Hepar.*
Compare: *Iodum,* and the iodides; *Mercur.*

IODUM.

Iodine.   *The element.*

Obtained principally from the ashes of seaweeds.

Provings by Hahnemann, Jorg, Hering, Macfarlan, Robinson, etc.   See
Allen's Encyclopedia, vol. 5, p. 119.

CLINICAL AUTHORITIES.—*Mania,* Spooner, N. E. M. G., vol. 4, p. 452;
Inflammation of brain, Schmid, Rück. Kl. Erf., vol. 1, p. 126; *Headache,* Alley,
N. A. J. H., vol. 7, p 395; *Acute hydrocephalus of scrofulous children,* Windelband,
B. J. H., vol. 36, p. 366; *Deafness,* Hughes, Raue's Rec., 1870, p. 119; *Catarrh of
Eustachian tubes,* Lobeth, Rück. Kl. Erf., vol. 1, p. 365; *Chronic nasal catarrh,*
Rosenberg, Rück. Kl. Erf., vol. 5, p. 166; *Eruption on nose,* Rosenberg, Rück. Kl.
Erf., vol. 5, p. 172; *Facial paralysis,* Chaffee, Raue's Rec., 1874, p. 271; *Ptyalism,*
Trinks, Rück. Kl. Erf., vol. 2, p. 120; *Diphtheria,* Goldman, Hirsch, Oehme's
Monog., p. 39; *Jaundice,* Hartmann, Rück. Kl. Erf., vol. 1, p. 696; *Dudgeon's*
B. J. H., vol. 22, p. 357; Moore, Times Retros., vol. 2, p. 170; *Affections of pan-
creas,* Reil, Rück. Kl. Erf., vol. 5, p. 331; *Tabes mesenterica,* Hale, N. E. M. G.,
vol. 10, p. 191; *Tuberculosis mesenterica,* Alvarez, T. H. M. S. Pa., 1880, p. 269;
Diarrhœa, Preston, Hom. Phys., vol. 7, p. 340; *Morning diarrhœa,* Jacobi, B. J. H.,
vol. 36, p. 366; *Urœmia,* Kafka, Raue's Rec., 1872, p. 168; *Chancre,* Gollman,
Rück. Kl. Erf., vol. 5, p. 559; *Hydrocele,* Black, Rück. Kl. Erf., vol. 2, p. 214;
Affection of testicles, Schwarze, Rück. Kl. Erf., vol. 2, p. 207; *Syphilitic affections,*
Lobeth, Rück. Kl. Erf., vol. 2, p. 120; *Galactorrhœa,* Selfridge, Hom. Obs., vol. 4,
p. 396; *Ovaritis,* Martin, Raue's Rec., 1874, p. 228; *Ovarian cyst,* Baldwin, Trans.
World's Hom. Con., 1876, p. 676; *Menorrhagia,* Sybel, Rück. Kl. Erf., vol. 5, p.
591; *Leucorrhœa,* Mauro, Rück. Kl. Erf., vol. 2, p. 363; *Spasm of glottis,* Dunham,
Raue's Rec., 1873, p. 90; *Membranous laryngitis,* Schlosser, N. A. J. H., vol. 7, p.
236; Sybel, Rück. Kl. Erf., vol. 5, p. 781; *Bronchitis,* Berridge, Raue's Rec., 1875,

p. 114; *Chronic bronchitis*, Schrön, Rück. Kl. Erf., vol. 3, p. 168; *Croup*, Hartmann,
Tietze, Rück. Kl. Erf., vol. 3, p. 132; (inhalation), Drake, N. A. J. H., vol.
10, p. 296; Koch, B. J. H., vol. 5, p. 297; Arnold, N. A. J. H., vol. 7, p. 236; Elb,
B. J. H., vol. 10, p. 537; Elb, Trinks, Fiedler, Rück. Kl. Erf., vol. 5, p. 758;
Hirsch, Rück. Kl. Erf., vol. 5, p. 240; *Membranous croup*, Bradford, T. H. M. Soc.
Pa., 1874, p. 350; *Cough*, Elb, Gross, Rück. Kl. Erf., vol. 3, p. 16; Miller, Rück.
Kl. Erf., vol. 5, p. 840; Lord, B. J. H., vol. 27, p. 314; Hirschel, B. J. H., vol. 31,
p. 242; Berridge, Hah. Mo., vol. 10, p. 112; *Whooping cough*, Syrbius, Rück. Kl.
Erf., vol. 3, p. 79; A. R., Rück. Kl. Erf., vol. 5, p. 720; *Asthma* (2 cases), Frank,
N. A. J. H., vol. 8, p. 96; *Tuberculosis*, Loebthal, Rück. Kl. Erf., vol. 3, p. 370;
Heart disease, Rockwith, Raue's Rec., 1872, p. 125; *Pneumonia*, Krummacher,
B. J. H., vol. 34, p. 161; (2 cases), De Gersdorff, N. E. M. G., vol. 1, p. 30; *Goitre*
(6 cases), Tietze, Kidd, Schepens, Trans. H. M. Soc. Pa., 1883, p. 200-3; Schepens
Raue's Rec., 1875, p. 88; Loebthal, Tietze, Gauwerky, Rück. Kl. Erf., vol. 4, p.
379; Mouremans, B. J. H., vol. 32, p. 720; *Chronic hydrarthrosis of knee joint*, Holt,
B. J. H., vol. 24, p. 184; *Scrofulous inflammation of knee*, Knorre, Griesselich, Rück.
Kl. Erf., vol. 3, p. 582; *Epilepsy*, Thompson, Raue's Rec., 1874, p. 268; *Scarlet
fever*, Helfrich, Rück. Kl. Erf., vol. 4, p. 51; *Small-pox*, Schmid, Rück. Kl. Erf.,
vol. 4, p. 112; Schmid, B. J. H., vol. 35, p. 154; *Gout*, Knorre, Rück. Kl. Erf., vol.
3, p. 51; *Primary syphilis*, Träger, Windelband, B. J. H., vol. 36, p. 365; *Syphilis*,
Guillemin, N. A. J. H., vol. 21, p. 425; *Serous cysts and dropsies* (17 cases), cured
by injection, Jousset, B. J. H., vol. 16, p. 259.

¹ **Mind.** ▮Feeling as of having forgotten something and does
not know what.

Fixed, immovable thoughts.

▮Must keep in motion day and night, brain felt as if it
was stirred up, felt as if going crazy.

Restless, inclined to move about, not permitting to sit or
sleep; thought she could tear everything to pieces.

▮Melancholy mood, low spirited.

▮Despondency, with disposition to weep.

Apprehends an accident from every trifle.

▮Fear of evil, with overcarefulness.

Fear and anxiety, shuns even the doctor.

▮Mind very sensitive during digestion, felt like crying.

▮Irritability and sensitiveness.

Cross, with excessive nervous excitability.

▮Excessive kind of impatience, she is running about all the
time and never sits down or sleeps at night.

▮Consequences of amorousness.

▮At night, especially when thinking of real or imaginary
wrongs, heart palpitates "like lightning," pulsations
being felt also at pit of stomach and in petrous portion of temporal bone, being especially violent in
latter locality; the violent palpitation and accompanying arterial excitement drives him out of bed; by use
of cold baths and friction obtains temporary relief; at
times most terrible thoughts take possession of him, and

he hardly dares go home for fear of doing some dreadful deed; on one occasion was seized with an* almost irresistible impulse to murder a woman who was acting as a guide for him, he having lost his way; these attacks of mania come on at most unexpected times; troubles all < by quiet and meditation; must be constantly in action, in some laborious occupation. θMania.

³ **Sensorium.** ⵏⵏConfusion of head, with great aversion to earnest work.

∎Vertigo: only on l. side, < from stooping; weakness in morning; with throbbing headache; very weak and tremulous; rising aggravates it, and produces faintness; with throbbing all over body; tremor at heart and fainting, < after just rising from a seat or bed, or on sitting or lying down after slight exercise; very sickly look of patient.

∎Goitre; hypertrophy of l. ventricle, with great congestions to head and face; hysteria and nervousness. θVertigo.

³ **Inner Head.** ⵏⵏSharp pressive pain in upper part of l. side of forehead.

∎Headache: l. side and top; as if a tape or band was tightly drawn around head; so violent it almost makes him crazy; with paralytic feeling of arms.

∎Pressure on a small spot above root of nose.

∎Pressive pains in vertex.

∎Congestions to and pulsations in head.

ⵏⵏThrobbing in head at every motion; < in warm air.

∎Brain feels as if stirred around with a spoon; must keep in motion day and night.

Violent aching at base of occiput, in afternoon.

∎Persistent, annoying, but not very violent headache; head feels heavy, as though a foreign substance was inside of brain, < by fatigue; oppressive, dull feeling, inclining head to seek a support.

∎Chronic headache; dizziness on active exertion; carelessly loquacious; languid, uneasy, and of fitful humor.

∎Chronic congestive headache, in old people with dark hair and eyes.

Headache <: in warm air; when riding a long time in a carriage; from walking fast.

∎During course of acute articular rheumatism inflammation in hands subsided and brain symptoms developed; became delirious and very restless, sat up in bed and then threw himself upon it.

ⵏⵏCholera encephalitica.

∎Acute hydrocephalus of scrofulous children.

Atrophy of brain; apoplexy.

⁴ **Outer Head.** Falling off of hair.

❘Nose runs a clear stream, hot fever, no appetite, hot, dry skin all day long, creepy sensation, face fiery red, pain in occiput and temples, teeth sticky with yellow phlegm.

❙❙Nasal catarrh thin, excoriating.

❙Ulceration of Schneiderian membrane; great fetor.

❙Small scab in r. nostril.

❙Small yellow scurf at each nostril and concha.

❙Chronic fetid discharge from nose; nose painful and swollen.

❙Large discharge of yellow mucus from nose.

❙Hard and red condition of mucous surfaces; scrofulous subjects; enlargement of cervical and subcutaneous glands. θNasal catarrh.

❙Nose bleeding.

⁸ **Upper Face.** Face: pale or alternately red; sallow, distressed; yellowish, or greenish; pale yellow or soon changing to brown.

Brown color of face, and copious and papescent stools; seems to be > after eating.

❙Coldness of face in very fleshy children.

❙Convulsive twitchings of facial muscles.

❙❙Facial paralysis following reduction of goitre.

❙Red, burning spot on nose; under eyes; itching protuberance on nose.

⁹ **Lower Face.** ❙Bluish lips, swelling of superficial veins.

❙Lips peel off.

❙❙Suppurating ulcer on l. cheek.

❙Swelling of submaxillary glands.

Pain from inner canthus to articulation of jaw.

¹⁰ **Teeth and Gums.** ❙Teeth yellow, covered with much mucus in morning, and more easily blunted than usual by vegetable acids.

❙Toothache, gums swollen and bleeding.

❙Little blisters form on gums.

❙Gums puffed, red, inflamed, painful to touch, bleed easily.

❙Softening and bleeding of gums.

❙❙Absorption of gums and alveolar processes.

¹¹ **Taste and Tongue.** Taste: salty; sourish; sweetish; on tip of tongue.

Soapy taste.

Tongue: dry; brown and dry; thickly coated; brown in centre, white at edges.

❙❙Tongue hypertrophied, painful, nodular or fissured.

¹² **Inner Mouth.** ❙Mouth filled with mucus on awaking in morning, with putrid taste, not > by washing mouth.

❙❙Increase of saliva; mercurial salivation.

❙Offensive odor from mouth.

\ ‖Aphthous ulcers in mouth with putrid smell; profuse
fetid ptyalism.

‖Gums red and swollen, receding from teeth, bleeding
slightly; small ash colored, painful ulcers; abuse of
mercury.

‖Croupous inflammation of pharynx, affecting also tonsils and softened gums; thick, grayish white deposit;
difficult deglutition; ptyalism; very offensive odor from
mouth.

‖Thick, brown, croup-like exudation in mouth and fauces.

Glands on inside of cheeks intensely painful as though he
had sharp vinegar in the mouth.

‖‖Discharge of mucus from posterior nares.

¹³·**Throat.** ‖Swelling and elongation of uvula.

‖Deglutition: so difficult that a considerable pause is required between each act; impeded from ulceration of
œsophagus.

‖Ulcers in throat, with swelling of glands of neck.

‖Mercurial cachexia; salivation and ulcers in the throat.

‖Follicular catarrh with ulceration.

‖Inflammation of throat, with burning pain.

‖Early stage of diphtheria; much glandular irritation;
disease threatens to attack larynx; formation of speck;
or patches of exudation, with sore throat; enlargement
of tonsils and of glands of neck; disinclination for food;
difficulty of breathing; cough and alteration of voice.

‖Velum palatinum and tonsils covered with thick, grayish white exudate; much pain in throat, painful swallowing; salivation; strong fetor oris. θDiphtheritis.

‖‖Pain in œsophagus increased by pressure.

‖Inflammation and ulceration of œsophagus.

¹⁴ **Appetite, Thirst. Desires, Aversions.** ‖Remarkable and
continued increase of appetite.

‖‖Suffers from hunger, must eat every few hours; gets
anxious and worried if he does not eat; feels > after
eating.

‖Eats too often and too much; loses flesh all the while.

‖‖Great longing for food, about 11 A.M.; can scarcely wait
for his meals.

‖‖Ravenous hunger, cannot be satisfied.

‖Alternate canine hunger and want of appetite.

‖‖Appetite for meat.

‖Thirst; desire for spirituous liquors.

¹⁵ **Eating and Drinking.** ‖Fasting causes pain in chest.

‖‖Most symptoms are better after eating.

‖‖Food distresses her.

Spasmodic pains in stomach > by eating.

¹⁶ **Hiccough, Belching, Nausea and Vomiting.** ‖‖Hiccough.

❚❚Empty eructations from morning till evening, as if every
  particle of food was turned into air.
❚Sour eructations, with burning therefrom.
❚Heartburn, after heavy food.
❚Qualmishness, nausea, with spasmodic pain in stomach.
❚Vomiting: of bile, with violent colic; of milk; first
  water, then food; of saltish tasting, oily or greasy sub-
  stances.
❚Violent vomiting renewed by eating.
¹⁷ **Scrobiculum and Stomach.** ❚Tenderness of epigastrium;
  pulsations in pit of stomach.
Spasmodic pains in stomach, renewed by eating.
❚❚Pains in stomach, gnawing or corroding, > after eating.
❚Dyspepsia with great weakness and loss of energy.
❚Gastric derangement, with constipation.
¹⁸ **Hypochondria.** ❚Region of liver sore to pressure.
❚Jaundice with much pain in liver through to shoulder-
  blade, no appetite, constant nausea; sluggish, clay colored stools, porter colored urine, debility, emaciation;
  skin brownish yellow; tenderness about hepatic region.
❚Pain in hepatic region, loss of appetite, emaciation, excessive weakness, diarrhœa; pressure and stitches in
  hepatic region, painful to touch.   θCirrhotic liver.
❚Jaundice: dirty, yellowish skin; great emaciation; depressed, irritable mood; yellow, almost dark brown color
  of face; thickly coated tongue; great thirst; nausea;
  constipation alternating with white diarrhœic stools;
  dark, greenish yellow, corroding urine; after abuse of
  mercury; in organic lesions of liver; dyscratic states of
  system accompanied by hectic fever.
❚Eyes, skin and nails completely jaundiced; nausea and
  vomiting after eating almost any kind of food; intense
  canine hunger; every third day attacks of gastrodynia;
  frequent eructations; heartburn; distension of stomach;
  pain when pressing on epigastrium; pain in r. hypochondrium; constipation; urine scanty, dark and turbid;
  menses absent six months.   θChronic jaundice.
❚Swelling and hypertrophy of liver.
❚❚Left hypochondriac region hard and acutely painful to
  pressure; enlarged spleen after intermittent.
❚Pressure in region of stomach, with much empty belching, occasionally vomiting of small quantity of tough,
  sour mucus; no actual pyrosis; constipation; ptyalism,
  constant expectoration; tongue moist, with mucous
  streak at sides; great thirst; appetite appeased by
  smallest quantity of food; urine scanty, brown; sallow
  face; depressed, irritable; constant profuse sweat; from
  pit of stomach to navel and in a corresponding region

in back, sensitiveness to pressure; pancreas enlarged; abdominal pulsations. *θ*Chronic inflammation of pancreas.

[19] **Abdomen.** ❚Swelling and distension, or emaciation and sinking in of abdomen.

❚Pulsations in abdomen; throbbing of abdominal aorta.

❚Incarceration of flatus in l. side of abdomen.

❚❚Rumbling in abdomen with gnawing hunger.

❚Swelling of mesenteric glands.

❚Marked irritability of mind; exceedingly cross, screamed in anger when simply looked at, talked to, or touched; large, tumid, doughy abdomen; loss of appetite; emaciation; diarrhœa, with copious, slimy, fetid stools. *θ*Tabes mesenterica.

❚Tabes mesenterica, with rapid emaciation, night sweats, slow fever, dry laryngeal cough and diarrhœa.

❚Inflammation and swelling of mesenteric glands, with bloating and distension of abdomen, which does not permit one to lie down; painful pressure and tension in abdomen, with incarceration of gas in l. side, < after eating; stools in beginning hard, knotty and dark; then alternate constipation and diarrhœa and finally profuse, frothy, bloody, even purulent diarrhœa, with itching and burning in anus, especially at night; ptyalism, constriction of throat, ulcers in mouth and putrid breath; constant and tormenting thirst with canine hunger, which cannot be satisfied; child wants to eat all the time; eats a large quantity and frequently without indigestion, yet becomes more and more emaciated; occasionally canine hunger is alternated with anorexia; burning heat after eating heavy food, with nausea or vomiting, pressure and hiccough. *θ*Tuberculosis mesenterica.

❚Swelling of inguinal glands.

[20] **Stool and Rectum.** ❚❚Brown color of face, with copious papescent stools.

❚Diarrhœa in morning; stools watery, foaming, whitish; pinching around navel and pressive pain in vertex.

❚Purulent stools, with cutting pains in intestines, nausea, vomiting and sour taste in mouth.

❚Stools: blackish, watery; brownish; frothy; bloody; whitish, mucous; thick, mucous; purulent; copious; fetid; of mucus and blood; whey-like; fatty.

❚Chronic diarrhœa of an exhausting character, with constant desire for change of place.

❚Morning: diarrhœa of scrofulous children.

❚Diarrhœa adiposa from pancreatic affections.

❚Summer complaint with swollen glands on neck.

⃗¹ Dysenteric mucous stools without feces.

∎ Discharges of thick mucus, or purulent matter; part of feces being retained.

∎ Constipation, alternating with diarrhœa.

∎ Stools hard, knotty, dark colored.

⃗ ⃗ Constipation with ineffectual urging > by drinking cold milk.

During stool: cutting pain in bowels; bearing down in genitals; painful pressure on vertex.

After stool: burning in anus; soreness in rectum; pressing in hypogastrium.

∎ Itching and burning of anus in evening.

∎ Piles protrude and burn; < from heat.

²¹ **Urinary Organs.** ∎ Uræmia; croupy exudation in mouth and fauces; tongue covered with thick brown, leather-like coating. θSenile hypertrophy and induration of prostate, stricture of urethra and ammonæmia.

∎ Bright's disease, with albuminous urine; much emaciation and debility.

⃗ ⃗ Obstinate retention of urine.

∎ Copious and frequent or involuntary micturition.

⃗ ⃗ Continued desire to urinate; nocturnal urination.

∎ Incontinence of urine in the aged.

∎ Urine: dark, thick, ammoniacal; dark yellowish green; acrid; milky; with a variegated cuticle on its surface; red and turbid.

²² **Male Sexual Organs.** ∎ Complete loss of sexual power; testicles atrophied.

∎ Bearing down, or twisting sensation in seminal cord.

∎ Aching, pressing or forcing pain in spermatic cords and testicles, after sexual dalliance.

∎ Testicles hypertrophied, with sexual excitement.

∎ Testicles swollen and hard, as large as hen's eggs, with pressure and tension extending into abdomen; on scrotum several swollen and inflamed openings, from which escapes a constant turbid, watery discharge; several of these openings penetrate through scrotum, others form canals running in different directions through skin.

∎ Painless swelling of testicles, with offensive sweat.

∎ Swelling and induration of testicles and prostate gland.

∎ After stool a milk-like fluid runs from urethra.

∎ Chancre with torpid, watery discharge.

∎ Hydrocele.

∎ Offensive sweating of genitals.

²³ **Female Sexual Organs.** ∎ Atrophy of ovaries and mammary glands, with sterility.

∎ Induration and swelling of uterus and ovaries.

∎ Pain commencing in r. ovary, passing down broad ligament to uterus.

∎Great sensitiveness of r. ovarian region during or after menses.

ⅠⅠPain in ovaries and back during menses.

∎Dull, pressing, wedge-like pain, as if a dull plug was driven from r. ovary toward womb.

∎Pain in lower part of abdomen; < l. ovarian region; comes on about 3 A.M.; > by motion and eating; likes acid things; l. ovary tender to pressure; pains before, during and after stool; leucorrhœa thick, yellow, burning; vertigo, staggering when walking; faint on getting up in morning; has to lie with head high on account of shortness of breath; menses too early; stoppage of urine, or it flows, stops, and flows again. θChronic ovaritis.

∎Abdomen as large as in pregnancy at sixth month from accumulation of fluid; rapid, irritable pulse; thirst; general prostration, able to sit up only part of day; loss of appetite; pain and tenderness in r. ovarian region, and fluid rapidly accumulating. θOvarian cyst.

∎Pressing, bearing down towards genitals; constipation; acrid leucorrhœa, corroding linen; dwindling and falling away of mammæ; strumous constitution. θOvarian dropsy.

∎Swelling and induration of uterus.

∎Uterine leucorrhœa with swelling of cervix, os uteri feeling hard and indurated; uterus enlarged; tendency to menorrhagia; corroding leucorrhœa, rendering thighs sore.

∎During course of inflammatory disease affecting uterus and surrounding parts; colliquative sweats; great emaciation and weakness; catarrh of chest, constantly growing more severe; sudden appearance of menses, very profuse and accompanied by severe abdominal pains, particularly in region of ovary.

∎Cancerous degeneration at neck of uterus.

∎Metrorrhagia: with acute pain in mammæ, or mammæ dwindle away and become flabby; at every stool, with cutting in abdomen, pain in loins and small of back; long lasting; after abuse of mercury. θCancer of womb.

∎Menses: sometimes too early, at others too late; premature, violent and copious.

∎Chronic menorrhagia in thin, delicate women, subject to corrosive leucorrhœa, with other indications of congested uterus and ovaries.

∎Premature and too copious menses, with goitre; dwindling away of breasts, and great weakness on going up stairs.

ⅠⅠViolent dysmenorrhœa with very scanty discharge.

❙Irregular menses; delaying eight days, with vertigo and palpitation of heart.

❙Chronic amenorrhœa of long standing.

Before menses: flashes of heat, with palpitation; tension and swelling of neck; abdominal pains.

During menses: pains in back and ovaries; lassitude; coughing up of blood; great weakness and loss of breath.

After menses: palpitation.

❙Thin, yellow leucorrhœa in scrofulous women, with induration and swelling of os uteri, and engorgement of vagina.

❙❙Chronic leucorrhœa most abundant at time of menses, rendering thighs sore and corroding linen.

❙Mammary hyperæsthesia.

❙❙Heaviness of mammæ, as if they would fall off.

❙Acute pain and soreness in mammæ, with metritis; cachectic state of system, with feeble pulse.

❙Bluish red nodosities, size of a hazel nut; in both mammæ; dry, black points at tips.

²⁴ Pregnancy. Parturition. Lactation. Abortion.

❙Excessive flow of very thin, watery milk; great weakness and rapid emaciation. *θ*Galactorrhœa.

❙Suppression of milk; atrophy and relaxation of mammæ.*

²⁵ Voice and Larynx. Trachea and Bronchia. ❙Voice: nasal, hoarse; has a deep, hoarse, rough sound, becoming continually deeper.

❙Hoarseness: in morning and insupportable tickling and tingling in larynx; lasts all day, phlegm in small quantities and tough, constant hemming and hawking.

❙Sensation of constriction (fulness or pressure) in larynx, with impeded deglution.

❙Tightness and constriction about larynx, with soreness and hoarseness.

❙Swelling and contraction of larynx.

❙❙Contraction and heat in larynx.

❙Spasm of glottis in rachitic children; cannot bear warmth.

❙Enlargement and induration of cervical and mesenteric glands; loss of appetite, utter indifference to food; scanty, high colored urine; clayey evacuations; emaciation; yellow skin; action of heart feeble and much increased by motion. *θ*Spasm of glottis.

❙Region of trachea smarting, accompanied by frequent lancinating pain.

❙Pains in larynx: with great hoarseness, or complete aphonia; with desire to cough; with discharge of hardened mucus.

---

* *Iodum* should not be given during lying-in period, except in high potencies. C. Hg.

∎Painful pressure mingled with stitches in region of
 larynx and sublingual glands, returning several times
 during day.

Roughness, painful pressure and stitches in larynx and
 pharynx, as if swollen; increased secretion of mucus in
 trachea; dry, short and hacking cough.

Soreness of throat and chest; wheezing; drawing pains in
 lungs; child grasps throat and chest with its hands.

∎Chronic laryngitis in scrofulous subjects; more or less
 hectic fever, especially serviceable when the trachea is
 implicated.

∎Intense membranous laryngitis; head and face hot; paroxysmal, dry, short, barking cough; respiration irregular, short and quick; active motion of alæ nasi.

∎Increased secretion of mucus in trachea; long lasting
 laryngeal catarrh.

Paralysis of throat.

∎Membranous croup, with wheezing and sawing respiration,
 dry, barking cough, especially in children with dark eyes
 and dark hair; child grasps throat with hand.

∎Violent attack of cough threatening suffocation, with
 whistling tone and great anguish. θMembranous croup.

∎Tracheal and bronchial croup, with tendency to torpor;
 extensive membrane; jerking breathing.

∎Cough is peculiar in that it has lost the metallic, loud
 timbre, so characteristic of croup, and has become muffled and indistinct; the more plastic the exudation, the
 more *Iodum* is indicated. θCroup.

∎Suffocating cough, can hardly get her breath for it; >
 by expectorating, sputa very scanty; weight and tightness at stomach after food; cough exhausts and chokes
 her, and causes retching and pain in forehead; < in a
 warm room; during day chilly, cold chills run up back;
 at night when in bed subjective dry heat, especially of
 head; bitter taste of solid food, not of drinks; burning
 pain below r. hip from back to front. θBronchitis.

∎Delicate constitutions, with quick pulse, tendency to
 bronchial and pulmonary congestion and hemorrhage;
 overgrown young people, with weak chest and dry
 cough, subject to spitting of blood and cardiac palpitation; swelling of cervical and bronchial glands; nocturnal sweats and progressive emaciation, notwithstanding
 good appetite and regular function of bowels; cough
 from every effort to expand chest; much dry cough;
 suffocative feeling; shortness of breath at least exertion.
 θBronchitis.

∎Chronic bronchitis in a scrofulous subject; dyspnœa at
 night, compelling him to sit up; raw sensation in l.

bronchus, particularly in morning; early in day cough dry, later transparent, occasionally grayish sputa; exacerbation after every cold.

²⁶ Respiration. ।।An effort to expand chest produced cough but no pain.

।Breath comes in wave-like expansions.

।Shortness of breath, palpitation and feeling of weakness on going up stairs.

।Tightness of respiration; out of breath from least exercise.

।Respiration, especially inspiration, difficult; constriction of throat prevents swallowing.

।Asthma, breathes heavily even when quiet.

।Rachitic children, swelling of bronchial glands; tightness and constriction about larynx, with soreness, hoarse voice; enlarged glands may cause paralysis of laryngeal, tracheal and bronchial nerves; mesenteric glands enlarged and indurated; tendency to marasmus; excellent appetite and yet grows thin, or indifferent to food; stools clayey; urine high colored, scanty; skin yellow; heart's action feeble and increased by any motion; unbearably irritable; well marked, painless goitre.

।Swelling and distension of abdomen; when assuming a wrong position he is threatened with suffocation (has to lie on back).

²⁷ Cough. ।।Dry morning cough, from tickling in larynx.

।Constant tickling, in trachea and under sternum, with inclination to cough.

।Unendurable tickling through whole chest, causing cough; during attack undulating inspiration; cough preceded by great anxiety and followed by depression; emaciation.

।Cough as from a feather in throat, especially in morning; sneezing; vomiting; stitches in chest and side, dyspnœa and great weakness. θLiver complaint.

।Annoying, tickling cough in phthisical persons.

।।Expansion of chest produces cough but no pain.

।।Dry cough, with stitches and burning in chest.

।Cough with copious collection of mucus in bronchi and inability to expectorate; moderate amount of fever.

।Dry, croupy cough, with titillation; sensation of soreness in larynx; barking, with gray or white salty, sweetish expectoration; shrill whistling and rattling in chest; sawing, hissing respiration; oppression; hoarseness, difficult speech; expectoration of tough mucus; soreness and pain extending to upper third of sternum.

।Cough moist but harsh as from tickling all over chest; wheezing, metallic cough; tough or slimy sputa; constriction of larynx; < in wet weather; < in morning.

।Cough often coming on in Fall, constant tickling in pit of

throat; < by expiration; frequent paroxysms of severe,
short, but continuous coughs, one rapidly following the
other, can scarcely utter a word; cough sounds as if
mucus was deep down in chest; expectoration of yellow
pieces, tasteless, or during day salty.

▮Cough caused and aggravated by tobacco; often accompanied by retching; could not lie down, sat bent forward.

Cough: after catching cold on damp day; > by expectoration; sputa very scanty; cough suffocating, can hardly
get breath; weight and tightness at stomach after food;
cough exhausts and chokes her, and causes retching and
pain in forehead; < in warm room; during day chilly,
cold chill runs up back; at night in bed subjective, dry
heat, especially of head; bitter taste of solid food, not of
drinks; burning pain below r. hip from back to front.

▮Chronic cough excited by pressure in throat, < at night,
in a very nervous, tall, thin and careworn old lady.

▮Dry, croupy cough; mucous membrane of larynx and
trachea dry; mucus hard and tough.

▮Croupy, hoarse cough, < in warm, wet weather.

▮Patients are weak, sallow, short of breath, emaciated and
have enormous appetites. θTussis convulsiva.

▮Great weakness with the cough.

During cough: tickling and burning pain in throat; oppression, pressing, burning and stitches in chest; rattling; anxiety; nausea; vomiting; sneezing.

▮Cough, with expectoration of large quantities of mucus,
frequently blood streaked.

▮Short, loose cough, with thick mucus and puriform expectoration, often bloody.

▮Cough < towards morning. θTuberculosis.

Dyspnœa, cough, palpitation and pains < by movement.

▮Expectoration: salty; sweetish; sourish; putrid; gray or
white; yellow; blood streaked.

⁸⁸ Inner Chest and Lungs. ❘❘A feeling of great weakness in
chest; can hardly walk up stairs.

❘❘Constriction of chest.

▮Sharp, quick, piercing pains in chest.

❘❘Itching: low down in lungs, behind sternum; causing
cough; extends through bronchi to nasal cavity.

▮Rattling in chest: yet nothing seems to loosen; with
roughness under sternum and oppression.

▮Tendency to bronchial and pulmonary congestion and
hemorrhage.

▮Violent chills, followed by fever and pain in chest; short,
anxious breathing, violent cough; lip and chin sore;
urine high colored and scanty; creaking, leathery noise
over middle and lower third of r. lung. θPneumonia.

∎Violent chill, followed by violent dry heat, pain in back
and r. side, from cough and dyspnœa; rust colored
sputum and fresh blood, crepitant râles, pulse 120, skin
hot and dry. θPneumonia.

∎Violent chill followed by great pressure on chest; respiration impeded, interrupted, imperfect and rapid;
pulse 110; urine scanty and red; frequent short cough,
with expectoration of tenacious, yellowish matter, occasionally tinged with blood; troublesome "cold sore"
on lips and nose; lower lobes of r. lung affected. θPneumonia.

∎Sensation of weakness in chest, with anxiety, oppression,
and burning, tearing, stabbing pains; sensation as if
something resisted expansion; cough, with dyspnœa
and blood streaked expectoration; also during third
stage, where slow suppuration sets in without marked
febrile symptoms in tuberculous patients, and causes a
slowly progressing hectic condition, entirely confined to
lungs. θCroupous pneumonia.

∎Continuous delirium; great dyspnœa; respiration 60;
unquenchable thirst, tongue dry; great prostration;
sputa gluey, rusty yellow, mingled with blood streaks,
is dislodged with difficulty and sticks fast to handkerchief. θPneumonia.

∎Pneumonia, when the disease localizes.

∎Pleuritic effusions.

∎Neck long and thin; clavicular region, particularly r. side,
sunken; empty percussion sound in upper portion of
chest, but especially on r. side; bronchial respiration on
r. side; chest flat, sunken; respiration short and ac-
complished only by lower portion of chest and diaphragm; strong impulse of heart; anæmic murmurs;
voice hoarse, toneless, weak; irritation in larynx; constant pressure and burning in throat; sensation of rawness in larynx and bronchial tubes extending into chest,
causing hawking and coughing; disagreeable tickling
in throat at night, causing severe and violent cough;
short, dry, irritating cough, < at night, followed in
morning by sweat; occasionally severe attacks of spasmodic cough, greatly prostrating patient, and causing
loss of breath and glowing heat in head and face; scanty,
tough, slimy expectoration, often streaked with blood;
pressure and heaviness on chest; loss of breath after
least exertion or talking. θConsumption.

∎Face pale, anxious, earthy; cheeks red, eyes languid,
appetite greatly impaired; pressure at stomach, particularly after eating; abdomen sunken; frequent colicky pains; diarrhœa, or scanty and delayed stool;

menses scanty and delayed; pulse small, frequent, particularly in evening; fever; every afternoon dry heat, thirst, confusion of head; restless and sleepless at night, sweat towards morning; skin dry, hot, pale, dirty gray in color; anæmia; great emaciation, lassitude and debility. θConsumption.

∎Voice weak, rough, hoarse; face pale; respiration impeded; pain in chest. θTuberculosis.

∎Tickling all over chest; tough, stringy, blood streaked sputa; hunger, yet emaciation; cannot bear a warm room. θPhthisis.

∎Phthisis pulmonalis, with constant tickling and inclination to cough, in trachea and under sternum; expectoration of transparent mucus streaked with blood; morning sweats; emaciation; wasting fever; rapid pulse; diarrhœa; amenorrhœa.

∎Emaciated almost to a skeleton; for several months has been compelled to stay in bed; decubitus; almost continual fever, remitting only for two or three hours in afternoon; profuse night sweats; continuous cough with copious expectoration. θConsumption.

∎For several years obstinate leucorrhœa, alternating with a cough which greatly reduced her strength and threatened to develop into consumption.

∎Advanced stage of tuberculosis, when glands and lymphatics are affected; much expectoration of blood, or even hemorrhages.

∎Swelling of cervical and bronchial glands.

²⁹ Heart, Pulse and Circulation. ∎Great præcordial anxiety, obliging constant change of position.

∎∎Sensation of weakness in heart.

∎Constant, heavy, oppressive pain, in region of heart.

∎Sharp, quick, piercing, and movable, but heavy, oppressive pain in region of heart.

∎∎Sensation as if heart was squeezed together.

∎Feeling as if heart was grasped by an iron hand.

∎∎Palpitation of heart: < from least exertion; with faintness.

∎∎Tumultuous, irregular or intermitting action of heart.

∎Cardiac action excessive. θExophthalmic goitre.

∎Pericarditis in complication with croupous pneumonia.

∎Mitral insufficiency and periodical attacks of pain about heart, following long fit of sickness with typhoid endocarditis; ventral dilatation of heart, with marked projection of l. second and third ribs; loss of strength; difficult breathing; violent palpitations.

∎Dilatation of heart, after scarlatina.

∎Darker color of skin, with sensation of heat; skin turns

brown, grows parchment-like, peels off, and shows
underneath the loosened scales a fatty transpiration;
thickening of epidermis; sudden turning of yellowish
color into brown, as if smoked; excessive weakness and
debility; muscular weakness and trembling; sadness
and depression of spirits; mental torpor; dulness and
pain in head; vertigo; nausea; violent, continuous
vomiting; violent, excruciating pain in stomach; constipation; frequent attacks of gastralgia; drawing and
pressing in region of kidneys; twitchings, convulsions;
epilepsy; paralysis; the formerly yellow face turns
brown; red hair turns to chestnut brown.   θAddison's
disease.

Pulse: large, hard and accelerated, with orgasm of blood
and beating in bloodvessels; rapid, but weak and
thread-like; small, very quick, irregular; weak, thread-
like; accelerated, by every slight exertion.

Extremely troublesome pulsations in larger arterial trunks.

Pulsation in arteries at every muscular effort.

Ebullition in chest and audible palpitation.

⁵⁰ Outer Chest. Burning stinging tension in integuments of
chest.

⁵¹ Neck and Back. Redness on neck and chest as if ecchymosed.

Yellow spots on neck.

Neck swells up when talking.

∎Swelling and induration of cervical glands.

∎Hard and red condition of mucous surfaces, scrofulous
subjects; enlargement of cervical and subcutaneous
glands.

∎Enlargement and induration of glands, cervical and
mesenteric; want of appetite; utter indifference to food;
scanty, high colored urine; clayey evacuations; emaciation; yellow skin; action of heart feebler and much <
by motion.

∎Gradual increase in size of neck, especially on r. side,
until it measured fourteen and a half inches over isth-
mus of thyroid body; soft and without any fluctuation.
θGoitre.

Marked increase of thyroid gland, which had been already
slightly enlarged; acute pain in gland upon pressure or
on slightest movement of head.

∎Non-lobulated tumor in anterior and median portion of
neck as large as a child's head; rosy red color heavy in
weight and of soft consistency; voice for past, two years
slightly rough, and respiration difficult, especially when
he lies on back.   θGoitre.

∎Hypertrophy of two lobes of thyroid gland; tumor becoming more swollen and painful at each return of
menses, which were irregular and painful.   θGoitre.

∎Sensation of constriction in goitre.

∎Goitre: recent and soft; with marked hardness; hard and nodulated.

ı ıLarge boil between scapulæ, with gangrene of legs.

Stitches in small of back; pains like rheumatism.

Pain in sacrum and coccyx.

∎Spinal complaints, with gressus vaccinus.

³³ Upper Limbs. ∎Swelling of axillary glands.

∎Hot, dark red, lymphatic swelling in r. axilla, size of a walnut, discharging a cheesy pus.

∎Weariness of arms, as if paralyzed, in morning, in bed.

∎Trembling of arms and hands.

∎Pain in bones of arm on which he lies at night.

ı ıSmall boil on posterior surface of r. upper arm.

ı ıTearing in l. elbow.

∎Pains in elbow.

∎Painful weakness in extensors.

ı ıSubsultus tendinum.

ı ıBack of l. hand painful, as if swollen, painful to pressure and when turning hand, not when closing fingers.

ı ıBrown discoloration on back of hand.

∎Sweating in palms of hands.

∎Coldness of hands and feet.

∎Fingers "go to sleep."

Round spot between thumb and index finger covered with two whitish vesicles.

³³ Lower Limbs. ∎Intermittent, sharp, tearing pains between l. hip and head of femur, < by moving joint; ear swellings; abuse of mercury.

ı ıJerking pain in legs each time after taking cold, following pressure in pit of stomach. *θ*Jaundice.

ı ıNumb feeling in thighs and legs.

∎Violent itching nettlerash on thigh and inside of l. knee.

Flat blister on knee looks as if full of bile.

∎After neglected injury, large, elastic and fluctuating swelling of knee; pale redness of skin upon which there are several very red, hot and painful spots; temperature at knee elevated; dull pain deep in knee-joint when lying quietly with leg stretched out, becoming very severe upon least motion or pressure; foot must be kept very quiet; febrile attacks; finally small opening over patella through which oozed laudable pus, later followed by a profuse, clear, yellow, serous discharge, particularly early in evening.

∎Knee greatly swollen, puffed and round on both sides; sensation of fluctuation; temperature elevated; pain when stretching leg or when attempting to stand; limps when attempting to walk and can only place tip of foot

upon floor; pressure upon patella causes great pain; no
pain during rest.

▮Hot, bright red, shining swelling of knee, with shooting.
stitches and burning; in several places, small, highly
inflamed openings through which oozes a watery,
bloody pus; least motion of body or foot, or least touch
or pressure upon swelling cause very severe pain.
θScrofulous inflammation.

▮Hot, bright red swelling of knee, with inflammation,
pricking and burning; < by touch or pressure.

▮White swelling of knee; dropsical swelling of knee joint.

▮Second and third stage; fistulous openings, discharging
a thin, watery ichor, and surrounded by pale, spongy
edges, which bleed easily; feverish; emaciation. θGo-
narthrocace.

▮Much swelling, with erratic tearing pains. θSynovitis.

▮Chronic hydrarthrosis of knee joint.

▮Violent itching nettlerash, particularly around knee; on
outer side of l. knee especially.

I ISubsultus tendinum of feet.

▮Œdematous swelling of feet.

▮Acrid, corrosive sweat of feet.

▮Painful corns.

³⁴ **Limbs in General.** Great weariness of arms and legs from
excessive debility.

Subsultus tendinum of both hands and feet.

▮Trembling of limbs.

▮Acute articular rheumatism, with violent pericarditis and
pleuro-pneumonia.

▮▮Chronic arthritic affections, with violent nightly pains
in joints, no swelling.

▮Subsultus tendinum of hands and feet; great drowsiness
and continual dreaming of eating, with great prostration
on rising from bed; picking of bedclothes and short,
dry cough.

▮Much coldness of hands and feet.

³⁵ **Rest. Position. Motion.** Rest: no pain in knee.

Lying down: < tremor at heart and fainting.

Lying quietly with leg stretched out: pain in knee.

Has to lie with head high on account of shortness of breath.

Pain in bones of arms on which he lies.

Has to lie on back: on account of swelling of abdomen.

When lying on back: respiration difficult.

Cannot lie down: on account of bloating and distension of
abdomen; on account of cough.

Sat up in bed, then threw himself upon it.

Able to sit up only part of day.

Is compelled to sit up: by dyspnœa.

Sitting: < tremor at heart and fainting; anxiety after mental labor >.

Stooping: < vertigo.

Hardly able to stand: chill two years old.

Attempting to stand: pain in knee <.

Head inclined to seek support: caused by oppressive, dull feeling in head.

Desire to change position continually.

Præcordial anxiety obliging constant change of position.

When assuming a wrong position he is threatened with suffocation.

Inclination to move about: not permitting one to eat or to sleep.

Grasps throat and chest with his hand.

Slightest movement of head: acute pain in thyroid gland.

Least motion: pain in knee <.

Least exertion: palpitation of heart <; accelerates pulse.

At every muscular effort: pulsations in arteries.

After slight exercise when lying down: tremor at heart and fainting <; out of breath.

Every motion: throbbing in head; increases heart's action.

Rising: < headache; produces faintness; tremor at heart and fainting <.

Rising from bed: great prostration.

When moving hip joint: pain <.

Stretching leg: pain in knee <.

When turning l. hand: painful.

Attempting to walk: knee causes limping; can only place tip of foot on floor.

Walking: vertigo, staggering.

Can hardly walk up stairs: weakness of chest.

Walking fast: < headache.

Active exertion: causes dizziness.

Running about, never sits down or sleeps at night.

Motion: > pain in lower part of abdomen; dyspnœa, cough, palpitation and pains <; action of heart feeble, much <.

Must keep in motion day and night.

Restless, inclined to move, not permitting her to sit or sleep.

Violent palpitations drive him out of bed.

³⁶ **Nerves.** ¹Excessive excitability; irritability and sensitiveness.

¹Restlessness, with inclination to move about, not permitting one to sit or to sleep.

¹¹Great weakness and loss of breath, on going up stairs.

¹Remarkable and unaccountable sense of weakness and loss of breath on going up stairs; leucorrhœa corroding the linen; food does not nourish or strengthen her.

¹Great debility; sweats, even from talking.

ㅣㅣTrembling of limbs or whole body.
❙Twitching of muscles.
❙Abdominal reflex chorea; the stomach, liver, pancreas, abdominal glands, being at fault.
❙Facial paralysis or epilepsy, following suppression of goitre.
³⁷ **Sleep.**   ❙Sleeplessness after midnight.
❙Restless sleep, with vivid or anxious dreams.
³⁸ **Time.**   Towards morning: cough <.
Morning: weakness; teeth yellow, covered with much mucus; much mucus in mouth; diarrhœa; faint on getting up; hoarseness, and tickling and tingling in larynx; raw sensation in l. bronchus; dry cough; cough as from a feather; cough moist but harsh; sweat following cough; weariness of arms; debilitating sweat.
From morning till evening: empty eructations.
3 A.M.: pain in lower part of abdomen.
11 A.M.: longs for food.
Early in day: dry cough.
During day: chilly; salty expectoration.
All day: hot, dry skin; hoarseness and tickling in larynx.
Afternoon: violent aching at base of occiput; for several hours fever remits.
Evening: sneezing; stoppage of nose; itching and burning of anus; pulse small and frequent; discharge from knee <.
Night: heart palpitates "like lightning;" pulsations felt at pit of stomach; watery, fluent coryza; burning and itching at anus; subjective dry heat; sweats; dyspnœa; chronic cough <; disagreeable tickling in throat; cough <; restless; sleepless; pain in bones of arms; pains in joints; cold feet; very profuse sweats.
After midnight: sleeplessness.
³⁹ **Temperature and Weather.**   Aggravation: warmth; wrapping up head; cannot bear hat on.
Amelioration: cold air; washing in cold water.
Rachitic children·cannot bear warmth.
Warm room: cough <; shaking chill.
Warm air: < throbbing in head.
Warm weather: great tendency to take cold.
External warmth: relaxed mammæ <.
Cannot bear warmth or a warm room.
Heat: < piles.
Inclination to uncover.
Open air: dry coryza becomes fluent.
Wet weather: cough <.
Damp day: caught cold, cough.
Drinking cold milk: constipation >.

IODUM. 226

Cold baths: < violent palpitations.
⁴⁰ **Fever.** Shaking chill, or chilliness, in a warm room.
Hands, nose, feet icy cold; cold feet the whole night.
Chill predominates, is cold most of the time.
∎Chill, frequently, alternating with heat.
∎Fever with dry skin, weak and rapid pulse, twitching of muscles, and more coldness than heat of skin.
∎Internal heat, with coldness of skin.
∣∣Flushes of heat; ebullitions and pulsations.
∣∣Heat or sweat, with inclination to uncover.
∎Burning heat of hands.
∎Quartan fever, with diarrhœa on days free from fever.
∎Sallow, distressed countenance. θIntermittent.
∎Left hypochondriac region hard and acutely painful to pressure. θIntermittent fever.
∎Intense pain in ileo-cæcal region; bloody, watery diarrhœa; great irritation of nervous system; picking at flocks; delirium. θTyphoid.
∎Palms of hands sweat continually.
∎Cold feet sweat easily; so acrid that it corrodes skin.
∎Debilitating, sour sweat in morning, with great weakness of limbs; much thirst.
∣∣Sweat with thirst.
∎Very profuse night sweat; profuse, cold, viscid sweat.
∎Profuse night sweats, with great emaciation and debility, and tendency to take cold, especially in warm weather.
⁴¹ **Attacks, Periodicity.** Frequent paroxysms of severe short but continuous coughs, one rapidly following the other.
Periodical attacks of pain about heart.
Occasional severe attacks of spasmodic cough.
Every time after taking cold: jerking pains in legs.
Every few hours: must eat.
For several hours in afternoon: fever remits.
Every afternoon: dry heat; thirst; confusion of head.
Several times during day: pressure in region of larynx.
Every third day: attacks of gastrodynia.
Menses delayed eight days.
At each return of menses: thyroid gland painful.
For several months: has been compelled to stay in bed.
Six months: menses absent.
Often in Fall: cough.
For several years: leucorrhœa alternating with cough.
⁴² **Locality and Direction.** Right: constant tearing pains around eye; small scab in nostril; pain in hypochondrium; pain in ovary; sensitiveness of ovarian region; tenderness and pain in ovarian region; burning pain below hip; creaking, leathery noise, over middle and lower third of lung; pain in side; lower lobes of lung

affected; clavical region sunken; empty percussion
sound on side of chest; bronchial respiration; increase
of size of neck; swelling of axilla; small boil on posterior surface of upper arm.
Left: vertigo on side; hypertrophy of ventricle; sharp,
pressive pain in upper part of side of forehead; headache on side; suppurating ulcer on cheek; hypochondriac region hard and acutely painful to pressure; incarceration of flatus in side of abdomen; pain in ovarian
region; ovary tender to pressure; raw sensation in
bronchus; marked projection of second and third ribs;
tearing in elbow; back of hand painful; sharp pain
between hip and head of femur; violent, itching nettlerash, inside of knee; outer side of knee nettlerash;
hypochondriac region painful to pressure and hard.
Hard boil on forearm near wrist.
From back to front: burning pain below r. hip.
[43] **Sensations.** Brain felt as if it was stirred up; as if going
crazy; as if a tape or band was tightly drawn around
head; brain feels as if stirred around with a spoon; as
though a foreign substance was inside of brain; like a
veil before eyes; pain in eyes as from excoriation; as if
alæ nasi were spread wide open; as though he had sharp
vinegar in mouth; as if every particle of food was
turned into air; as if a plug was driven from r. ovary
to womb; as if mammæ would fall off; pharynx as if
swollen; cough as from a feather in throat; as if something resisted expansion in chest; as if heart was
squeezed together; as if heart was grasped by an iron
hand; arm as if paralyzed; l. hand as if swollen;
blister on knee looks as if full of bile.
Pain: in eyes; in occiput and temples; from inner canthus to articulation of jaw; in throat; in œsophagus;
in chest; in liver through to shoulder blade; in hepatic
region; in r. hypochondrium; in r. ovary passing down
broad ligament to uterus; in ovaries and back during
menses; in lower part of abdomen; in l. ovarian region;
in r. ovarian region; in loins and small of back; in
larynx; in forehead; extending to upper third of
sternum; in r. side, about heart; in head; in sacrum
and coccyx; in bones of arm on which he lies; in elbows; in bones.
Violent, excruciating pain in stomach.
Intense pain: in ileo-cæcal region.
Acute pain: in mammæ; in thyroid gland.
Violent nightly pain: in joints.
Great anguish: with cough; præcordial.
Sharp. tearing pain: between l. hip and head of femur.

Constant tearing pain: around r. eye, passing backwards
from inner canthus to articulation of jaw.
Tearing: in l. elbow; in chest.
Lancinating pain: in region of trachea.
Sharp, quick, piercing pains: in chest; in region of heart.
Cutting pains: in intestines; in abdomen.
Erratic tearing: in knee.
Stabbing: in chest.
Shooting stitches: in knee.
Stitches: in hepatic region; in region of larynx; in region
of pharynx; in chest and side; in small of back.
Sharp, pressive pain: in upper part of side of forehead.
Throbbing pain: in head.
Burning pain: in throat; in chest; below r. hip.
Burning, stinging tension: in integuments of chest.
Corroding pains: in stomach.
Severe abdominal pain: in region of ovary.
Violent colic and colicky pains.
Drawing pains: in lungs; in region of kidneys.
Gnawing pains: in stomach.
Jerking pains: in legs.
Spasmodic pains: in stomach.
Forcing pain: in spermatic cord and testicles.
Pinching: around navel.
Pricking: in knee.
Dull, pressing, wedge-like pain: from ovary to womb.
Dull pain: deep in knee joint.
Pain like rheumatisms: in back.
Violent aching: at base of occiput.
Aching, pressing pain: in spermatic cords and testicles.
Pressive pains: in vertex.
Heavy, oppressive pain: in region of heart.
Painful pressure: in abdomen; in vertex; in region of
larynx; of pharynx.
Smarting: in eyes; in region of trachea.
Soreness: in rectum; of mammæ; about larynx; of
throat and chest; in larynx; extending to upper third
of sternum; of lip and chin.
Burning heat: of hands.
Glowing heat: in head and face.
Burning: in anus; in piles; in throat; in chest; in knee.
Heat: in larynx.
Bearing down: in genitals; in seminal cord.
Painfulness: of tongue; of ulcers on gums; in corns.
Painful weakness: of extensors.
Intense painfulness: of glands on inside of cheek.
Sensitiveness: of r. ovarian region.
Raw sensation: in l. bronchus; in larynx and bronchial
tubes to chest.

Tenderness: of epigastrium; about hepatic region.

Dull pressure in frontal sinuses.

Dulness: in head.

Pressure: on a small spot above root of nose; in hepatic region; in region of stomach; in testicles extending to abdomen; in throat; on chest; in region of kidneys; in pit of stomach.

Oppressive, dull feeling: in head; in chest; under sternum.

Heaviness: of both mammæ; on chest.

Confusion: of head.

Twisting sensation: in seminal cord.

Tightness: about larynx; at stomach.

Tension: in abdomen; in testicles; of neck.

Constriction: about larynx; of throat; of chest; in goitre.

Contraction: of larynx.

Throbbing: all over body; in head at every motion; of abdominal aorta.

Palpitation: felt at pit of stomach.

Pulsations: in pit of stomach; in abdomen.

Sensation of fluctuation: in knee.

Unendurable tickling: through whole chest.

Continual tickling: in middle of chest.

Tingling: in larynx.

Tickling: in larynx; in throat; in pit of throat.

Irritation: in larynx.

Roughness: under sternum.

Numb feeling: in thighs and legs.

Paralytic feeling: of arms.

Great weariness: of arms and legs.

Great weakness: in chest; in heart.

Weight: at stomach.

Creepy sensation: in skin.

Violent itching nettlerash on thigh and inside of l. knee.

Itching, stinging: in front part of septum narium; in protuberance on nose; of anus; low down in lungs behind sternum, extending to bronchi and nasal cavity; of scars.

" **Tissues.** Gradual or rapid emaciation, almost to a skeleton.

Atrophy of children, with inordinate appetite; restless; desires to change position continually; face yellow, or brownish and shrunken; copious and papescent stools; glands swollen and painless, especially mesenteric ones.

Marasmus with intolerable irritability, child will be approached by no one.

Scrofulosis with emaciation, in spite of necessity of eating every few hours; swelling and induration of glands, the whole of lymphatic system being involved; rachitic affections; inflammation of eyes and eyelids; otitis and otorrhœa; swelling of mesenteric glands; frequent catarrhs; bronchocele; scrofulous women with dwindling of and falling away of mammæ.

∎A colored child, two years old, with the face of an old man, dry skin, large head and stomach, very large genitals, thin arms and legs, is hardly able to stand, sits by preference out doors in the burning sun of the tropics; is always hungry; has a blood boil on l. forearm near the wrist; *Iodum* was followed by a fine eruption, resembling itch when the child began to improve and got well.

∎Low cachectic state of the system, with feeble pulse.

∎In strumous habits, if expectoration or leucorrhœal discharge corrode the linen.

Syphilis: mercurial cachexia; salivation; ulcers in throat; skin and muscles lax; nightly bone pain; very hard chronic buboes.

∎Arthritic affections.

∎∎Hypertrophy and induration of glands.

Inveterate cases of goitre; the harder they feel, and the more other symptoms are wanting, the better indicated.

∎Felons.

∎Bleeding ulcers, destitute of feeling; hard, spongy, and sensitive ulcers, with feeling of tenseness and soreness; pus copious, bloody, and corroding, or thin, watery, and yellow.

∎Very profuse suppuration; enormous quantities of pus with hectic.

"Touch. Passive Motion. Injuries. Touch: gums painful; hepatic region painful; knee <.

Pressure: < pain in œsophagus; region of liver sore; epigastrium painful; l. hypochondriac region very painful; from pit of stomach to navel and in corresponding region in back sensitiveness; l. ovary tender; causes acute pain in thyroid gland; back of l. hand painful; pain in knee <; on patella causes great pain; l. hychondriac region painful.

Friction: > violent palpitations.

When riding long time in open carriage.

After neglected injury: large swelling of knee.

" Skin. ∎Skin: rough; dry; dirty yellow; clammy; moist; cool.

Eruption: furfuraceous; humid; like scarlet rash; herpes; ringworm ; acne; urticaria; inveterate impetigo scrofulosa.

∎High fever with great weakness; for some days slight eruption, not distinctly characteristic; frequent attacks of anxiety and oppression of breathing, with faintness,

especially in night; weakness always increasing, so that
fatal paralysis of heart was apprehended; developed the
eruption.   θSmall-pox.

∎Scarlatina: ulcers in throat; glands swollen, suppurating;
everything appears bright blue to him in the distance.

Small, dry, red pimples on arms, chest and back.

∎Scars itch, break open, or pimples break out on them.

∎Tendency to papulæ, small boils and abscesses.

∎Nodosities.

∣∣Morbus maculosus.

Fungus articularis after measles.

Tertiary syphilis, with ulceration of skin.

⁴⁷ **Stages of Life, Constitution.** ∎∎Dark hair and eyes.

∎Overgrown boys with weak chest; aged persons.

∎∎Scrofulous diathesis.

∎∎Low cachectic condition with profound debility and
great emaciation.

Boy, æt. 6 months, affection of eyes; hydrocele.

Infant, æt. 10 months, early in life had marasmus; spasms
of glottis.

Boy, æt. 14 months, dark eyes, light hair, rickets; laryngismus stridulus.

Colored boy, æt. 2, old face and wise look; marasmus.

Girl, æt. 2½, vigorous constitution; membranous laryngitis.

Boy, æt. 4; diphtheria.

Boy, æt. 8, scrofulous; inflammation of knee.

Girl, æt. 10, scrofulous, had swollen submaxillary glands
for several months; diphtheritis.

Girl, æt. 10, scrofulous; croupous inflammation of pharynx.

Girl, æt. 11; inflammation of knee.

Girl, æt. 12, lymphatic temperament, fair complexion,
delicate constitution, general health feeble, and menses
not yet appeared, suffering one year; goitre.

Girl, æt. 12, during attack of rheumatism; threatened inflammation of brain.

Girl, æt. 16, bilious-lymphatic temperament, suffering one
year, since date of first menstruation; goitre.

Girl, æt. 18, slender form, after exposure on ice, while
skating; pneumonia.

Girl, æt. 18, brunette, features regular but pale, mild, peace-
ful disposition, almost phlegmatic, menses regular for
some years and of general good health; goitre.

Girl, æt. 20, after neglected injury; inflammation of knee.

Girl, æt. 20, large, thin, phthisical habits; threatened
tuberculosis.

Woman, æt. 20, after a long illness; heart disease.

Miss L., æt. 21; deafness.

Man, æt. 21, tailor, poor and ill nourished, lymphatic

temperament and scrofulous, suffering several months; goitre.

Woman, æt. 22, medium height, blue eyes, light auburn hair, sanguine-nervous temperament, predisposed to consumption; galactorrhœa.

Young man, lymphatic temperament, full habit, suffering two years; headache.

Young man, swollen nose, enlarged thyroid; chronic bronchitis.

Girl, æt. 22, of phthisical family; consumption.

Woman, æt. 25, married for three months, general health good, sudden attack; goitre.

Man, æt. 27, after muscular exertion and subsequent exposure to cold; pneumonia.

Man, slender, nervous-bilious temperament, of strong likes and dislikes; mania.

Woman, æt. 28, after being delivered of a healthy child, was found to be as large as at full term, from dropsical effusion; a month afterwards four and a half gallons of a thick, dark and highly albuminous fluid were removed by ordinary paracentesis; about a year afterwards, at seventh month of a second pregnancy, four and a half gallons of fluid were drawn off, and six weeks later a normal labor occurred, and again, in about three months, four gallons of fluid were removed by aspiration; the effusion, however, continued, and ovariotomy was believed to be the only remedy; ovarian cyst.

Pregnant woman, æt. 30; small-pox.

Man, æt. 32, small and weak, dark hair, mild disposition, works much in cold water; has suffered from cardiac and hemorrhoidal troubles; affection of testicles.

Man, æt. 34; pneumonia.

Woman, suffering for one and a half years; chronic jaundice.

Man, æt. 40, innkeeper; affection of pancreas.

Colored woman, æt. 42, suffered for twenty years; chronic ovaritis.

Woman, æt. 50, has suffered very much for several years; leucorrhœa.

Man, æt. 58, general health good, could not remember when tumor first came; goitre.

Man, æt. 58, suffering 15 years; goitre.

Man, æt. 62, six years ago had itch; inflammation of knee.

Man, æt. 64; jaundice.

Woman, æt. 70, two months ago caught cold on a damp day; bronchitis.

Woman, æt. 70, after catching cold; cough.

" Relations. Antidoted by: starch or wheat flour mixed

with water in case of large doses; small doses by: *Ant. tart., Arsen., Bellad., Camphor., Cinch. sulph., Cinchona, Coffea, Hepar, Opium, Phosphor., Spongia, Sulphur.*

It antidotes: *Mercur.*

Compatible: after *Mercur.*, after *Hepar* in croup, after *Arsen.; Acon., Argent. nitr., Calc. ostr., Merc. sol., Phosphor., Pulsat.* frequently follow well.

Compare: *Bromine, Cactus, Caustic., Conium, Digit., Kali bich., Phos. ac.*

Complementary: *Lycop.*

IPECACUANHA.

Ipecac.   *Rubiaceæ.*

A plant native to Brazil. The tincture is prepared from the dried and finely powdered root.

Provings by Hahnemann and his provers. See Allen's Encyclopedia, vol. 5, p. 137.

CLINICAL AUTHORITIES.—*Hypochondriasis,* Hufeland, B. J. H., vol. 27, p. 621; *Apoplexy,* Rummel, Rück. Kl. Erf., vol. 1, p. 92; *Choroiditis,* Tamhayn, B. J. H., vol. 18, p. 252; *Ophthalmia,* Jousset, B. J. H., vol. 28, p. 19; Turrel, Hom. Clin., vol. 3, p. 30; *Nasal catarrh,* Bigel, Rück. Kl. Erf., vol. 1, p. 388; *Influenza,* Gerner, Rück. Kl. Erf., vol. 3, p. 42; Rückert, B. J. H., vol. 26, p. 569; *Vomiting,* Lobeth, Genzk, Diez, Rück. Kl. Erf., vol. 1, p. 557; Hughes, B. J. H., vol. 18, p. 38; *Nervous vomiting,* Jousset, B. J. H., vol. 27 p. 622; *Chronic vomiting,* Hughes, B. J. H., vol. 23, p. 677; Smith, Allg. Hom. Ztg., vol. 109, p. 32; *Hæmatemesis,* (5 cases), Goullon, Nunez, Rück. Kl. Erf., vol. 5, p. 265; Goullon, B. J. H., vol. 26, p. 583; *Melæna,* Pomeroy, Raue's Rec., 1872, p. 151; *Diarrhœa,* Kafka, Rück. Kl. Erf., vol. 5, p. 418; Huber, Rück. Kl. Erf., vol. 5, p. 418; Knorre, Goullon, B. J. H., vol. 27, p. 632; Lobethal, Bœnninghausen, Müller, B. J. H., vol. 27, p. 630; Jahr, Hom. Clin., vol. 1, p. 195; *Dysentery,* Henke, B. J. H., vol. 27, p. 627; (2 cases), Drysdale, B. J. H., vol. 33, p. 738; Thayer, Raue's Rec., 1872 p. 43; *Cholera infantum,* Miller, Raue's Rec., 1874, p. 196; *Cholerine,* Goullon, Kafka, B. J. H., vol. 27, p. 632; *Cholera,* Drysdale, B. J. H., vol. 8, p. 161; Widman, Rupprig, Roth, Rück. Kl. Erf., vol. 1, p. 948; *Hæmaturia,* Gaspary, B. J. H., vol. 26, p. 583; *Uterine hemorrhage,* Hawkes, Organon, vol. 2, p. 132; Teller, B. J. H., vol. 26, p. 580; Hartmann, Kallenbach, Gaspar, Rück. Kl. Erf., vol. 2, p. 312; *Menorrhagia,* Patzak, Rück. Kl. Erf., vol. 2, p. 235; *Nausea and vomiting of pregnancy,* Müller, Schreter, Wolf, Knorre, Rück. Kl. Erf., vol. 2, p. 382; Müller, Rummel, Schreter, Rau, Knorre, B. J. H., vol. 27, p. 622; *Hemorrhage with abortion,* Käsemann, Kallenbach, B. J. H., vol. 26, p. 582; *Eclampsia,* Rummell, B. J. H., vol. 28, p. 10; *Post-partum hemorrhage,* Raue's Rec., 1870, p. 271; Miller, Raue's Rec., 1873, p. 183; Bell, Hah. Mo., vol. 4, p. 405; *Laryngismus stridulus,* B. J. H., vol. 12, p. 457; *Laryngitis, spasm of cords*, Pemerl, Raue's Rec., 1870, p. 156; *Emphysema*, Meyer, Petroz, Müller, B. J. H., vol. 26, p. 567; *Asthma*, Frank, N. A. J. H., vol. 8, p. 96; Kreuss, Sonnenburg, Kämpfer, Bethmann, Rück. Kl. Erf., vol. 3, p. 189; Müller, Meyer, Rück. Kl. Erf., vol. 5, p. 799; *Cough*, Hughes, B. J. H., vol. 18, p. 39; Knorre, Lobethal, Bernstein, Hering, Käsemann, Hirsch, B. J. H., vol. 26, p. 568–9; Knorre, Lobethal, Bernstein, Käsemann, Hering, Bigel, Hirsch, Rück. Kl. Erf., vol. 3, p. 16; Hartmann, Schrön, Käsemann, Schelling, Bethmann, Rück. Kl. Erf., vol.3, p. 79; *Whooping cough* Meyer, B. J. H., vol. 15, p. 43; Müller, Kafka, B. J. H., vol. 26, p. 570; *Hæmoptysis*, Chalmers, Raue's Rec., 1870, p. 195; Eidherr, Rück. Kl. Erf., vol. 5, p. 805; *Hysteria*, Rummel, Rück. Kl. Erf., vol. 2, p. 286; *Hysterical spasms*, Attomyr, Rück. Kl. Erf., vol. 4, p. 574; *Spasms*, Jahr, Rück. Kl. Erf., vol. 4, p. 674; Schreter, Nenning, Rück. Kl. Erf., vol. 4, p. 574; *Spasmodic conditions*, Rummel, Rück. Kl. Erf., vol. 4, p. 573; *Tetanus, Trismus*, Schneider, Hahnemann, Ackerman, Bogel, B. J. H., vol. 28, p. 11; *Epilepsy*, Tietzer, Rück. Kl. Erf., vol. 4, p. 573; *Ague*, Hering, Loebthal, Nagel, Tripl, Escallier, Hencke, Hirsch, Bürkner, Vehseman, Müller, Horner, Thorer, Neumann, Szontagh, Käsemann, Baertl, Rück. Kl. Erf., vol. 4, p. 928–40; Lobethal, Ecallier, Wurmb, Caspar, Hencke, B. J. H., vol. 28, p. 4; (34 cases), Muller, N. A. J. H., vol. 4, p. 271–273; Hawkes, Organon, vol. 2, p. 114; Allen, Organon, vol. 2, p. 239; Hoffman, Organon, vol. 3, p. 112; Morrison, Allen's Int. Fever, p. 152; *Intermittent fever*, Stow, Raue's Rec., 1871, p. 196; Edmundson, Raue's Rec., 1874, p. 279; Frost, Raue's Rec., 1875, p. 272; Carr Organon, vol. 2, p. 204; *Measles*, Hartmann, Rück. Kl. Erf, vol. 4, p. 97; *Scarlet fever*, Hahnemann, Trinks, Rück. Kl. Erf., vol. 4, p. 53; *Yellow fever*, Taft, Rück. Kl. Erf., vol. 4, p. 665; *Anæmia*, Hanbold, Rück. Kl. Erf., vol. 5, p. 604; *Opium poisoning*, Korndœrfer, Hom. Clin., vol. 1, p. 266.

[1] **Mind.** Is awkward and stumbles against everything.

Wrapt in thought; taciturnity.

I I Full of inexpressible desires.

I Moaning and sighing with the fever. θIntermittent.

I Child cries and screams violently and incessantly; sticks fist into mouth; face pale, body cool.

I Every 6 or 8 weeks anorexia and hypochondria, with pressure and tension, •and tympanitis of epigastrium; constipation, with disgust and impatience of labor; attacks preceded by nausea, and tendency to diarrhœa. θHypochondriasis.

I I Dejected mood, morose, enjoys nothing.

I Peevish; irritable; impatient; morose, scornful mood.

I Ill humor, despises everything.

I I Fretfulness. θIntermittent. θCholera infantum.

I I Extremely impatient.

I I Morose mood that scorns everything, and desires also that others shall not appreciate or value anything.

I I Ailments from vexation and reserved displeasure.

[2] **Sensorium.** I Apoplexia nervosa et serosa; vertigo; drooping of lips; impaired speech; dribbling of saliva from mouth; paralysis of extremities.

I Vertigo when walking and when turning.

³ Inner Head. ▮Lacerating pain in forehead, excited and aggravated by feeling the heart, or by stooping.

▮Aching in forehead; fine stinging pains in forehead.

▮Headache over l. eye.

Stitches in vertex, or forehead.

▮Lancinating in head.

▮▮Short paroxysms of fine and violently stinging pains in head, increasing to an aching.

▮Stinging headache, with heaviness of head, also with drowsiness.

▮▮Headache, as if bruised, all through bones of head and down into root of tongue; nausea, vomiting; > outdoors.

▮▮Headache as of a bruise of brain and skull, which pierces through all the cranial bones into roots of teeth, with nausea.

▮Headache as though brain were mashed, with nausea and vomiting; miliary eruptions on forehead and cheeks by spells; pale face, and pale mucous membranes; scanty and short menses; weak pulse, cold hands; morose, enjoys nothing. θChlorosis.

▮Lacerating headache, from morning till noon.

▮▮Dull drawing in head, to and fro.

▮Beating pain in head and pit of stomach after coughing.

▮Heat and throbbing in head, with red cheeks.

▮Semilateral headache, with nausea and vomiting.

▮▮Tensive headache in occiput and nape of neck, extending as far as shoulders.

▮Pain in occiput and nape of neck.

▮▮Gastric headaches, occurring in nervous, sensitive persons, commencing with nausea and vomiting.

▮Malarial headache; loss of appetite and vomiting.

▮Hydrocephaloid: fontanelles open; painful soreness of occiput and neck; blue rings under eyes; frequent nosebleeding; pale face; nausea and vomiting; green, putrid discharges from bowels.

⁴ Outer Head. ▮Cold sweat on forehead. θDiarrhœa.

▮Open fontanelles; occiput and neck sore. θHydrocephaloid.

⁵ Sight and Eyes. ▮Worse from light, especially of a candle.

▮Blue and red halo around light.

▮Optical illusions in bright colors.

▮Obscuration of sight; eyes inflamed.

▮▮Eyes sunken; blue margins around them. θCholera infantum.

▮▮Dilated pupils.

▮Severe shooting pains through eyeballs, profuse lachrymation on looking steadily; blue and red halo around flame, pupil normal and mobile, with no external inflammation or lesion, except slight palpebral conjunctivitis. θChoroiditis.

❙Phlyctenules and ulcers of cornea or conjunctiva, especially if there is much photophobia; cornea may be
vascular; redness of conjunctiva, lachrymation and pain
and nausea.

❙Pustular inflammation of cornea and conjunctiva.

❙Child after catching cold: lids red and swollen; photophobia, lids being kept tightly closed; copious, purulent
discharge, < at night; conjunctiva injected and swollen,
especially on r. side, where engorgement was so severe
that pupil appeared buried in a circular depression; discharge from eyes so copious that it soiled hair and ears;
continual copious, green, diarrhœic stools, with colic;
great emaciation; sleepless day and night; edges of lid
red, without œdema; r. imbedded cornea ulcerated, also
l., but in a less degree.

❙Inflammation of eyes; on opening r. lids, which were
swollen, copious gush of tears; conjunctiva of bulb injected and infiltrated, and on close examination number
of small depressions were noticed; intense tearing or
tensive pains in eyes; great photophobia.

❙Scrofulous ophthalmia when there is keratitis with ulceration or infiltration of cornea; redness of eye, extreme
photophobia, pain in temples and forehead.

❙Catarrhal conjunctivitis with profuse yellow discharge
and chemosis.

❙Scleroticæ yellow.

❙❙Hardened mucus in external canthi.

❙Twitching of eyelids.

⁶Hearing and Ears. ❙Cannot endure the least noise.

❙Ears cold during febrile heat.

⁷Smell and Nose. Coryza: dry; with stoppage of nose; loss
of smell; nausea; epistaxis.

❙Stoppage of nose; loss of smell; heaviness of head; dry
cough, particularly at night coming on in long lasting
paroxysms, with painful shocks in head and stomach;
nausea followed by vomiting, general sweat and great
weakness. θChronic catarrh.

❙❙Nosebleed, blood bright red; face pale.

Nose itches; when nausea is over, violent hunger.

⁸Upper Face. ❙Face: pale and puffed; pale, and body cool;
sunken; deathly pale, sunken eyes with blue margins;
livid, yellowish.

❙Convulsive twitches in muscles of face and lips.

❙Rash.

⁹Lower Face. ❙❙Skin around the mouth red.

Smarting eruption and·aphthæ on margin of lips.

❙Lips: blue, during chill; white, during hemorrhage.

¹⁰Teeth and Gums. ❙Child thrusts its fist into mouth; screams

violently; face pale; body cool; vomiting and watery
stools; prostration; spasms. *θ*Dentition.

I I Pain in a hollow tooth when biting on it.

I I Pain in molars > while eating; < in afternoon and
still more at night.

∎Teeth chatter, with chill. *θ*Intermittent.

¹¹ Taste and Tongue. I I Loss of taste.

Taste: bitter; sweetish, bloody; like rancid oil, when swallowing; earthy; flat, with white, thickly coated tongue.

∎Tongue: clean; yellow or white; pale.

∎Disinclined to talk; tongue dry.

¹² Inner Mouth. ∎∎Profuse accumulation of saliva; is constantly obliged to swallow it.

∎Smarting in mouth and on tongue.

¹³ Throat. ∎Fauces dry, sore, rough, stinging.

∎Spasmodic contractive sensation in throat and chest;
difficult deglutition.

∎Pressure in throat, with pains in diaphragm.

I I Deep red color of tonsils and pharynx.

I I Rapid congestion of mucous membrane of pharynx;
secretion of a thick, plastic, whitish, nauseous humor,
appearing at first under form of small white or grayish
points, either on tonsils or velum palati or pharynx.

¹⁴ Appetite, Thirst. Desires, Aversions. I I Thirst or thirstlessness.

∎Desire for dainties and sweets.

∎∎Averse to all food, no appetite; earthy taste; stomach
feels relaxed; nausea.

∎∎Great disgust and loathing of any sort of food.

¹⁵ Eating and Drinking. ∎Indisposition from indigestible
substances, lemon peel, berries, raisins, sweets, cake,
pastry and unripe fruit, salads, pork, fats, sour beer, etc.

After eating: nausea; vomiting; stool.

∎Colic, with nausea and vomiting, after cold drinks or ice
cream.

¹⁶ Hiccough, Belching, Nausea and Vomiting. ∎Hiccough:
with nausea; of children.

∎Eructations every eight to ten minutes; with rumbling
in abdomen.

∎Waterbrash.

∎∎Nausea: distressing; constant, with almost all complaints; as if from stomach; with empty eructations;
accumulation of much saliva; qualmishness, and efforts
to vomit.

∎Nausea and retching from smoking; primary effects of
tobacco.

∎Faintness, nausea, retching. *θ*Post-partum hemorrhage.

∎Inclination to vomit without nausea.

‖Nausea, profuse saliva; vomiting of white, glairy mucus; < stooping.

‖‖Nausea, with distension of abdomen and dryness in throat; after vomiting inclined to sleep.

‖Constant but unavailing desire to vomit; or immediately after vomiting wishes to do so again.

‖Incessant retching with vomiting of watery fluids and cutting pain in belly.

‖Constant nausea and vomiting of yellowish mucus.

‖Vomiting: of ingesta; of bile; of grass green mucus; bilious, putrid; copiously of jellylike mucus; of blood, or of a pitchlike substance; of a dark colored liquid, with or without blood; of a sour fluid; of large quantities of mucus; always with nausea; during pregnancy; with thirst, sweat, bad breath; with diarrhœa, colic, distended abdomen; with clean tongue.

‖‖Vomiting causes great pain in loins and hips.

‖Nervous vomiting, frequent and with constant nausea.

‖Vomiting due to irritability or other abnormal condition of nerves of stomach, particularly when tongue is clean, and persons are weak and nervous, and of large build; constant nausea and retching of hysterical women; morning vomiting in weakly persons who are affected by worms; nausea in nervous fevers and that which remains after an attack of indigestion.

‖Vomiting of food soon after eating, tasting very sour and accompanied by much retching; tongue coated in middle, edges red; region of stomach and hypochondria sensitive to pressure; three or four stools daily; general weakness; menses irregular; urine dark, depositing urates.

‖Vomits everything taken; food causes pain during short time it remains in stomach; tongue brown and cleft; bowels regular; urine thick. θChronic vomiting.

‖Loss of appetite nine months ago, without assignable cause; then followed vomiting of all food, with great debility; bowels much relaxed; smarting of eyes; catamenia regular.

‖Vomiting almost constantly for days. θRemittent fever.

‖Emaciated, scrofulous child, suffering from disease of mesenteric glands, vomited everything taken and cried the whole day; the vomited matter and accompanying chopped stools smelt very sour.

‖‖Constant nausea often with vomiting large masses of mucus, generally green. θDiarrhœa of children.

‖Tormina and bilious vomiting, coming on at first every fourth day, but latterly every Saturday; nausea with extreme weakness and repeated fainting; frequent at-

tacks of violent, bilious vomiting, obliging her to keep
in bed all day; on other days perfectly well.
▮Vomiting of infants at the breast.
▮Stooping causes vomiting.
[17] **Scrobiculum and Stomach.** ▮▮Uncomfortable· feeling in
epigastrium.
▮Violent distress in pit of stomach; attacks of pain;
beating.
▮▮Indescribable sick feeling in stomach.
▮▮Sensation as if stomach hung down relaxed.
▮▮Pressure in stomach; clutching pains; beating.
▮Cardialgia; typical form.
▮▮Pain most severe in front of abdomen, extending to l.
hypochondrium, to sides, to back, and base of chest, with
swelling of stomach; great agitation; constant nausea
proceeding from stomach, with empty eructations and
accumulation of much saliva; easy vomiting; diarrhœa.
▮Stomachal catarrh, with abhorrence of all food, and
tobacco; with nausea, vomiting, colic and diarrhœa;
tongue always clean.
▮Gastric catarrh from indigestible food or ice cold things;
pain and mucous vomiting.
▮After eating fat pork, headache, loss of appetite, nausea,
vomiting; prostration and debility; pain in forehead;
pale, bloated face; photophobia without redness of eyes;
flat taste, slimy coated tongue; great thirst; frequent
vomiting preceded by pressure and pain in stomach;
frequent, offensive, flocky stools; slight, dry cough; occasional twitchings of muscles of face, lips and eyelids;
restless sleep with frequent startings.
▮Indigestion, from overloading stomach.
▮Dyspepsia every day, or every other day, at same hour.
▮After slight digestive disturbance, sudden vomiting of
blood, occurring three times within seven days; blood
at first dark and coagulated, in subsequent attacks fluid
and bright red, followed by bloody stools; great prostration; frequent fainting fits; dimness of sight; slightest motion or cough causes nausea; tongue brown, dry,
like earth; unquenchable thirst; obstinate constipation.
▮After chagrin, constant pressing pain in pit of stomach,
loss of appetite, frequent nausea; eight days after this,
in consequence of anger, sudden vomiting, first of clotted,
then of fluid blood, amounting to about two pounds;
deathly pale; almost pulseless; faintness.
▮Acute distress in epigastric region; forcibly vomiting immense quantities of black, tarlike matter, gushing from
nostrils as well as mouth; extremities cold; hippocratic
countenance; pulse almost imperceptible; cold, clammy
sweats; extreme prostration and exhaustion. θMelæna.

¹After long continued, pressing pain in stomach, which alternated with toothache, sudden vomiting of blood, with great faintness; blood dark, thin, about one pound in quantity; pulse full; a second attack with great faintness, anxiety, feeble pulse, pale, cold face and cold hands.

ᴵPale, anæmic girl, subject to pains in stomach and irritable conditions of mind, was suddenly seized with vomiting of blood after indulging in strong coffee; blood at first brownish black, then black and half coagulated, escaping in great quantities; between each attack of vomiting, which occurs about every half hour, anxiety, pressure in stomach, fainting; pulse small and feeble; face and hands pale and cold; thirst and internal heat.

ᴵAfter exposure to cold and wet, rigors and dyspnœa, followed by copious spitting of blood; cannot speak; sits on a chair, gasping, and every few seconds brings up a large mouthful of bright colored, frothy blood; pulse small and frequent; respirations short and very frequent; face livid and expressive of anxiety. *θ*Hæmoptysis.

ᴵSudden attack; blood dark, black, sour; paleness; coldness; pulse scarcely perceptible; fainting; anxiety; pressure in stomach; great thirst; oppression of breathing. *θ*Hæmatemesis.

ᴵHæmatemesis of children.

¹⁸ **Hypochondria.** ᴵPinching pain in both hypochondria and in region of pit of stomach.

ᴵPain in l. hypochondrium.

ᴵDiaphragm feels as if pressed between two millstones, front to back.

¹⁹ **Abdomen.** ᴵᴵDistressing feeling in abdomen, as though stomach were hanging down, relaxed.

ᴵSore feeling in abdomen.

ᴵᴵGriping, as from a hand, each finger sharply pressing into intestines; > during rest, much < by motion.

ᴵClutching and squeezing in abdomen.

ᴵᴵFlatulent colic about navel, as though bowels were grasped with hand. *θ*Dysenteric diarrhœa.

ᴵᴵCutting colic near umbilicus; sometimes shivering.

ᴵᴵTenderness and pain about umbilicus, towards uterus.

ᴵStitches from navel to uterus.

ᴵCutting pain almost constantly running from l. to r. with every movement.

ᴵParoxysms of shooting across abdomen from l. to r., causing nausea and vomiting, vomits froth and bile with difficulty; when vomiting, coughs to bring it up; sweats; offensive black stools; vomiting causes great pain in loins and hips, as if all the bones in body were being torn to pieces.

∎Severe pains in abdomen, radiating to all sides.

∎Flatulent colic, with frequent loose stools.

∎Colic of children: with diarrhœa, uneasiness, screaming and tossing about; from indigestion; after acid or unripe fruit, beer, etc.

∎Inguinal hernia, readily reducible, or strangulated.

²⁰ Stool and Rectum. Stool: bloody; as if fermented; consistence and appearance of fermented yeast; spurting out with much flatus; very offensive; light yellow; lemon colored; green as grass; greenish mucus; lumpy, greenish watery; white mucous, bloody; yellow, liquid, covered with bloody mucus; pitchlike or like frothy molasses; slimy, bloody, offensive, followed by tenesmus; putrid smelling; containing blood and matter.

∎Diarrhœa of teething children, yellow, white or green discharges, no pain or emaciation, but serious because of its long continuance; particularly indicated at period of weaning when food disagrees.

∎Diarrhœa: with pain, causing unceasing screaming and tossing about, in children; from taking cold; from disordered stomach, after late suppers; of infants, with vomiting of green or whitish matter; due to chill or to mental emotions; after overloading stomach with sweets, or fat pastry; in the Autumn.

∎Summer complaint of children, with crying, tossing, large abdomen, frequent, small, yellow, fermented stools.

∎Colliquative diarrhœa of dark colored stools, or of greenish matter, with particles having appearance of coagula.

∎Chronic diarrhœa, of miasmatic origin; clean tongue and frequent nausea, constant pain at umbilicus.

∎Acute internal catarrh.

∎Epidemic dysentery, with nausea, vomiting, pain in epigastrium; pressive frontal headache, loaded tongue, tenesmus, mucous fetid diarrhœa, < at night.

∎Dysentery: stools frequent, slightly tinged with blood, and often entirely composed of blood and slime; in the Fall, with vomiting of bile, tenesmus after stool and simultaneous affection of cœliacus; stools almost black, and fermented like frothy molasses; of children; cold nights after hot days.

∎Cholera infantum: nausea, vomiting, colic, diarrhœa; especially in fat, pale children; nausea and vomiting of yellowish mucus; lumpy, greenish, watery stools; paleness of face; blue margins around eyes; wants to lie down, ill humor; copious, fermented, flatulent, lemon colored stools, with thirst, fever and fretfulness.

∎Stools light green or an arsenic green.

∎First symptoms of cholera Asiatica; the nausea and vomiting predominates, headache and tightness of chest.

‖Vomiting after all ingesta, and as often as every quarter of hour, without cause; vomiting copious, preceded by shivering all over; no coldness or cramps; pulse slow; tongue furred. θCholera.

Before stool: colic, nausea, vomiting.

During stool: colic, nausea, vomiting; violent tenesmus; lassitude, coldness, paleness of face.

After stool: lassitude; tenesmus; twitching of face.

‖Hemorrhoids bleeding very profusely.

‖Itching at anus.

²¹ **Urinary Organs.** Urine: scanty, dark red; turbid, with red sediment.

‖Yellowish red sediment in urine. θQuotidian ague.

‖Unsuccessful urging to urinate.

‖Ischuria, with convulsions.

‖Hæmaturia: with cutting in abdomen and urethra; from suppressed itch; with vesical spasm.

‖After becoming chilled, felt ill all over; very weak; could hardly move about from vertigo; confused ideas; severe pain in kidneys, with heat in lower bowels as if hot water was poured into them; towards evening violent pain in abdominal region and bladder, with desire to urinate, with passage of scalding urine and blood, fluid and clotted; next day, too weak to stand; feet quite cold, and as if paralyzed; head stupefied, could not sit up; more blood, followed by swoon, with deadly pallor, hardly perceptible pulse, and cold extremities; could hardly speak; heaviness of head, uneasiness and inclination to vomit, pressure on pit of stomach, pain in lower bowels and kidneys, weight and coldness of feet; frequent micturition. θHæmaturia.

‖During urination: burning in urethra; pains in back and epigastrium.

²² **Female Sexual Organs.** ‖Prolapsus and hemorrhage; profuse, clotted blood, with heavy, oppressed breathing; constant flow of bright red blood, with cutting about umbilicus; constant nausea and vomiting; feels cold and is very pale; dizziness and headache; chill and coldness of body while internal heat rises up into head, with a bearing down pressure to uterus and anus; fainting; blood spitting, hæmatemesis; faintness with convulsions.

‖Great debility and leucorrhœa during intervals of menses.

‖Continual discharge of bright red blood.

Profuse menstruation, with constant nausea, not a moment's relief, not even after vomiting; nausea proceeds from stomach, and the discharge of bright red blood is increased with every effort to vomit, and flows with a gush; violent pressure over uterus and rectum, with shuddering and chilliness; heat about head and debility; gasping for breath, faintness; after childbirth, after removal of placenta or after miscarriage; < when getting out of bed. θUterine hemorrhage.

∎Menses appeared four times in seven weeks, and last time so seriously that blood passed in large clots, and such a quantity of black fluid that it brought on swooning, loss of consciousness; vomiting of mucus, with cold skin looking like wax, blue lips, small, scarcely perceptible pulse. θCongestive menorrhagia.

∎Menses: too early and too profuse; blood bright red; menses return every two weeks; great weakness after menses; peevish humor; aching in head; lancinating in forehead; pale face; blue rings around eyes; vomiting of ingesta; distress in umbilical region.

∎Profuse menstruation, with constant nausea; not a moment's relief, not even after vomiting.

∎Discharge of blood before the proper period.

ı ıScanty or short menses.

Dysmenorrhœa.

∎Severe pain about umbilicus, extending towards uterus, most distress about navel, but it runs off into uterus

∎With every movement a cutting pain, almost constantly running from left to right.

∎Uterine pains running down.

∎Pain extending towards and passing off into uterus.

** Pregnancy. Parturition. Lactation.** ııVomiting of pregnancy; in some cases more nausea than vomiting.

ı ıVertigo in pregnancy, with pale, bluish, puffed face, blue lips and nails; undulation of jugular veins.

∎Threatened abortion, often with a sharp or pinching pain around umbilicus, which runs downward to uterus, with constant nausea and discharge of bright red blood; convulsions.

∎In sixth week of pregnancy seized suddenly with abdominal pains, heat in epigastrium and vertigo; flooding soon followed by shooting in kidneys, weakness and heaviness of thighs and general debility; flooding increased hourly, soon passing through mattrass, and flowing in abundance under bed; colic increased, face pale and ' eyes encircled with blue; miscarriage followed, accompanied by acute pain; hemorrhage became more serious; pains in heart followed by dryness of mouth and great thirst; great exhaustion, could hardly speak.

∎After abortion occasional slight loss of blood, for four months, when an alarming hemorrhage took place with the usual symptoms, besides vomiting after least drink.

∎Incessant flooding; complete prostration; breathing heavy; oppression; colorless face and lips; ringing in ears; faint on raising head from pillow; flow bright red; much persistent nausea; pain in umbilical region, running down to uterus.

∎During labor pains great hemorrhage, apparently from placenta.

∎Labor pains spasmodic; cutting across from l. to r.; nausea; clutching about navel.

∎∎Uterine pains accompanied by severe cutting pains in umbilical region, interfering with true pains; faintness and nausea.

∎Uterine pains running downward.

∎∎Stitches darting off from umbilicus towards uterus.

∎After removal of placenta, sudden and alarming distension of abdomen in region of atonic uterus; face and tongue pale; sighing respiration; faintness, nausea, retching; cutting pains about umbilicus. θPost-partum hemorrhage.

∎Arterial bleeding from partial separation of placenta.

∎Post-partum hemorrhage; placenta attached; hemorrhage frightful, very fluid and gushing.

∎Metrorrhagia, often after confinement, heralded by slow pulse, nausea, etc.; steady flow of bright, red blood.

∎Nausea and vomiting in nursing women.

²⁵ **Voice and Larynx. Trachea and Bronchia.** ∎Voice hollow.

∎Spasm of cords; constant, alternate contraction and relaxation of cords, following each other in rapid succession.

∎Contraction accompanied by a sensation of tickling at entrance of trachea.

∎Spasm of glottis; blueness of face and coldness of extremities.

∎Inflammation of fossa; very little œdema. θLaryngitis.

∎∎Rattling in bronchi, when drawing a long breath; large accumulation of mucus in bronchi, difficult to raise.

∎∎Rattling noises in air passages during respiration.

∎Suffocative attacks from foreign substances in windpipe.

∎Bronchitis, with loud mucous râles; difficult expectoration; cough with nausea, even vomiting, or oppression, > by abundant expectoration.

²⁶ **Respiration.** ∎Oppression of chest in forenoon, with shortness of breath, as from inhaling dust.

∎Breathing: anxious and hurried; short and hurried; short and panting; heavy.

∎Rattling noise in bronchi when drawing breath.

∎Breath fetid, with vomiting and sweat.

▮▮Difficulty of breathing from least exercise.
▮▮Pain in diaphragm takes away breath.
▮▮Violent degree of dyspnœa, with wheezing, and great
weight and anxiety about præcordia.
▮▮Attacks of suffocation; $>$ in open air; $<$ from least
motion; constriction in throat and chest.
▮Threatened suffocation from accumulation of mucus.
▮Cough impedes respiration, even to suffocation.
▮Loses breath with the cough, turns pale in face and
stiffens. θWhooping cough.
▮Suffocative cough with dyspnœa, nausea vomituritio, at
end of attack. θWhooping cough.
▮Urgent dyspnœa, with sense of constriction across chest,
accompanied by violent and convulsive cough.
▮Dry, spasmodic, shattering cough; during attack arrest
of breathing, patient falling senseless to floor; each attack threatens to end fatally, and can only be overcome
by use of cold water.
▮Difficult expiration.
▮Severe and convulsive paroxysm of asthma.
▮Violent constriction of throat and chest, peculiar, panting
sound; gasps for air at open window; face pale; scarcely
perceptible pulse; $<$ from least motion; threatened suffocation. θAsthma.
▮Spasmodic asthma: with great constriction in throat and
chest; with peculiar wheezing noise; with danger of
suffocation; with bronchial catarrh; of adults; in hysterical subjects; after suppressed miliary eruptions.
▮Asthma, cyanosis supervening during fit, with frequent
dry cough, cold sweat on face and extremities, constitutional vomiturition, nausea or even vomiting after cough.
▮Nightly suffocative fits. θAsthma.
▮Asthma Millari, with tickling in larynx, retching and
vomiting.
▮Asthma of emphysematous subjects, when auscultation
detects considerable quantity of mucus accumulated in
bronchi, which patient cannot by any effort throw up in
sufficient quantity; coughing brings on nausea.
" **Cough.** ▮Dry cough, caused by tickling in upper part of
larynx.
▮Cough caused by a constrictive tickling from upper portion of larynx to lowest extremity of bronchi.
▮Cough dry, spasmodic, capricious, provoked by tickling
and irritation of larynx, after coryza, at first dry, then
fluent.
▮Spasmodic or catarrhal titillating cough, or suffocating
cough with dyspnœa, nausea, vomiturition, especially
at end of paroxysm, or with expectoration of scanty,

albuminous, nauseous mucus; mucous râles and vomiting of food.

▮Violent spasmodic cough, cannot cough soon enough at first; covers mouth with hand, in order not to inhale too much air.

▮Frequent attacks of spasmodic cough, shaking, racking, hollow; quickly following coughs from tickling in upper part of larynx, as from vapor of sulphur; expectoration of blood and mucus in morning.

▮Spasmodic cough with tendency to vomit, or with vomiting of whitish mucus; mucosity is easily produced in chest, and cough produces sonorous and bubbling râles.

▮Dry, spasmodic cough without vascular excitement.

▮Dry, spasmodic cough of old persons, coming on in fits, particularly at night after going to bed, or after dinner; tends to emphysema.

▮Cough with pain in abdomen, especially about navel, or pressure on bladder, hindering passage of urine; beating in head, or in pit of stomach; sense of excoriation in chest; after paroxysm of coughing respiration continues short, and forehead streams with perspiration; < in open air.

▮Cough coming on after a meal, especially P.M.; cough excited by each inspiration; tickling and constriction of upper part of trachea, coming on in open air; sudden precipitate fit of coughing; failure of breath; danger of asphyxia from mucus; anguish from choking; eyes starting out of head; face bluish red; buccal and nasal hemorrhage; efforts at vomiting; fit, ending with vomiting of food; swooning during fit. θInfluenza.

▮Suffocative, racking, very exhausting cough, lasting an hour, towards evening.

▮▮Suffocating cough, whereby child becomes quite stiff and blue in face.

▮▮Loses breath with cough, turns pale in face, and stiffens.

▮Suffocative evening cough; continuous cough, with sweat on forehead, shocks in head, retching and vomiting.

▮Strangling with cough till blue in face. θPertussis.

▮Incessant and most violent cough with every breath.

▮▮Cough causing inclination to vomit without nausea.

▮Cough, with retching, much mucous expectoration and considerable dyspnœa.

▮Cough causes gagging, vomiting is followed by relief.

▮Cough with expectoration of blood.

▮Convulsive evening cough, expectoration having a repulsive metallic taste.

▮Cough especially at night, with loathing and vomiting.

▮Croupy coughs occurring at night.

❙Cough: nervous, spasmodic; rough, shaking; dry, from titillation in upper part of larynx; with every breath; returning after exertion; < from cool air; with inclination to vomit; with spitting of blood from least effort; constant, no phlegm yields, though chest seems full; strangling, so much mucus seems accumulated in bronchia; croupy, at night; fat children; in hysterical women; in teething children.

During cough: headache; sore pain in chest; paroxysms of suffocation, with rigidity of body; painful concussions (shocks) in stomach and head; pains in epigastrium and umbilical region; bleeding from mouth and nose; nausea, retching, vomiting; perspiration of forehead; blueness of face; jarring of body; loss of consciousness and falling down.

❙Spasm of glottis before paroxysm; bleeding from nose and mouth during coughing fits; vomiting of mucus or food; convulsions and stiffening of body backwards; vomiting of food without coughing; rattling of mucus in bronchial tubes; rash, eruption. θWhooping cough.

❙Convulsion of glottis continuing so long that child remains for a time without respiring; cough dry, vomiting after the fit without expelling much mucus; dyspnœa; fine râles in back at lower part of thorax. θWhooping cough.

❙Violent, shattering, hollow coughs, following each other in quick succession, and do not admit recovery of breath; expectorates mornings some light red blood, mixed with mucus, of a putrid, sweetish taste. θTussis convulsiva.

❙❙Whooping cough: with nosebleed; bleeding from mouth; vomiting; loses breath, turns pale or blue, and becomes rigid.

❙Febrile cough (principally after *Pulsat.* and *Nux vom.*), in women and children; irregular periods of heat, during which the dry cough gets worse.

❙Tussis abdominalis, with vomiting which relieves.

❙❙Phlegm rattling on chest, sometimes vomited, with young children.

Expectoration of mucus with metallic taste.

❙❙Sputa scanty, albuminous.

❙Expectoration: mornings, of a light red blood, mixed with mucus, or of ropy mucus, often vomited; of blood from least effort.

※ **Inner Chest and Lungs.**   ❙Spasmodic tightness of chest, with contraction of throat and panting breathing.

❙Great oppression of chest, can hardly breathe. θIntermittent fever.

∎Acute catarrh of children; suffocating cough, with congested and bluish face, and loss of breath, or when cough is accompanied by nausea and vomiting, or provoked by a tickling in larynx, with throbbing of head and heart and longing to pass water.

∎Rattling of large bubbles; fever, but face rather pale; cough and gagging.

∎Collection of mucus which is difficult to expectorate; expectoration gives but temporary relief.

∎∎Strangling as if from mucus in chest.

∎Bronchitis: of children; with accumulation of phlegm, which threatens to suffocate; spasmodic cough; rash on chest.

∎Fine, rattling noises in chest, spasmodic cough; nausea; œdema pulmonum.

∎Pulmonary congestion and simple pneumonia, consequent upon repercussion of scarlatinal eruption.

∎Infantile pneumonia; respiration rapid, difficult; surface blue; face pale.

∎Profuse hemorrhage, of a bright red color, provoked by a dry, tickling, racking cough, or even by a little hawking, < from least exertion; preceded by a sense of bubbling in chest and accompanied by nausea, chills, heavy breathing, oppression, livid face, small and frequent pulse, anxiety and debility; cannot utter a word; protracted taste of blood in mouth.

∎Hemorrhage from lungs after venesection, especially if bleeding is scanty, constituting an expectoration of blood streaked mucus; or a blood spitting, from least effort, without cough.

∎Blood frothy and bright colored; gasping for breath pulse small and frequent; face livid and anxious.

∎∎Hemorrhage from lungs: bright red; coming up with slight effort; < from least exertion; frequent hacking, with expectoration of blood streaked mucus; with or without cough; after disturbed catamenia; after mechanical injuries; after former bleedings have weakened lungs; with dry cough in phthisis.

∎Hæmoptysis; recent cases.

∎Vomiting and complication of asthma in emphysematous subjects. θInfluenza.

∎Cyanotic symptoms with spasms of chest and dyspnœa.

∎Spamodic affections of chest.

∎Shooting pain with remissions, not inflammatory, cannot breathe, puts both hands down, bends forward, opens windows, gasps for breath; attacks < at night.

∎Emphysema of old people

²**Heart, Pulse and Circulation.**   Pulse: large and soft: accelerated but weak; sometimes imperceptible.

³¹ Neck and Back. ❙Swelling and suppuration in throat pit.
❙Cramp between scapulæ during motion.
Much pain in back, at same time in limbs.
❙Shooting pains, from r. kidney down thigh to knee, like
    cramp.
³² Upper Limbs. ❙Coldness of one hand, while the other is hot.
❙Cold hands.
³³ Lower Limbs. ❙Sensation in femur, as if dislocated, on sit-
   ting down.
❙Cramps in thighs, at night, with lumps in thighs.
❙Convulsive twitchings of legs and feet. θHemorrhage.
❙❙Itching of calves.
❙❙Ulcer with black base on foot.
³⁴ Limbs in General. Sensation as if joints had gone to sleep.
❙❙Pain in joints, as is usual when limb goes to sleep.
❙❙Pain, as if bruised, in all the bones.
❙Cold hands and feet.
³⁵ Rest. Position. Motion. Rest: griping in intestines >.
Restless, tosses about from side to side.
Hands clenched and arms thrown violently forward.
Puts both hands down, bends forward: on account of
    shooting pain in chest.
Sitting down: sensation in femur as if dislocated.
Sits on a chair gasping: after blood spitting.
Could not sit up: after pain in abdomen.
Falling down: during cough, with unconsciousness.
Wants to lie down: cholera infantum.
Lies upon back unconscious: during spasms.
Head thrown back: during spasms.
Body bent backwards: during hysterical spasm.
Body rigid, stretched out, jerking of arms.
Body violently bent backwards and drawn in same direc-
    tion by spasmodic jerks.
Slightest motion causes: nausea, cutting pain in abdomen;
    attacks of suffocation; constriction of throat <; cutting
    pain from l. to r. through uterus.
Motion: griping in intestines <; sweat <; cramp be-
    tween scapulæ; sweat <.
Least effort: difficulty of breathing; spitting of blood;
    profuse hemorrhage.
Exertion: cough returns.
On raising head from pillow: faintness.
Getting out of bed: vertigo and weakness of knees; men-
    struation <.
Tossing about: from diarrhœa.
Tossing up body: during spasm.
³⁶ Nerves. ❙Oversensitive to heat or cold.
❙Restlessness with the fever. θIntermittent.

. ❙Very weak, averse to all food; nausea; sudden prostration.

❙Extreme prostration and exhaustion; seemingly the last straits of vitality are reached. *θ*Melæna.

❙❙Wants to lie down. *θ*Cholera infantum.

❙Awkward, stumbles against everything.

❙Fainting; convulsions; apoplectic sopor.

❙Hysterical spasms, coming on several times a day, and gradually growing more severe; body bent backwards; muscles of face distorted; groaning.

❙Hysteria; every fresh development of hysterical symptoms brings on a sensation of continual nausea.

❙Nervous attacks with feeling of suffocation.

❙Convulsive twitching in limbs, a painful tremor.

❙Spasms without loss of consciousness.

❙Tetanic rigidity of body with bluish redness of face.

❙Body rigid, stretched out, spasmodic jerking of arms.

❙Body violently bent backwards and drawn in same direction by spasmodic jerks. *θ*Tetanus.

❙Spasms after catching cold during purpura; lies upon back unconscious; face pale and swollen; eyes at one time closed, again open; horrible twitching of muscles of face, lips and eyelids; spasms of arms and legs often tossing up the body; attacks come on every five minutes, lasting ten to fifteen minutes, and are followed by great prostration; occasional retching.

❙Clonic or tonic spasms in children and hysterical women; head thrown back; loss of consciousness; outcries; pale, puffed face; distortion of muscles of face and of half closed eyes; convulsive twitchings of muscles of face, lips, eyelids and limbs; asthma; nausea; vomiting.

❙Awoke from sleep in evening with wide open, staring eyes; hands clenched and arms thrown violently forward; lies quiet several minutes, then gasps and groans; constant staring with spasmodic contraction of r. arm; eleven attacks in twenty-four hours.

❙Frightful spasms affecting whole of l. side, followed by paralysis; eyes fixed and turned to right; pupils dilated and insensible; frequent opening and shutting of lids; slight contractions of r. corner of mouth; at times regular movements of r. arm and hand; pulse frequent and feeble; tracheal râle, as in paralysis of lungs; discharge of brown mucus from mouth; respiration irregular; inspiration short, followed by slow, sighing expiration; skin hot, but r. ear cold. *θ*Eclampsia.

❙Eclampsia in pregnancy or childbed; violent cutting around navel; vomiting; pale face.

❙Fainting, summer heat or hot rooms, with nausea.

❙Convulsions: in whooping cough; from suppressed exanthema; from indigestible food, etc.

❚❚Tetanic spasms from swallowing tobacco.

❙❙Tetanic spasms in old lady, with starting, twitching; coughs up bloody phlegm.

❚Tetanus; trismus.

❙Opisthotonos and emprosthotonos.

❙Catalepsy.

❙Epileptiform spasms, with shrieks; opisthotonos; face pale, puffed; gastric derangement.

❙Epilepsy of children or secondary epilepsy, when its starting point is the pneumogastric nerve.

³⁷ Sleep. ❙Yawning and stretching.

❙Shocks on falling asleep.

❙Sleep, with half open eyes; moaning, groaning.

❙❙Starts up in sleep.

❙❙Sleepless.

❙When deprived of sleep: nausea and languor.

³⁸ Time. Morning: vomiting; expectoration of blood and mucus; expectorates light red blood with mucus; paroxysms of chill lasting half an hour, heat lasting two hours; bitter taste in mouth.

From morning till noon: lacerating headache.

9 A.M.: chill.

11 A.M.: chill.

Forenoon: oppression of chest.

Day: sleepless.

All day: cried continually; obliged to keep in bed on account of bilious vomiting.

Afternoon: pain in molars <; severe chill; yawning with chilliness.

Till 2 P.M.: nausea and vomiting.

3 P.M.: severe chill lasting one hour.

Towards evening: lasting one hour, suffocative, racking, very exhaustive cough; violent pain in abdominal region and bladder.

Evening: suffocative cough; anxious, dry heat; sensation of great weakness; awoke from sleep with wide open, staring eyes; general heat; dry heat very troublesome.

Lasts till 7 P.M.: fever.

Night: discharge from eyes <; sleepless; dry cough <; pain in molars <; dry, spasmodic cough; croupy cough; attacks of shooting in chest <; very profuse sour sweat; disagreeable heat; epidemic dysentery <; cramp in thighs; irritable, irascible; fever <.

³⁹ Temperature and Weather. ❙Oversensitive to heat and cold.

Worse in winter and in dry weather.

❙Worse in warm, moist wind, south winds; catarrhs; asthma, etc.

Warm room: chill <.
Summer heat or hot room: fainting.
External heat: < chill.
Oversensitiveness to heat or cold.
Out of doors: headache >; sweat <.
Open air: suffocation >; cough <; cough comes;
   chill <; chill >.
Covers mouth with hand not to inhale too much air.
Gasps for air at open window: constriction of throat.
Cool air: nervous cough <.
After exposure to cold and rain: hemorrhages <.
After exposure to cold and wet: rigors and dyspnœa, then
   spitting of blood.
After catching cold: lids red and swollen.
Drinking: chill >.
After cold drink or ice cream: colic.
Cold water: > spasmodic cough.

⁴⁰ **Fever.** ▮Paroxysm begins with an internal chill, made < by
   external heat.
▮Chilliness, cold hands and feet, which are moist or drip-
   ping with cold sweat.
▮Coldness of upper part of body.
▮Chill but slight with many gastric ailments.
▮Chill: preceded by violent retching; mostly with thirst
   but also without; with great oppression of chest; with
   nausea and vomiting; with diarrhœic stools; < in a
   warm room or from external heat; > by drinking, and
   in open air; at 9 A.M.; every other day at 11 A.M.; of
   short duration soon changing to heat; with great lassitude and weariness.
▮▮After a short chill, dry heat, with parchmentlike skin.
▮Severe chill in afternoon with nausea, followed by heat
   with sweat of several hours' duration, and ending with
   sour sweat; during apyrexia, coated tongue; pressure at
   stomach. θQuartan ague.
▮Great nausea before chill and during whole paroxysm,
   cannot stir eyes without nausea, but no vomiting; great
   thirst during chill, none during fever or sweat; very
   nervous, trembling, during chill shook inside; intense
   headache during paroxysm, and in a modified degree
   during apyrexia, extending down to root of nose and
   throat; sweat like rain; paroxysms irregular. θAgue.
▮Chill irregular, light and short; fever long, but not very
   violent; no thirst during chill, but much thirst all
   through heat; thick, white, pappy coating on tongue;
   complete loss of appetite; great weakness and prostration during apyrexia; constant nausea and occasional
   vomiting.

▮Chill from 9, A.M. to 3 P.M., with intense aching in back
  and bones; nausea and vomiting after chill; intense
  fever with thirst and throbbing frontal headache; becomes unconscious during fever, which lasts till 8 P.M.,
  when sweat comes on for about one hour, together with
  great shaking all over, and great thirst; continued
  jumping headache, very thirsty all the time with anorexia. θAgue.
▮In afternoon yawning with chilliness, extending from
  back, soon followed by coldness of extremities, internal
  shaking, trembling and cramps in chest; in evening,
  general heat accompanied by great impatience and despondency; great heat, particularly in head and face,
  cheeks red, pulse soft, small, slightly increased; pain in
  limbs as if they were broken; heat followed by sweat;
  no thirst during fever; loss of appetite; escape of saliva
  from mouth during sleep; next day lassitude, headache,
  flat taste, several diarrhœic stools, with cutting pains in
  abdomen. θAgue.
Paroxysm at 10 A.M.
▮Aching in bones and pain through temples, with heaviness in forehead; chills up and down back, with great
  thirst, lasting fifteen minutes, was not a "regular
  shake," accompanied by great languor and weakness,
  so that "he fell down in a bunch," then came nausea
  and vomiting, followed by a burning fever, which lasted
  until 2 P.M.; thirst and throbbing headache during
  fever, followed by profuse sour sweat; paroxysms postponing. θAgue.
▮Chill at 9 A.M.; teeth chatter; nails and lips blue; no
  thirst; next fever, slight thirst, moaning, sighing;
  slight heat; restlessness; pulse large and soft; tongue
  coated white and thick; frontal headache; diarrhœa,
  stools yellow and painless; internal heat, with external
  coldness; drinks little; much nausea and vomiting; al-
  buginea yellow; perspiration stains linen yellow.
▮External coldness with internal heat.
▮Sudden attacks of general heat, with cold hands and feet.
▮One hand cold, the other hot.
▮Hands and feet icy cold and bathed in cold sweat, with
  redness of one cheek and paleness of the other.
▮Heat all over, with alternate coldness and paleness of
  face; cold sweat on forehead.
▮Heat with nausea and vomiting; anxious, oppressed
  breathing; dry, hacking cough, often exciting nausea
  and vomiting.
▮Anxious dry heat in evening.
▮Heat, with or without thirst.

∎Sweat: hot, sudden attacks in room; partial, cold; on upper part of body; < by motion; pungent, sour smelling; stains yellow; < out of doors; cold, clammy.

∎Sour sweat with turbid urine.

∎Very profuse sour sweat, mostly during night.

∎Profuse sweat after abuse of quinine.

∎Paroxysm sets in with yawning, stretching, and a collection of saliva in mouth; chill generally of short duration, soon passing over into heat; internal chill, as if under skin, < by hot applications, > by drinking and in open air; no thirst or but little during chill; violent thirst for large quantities during heat. θIntermittent.

∎In evening sensation of great weakness; restless, tosses about from side to side; slowly opens eyes and then closes them again; speaks in a low voice of things which have occurred previous day; spasmodic stretching and yawning; cold feet; paroxysm lasts one to two hours followed by sleep, after which patient is not aware of having had attacks. θQuotidian ague.

∎Paroxysms occur in morning and consist of moderate chill lasting about half an hour, followed by scarcely perceptible dry heat, lasting about two hours, during which pulse is full, soft and moderately frequent; with chill severe raging headache, brings tears to patient's eyes; nausea, pain in stomach, and short dry cough; headache continues until evening; during apyrexia, vertigo, loss of appetite, pain in small of back and limbs. θQuotidian ague.

∎Shivering, with gooseflesh, followed by flying heat, both of short duration; loss of appetite; tongue white; stool scanty and hard; heat in stomach and sensation of hunger; bitter taste in mouth in morning; waterbrash and retching; red, itching spot on r. chest, burning after scratching. θQuotidian ague.

∎Severe chill 3 P.M. without thirst, lasting one hour, followed by heat with stupefying headache and great thirst; sweat long and profuse with thirst; during apyrexia great weakness and lassitude; on getting out of bed vertigo and weakness of knees; disagreeable heat at night; restless, unrefreshing sleep; anorexia; bitter taste; white tongue; thirstlessness. θQuotidian ague.

∎Tertian ague anteponing half hour; chill one and a half hours' duration; high fever with sweat, lasting rest of day; during whole attack great thirst, water taken being soon vomited; headache with the fever; during apyrexia, earthy taste, pressure in stomach, debility.

∎Chilliness with yawning and vomiting; after an hour heat in head and redness of face, hands and feet being scarcely warm, followed by sweat on face; during apyrexia despondent, will not play, lies about a good deal, loss of appetite, grayish yellow diarrhœa, scanty red urine, restless sleep. θTertian ague.

❚Hard chill every other day, at 1 or 2 P.M.; continual nausea and vomiting of bitter, bilious matter, and of everything taken into stomach; chill very violent, with great thirst, and drinking only a little at a time; towards the last has chills and flushes of heat, then great heat and profuse sweat.

❚Chill every other day, at about 11 A.M.; shivers awhile, then shakes for twenty minutes; headache; hands first cold; nausea all the time; no thirst with the chill, but with the heat; chill followed by fever; sweat after fever. θIntermittent.

❚❚Backache, short chill, long fever; heat, usually with thirst, headache, nausea and cough.

❚❚Recent cases, occurring in young, previously healthy persons; paroxysms violent and regular, generally of tertian type. θAgue.

❚Predominance of gastric symptoms during paroxysm as well as during apyrexia. θIntermittent.

❚Relapses from improprieties in diet.

❚❚Paroxysms suppressed by quinine.

❚Intermittent fevers after abuse of quinine; also in beginning of irregular cases, especially if there is much nausea.

❚Worse during sweat; better after it.

Type: quotidian; tertian; quartan; apt to postpone and become irregular.

Prodroma: nausea; violent retching; yawning, stretching, backache, headache, and profuse flow of saliva.

Apyrexia: never clear; disturbed by gastric troubles; pale face; herpes labialis; anorexia; taste of insipid water, salivation; sense of emptiness and weakness of stomach, nausea; loose stools; bruised feeling of limbs; restless sleep; difficulty in collecting one's thoughts; sadness.

❚Infantile remittent fever.

❚Yellow coating on tongue, with dry mouth; loathing of food, with desire to vomit; fetid odor from mouth; bitter taste in mouth, and of food; nausea, with regurgitation of ingesta, and vomiting of undigested food; pressure and painful fulness in pit of stomach; colic; diarrhœic, yellowish stools, or fetid, putrid stools; pale, yellowish color of skin; headache, especially in forehead; febrile heat, with thirst or shivering. θBilious fever.

❚Yellow fever, in first stage; dizziness, chilliness, pain in back and limbs, uncomfortable feeling in epigastrium, with nausea, vomiting and great weakness.

∎Dry and extremely troublesome heat, especially in evening, with thirst; great restlessness, burning in palms of
hands and night sweats; parchmentlike skin; desire
for dainties only; very listless. θHectic fever.

∎Worm fever, with retching, blue rings around eyes, vomiting with a clean tongue.

" Attacks, Periodicity. ∎Attacks of illness, with loathing
of food.

Paroxysms: of abdominal pains; of great weakness, last
one to two hours; of suffocation; intermittent.

Fits: of dry, spasmodic coughing.

Following each other in quiet succession: violent shattering, hollow cough.

Sudden attacks: of general heat.

For a time: child remains without respiring; during
whooping cough.

Every few seconds: brings up a mouthful of bright colored
frothy blood.

Every five minutes: lasting ten to fifteen minutes; spasms.

Every eight to ten minutes: eructations.

Evening, 10, 15 minutes: attacks in pit of stomach.

Every quarter of an hour: vomiting.

Fifteen minutes: chill lasts.

Twenty minutes: shakes.

Half hour: tertian ague anteponing; attacks of vomiting
of blood.

One hour: chill lasts; heat in head; sweat after chill.

Eleven attacks in twenty-four hours: of spasms.

After a meal, especially P.M.: cough.

After dinner: dry, spasmodic cough.

Three or four stools a day.

Chill irregular.

Several times a day: hysterical spasms.

Every day at same hour: dyspepsia.

Every night: suffocative fits.

Every other day at same hour: dyspepsia.

Every fourth day: tormina and bilious vomiting.

For days: constant vomiting.

Every Saturday: tormina and bilious vomiting.

Every two weeks: menses.

Every six or eight weeks: anorexia and hypochondria.

Sixth week of pregnancy: abdominal pains, heat in epigastrium and vertigo.

Four times in seven weeks: menses.

For four months: occasional slight loss of blood.

In Autumn: diarrhœa; dysentery.

" Locality and Direction. Right: eye <; imbedded cor-
nea, ulcerated; opening lid gush of tears; shooting

pain from kidney down thigh to knee; spasmodic contraction of arm; slight contraction of corner of mouth; regular movements of arm and hand; ear cold.

Left: headache over eye; cornea ulcerated; pain in hypochondrium; frightful spasms affecting side.

Downwards: pain from umbilicus to uterus.

From l. to r.: cutting pain in abdomen shooting across.

Turned to right: eyes.

From front to back: diaphragm feels as if pressed between two millstones.

Backwards: stiffening of body.

Down: uterine pains running.

⁴³**Sensations.** Pricking burning pains.

Headache, as if bruised, through bones of head and down to root of tongue; as of a bruise of brain and skull; as though brain was mashed; as if stomach hung down relaxed; diaphragm feels as if pressed between two millstones; griping, as from a hand, each finger sharply pressed into intestines; as though bowels were grasped with hand; as if all the bones in body were being torn to pieces; strangling, as if from mucus in chest; oppression of chest as from inhaling dust; tickling in upper part of larynx, as from vapor of sulphur; as if hot water was poured into bowels; feet as if paralyzed; as if blood was vomited up; sensation in femur as if dislocated; as if joints had gone to sleep; pain in bones as if bruised; as if limbs were broken; as if chill was under skin; as if forehead was being crushed; as if all the bones were being torn to pieces.

Pain: over l. eye; in occiput and nape of neck; in temples and forehead; in hollow tooth; in molars; in diaphragm; in loins and hips; in stomach; most severe in front of abdomen; extending to l. hypochondrium to sides, to back and base of chest; in teeth; in l. hypochondrium; about umbilicus toward uterus; in abdomen; in heart; in uterus; in small of back; in limbs; at umbilicus; in epigastrium; in lower bowels and kidneys; in joints.

Violent pain: in abdominal region and bladder.

Intense tearing pains: in eyes.

Intense headache: extending to root of nose and throat.

Severe raging headache.

Acute pain: after miscarriage.

Violent distress: in pit of stomach.

Severe pains: radiating in abdomen; in kidneys; about umbilicus.

Cutting pain: in belly; near umbilicus; through abdomen from l. to r.; in abdomen and urethra.

Anxiety: about præcordia.

Piercing pain: through all cranial bones into roots of teeth.
Pinching pain: in both hypochondria and region of pit of
stomach; around umbilicus downward to uterus.
Shooting pain: through eyeballs; from r. kidney down
thigh to knee; across abdomen; in kidneys; in chest.
Stitches: in vertex or forehead; from navel to uterus.
Fine and violently stinging pains: in head.
Stinging pain: in head; in fauces.
Beating pain: in head; in pit of stomach; in stomach.
Throbbing: in head; of heart; frontal headache.
Jumping headache.
Painful concussions: in stomach and head.
Clutching pains: in stomach; in abdomen.
Cramp: between scapulæ; in thighs; in chest.
Griping: in intestines.
Squeezing: in abdomen.
Stupefying headache.
Pressing pain: in stomach.
Intense aching: in back and bones.
Aching: in forehead; in head; in bones.
Pressive frontal headache.
Constant pressing pain: in pit of stomach.
Bearing down pressure: to uterus and anus.
Tensive pain: in occiput and nape of neck, extending to
shoulders; in eyes.
Sense of excoriation; in chest.
Painful soreness: of occiput and neck.
Burning: in urethra; in palms of hands.
Smarting: eruption on margin of lips; in mouth and on
tongue; of eyes.
Sore pain: in chest.
Sore feeling: in abdomen.
Soreness: of fauces.
Bruised feeling: of limbs.
Tenderness: about umbilicus.
Painful fulness: in pit of stomach.
Violent pressure: over uterus and rectum.
Indescribable sick feeling: in stomach.
Heat: in head; in epigastrium; in stomach; dry and ex-
tremely uncomfortable.
Dull drawing: in head to and fro.
Dryness: of fauces; of mouth.
Distress: about navel.
Sense of emptiness: of stomach.
Pressure: in throat; in stomach; in bladder; in pit of
stomach.
Uncomfortable feeling: in epigastrium.
Constriction: in throat and chest.

Oppression: of chest.
Heaviness: of head; of thighs; in forehead.
Strangling: with cough.
Spasmodic tightness: of chest.
Contractive feeling: in throat and chest.
Tickling: at entrance of trachea; from upper portion of
    larynx to lower extremity of bronchi.
Bubbling: in chest.
Weakness: of thighs.
Trembling: internal.
Coldness: of upper part of body; of feet; of extremities; of
    one hand.
Internal chill.
Itching: spot on r. chest; at anus; of calves.

" **Tissues.** ∎Muscular awkwardness.
  ∎∎Hemorrhages: bright red, from all the orifices of body;
    after mechanical injuries.
  After exposure to cold and rain.
  ∎Plethora, fat children.
  ∎Skin and mucous membranes pale; pulse small, soft;
    chilliness; little appetite; constipation; marked anæmic
    murmurs; great debility and weakness; finally could
    hardly eat anything; nausea and vomiting following
    slightest amount of food; great emaciation; headache,
    as if forehead was being crushed, with nausea; erup-
    tion on forehead and cheek; scanty menses; querulous,
    not pleased with anything; hands cold; hysterical.
  ∎Cholerose gastric symptoms, nausea, vomiting, diarrhœa.
  ∎Dropsy in internal parts.
  ∎Skin and muscles lax.
  ∎Pain as if bruised in all the bones.
  ∎Pains as if all the bones were being torn to pieces; with
    vomiting and pains in bowels.
  ∎Icterus; rickets; atrophy:
  ∎Has an unmistakable relation to the voluntary muscles;
    in every kind of convulsions in children, in tonic, and
    especially in clonic convulsions, from the distortion of
    face, rolling of eyes and clenching of thumbs to the most
    severe epileptic spasms, particularly if there is nausea.

" **Touch. Passive Motion. Injuries.** Pressure: stomach
  and hypochondria sensitive.
  When biting on hollow tooth: pain in it.
  After mechanical imjuries: hemorrhage from lungs.

" **Skin.**   ∎∎Itching, unchanged by scratching.
  ∎Itching of skin, with nausea; has to scratch till he vomits.
  ∎Miliaria rubra, with dyspnœa, colic and nausea.
  ∎Miliary rash on forehead, temples and cheek.
  ∎Rash of the lying in.

❙Suppressed eruption with cool skin.

❙Eruptions suppressed, or tardily appearing, with oppression of chest; vomiting and tickling cough.

Herpetic eruption at wrist joint and anus, with red blotches after scratching.

❙Erysipelas, the redness leaves too soon, with renewed vomiting.

❙Reaction so weak that eruption developes tardily or does not appear at all; anxious oppression, or constriction of chest; irascible, irritable, particularly at night, preventing sleep, and causing great anxiety; severe tickling cough, with blueness of face and dyspnœa. *θ*Measles.

❙Fever, < towards night; sleeplessness; complete loss of appetite; nausea; despondent and lachrymose; groaning. *θ*Scarlet fever.

❙Vascular erethism with tardy development of eruption; anxious constriction of chest; restless tossing about. *θ*Scarlet fever.

❙Delayed eruption in scarlatina, with vomiting, diarrhœa, oppression and anxiety.

ᵃ **Stages of Life, Constitution.** Women and children; emphysematous individuals.

Girl, æt. 6 weeks, eight days after birth caught cold; inflamed eyes.

Girl, æt. 3 months, after receiving eight drops of laudanum; opium poisoning.

Child, æt. 17 weeks, scrofulous; vomiting and diarrhœa.

Child, æt. 22 weeks; spasms.

Child, æt. 30 weeks, pale, fat; spasmodic cough.

Boy, æt. 3, after overloading stomach; diarrhœa.

Boy, æt. 4; ague.

Boy, æt. 4; eclampsia.

Boy, æt. 10, sanguine, scrofulous, after eating pork; diarrhœa.

Girl, æt. 11, black hair and eyes, subject to attacks of ague for which quinine was taken; intermittent.

Boy, æt. 14; chronic vomiting.

Girl, æt. 15; ague.

Girl, æt. 16; melæna.

Man, æt. 17, sanguine temperament, suffering from purpura, after catching cold; spasms.

Girl, æt. 18, graceful, menses profuse; ague.

Man, æt. 20, weak, brunette, melancholic; ague.

Woman, æt. 21; ague.

Woman, æt. 22; ague.

Woman, æt. 23, small, pale, irritable, brown hair, menses appeared at 17 but were very scanty; anæmia.

Woman, æt. 23, blonde; hæmatemesis.

Women, æt. 24, strong, good constitution, married three months, pregnant six weeks; uterine hemorrhage, with abortion.

Woman, primipara, after tedious labor, terminated by instrumental delivery; hemorrhage from uterus.

Woman, suffering four weeks; flooding.

Woman, æt. 24; hysterical spasms.

Girl, æt. 25, strong; hæmatemesis.

Man, æt. 25; chronic nasal catarrh.

Woman, æt. 26, large, robust, fair complexion, has suffered four years; tormina and bilious vomiting.

Swedish girl, æt. 26, ill for three years, has taken much quinine; intermittent fever.

Woodcutter, suffering for years, every spring and fall; ague.

Man, suffering some weeks; ague.

Girl, æt. 28, anæmic; hæmatemesis.

Man, æt. 28; cholera.

Woman, æt. 30, blonde, weak; ague.

Soldier, æt. 34; dysentery.

Negro, after piercing sole of foot by stepping upon a fish bone; tetanus.

Woman, æt. 35, ill two weeks; ague.

Woman, æt. 35; ague.

Woman, æt. 38; cough.

Woman, æt. 38, has taken quinine; intermittent fever.

Man, æt. 39, tuberculous, after exposure to wet and cold; hæmoptysis.

Woman, æt. 39, married; vomiting.

Woman, æt 40, four months after abortion; hemorrhage.

Woman, æt. 42, suffering 2½ years; vomiting.

Man, æt. 44, ague.

Man. æt. 45, suffering four weeks; constant vomiting.

Woman, æt. 47, suffering six weeks; choroiditis.

Man, æt. 54, suffering three months; chronic vomiting.

Woman, æt. 54, good constitution, menstruation ceased six months ago without inconvenience, after taking journey during which she became chilled; hæmaturia.

Widow, æt. 54, since attack of cholera four years ago, continual suffering in abdomen; dysentery.

Man, æt. 62; ague.

Woman, æt. 72, melancholic temperament, brunette, thin, tendency to hemorrhoids and abdominal affections; spasmodic cough.

Relations. Antidoted by: *Arnica, Arsen., Cinchona, Nux vom., Tabac.*

It antidotes *Alum., Arnica, Arsen., Cinchona,* vapors of copper, *Dulcam., Ferrum, Lauroc., Opium, Sulph. ac., Tabac., Tart. em.*

Compatible: is followed well by *Arsen.* (cholera infantum, debility, colds, croup, chills), *Bellad., Bryon., Cadmium sulph.* (yellow fever), *Calc. ost., Chamom., Cinchona, Cuprum, Ignat., Nux vom., Phosphor., Pulsat., Sepia, Sulphur, Tart. em., Tabac., Veratr.*
Complementary: *Cuprum.*

IPOMŒA.

Morning Glory.   *Convolvulaceæ.*

Fragmentary provings by Jeanes from tincture of leaves, 2d dil., in 1843 (marked l.), and from preparing tincture of seed in 1845 (marked s.).

CLINICAL AUTHORITIES.—*Renal calculus,* Farrington, A. H. Z., vol. 101, p. 184.

¹ Sensorium.   Vertiginous affection, immediately; s.
³ Inner Head.   Pain first in r. then in l. temple; s.
   Pain in r. temple and eye; l.
   Pain in l. temple, jaw and eye; l.
   Great heaviness of head; s.
⁴ Outer Head.   Itching of scalp; s.
⁵ Sight and Eyes.   Smarting of eyes; s.
   Itching of internal canthus of l. eye; l.
   Pain in r. eye and temple; l.
⁷ Smell and Nose.   Very acute sense of smell; s.
   Smarting and dryness in nostrils; s.
   ▌Purulent discharge from nose; s.
⁸ Upper Face.   Pain in l. upper jaw, eye and temple; l.
¹³ Throat.   Pain in l. tonsil; l.
¹⁷ Scrobiculum and Stomach.   Rumbling and grumbling in epigastric region; l.
¹⁹ Abdomen.   Sharp cutting pain in abdomen above umbilicus; l.
   Rumbling of flatus: with pain in l. superior flexure of colon, followed by speedy discharge of flatus; in transverse colon; in region of sigmoid flexure; s.
   Pain in region of descending colon; l.
   Shooting reports of flatus in abdomen; s.
   Grumbling in lower bowels; l.
   Great distension of abdomen; l.
   Flashing heat in superior abdomen and stomach; l.
²¹ Urinary Organs.   ▌Severe pains in l. kidney, with paroxysms of pain running along ureter and in back; nausea and occasional vomiting.   θRenal calculus.
   Diminution of contractile power of bladder; l.

‖Kidney disorders or gravel with pain in back.

²⁷ Cough. Disposition to cough; sneezing; l.

³¹ Neck and Back. ‖Pain in first dorsal vertebræ; l.
Itching over l. scapula; s.
Pain in lumbar region; l.
Pain in l. lumbar region; l.
Pain in region of lumbar vertebræ; l.

³² Upper Limbs. Aching in top of r. shoulder; s.
Pain in r. biceps flexor cubiti near elbow; s.
Pain in l. shoulder and arm; s.

⁴⁰ Fever. Backache alternating with chilliness; l.
Flushing of heat followed by copious sweats.

⁴² Locality and Direction. Right: pain in temple; in eye;
aching in top of shoulder; pain in biceps flexor cubiti
near elbow.

Left: pain in temple, jaw and eye; itching of internal
canthus of eye; pain in upper jaw; pain in tonsil; pain
in superior flexure of colon; severe pain in kidney;
itching over scapula; pain in lumbar region; pain in
shoulder and arm.

⁴⁵ Sensations. Pain in r. then in l. temple; in eye; in jaw; in
r. eye and temple; in l. upper jaw, eye and temple; in
l. tonsil; in l. superior flexure of colon; in region of
descending colon; along ureter and back; in first dorsal
vertebræ; in lumbar region; in l. lumbar region; in
region of lumbar vertebræ; in r. biceps flexor cubiti
near elbow; in l. shoulder and arm.

Severe pain: in l. kidney.
Sharp cutting pain: in abdomen above umbilicus.
Aching: in top of r. shoulder.
Backache: alternating with chilliness.
Smarting: of eyes; in nostrils.
Dryness: in nostrils.
Heaviness: of head.
Great distension of abdomen.
Flushing heat: in superior abdomen and stomach.
Itching: of scalp; of internal canthus of l. eye; over l.
scapula.

IRIDIUM.

The metal.   *Ir.*

One of the metals of the platinum group, among the heaviest of known sub-substances and almost indestructible.

Introduced by Hering in 1853.

The precipitate made by Genth was triturated by Boericke ; one ten thousandth part of it produced a vivid black.

Twenty grains of the 3d trituration were taken by A. J. Tafel when in a state of perfect health. It is the only proving of Iridium and not contained in Allen's Encyclopedia. All the symptoms were experienced within two hours.

⁴ **Outer Head.** Pain in middle of occipital bone.

⁵ **Sight and Eyes.** A feeling as if the eyes were being affected from below upward.

⁶ **Hearing and Ears.** Feeling of numbness in ears and throughout the body, lasting but a short time.

⁸ **Upper Face.** Pain in l. malar bone, a kind of stinging; from this place a kind of warmth spreads over the whole face; the pain is also felt in r. malar bone like a pressure.

Feeling as of a triangle in face, the base is formed by the two malar bones, the apex in the vertex.

¹² **Inner Mouth.** Increased saliva with sensation in malar bones which is more perceptible on l. side.

¹² **Upper Limbs.** A transient pain on inner side of wrists, particularly the left, also in bend of knee joint.

²² **Lower Limbs.** Pressing in anterior portion of l. thigh in middle of upper half, followed by pressing in groin.

While walking, feeling of tension in both thighs, particularly in l.; then a dislocated feeling in l. hip joint, and a dull pain tending toward l. gluteal region.

Cramp-like contraction in r. calf and middle of sole of foot.

³³ **Rest. Position. Motion.** While walking : feeling of tension in both thighs.

⁴³ **Locality and Direction.** Right : pain in malar bone; cramp-like contraction in calf.

Left : pain in malar bone; sensation more perceptible in malar bone; transient pain in wrists, < l.; pressing in anterior portion of thigh; feeling of tension in thigh; dislocated feeling in hip joint; dull pain tending towards gluteal region.

From below upward : eyes affected. ·

⁴³ **Sensations.** As if the eyes were being affected from below

upwards; as of a triangle in face, the base formed by the two malar bones, the apex in the vertex.

Pain: in middle of occipital bones.

Stinging pain: in l. malar bone.

Cramp-like contraction: in r. calf and middle of sole of foot.

Pressure-like pain: in r. malar bone.

Dull pain: tending toward l. gluteal region.

Transient pain: on inner side of wrists; in knee joints.

Pressing: in anterior portion of l. thigh, in middle of upper half; in groin.

Dislocated feeling: in l. hip joint.

Feeling of tension: while walking, in both thighs.

Numbness: in ears and throughout whole body.`

IRIS VERSICOLOR.

Blue Flag.   *Iridaceæ.*

Provings by Rowland, Burt, Holcombe, Berridge, Croker, Wesselhœft, etc. See Allen's Encyclopedia, vol. 5, p. 153.

CLINICAL AUTHORITIES.—*Headache,* Palmer, Raue's Rec., 1871, p. 179; Warren, A. H. O., vol. 1, p. 109; *Sick headache,* Kitchen, N. A. J. H., vol. 1, p. 464; Williamson, Raue's Rec., 1871, p. 16; Wesselhœft, Raue's Rec., 1870, p. 287; *Bilious headache,* Blake, A. H. O., vol. 9, p. 411; *Tinea capitis,* Burt, A. H. O., vol. 3, p. 257; *Inflamed eyelids,* Kitchen, N. A. J. H., vol. 1, p. 466; *Prosopalgia* (3 cases), Holcombe, B. J. H., vol. 24, p. 512; *Salivation,* Stevenson, Raue's Rec., 1871, p. 70; B. J. H., vol. 29, p. 429; Claude, B. J. H., vol. 36, p. 183; *Vomiting,* Kitchen, N. A. J. H., vol. 1, p. 462; *Colic,* Kitchen, N. A. J. H., vol. 1, p. 465; Sanford, B. J. H., vol. 25, p. 671; *Bilious colic,* Hawkes, Raue's Rec., 1875, p. 162; *Diarrhœa,* Oehme, Times Retros., vol. 3, p. 27; (2 cases), Casseday, Hah. Mo., vol. 15, p. 604; Kitchen, N. A. J. H., vol. 1, p. 463; *Autumnal diarrhœa, cholera,* Lade, Hom. Rev., vol. 10, pp. 28, 503; *Dysentery,* Kitchen, N. A J. H., vol. 1, p. 464; *Constipation,* Claude, B. & S.; *Cholera morbus* (2 cases), Casseday, Hahn. Mo., vol. 15, p. 604; Kitchen, N. A. J. H., vol. 1, p. 462; (Irisin) Lade, N. A. J. H., vol. 15, p. 476; *Menorrhagia,* Wesselhœft, Raue's Rec., 1870, p. 25; *Vomiting of pregnancy,* Clark, Raue's Rec., 1872, p. 183; *Cough,* Wesselhœft, Raue's Rec., 1870, p. 180, *Sciatica,* Payne, Hah. Mo., vol. 4, p. 405; Wesselhœft, Raue's Rec., 1870, p. 293; *Neuralgia,* Kitchen, N. A. J. H., vol. 1, p. 467; *Typhoid fever,* Kitchen, N. A. J. H., vol. 1, p. 467; *Itch* (2 cases), Burt, A. H. O., vol. 3, p. 257; *Eczema,* Palmer, Raue's Rec., 1871, p. 210; *Impetigo,* Buck, B. J. H., vol. 24, p. 508; *Felon,* Gilchrist's Surg., p. 98.

¹ **Mind.** Low spirited; discouraged.

Fears approaching illness.

Easily vexed.

Dulness of mental faculties; cannot fix mind on studies.

Muttering.

¹ Sensorium. Head full, heavy.

³ Inner Head. Constriction around forehead.

Sensation as of a band around head.

❚ Dull, heavy frontal headache with nausea. ➤

❚ Severe frontal headache, constant nausea and occasional vomiting; sleepless from pain; no appetite; great weakness.

❚ Headache in forehead and eyes, < r. side; with distressing nausea and vomiting of intensely sour or bilious matter; < in rest.

❚❚ Dull throbbing or shooting in r. side of forehead; nausea; < toward evening, from rest, from cold air, or coughing; > from moderate motion.

❚ Habitual headache; violent throbbing on either side of frontal protuberance, < in evening or after exertion.

❚ Chronic frontal headache; < sitting down, studying or sewing; > standing up or working; could not attend school.

❚ Headache with violent pains over eye, in supraorbital region, on either side, but only on one side at a time.

❚ Severe pain in head, through temples and over eyes, with vertigo, nausea and vomiting.

❚ Shooting pains in temples, generally right, with constricted feeling in scalp.

❚ Headache affecting r. side, < at rest, > by constant motion, accompanied by nausea, vomiting and low spirits.

❚ Hemicrania of r. hemisphere.

❚ Pain shoots like an electric shock from r. temple to l. side of occiput; depression of spirits, debility.

❚ Slight dull pain at situation of posterior fontanelle.

❚ Severe pain in occiput, < r. side.

❚❚ Stitches in lower cerebellum, r. side.

❚ Violent, stunning headache, with facial neuralgia, followed by copious, limpid urine and vomiting.

❚ Sick headache, every eighth day.

❚❚ Sick headache, of gastric or hepatic origin, always beginning with a blur before eyes.

❚ Sick headache, seemingly the result of intense gastric and abdominal disturbance; dull, throbbing, or hammering, and also shooting or acute boring pains in one side of forehead, generally left, or passing from r. to l., with nausea; pain begins in morning and grows more violent towards afternoon and night; < from violent motion; > from moderate exercise in open air; sometimes paroxysmal, through day, or at intervals of many days,

so as to become periodical; $<$ in cold air and from
coughing.

❚Headache, vomits sweetish mucus, occasionally with a
trace of bile.

❚Sick headache in bilious subjects, with gastric derangement and dyspepsia, tenderness in region of stomach and
liver.

❚Headache reflex from acid stomach, or irritation of that
organ from acid secretions.

❚Neuralgia, facial or cephalic, with nausea and vomiting.

❚Neuralgia of head, eyes and temples; pains cutting, of
short duration, with acid vomiting; bilious vomiting,
or vomiting of sweetish water; great despondency.

❚Tired headache, from mental exhaustion.

❚Chronic headaches with asthenopia and fulness in
stomach.

❚❚Sharp, cutting pains of short duration, changing often.

⁴ **Outer Head.** ❚Shooting in temples, mostly right, with constrictive feeling of scalp.

❚Pustular eruptions on scalp in children.

· ❙❙Twenty-six pustules on top of head, some as large as a
three cent piece.

❚Whole top of head one complete scab, yellow matter
oozing from under crust, which has matted hair together;
l. ear covered with eruption, it also gathers every two
weeks and discharges a yellow greenish pus; numerous
yellow pustules scattered over scalp, each pustule containing a hair. *θ*Tinea capitis.

⁵ **Sight and Eyes.** ❚Redness of conjunctiva, as from a
cold; eyes feel dull, with neuralgia; burning in internal
canthus, with effusion of tears.

❚Inflamed eyelids; simple palpebral inflammation, apparently arising from cold.

❚Chronic inflammation of eyelids.

⁷ **Smell and Nose.** ❙❙Constant sneezing; sharp pains in
centre of temples; tickling cough; light, mushy stools.

⁸ **Upper Face.** ❚Sunken eyes with blue circles.

❚Neuralgia, involving supra and infraorbital, superior
maxillary and inferior dental nerves; begins after breakfast every morning, with a stupid, stunning headache;
copious urine; disposition to stool; burning at anus.

❙❙Neuralgia in head, temples and eyes, attended with most
distressing vomiting of sweetish mucus, and occasionally,
when much straining, with a trace of bile.

❚Waked with neuralgic pains in r. side of face; darting
stitches in two carious teeth; infraorbital nerves especially affected.

⁹ **Lower Face.** ❙❙Dry, cracked lips.

‖Pustular eruptions on face, around nose, lips and cheeks, secreting a sanious, irritating matter.

¹⁰ Teeth and Gums. ‖Toothache in warm room; dental neuralgia.

¹¹ Taste and Tongue. Taste: lost; flat; bitter or putrid.
‖Tongue feels as if scalded; greasy feeling on arising in morning.
‖Tongue white.

¹² Inner Mouth. ‖Burning in mouth and fauces, as if on fire.
‖‖Mouth and tongue feel as though they had been scalded.
‖Salivation after diphtheria, with swelling of parotids.
‖‖Profuse flow of saliva.
‖Constant discharge of ropy saliva, dropped from mouth during conversation.
‖Salivation, first of tough mucus hawked from throat, which presented a dark appearance, and afterwards a profuse, watery discharge from whole buccal cavity; clammy, greasy sensation in mouth, with bilious coating on root of tongue; lethargy; hunger, with inability to eat; general "bilious" condition; constipation, succeeding a profuse, watery, offensive pancreatic diarrhœa.
‖Salivation with profuse flow; gums and tongue feel as though covered with a greasy substance.
‖Stomatitis, with painful burning in mouth and fauces.
‖Ulcers on mucous membrane of cheeks.

¹³ Throat. Pain in tonsils, shooting into ears.
‖Smarting, burning sensation, with feeling of enlargement, like a burning cavern, while throat is dry injected, and of bright red color.
‖Peculiar irritability of throat, palate and pharynx, coming on without any appearance of inflammation, and sometimes attended with cough.
‖Spasms of pharynx while swallowing food.

¹⁴ Appetite, Thirst. Desires, Aversions. ‖Loss of taste and appetite, nausea and empty eructations.

¹⁵ Eating and Drinking. ‖Headache after breakfast; aching in stomach before breakfast and after a cold drink.
‖Chronic indigestion of milk; it sours and is vomited.

¹⁶ Hiccough, Belching, Nausea and Vomiting. Eructations: of tasteless gas; of wind from stomach with considerable force; tasteless; acid; of sour food.
‖Heartburn.
‖Nausea: from riding, from overexertion or from irregularities of diet; and retching.
‖‖Nausea and vomiting: of sour food, whole person smells sour; of thin, watery fluid of an exceedingly sour taste.
‖Vomiting: an extremely sour fluid which excoriates throat; with burning in mouth, fauces, œsophagus and

stomach; of sweetish water; of ingesta; of soured milk
in children; of food an hour after eating; of bile, with
great heat and sweat.

∎Bilious vomiting, with great heat of head and perspiration.

∎Violent pain with every fit of vomiting.

∎Periodical vomiting spells, coming on once every month
or six weeks, lasting two or three days.

∎Vomiting of ingesta, then sour fluid, and at last bile yellow and green, with great heat of head, some general
fever, and great prostration; perspiration warm, caused
by efforts of straining and vomiting.

[17] **Scrobiculum and Stomach.** ∎Great burning distress in epigastrium; can hardly endure it.

∎Violent pains in epigastric region, coming on at intervals.

∎Gastralgia.

∎∎Pain in stomach before breakfast, and from drinking
water.

Beating, throbbing, in and about heart and sternum, then
fearful cramps or spasms from middle of sternum to pit
of stomach, with repeated vomitings.

Everything sours in stomach.

∎Dyspepsia; food vomited an hour or so after meals.

∎Gastric symptoms predominate with headache.

∎Burning distress in stomach and pancreas, with watery
diarrhœa and great prostration.

∎Burning distress in pancreas, sweetish vomit.

∎Shocks of pain in umbilical region up to epigastrium;
nausea, straining and belching of wind.

[18] **Hypochondria.** ∎Cutting in region of liver.

∎Pain in r. hypochondriac region; < from motion.

∎Acute and chronic disorders of liver.

∎Increase of bile, then deficiency of, with jaundice.

∎Anxious look; vomits almost constantly a greenish yellow
matter, very bitter; great tenderness in region of liver;
urgent desire for stool; bowels torpid; pulse 130, temperature, 103.2; great pain in abdomen, < on pressure;
tongue dry, coated on each side, red streak in centre;
dull and stupid. θBilious colic.

∎Acute affections of pancreas, inflammation or salivation.

∎Pains above crest of ilium, right side, then left.

[19] **Abdomen.** ∎Colicky pains, intermittent about navel, before
each spell of vomiting or purging.

∎Pains in umbilical region and loud rumbling in bowels.

∎Pain in region of umbilicus, < from motion; diarrhœa
threatening or actually existing; general headache, < in
anterior half, in individuals subject to headache; nausea
and vomiting.

∎Sharp, griping pains in bowels.

▮Colicky pains, must bend forward for relief; > after discharges of flatus.

▮Great prostration; pulse frequent and feeble; expression of great anguish in face; much mental depression; frequent and violent efforts to vomit, resulting, however, in little more than an enormous discharge of air, which seemed to roll off her stomach with great force; intense pain in umbilical region, passing in successive shocks, like effects of a galvanic battery, upward to epigastric region, followed or accompanied by nausea, straining and belching of wind; great commotion and rumbling of bowels above seat of pain, little or none below; no desire for stool. *θ*Colic.

▮Abdomen very prominent; severe rumbling of gas; excessive watery discharges, preceded by soft and more substantial evacuations and intense aching, cramplike pains; excessive nausea and vomiting.

▮Rumbling and cutting pain in lower part of abdomen, > by pressing flatus.

▮Periodical night colic, > by two or three free discharges before morning.

▮Colic of infants with flatulency and constipation.

▮Abdominal complaints of children occurring in Spring and Autumn.

▮Syphilitic sinus in l. groin, result of a bubo, discharge ichorous.

²⁰ **Stool and Rectum.** Diarrhœa: with colic and rumbling in bowels; with pain in bowels, with or without vomiting; cramps in bowels; thin, watery; with frequent bilious stools; brown and very offensive, with cutting, colicky pains, nausea and vomiting.

▮Stool: thin, watery, tinged with bile, copious, in a continuous stream; green, undigested; mushy, pappy, with fetid flatus; bloody mucus, with great straining; black, with fever, hot sweat, white tongue, severe headache, despondency; yellow, watery, corrosive; copious, watery, with or without tenesmus; frequent, very green and watery; watery, mixed with mucus; thin, yellow, fecal; fetid or coppery smelling; containing undigested food.

▮▮Watery stool; anus feels on fire; disposition to strain and bear down; great burning in anus.

▮Watery diarrhœa and colic pains precede the bloody, mucous discharges.

▮Bloody, mucous discharges, with severe tenesmus and rectal prolapsus.

▮Very soft, yellow stools, with great rumbling in bowels.

▮Stool of scybalous matter, together with fluid mucoid feces of offensive, putrid and coppery odor.

Before stool: rumbling in abdomen; cutting in lower part
of abdomen.

During stool: cutting; severe cramplike pains; tenesmus;
burning at anus; fetid, coppery smelling flatus.

After stool: pricking as of points in anus; burning of anus,
as though on fire; prolapsus of rectum.

∎Periodical spells of diarrhœa, always at night about two
or three o'clock.

∎Burning from mouth to anus. θDiarrhœa.

∎∎Acute mucous enteritis.

∎Stools brown, slimy, or watery, frequent and generally
very offensive; attacks sudden and characterized by
• uncommonly severe tenesmus, prolapsus of rectum,
frequently piles, and very intense feeling of exhaustion
from very commencement; appetite not much affected;
generally no pain in bowels. θDiarrhœa.

∎Cholera infantum, with profuse, sour discharges from
stomach and bowels, and pain in head.

∎Cholera morbus: occurring in hottest part of season; vomiting; grumbling pains in bowels, watery, green stools.

∎Severe pain in bowels, with much rumbling; constant
nausea; vomiting and purging every few moments; limbs
and body cold; occasional cramps in lower extremities;
vomited matter was glairy mucus with some bile at
times; stools thin and colorless. θCholera morbus.

∎∎Autumnal bilious diarrhœa.

∎Bilious dysentery; body cold; skin blue; vomiting with
prostration.

∎Constipation: succeeded by thin, watery diarrhœa; with
flatulent colic; migraine; nervousness; irregular menses;
colic and sick headache; headache affecting forehead
and eyes; hemorrhoids.   .   . .

∎Prolapsus of rectum.

∎∎Anus feels sore, or as if sharp points were sticking in it.

∎Premonitory diarrhœa for two or three days, then purging suddenly became <, with vomiting, cramps in body
and lower limbs; two hours later diarrhœa profuse and
involuntary, evacuations being wholly of rice water
character; vomiting frequent and severe, the matter
ejected consisting principally of small white flocculent
bodies, with bodies of undigested food; crampy pains in
abdomen and lumbar region, also less severely in legs;
intense and urgent thirst; difficulty and oppression of
breathing; choleraic expression; face limbs and body
cold; tongue slightly bluish, furred and icy cold to
touch. θCholera.

∎Asiatic cholera, with rice water discharges, cramps, etc.

²¹ **Urinary Organs.** Cutting and pricking in urethra while
urinating.

Urine: scanty, red; burning length of urethra after passing it; clear, profuse; copious, watery in nervous headache; very high colored and scanty.

²² Male Sexual Organs. ❙Nocturnal emissions, with amorous dreams.

❙Coldness and itching of parts.

❙❙Excitement of generative organs reflex from an excessively acid stomach.

❙❙Heavy, dragging gait and excitable sexual desire.

❙❙Coldness and relaxation of scrotum.

❙Spermatorrhœa, with pale face, sunken eyes; depression.

❙Secondary gonorrhœa or gleet; syphilis; mercurial syphilis.

²³ Female Sexual Organs. ❙Neuralgia and rheumatism of uterus.

❙Metrorrhagia.

❙Menses regular but excessive.

❙Uterine leucorrhœa.

²⁴ Pregnancy. Parturition. Lactation. ❙Morning sickness during pregnancy; vomit sour or bitter.

❙Protracted nausea and vomiting during pregnancy; profuse flow of saliva.

❙Inflammation and soreness of uterus, very sensitive to touch; pain across umbilicus, with severe griping at short intervals; nausea and vomiting of green or yellow bile, with eructations of a great deal of flatus during and between times of vomiting; diarrhœa of a yellow, bilious character. θMiscarriage.

²⁵ Voice and Larynx. Trachea and Bronchia. ❙Dry, tickling cough, with smarting burning in throat.

²⁷ Cough. ❙Short, dry cough, excited by excessive tickling in larynx, preceded or accompanied by dry, smarting, or burning sore throat.

²⁸ Inner Chest and Lungs. ❙Pain in l. side of chest, as if ribs were pressing against lungs.

³¹ Neck and Back. Crampy pain in r. lumbar region.

³² Upper Limbs. ❙Acute rheumatic pain r. shoulder < from motion, especially on raising arm.

❙Shooting burning pain in r. shoulder; gastralgia or enteralgia.

❙Pains shift rapidly in phalanges and metacarpal bones.

❙❙Fingers pain on writing.

³³ Lower Limbs. ❙Slight coxalgia in l. hip.

❙Sciatic pains, as if l. hip joint was wrenched.

❙Painful drawing and lameness behind l. trochanter, extending down to popliteal space.

❙Shooting, burning, laming pain, affecting posterior femoral muscles; shooting along l. sciatic nerve to foot, < by motion; moderate motion aggravates, violent motion makes no difference; shooting, burning pains in r. shoulder.

❙Pain confined to l. leg, shooting, burning, laming, affecting posterior femoral muscles, and shooting along l. sciatic nerve to foot; < by motion. θSciatica.

³⁴ Limbs in General. ❙Shifting pains in r. hip, both knees, < r. and in r. foot, especially, and first joint of great toe.

❙❙Tearing, shooting and rapidly shifting pains in joints and extremities, especially smaller joints, but more particularly in r. shoulder.

³⁵ Rest. Position. Motion. Rest: headache <.

Sitting down: chronic frontal headache <.

Must bend forward for relief: from colicky pains.

Standing up: chronic headache >.

Raising arm: pain in shoulder <.

After exertion: headache <.

Overexertion: causes nausea.

Constant motion: headache >.

Motion: pain in r. hypochondriac region <; pain in region of umbilicus <; pain in shoulder <; pain along sciatic nerve <.

Moderate motion: headache >.

Violent motion: sick headache <; pains along sciatic nerve not affected.

³⁶ Nerves. ❙Great debility; faint, weak knees, trembling; sunken eyes; after protracted or severe serous or bilious stools, as in summer diarrhœa.

³⁷ Sleep. ❙❙Sleeplessness; starts in sleep.

³⁸ Time. Aggravation in evening and at night; from rest, also from motion; > from continued motion.

Morning: pain in head grows more violent towards afternoon and night; sickness.

Towards evening: headache and nausea <.

Evening: headache <; much itching of eruption.

Night: emissions; chilliness; great itching of eruption; great itching of eczema.

³⁹ Temperature and Weather. Warm room: toothache.

Open air: headache >.

After cold drink: aching in stomach.

Cold air: headache and nausea <.

⁴⁰ Fever. ❙❙Chilliness all night.

❙❙Chills, with sleepiness.

Head and face cold.

❙Heat followed by chill, with cold hands and feet.

❙Chills over whole body, even when well covered; fever with muttering delirium and bilious diarrhœa.

Skin hot; dry, black stool.

▮Sweat over whole body, particularly in groin.

▮Bilious fever after *Bryon.* or *Acon.*

▮Typhoid fever, with symptoms similar to *Baptis.*

▮Muttering delirium; yellow, watery, stinking diarrhœa; involuntary passage of urine and feces; coated tongue, dry, brown, crusty, edges red, sordes on gums and teeth, and foul breath. *θ*Typhoid.

▮Fever; stupor; black, stinking, involuntary diarrhœa, tongue dry and brown; fetid breath. *θ*Typhoid.

▮Fever, intense headache, pain in small of back, black dysenteric passages, nausea and efforts to vomit. *θ*Typhoid.

⁴¹ **Attacks, Periodicity.** Paroxysmal: headache through day.
Every few moments: vomiting and purging.
At short intervals: severe griping in abdomen.
An hour after eating: vomiting of food.
After breakfast every morning: neuralgia of face; head-ache; pain in stomach.
Periodical nightly colic, diarrhœa 2 or 3 A.M.
Every eighth day: sick headache.
At intervals of many days, so as to become periodical: headache.
Every two weeks: ear gathers and discharges.
Once every month or six weeks: periodical vomiting spells, lasting two or three days.
Spring and Autumn: abdominal complaints.

⁴² **Locality and Direction.** Right: headache in forehead and eyes <; dull throbbing or shooting in side of fore-head; shooting in temple; hemicrania; severe pain in occiput <; stitches in lower cerebellum; neuralgic pain side of face; pain in hypochondriac region; crampy pain in lumbar region; acute rheumatic pain in shoul-der; shooting, burning pain in shoulder; shifting pains in hip, in foot; herpes zoster on side of body.
Left: acute, boring pains on side of forehead; ear covered with eruption; syphilitic sinus in groin; pain in side of chest; slight coxalgia in hip; sciatic pain in hip joint; painful drawing and lameness behind trochanter; pain along sciatic nerve to foot; in leg vesicular erup-tion on knee.
From r. to l: pain shoots like an electric shock from temple to occiput; acute, boring pains through forehead; pain above crest of ilium.

⁴³ **Sensations.** As of a band around head; tongue feels as if scalded; as if mouth and fauces were on fire; mouth as if it was scalded; gums and tongue feel as though cov-ered with a greasy substance; feeling of enlargement like a burning cavern in throat; pain like effects of a

galvanic battery upward to epigastric region; arms feel
as if on fire; pricking as of points; as if ribs were pressing against lungs; as if l. hip joint was wrenched.

Pain: in head, in forehead and eyes; in tonsils; in stomach; in r. hypochondriac region; above crest of ilium,
r. side, then l.; in umbilical region; in bowels; across
umbilicus; in l. side of chest; shifts rapidly in phalanges and metacarpal bones; in fingers; in l. leg; in
small of back.

Pain: like an electric shock from r. temple to l. side of
occiput.

Intense pain: in umbilical region.

Violent pain: over eyes; in supraorbital region on either
side, but only on one side at a time.

Violent pain: with every fit of vomiting; in epigastric
region.

Great pain: in abdomen.

Severe pain: in head, through temples and over eyes; in
occiput < r. side; in bowels.

Severe frontal headache.

Violent stunning headache with facial neuralgia.

Great burning distress: in stomach; in epigastrium; in
pancreas.

Fearful cramps: from middle of sternum to pit of stomach;
in bowels.

Sharp, cutting pains of short duration in head.

Cutting: in head; in region of liver; in lower part of abdomen; in urethra.

Tearing, shooting and rapidly shifting pains in joints and
extremities, especially smaller joints, but more particularly in r. shoulder.

Shooting, burning pain: in r. shoulder; affecting posterior femoral muscles.

Shooting pains: in temples; into ears; in r. shoulder;
along sciatic nerve to foot.

Acute, boring or shooting pains: in one side of forehead,
generally left.

Sharp pains: in centre of temples.

Darting stitches: in two carious teeth.

Stitches: in lower cerebellum, r. side.

Violent throbbing: in either side of frontal protuberance. '

Beating, throbbing: in and about heart and sternum.

Dull throbbing or shooting: in r. side of forehead.

Dull throbbing or hammering: in forehead.

Severe griping: in abdomen.

Sharp, griping pains: in bowels.

Intense aching, cramplike pains: in abdomen.

Colicky pains: about navel.

Neuralgic pains: in r. side of face.
Neuralgia: facial or cephalic; of head, eyes and temples; involving supra and infraorbital, superior maxillary and inferior dental nerves.
Acute rheumatic pain: in r. shoulder.
Sciatic pains: in l. hip joint.
Shifting pains: in r. hip, both knees, in r. foot and first joint of great toe.
Grumbling pains: in bowels.
Shocks of pain: in umbilical region, up to epigastrium.
Habitual headache.
Chronic headaches with asthenopia.
Chronic frontal headache.
Slight dull pain: at situation of posterior fontanelle.
Dull, heavy frontal headache.
Sick headache: of gastric or hepatic origin.
Cramps: in lower extremities; in body.
Crampy pains: in abdomen and lumbar region; in r. lumbar region.
Aching: in stomach.
Pricking: in urethra.
Smarting burning: in throat.
Burning: in internal canthus; at anus; in mouth and fauces; œsophagus and stomach; from mouth to anus; in urethra.
Soreness: of uterus.
Painful drawing and lameness behind l. trochanter, extending down to popliteal space.
Tenderness: in region of stomach and liver.
Tired headache.
Full, heavy feeling in head.
Fulness: of stomach.
Greasy feeling: in mouth.
Very intense feeling of exhaustion.
Constriction: around forehead.
Constricted feeling: in scalp.
Great heat: of head.
Tenderness: in region of liver.
Excessive tickling: in larynx.
Coldness: of male sexual organs.
Itching: of male sexual organs; of eruption.
" **Tissues.** Excites secretion of glands, salivary, pancreatic, intestinal, etc.
Acts powerfully on gastro-intestinal mucous membrane.
Ascites and anasarca of hepatic origin.
Scrofula; eruptions on skin; glandular swellings.
▮Will abort felon.
" **Touch. Passive Motion. Injuries.** Touch: uterus very sensitive.

Pressure: great pain in abdomen. < •

Riding: causes nausea.

" Skin. Small bloodboils on face, hands and back.

I I Fine eruption, showing black points after scratching, great itching at night.

I I Herpes zoster on r. side of body.

I Vesicular eruption, becoming pustular, on arms, abdomen, back, nates and l. knee; much itching in evening.

I Vesicular eruption, becoming pustular.

I Pustular eruption on scalp, face, around mouth and other parts of body.

I Eczema, with great itching, especially at night; small, fine eruptions, which show black points after scratching.

I Irregular patches on knees, elbows and body, with shining scales, edges slightly raised. θPsoriasis.

I Psoriasis in relievo, skin fissured and irritable.

I Tinea capitis; crusta lactea; porrigo; eczema of face.

I Impetigo capitis, with gastric complaints, nausea and vomiting.

I Impetigo figurata, eruption dry, distinct and of dark .hue.

I Obstinate lepra vulgaris on arms.

" Stages of Life, Constitution. Scrawny, scrofulous child, few weeks after birth; impetigo.

Baby, æt. 5 months; diarrhœa.

Baby, æt. 8 months, suffering for two months; diarrhœa.

Baby, frequently troubled with boils, mother had itch; tinea capitis.

Girl, æt. 11, suffering for three or four years; headache.

A boy, æt. 12; typhoid fever.

Man, æt. 20, has had syphilis and taken mercury, suffering three months; syphilitic sinus.

Woman, æt. 20 ; cholera morbus.

Woman, æt. 30; bilious colic.

Woman, æt. 30, nervo-sanguine, suffering from phlegmasia alba dolens succeeding an abortion; salivation.

Lady, æt. 31, debilitated by overlactation; cholera.

Man, health good, subject to sudden and often unaccountable attacks; diarrhœa.

Widow, æt. 42, tall, light complexion and hair, blue eyes, suffering three weeks; sciatica.

Woman, æt. 43, small in stature, black hair, blue eyes, active disposition, slight icteric taint, uses strong tea and coffee to excess; constipation.

Middle aged woman; typhoid.

Woman, æt 60; cholera morbus.

Woman, æt. 65, nervous bilious temperament, wife of farmer, works very hard; colic.

A woman, æt. 83: typhoid.

⁴⁸**Relations.** Antidoted by *Nux vom.*

   Antidotes: *Mercur., Nux vom., Phytol.*

   Compare: *Ant. crud., Ant. tart.; Arsen., Colchic., Eupator. perf., Ipecac., Juglans cin., Leptandra, Mercur., Pulsat., Sanguin., Veratr.*

JABORANDI.

Jaborandi.   *Rutaceæ.*

A tree attaining a height of more than twenty feet, native to Brazil. The blossoms, which appear in September, are large and violet colored; it is from them the alcoholic tincture is prepared. The Jaborandi " is used by South American Indians as antidote to the bite of serpents of the Trigonecephalus group."

The substance contains an alkaloid passing under the name of Jaborandine, or Pilocarpia, and is used by the old school as a diaphoretic.

Physiological effects from infusions, extracts and powdered leaves have been reported by Gubler, Coutinho, Robin, Ringer, Gould, Martindale, Smith, Green, Craig, Strumpf and Lewi.

Watkins and Thayer have made provings with the first to fifth dilutions, 5 to 100 drops. See Allen's Encyclopedia, vol. 5, p. 165.

CLINICAL AUTHORITIES.—*Hyperopia et spasmus musc. cil ; Cataracta dura immat. et asthenopia ; Torpor retinæ squint;* Deady, Buffum, Norton's Ophth. Therap., p. 98 ; *Night sweats,* Chase, N. E. M. G., vol. 11, p. 152.

³**Inner Head.** Headache.
⁴**Outer Head.** : Alopecia.
⁵**Sight and Eyes.** ❚Dim vision, twitching of lids and pain in eyeballs.

   ❚For many months could not read more than five minutes without the eyes tiring; nausea on looking at moving objects. *θ*Hyperopia cum asthenopia.

   ❚Hyperopia et spasmus musc. cil.; everything becomes black before· eyes on stooping; aching of eyes on reading and spots before vision; V $\frac{20}{30}$; with concave 42, V $\frac{20}{20}$.

   ❚Hyperopia et spasmus musc. cil.; constant pain in eyes even upon using for distance.

   ❚Everything at a distance appeared hazy, and although he could read moderate sized type at one foot, at two feet it was indistinct.

   ❚Blue before eyes at times, especially on looking in the distance.

■After constant and close application to fine work; retinal images retained for several minutes; vision impaired and finally unable to use eyes at all for work; R. V., $\frac{2\theta}{6\theta}$; L. V., fingers at eighteen feet; convex 42, R. V., $\frac{2\theta}{4\theta}$; insufficiency of each internal rectus; sharp pains in eye shooting back into head, with general dull ache of head; light is painful. θTorpor retinæ.

■Eyes very weak, could not use them even a few minutes without smarting and pain in them, with nausea; pain and nausea also experienced when looking steadily at a distance; much vertigo, as if head was too light, especially on moving or looking at objects; constant dull pain in eyes, or occasional sharp pain. θCataracta dura immat. et asthenopia.

■Serous choroiditis.

■Tension of accommodative apparatus of eye, with approximation of nearest and farthest points of distinct vision.

■State of vision constantly changing, becoming suddenly more or less dim, every few moments.

■Spots before vision and aching of eyes upon using. θSpasmus musc. cil.

■Spasm or irritability of ciliary muscles.

■Contraction of pupil.

▮Heat and burning in eyes upon using.

■Eyes tire easily and are irritable, especially on moving.

▮Headache upon using eyes; smarting and pain in globes.

■Periodic convergent squint; strabismus of recent date not dependent upon weakness of opposing muscle; tendency to recurrence of squint after an operation.

[7] **Smell and Nose.** Coryza with feverishness; free flow of saliva; discharge from nostrils; eyes weeping; headache; soreness in nostrils and bones; profuse perspiration; dimness of sight; dulness alternating with hilarity without cause; diarrhœa or constipation.

[8] **Upper Face.** ▮Face flushed.

[12] **Inner Mouth.** ▮▮Profuse salivation. θDiphtheria.

: Mumps with metastatic orchitis; testicle swollen twice natural size and very painful.

[14] **Appetite, Thirst. Desires, Aversions.** ▮Loss of appetite, with bitter taste.

▮Intense thirst.

[16] **Hiccough, Belching, Nausea and Vomiting.** Eructations. Great nausea and retching, often attended with hiccough, and sometimes terminating in vomiting.

[17] **Scrobiculum and Stomach.** Distress in stomach, >by eating.

[19] **Abdomen.** Empty, gone feeling in abdomen.

[20] **Stool and Rectum.** Thin, watery, copious diarrhœa, with slight nausea.

Yellow, watery, painless, gushing diarrhœa; goneness and emptiness from diarrhœa, but no pain; eructations and hiccough; nausea and sudden vomiting.

Thin, yellow, watery, undigested stools.

²¹ Urinary Organs. :Renal dropsy, after scarlatina, or Bright's disease.

: Diabetes insipidus.

❙Urine dark, scanty; profuse.

²² Male Sexual Organs. :Orchitis: with incipient bronchial trouble (relieved pain and cough); metastasis of mumps.

²³ Female Sexual Organs. Flushings at climacteric period.

²⁴ Pregnancy. Parturition. Lactation. :Œdema of pregnancy; swelling of face, labia, extremities.

: Puerperal convulsions; symptoms of suffocation, patient in her stupor, being unable to swallow the great secretion of saliva (three cases).

: Galactorrhœa.

: Deficient secretion of milk.

²⁷ Cough. :Humid asthma with profuse expectoration; bronchitis with abundant non-purulent expectoration.

²⁸ Inner Chest and Lungs. Stitching pain in chest.

: Hydrothorax; pleuritic effusions.

²⁹ Heart, Pulse and Circulation. Heart's action irregular, intermittent and increased.

: Cardiac dropsy.

Rapid pulse, with visible throbbing of arteries.

³⁶ Rest. Position. Motion. Stooping: everything becomes black before eyes.

On moving: much vertigo; eyes tire easily.

³⁷ Sleep. ❙❙Profound, heavy sleep.

³⁸ Time. Night: sweats.

⁴⁰ Fever. ❙❙Profuse sweat.

❙Copious sweating and salivation; profuse secretion from most of glandular structures of body; perspiration starts on forehead and face and then spreads all over body, most profuse on trunk; profound prostration after sweating; unilateral l. sided sweat.

❙Excessive perspiration either during convalescence from diseases, or in course of chronic diseases, as in phthisis.

❙Colliquative sweating of phthisis, very profuse, causing great prostration.

❙Profuse night sweats.

⁴¹ Attacks, Periodicity. Every few moments: state of vision changing.

For several minutes: retinal images retained.

For many months: could not read more than five minutes without the eyes tiring.

At climacteric period: flushings.

Locality and Direction. Left: unilateral sided sweat.
Sensations. As if head was too light.
    Pains in eyeballs; in globes; in head.
    Stitching pain: in chest.
    Sharp pains: in eye shooting back into head.
    Constant pain: in eyes.
    Aching: of eyes on reading.
    Dull ache: of head.
    Heat and burning: in eyes.
    Smarting: in eyes; in globes.
    Soreness: in nostrils and bones.
    Distress: in stomach.
    Empty gone feeling: in abdomen.
Tissues. : Dropsical effusions, especially of pleura and lungs.
    : Ascites.
Skin. : Prurigo.
Stages of Life, Constitution. Boy, æt. 9, suffering seven
    years; recurrent squint after operation.
    Boy, æt. 14, after constant and close application to fine
    work on cardboard one year ago; torpor retinæ.
    Boy, æt. 17; hyperopia and spasm of ciliary muscle.
    Girl, æt. 22; spasm of ciliary muscle.
    Man, æt. 28, for seven years writing in poor light all day;
    myopia and spasm of ciliary muscle.
    Man, æt. 32; hyperopia and spasm of ciliary muscle.
    Man, æt. 32; spasm of ciliary muscle.
    Miss ——, æt. 40, suffering many months; hyperopia and
    asthenopia.
    Mrs. ——, æt. 52, suffering four years; cataracta dura
    immat., et asthenopia.
Relations. Compare: *Amyl nit., Atrop., Physos.*

JACARANDA CAROBA.

Caroba. *Bignoniaceæ.*

A tree common to Brazil. The tincture is prepared from the flowers.
Provings by Mure. See Allen's Encyclopedia, vol. 5, p. 176.
CLINICAL AUTHORITIES.—Schüssler, Gilchrist's Surg., p. 572.

[3] **Inner Head.** Fulness: in head; first in r., later in l. temple,
going to nape of neck, where it disappears.
Pain, as if a plug was pressing on r. side of forehead.
Dull pain between forehead and r. temple, shifting to other
side and then disappearing.

[6] **Hearing and Ears.** Flapping in ears, as of wings.
Stoppage and heat in l. ear, with burning, digging pain,
extending to l. nostril.

[7] **Smell and Nose.** Sneezing and fluent coryza.
Coryza, with heaviness and weariness at vertex, forehead
and eyes.

[11] **Taste and Tongue.** Food tastes flat or acid.
Raw pain at l. side of tongue.

[12] **Inner Mouth.** Dry mouth in morning in bed.
Mouth dry and clammy.

[13] **Throat.** Sore throat, with constriction of pharynx and difficult deglutition.
Constrictive sensation at throat.

[16] **Hiccough, Belching, Nausea and Vomiting.** Nausea
when eating.

[17] **Scrobiculum and Stomach.** Fulness at pit of stomach,
with hurried breathing.
Pressure at pit of stomach.
Sensation as if heart beat in pit of stomach.

[19] **Abdomen.** Painful stitch: between pit of stomach and um-
bilicus; in l. side of navel.
Acute pain at hypogastrium when pressing upon it.
Swelling of r. groin painful to touch.

[20] **Stool and Rectum.** Constipation.
Acute pain, with lancination in anus.
Pricking around anus.
Excrescence at anus.
Itching at anus while sitting.

[21] **Urinary Organs.** ││Contact of urine with chancre causes
tearing pains, which affect whole organism. θSyphilis.

²² Male Sexual Organs. Heat and pain in penis.

Orifice of urethra looks like two inflamed lips, itching on being touched.

Discharge of yellowish white liquid from prepuce.

Prickling in prepuce.

Pain in prepuce, as if a small bundle of fibres was seized. Phimosis.

Suppuration between glans and prepuce.

Itching and pricking at margin of prepuce.

Itching pimple at glans, suppurating like a chancre, and leaving a red point when dry.

Acute pain in l. testicle when walking.

Heat and swelling of scrotum.

Painful erections caused by swelling of prepuce.

❙Prepuce much swollen, could not be drawn over glans; on attempting to do so, copious discharge of yellowish green pus. θSecondary syphilis.

❙❙Chordee in gonorrhœa.

²⁹ Inner Chest and Lungs. ❙❙Dull pain under sternum on raising head and drawing breath.

Prickings under sternum.

²⁹ Heart, Pulse and Circulation. Lancinating pain in region of heart.

Painful stitch at heart, extending to r. side.

Stitch at heart, which seems to beat slowly.

³² Upper Limbs. Rheumatic pains in l. arm in morning.

Pain from l. elbow through forearm.

Red spot with a yellowish pellicle on wrist.

³³ Lower Limbs. Ulcers on legs.

Rheumatic pain in r. knee, disappearing on motion.

³⁵ Rest. Position. Motion. Sitting: itching at anus.

Raising head: dull pain under sternum.

Motion: > rheumatic pains in r. knee.

Walking: acute pain in l. testicle.

³⁷ Sleep. Restless sleep with frightful dreams.

³⁸ Time. Morning: dry mouth; rheumatic pain in arm.

⁴⁰ Fever. Internal chill.

Dry, pricking heat all over.

⁴² Locality and Direction. Right: fulness in temple; pain on side of forehead; swelling of groin; painful stitch from heart to side; rheumatic pain in knee.

Left: fulness of temple; stoppage and heat in ear; burning in nostril; raw pain on side of tongue; painful stitch on side of navel; acute pain in testicle; rheumatic pain in arm; pain from elbow through forearm.

⁴⁵ Sensations. As if a plug was pressing on r. side of forehead; flapping as of wings in ears; as if heart beat in pit of stomach; as if a small bundle of fibres was seized.

Pain: from l. elbow through forearm.

Acute pain: at hypogastrium; in anus; in l. testicle.

Tearing pains: when urine comes in contact with chancre.

Lancination: in anus; in region of heart.

Rheumatic pains: in l. arm; in r. knee.

Painful stitch: between pit of stomach and umbilicus; in l. side of navel; at heart, extending to r. side.

Raw pain: at l. side of tongue.

Pricking: around anus; under sternum.

Prickling: in prepuce.

Soreness: of throat.

Heat and pain: in penis.

Dry pricking heat: all over.

Dull pain: between forehead and r. temple, shifting to other side, then disappearing; under sternum.

Painful erection.

Constriction: of pharynx; at throat.

Stoppage and heat in l. ear, with burning, digging pain, extending to l. nostril.

Pressure: at pit of stomach.

Fulness: in head, first in r., later in l. temple, going to nape of neck; at pit of stomach.

Heaviness and weariness: at vertex; forehead and eyes.

Itching: at anus; at orifice of urethra; at margin of prepuce; pimple at glans.

" **Tissues.** Gonorrhœal rheumatism.

Syphilis; Hunterian chancre.

" **Touch. Passive Motion. Injuries.** Touch: groin painful; causes itching on urethra.

" **Relations.** Compare: *Coral. rub.* in red and sensitive chancres or chancroids; *Thuja* in gonorrhœal rheumatism.

JACEA. (Viola tricolor.)

Pansy; Heart's ease.   *Violaceæ.*

The tincture is prepared from the fresh plants gathered when in flower.
Proved by Hahnemann and his provers. See Allen's Encyclopedia, vol. 10, p. 132.

CLINICAL AUTHORITIES.—*Eczema,* Bigler, Hahn. Mo., vol. 15, p. 86; *Crusta lactea,* Toothaker, Org., vol. 3, p. 872.

[1] **Mind.** Great dulness of intellect.
Low spirited about domestic affairs.
Great indifference.
Bad, morose humor, with disinclination to talk.
Very sensitive and inclined to scold.

[2] **Sensorium.** ▮Vertigo when walking.
Heaviness of head when raising it, disappears by stooping.

[3] **Inner Head.** ▮Pressing headache, chiefly in forehead and temples.

[4] **Outer Head.** ▮Scurfs on head, unbearable burning, < at night.
▮Tinea capitis, with frequent involuntary urination.
Burning stitches in scalp, especially in forehead and temples.
▮Impetigo of hairy scalp and face.
▮Crusta lactea: with violent cough and excessive oppression; with children recently weaned; syphilitic.
▮Thick incrustations, pouring out a large quantity of thick, yellow fluid, which agglutinates hair.
▮Crusta lactea; hair falls off, scabs dry, of a light cream color, and without discharge.
▮▮Plica polonica.

[5] **Sight and Eyes.** Smarting in eyes.
Eyelids sink down as from sleepiness.
Contraction and closing of lids.
▮Scrofulous ophthalmia with crusta lactea; lids much swollen, and soft parts around so much inflamed that lids cannot be opened; face covered with a raw looking, excoriating eruption.

[6] **Upper Face.** Heat of side of face not lain on, evening in bed.
Induration of skin of face.
▮Milk crust, burning, itching, especially at night, with discharge of viscid yellow pus.
▮Impetiginous exanthem on forehead.
Tension in integuments of face and forehead.

⁹ Lower Face. ▌Pustular eruption on whole upper lip and chin, a thick, yellow, friable, semi-transparent incrustation; acne rosacea on chin.

¹¹ Taste and Tongue. Taste bitter, tongue coated with white mucus.

¹² Inner Mouth. Sensation of dryness, yet with much saliva in mouth.

¹³ Throat. ▌Much phlegm in throat, causes hawking, at 11 A.M. ▌Swallowing difficult and very painful. *θ*Syphilis.

▌Very prominent yellow greenish ulcer with adherent pus, in l. side of throat, extending from velum palati over entire l. tonsil. *θ*Syphilis.

▌Chancroid ulcer on posterior surface of fauces and soft palate. *θ*Syphilis.

¹⁵ Eating and Drinking. While eating, hot sweat.

Immediately after eating: dyspnœa; anxious heat.

¹⁸ Hypochondria. Pressing stinging in diaphragm.

▌Pain in r. side of diaphragm.

¹⁹ Abdomen. Cutting pains in abdomen, with urging to stool, crying and lamentations, followed by profuse discharge of flatus, with large lumps of mucus.

²⁰ Stool and Rectum. Diarrhœa with flatulency.

Stool: soft, as if minced; of mucus, with much flatus.

²¹ Urinary Organs. Urging to urinate, with profuse discharge of urine.

Urine: offensive, smelling like cat's urine; very turbid.

Stitches in urethra.

Frequent and profuse emission of urine.

²² Male Sexual Organs. ▌Involuntary seminal discharges, with lewd dreams.

▌Nocturnal emissions, accompanied by vivid dreams, not very exhausting, but causing weariness of mind; loss of seminal fluid at stool and in urine; trembling; feels dull, sleepless, poor appetite.

▌Suppression of gonorrhœa; induration of testicle.

▌Venereal ulcers.

▌Swelling of prepuce, with itching.

▌Stitches in penis or pressing in glans; burning of glans.

▌▌Itching stitches in scrotum.

²³ Female Sexual Organs. Leucorrhœa: with stitching pain in mons veneris; in children; in syphilis.

▌Painful pustules on labia. *θ*Syphilis.

²⁴ Pregnancy. Parturition. Lactation. ▌▌Chancroid ulcers about breasts. *θ*Syphilis.

²⁵ Voice and Larynx. Trachea and Bronchia. ▌▌Hoarseness. *θ*Syphilis.

²⁶ Inner Chest and Lungs. Stitches in l. side of chest, < during inspiration and expiration.

²⁹ **Heart, Pulse and Circulation.** Oppression and stitches in heart, on bending forward when sitting.

Anxiety about heart while lying, with beating like waves.

Pulse accelerated.

³⁰ **Outer Chest.** Stitches in chest and ribs, sternum and intercostal muscles.

ǁSyphilitic ulcers on clavicles.

³¹ **Neck and Back.** Tension between shoulder blades, with cutting and tingling in skin.

Swelling and induration of cervical glands.

³² **Upper Limbs.** Stitches in shoulder joints, elbows, forearms and fingers.

ǁPainful pustles in axillæ. θSyphilis.

³³ **Lower Limbs.** Stitches in patella, tibia and feet.

Pustulous and ichorous exanthema on feet.

³⁵ **Rest. Position. Motion.** Lying: anxiety about heart.

Raising head: heaviness.

Stooping: > heaviness of head.

Bending forward when sitting: oppression and stitches in heart.

Walking: vertigo.

³⁶ **Nerves.** ǀNervous paroxysms from suppression of milk crust.

³⁷ **Sleep.** ǀYawning.

Sleepless; frequent waking.

Goes to sleep late on account of ideas crowding his mind.

The child twitches with his hand in his sleep, with clenched thumbs, general dry heat and red face.

Dreams pleasant, or amorous.

³⁸ **Time.** 11 A.M.: much phlegm in throat, causing hawking.

Forenoon: chilliness.

Evening in bed: heat of side of face not lain on.

Night: burning and itching of milk crust; dry heat; itching of eruption <.

³⁹ **Temperature and Weather.** Aversion to the open air.

Open air: chilliness.

Worse in winter, when walking out in cold air.

⁴⁰ **Fever.** Chill or chilliness in forenoon, and in open air.

Dry, anxious heat at night in bed, with red face.

Night sweats.

⁴² **Locality and Direction.** Right: pain in side of diaphragm.

Left: yellow greenish ulcer in side of throat, extending over entire tonsil; stitches in side of chest.

⁴³ **Sensations.** Pain: in r. side of diaphragm.

Cutting pain: in abdomen; between shoulder blades.

Burning stitches: in scalp, forehead and temples.

Stitches: in urethra; in penis; in l. side of chest; in heart; in ribs; sternum; intercostal muscles; in shoulder joints, elbows, forearms and fingers; in patella; tibia; in feet.

Stitching pain: in mons veneris.
Pressing stinging: in diaphragm.
Pressing pain: in forehead and temples.
Anxiety: about head.
Unbearable burning: in scurfs on head.
Burning: of glans.
Smarting: in eyes.
Beating, like waves: about heart.
Painful pustules: on labia; in axillæ.
Heaviness: of head.
Dryness: of mouth.
Tingling: in skin.
Itching stitches: in scrotum.
Violent itching: of eruptions.
Itching: of milk crusts.

"Tissues. Swelling of glands; eruptions; syphilis.
Rheumatic affections of muscles.
Rheumatism or gout.
Articular rheumatism, with itchlike eruption around joints.
Impetiginous and eczematous diseases, especially crusta lactea.

"Touch. Passive Motion. Injuries. Worse from pressure on side opposite to painful side.
Worse lying on unpainful side.

"Skin. Cutting, or stinging in skin.
Stinging, biting rash.
Miliary eruption all over body.
Eruption: burning, dry, stinging; violent itching, < at night; crusty; scurfy.
|Squamous spots on skin.
|Dry scabs over body, exude yellow water when scratched.
|Acute eruption, confined principally to face, though it may extend to scalp, tends rapidly to pustular form; yellowish brown crusts; much itching in all stages, temporarily > by rubbing; sometimes there is a rather thin white nasal discharge, or a loose catarrhal cough. θEczema of children (tea of dried herb).
|Milk crust.
|Impetigo, recent cases in adults.
||Large boils all over body.
||Painful pustules secreting yellowish green fetid pus.
||Ichorous ulcers with violent itching.
||Burrowing ulcers.
|Skin eruptions of scrofulous children.
|Consequences of suppressed eruptions.
||Skin difficult to heal.

"Stages of Life, Constitution. Scrofulous children.
A nursing infant, æt. 1 (mother, æt. 42), covered with chancroid ulcers.

Young girl, after suppression of milk crust; nervous par-
oxysms.
⁴⁸ **Relations.** Antidoted by: *Camphor., Mercur., Pulsat., Rhus tox.*
Compatible: *Pulsat., Rhus tox., Sepia, Staphis.*
Compare: *Clemat., Graphit., Hepar, Mezer., Oleand., Petrol.,
Staphis., Vinca minor.*

JALAPA.

Jalap.   *Convolvulaceæ.*

Native to Mexico, from whence the first roots were brought by Coxe, in 1827.
The flowers are large and lilac purple, the roots tuberous. The tincture is prepared from the dried and finely pulverized root.

It has been much used by the Old School as an active cathartic, generally in
connection with other drugs. Its action was found to be violent, and in overdoses
dangerous.

The symptoms contained in Allen's Encyclopedia are from Noack and Trinks'
Materia Medica, to which we add a small proving by Jeanes, made with the fourth
dilution, in 1844.

¹ **Mind.** ❙Great restlessness with anxiety.
³ **Inner Head.** Violent headache.
   Pain in head; smarting in skin of forehead.
⁶ **Hearing and Ears.** Humming in ears.
⁹ **Lower Face.** Dryness of lips.
¹¹ **Taste and Tongue.** Biting and smarting of tongue.
¹² **Inner Mouth.** Stinging on tongue and in fauces.
¹⁶ **Hiccough, Belching, Nausea and Vomiting.** Flatulent
   and frothy eructation with abatement of pain.   •
   Nausea and vomiting.
¹⁸ **Hypochondria.** Pain in r. hypochondrium.
¹⁹ **Abdomen.** ❙❙Severe griping, cutting pain in bowels, < at
   night.
   Pain in middle of abdomen and in region of l. superior
   flexure of colon.
   Pain in cæcum.
   Flatulent rumbling in bowels.
   Colic; violent pains in small intestines, as if abdomen
   would be cut to pieces.
   Inflammation of intestines.
²⁰ **Stool and Rectum.** Stools: violent, excessive; bloody;
   VOL. VI.—19.

watery, with weak pulse; sour smelling; with great
restlessness and anxiety.

Before and during stool: cutting colic.

Pain in sigmoid flexure of colon.

Soreness of anus.

■Diarrhœa in infants: child is quiet all day, but screams
and tosses about all night.

❘❘Infantile diarrhœa, general coldness, blueness of face.

²¹ Urinary Organs. Pain and pressure in region of bladder.

²² Male Sexual Organs. Thrilling sensation in urethra
whilst urinating.

³¹ Neck and Back. Severe pain about superior margin of l.
scapula.

³² Upper Limbs. Pain in thighs.

³³ Lower Limbs. Smarting on inside edge and at root of l.
great toenail, with heat, tearing and pulsation.

Pain in large joint of great toe.

Burning of soles of feet.

³⁴ Limbs in General. Aching in arms and legs, most r. side.

³⁷ Nerves. Fainting fits; weakness.

Excessive uneasiness and tossing about of limbs.

³⁸ Time. Night: severe cutting, griping pain in bowels <;
child screams and tosses.

⁴⁰ Fever. Febrile attacks.

Great disposition to perspiration of head and superior
parts of body.

⁴² Locality and Direction. Right: pain in hypochondrium;
aching in arm and leg.

Left: pain in superior flexure of colon; severe pain about
superior margin of scapula; smarting on inside edge
and at root of great toenail.

⁴³ Sensations. As if abdomen would be cut to pieces.

Pain: in head: in r. hypochondrium; in middle of abdomen: in region of l. superior flexure of colon; in region
of bladder; in thigh; in large joint of great toe.

Violent pains: in head; in small intestines.

Severe pain: about superior margin of l. scapula.

Tearing: at root of great toenail.

Severe griping, cutting pain: in bowels.

Cutting colic.

Aching in arms and legs.

Stinging: on tongue and in fauces.

Biting: of tongue.

Smarting: in skin of forehead; of tongue; on inside edge
and at root of l. great toenail.

Burning: of soles of feet.

Soreness: of anus.

Pressure: in region of bladder.

Pulsation: in great toe.
Thrilling sensation: in urethra.
Dryness: of lips.
⁴⁸ Relations. Compare: *Camphora* (diarrhœa with coldness),
Coloc. (colic).

JAMBOS EUGENIA.

Malabar Plum tree ; Rose apple.   *Myrtaceæ.*

A tree native to the tropics, never without flowers or fruit. The tincture is
prepared from the fresh seeds, which are considered poisonous.
Introduced and proved by C. Hering. See Allen's Encyclopedia, vol. 5, p. 231.

CLINICAL AUTHORITIES.—*Epidemic catarrhal affections of respiratory passages*,
Hrg., Bück. Kl. Erf., vol. 3, p. 13; *Acne*, C. Hg. and others, MSS.

¹ **Mind.**   Constantly desirous of sitting alone and reflecting.
Nothing seemed right, when sitting, he wanted to lie ;
when lying, he wanted to rise again.
Slight but long continued drunkenness, which made him
very talkative, but indolent.
Sudden, great change in him after micturition, everything
seems more beautiful and bright, sky and trees more
joyous and clear; but after quarter of an hour everything became gloomy again.
² **Sensorium.**   Whirling in head while sitting; houses at a
distance seem to turn bottom upwards.
Vertigo after rising from lying down, caused by rush of
blood to head.
Looking inattentively objects waver or tumble one over
the other, on looking sharp all is right.
Confusion of head, and slight sticking in it.
Dulness and slight ticking in head.
Dizzy and nauseated, in evening.
³ **Inner Head.**   Pressive, pinching pain in small spot deep in
forehead.
❙Neuralgia in l. forehead over eye.
Headache on r. side, deep in, as if a heavy board was lying
there.
Headache as from a sticking from all sides at once, or as
if everything was drawn together from within, recurring like a slow pulsation.
Headache, as if something was rolling in head, with burn-
ing in it coming out at eyes, with lachrymation; no re-

lief from cold water; at last he became nauseated, was obliged to vomit, but headache was made < thereby; in evening lasting into night.

In evening, headache, nausea, vomiting, with subsequent bitterness of mouth, much thirst for cold water, and perspiration after drinking.

Whole night, headache, burning in eyes, great thirst, and much micturition.

Pressive pinching pain on vertex.

⁵ **Sight and Eyes.** Darkness before eyes, everything seems double; on looking intently double vision disappears.

On looking intently at anything everything is in order, but if he only looks ahead of him, everything wavers before eyes and becomes confused.

Whirling before r. eye, as if it would become dark; eye becomes inflamed.

After micturition, suddenly bright before eyes.

Eyes look sleepy and drunken.

Red vessels from inner canthus to cornea.

It seems as though fire came out of eyes, and tears ran out of them in streams in evening and night.

Suddenly, biting in eyes, as from pepper.

Contractive, pinching pain in eyeball in small spot above r. inner canthus.

Right eye inflamed; needle-like stitches in inner canthus.

Unable to look at sun, eyes fill with water.

Unable to close eyes in evening on account of burning in them; this also prevents sleeping at night.

Violent internal itching in eyes and nose in evening.

⁸ **Hearing and Ears.** ι ιCatarrhal otitis.

⁹ **Upper Face.** ι ιPimples on face, painful for some distance about them. θAcne rosaceæ.

¹⁰ **Teeth and Gums.** Gums about hollow teeth inflamed and painful.

¹¹ **Taste and Tongue.** Pain on very small spot in region of l. corner of hyoid bone, also when swallowing.

¹² **Inner Mouth.** Frothy saliva in mouth when talking.

Mouth full of frothy, tenacious saliva; spits and hawks whole day.

Tenacious, yellowish, bloody mucus in mouth after midday nap.

¹¹ **Throat.** At night, burning in eyes, violent thirst from dryness, low down in throat, so that he did not feel the drink, which also did not > the dryness.

Pain in a very small place in region of l. corner of hyoid bone, also on swallowing.

ιThroat inflamed. θCatarrhal fever.

Cough felt in whole chest, but especially in pit of throat.

Mucus goes from nose into throat.

[14] **Appetite, Thirst. Desires, Aversions.** Eats and drinks
    with a very good appetite, so that he takes too much;
    greater relish for tobacco.

Much thirst for cold water, with perspiration, in morning;
    on awaking.

Wants to do nothing but smoke all day.

[16] **Hiccough, Belching, Nausea and Vomiting.** Hiccough
    when eating, more like eructations than loud hiccough.

Heartburn at night.

Nausea, going off by smoking.

I I Vomiting.

[17] **Scrobiculum and Stomach.** Sticking in pit of stomach.

Pain in r. side near pit of stomach, under ribs as if it
    would be drawn inward.

Pressure and sticking in l. side under ribs, near pit of
    stomach.

Contractive, pinching sensation deep in stomach.

Sensation as of cramp in orifice of stomach, which results
    in nausea.

Nausea commences deep in stomach and rises up from end
    of œsophagus.

[19] **Abdomen.** Flatulence, rumbling in bowels.

Drawing about navel as from a purge.

Confused feeling in upper abdomen like a coldness in it.

Burning in abdomen, as after drinking brandy, at first
    transversely across abdomen, then becoming general.

Colic, with laborlike pressing downward, much urging to
    stool and to urinate, with scanty discharge.

I I Colic.

I I Inguinal hernia from a fall.

[20] **Stool and Rectum.** Urging to stool and colic; now and
    then a somewhat diarrhœic discharge is forced out
    as with a syringe.

Diarrhœa: with much pressure backward.

Diarrhœic discharge followed by vomiting.

Several stools a day with burning in abdomen and sput-
    tering, fetid discharge.

I I Offensive, sputtering stool, without much urging.

Several small stools, with burning in abdomen.

Only wind is passed instead of stool.

I Scanty, hard stool, after much pressing, with spasmodic
    closure of anus after evacuation.

Very scanty, pasty, gritty stool.

Pressure as in diarrhœa, at first a hard, then a pasty stool.

After stool, stitching in abdomen from above downward.

It seems as if a ten pound weight was hanging upon rec-
    tum, and as if everything below would fall out.

Cramp or pinching pains in rectum.

I I Tenesmus.

❙Bleeding hemorrhoids, copious for days, with great relief of mind and body.

❝ **Urinary Organs.** ❙❙Tenesmus in bladder, ischuria.

Burning during micturition.

❙Frequent urination during night.

❝ **Male Sexual Organs.** Violent erections with sexual desire, after midday nap.

Painful erections, with inward itching, without sexual desire.

Seminal discharge: too soon and almost without excitement in morning; retarded; the orgasm subsides several times before it leads to an ejaculation.

During coition no seminal discharge; penis relaxed.

No erections in morning.

❙Impotence.

Glans penis remains sensitive a long time after coition.

Much turning and twisting in scrotum.

❝ **Voice and Larynx. Trachea and Bronchia.** Sensation as if larynx was narrowed; it prompts to a deep inspiration, whereby tightness is still more felt, it makes him hoarse.

❙Inflammatory affection of trachea. θCatarrhal fever.

❝ **Cough.** Cough: from throat; in coughing, pain principally in throat pit; more frequent in evening and at night; not the least expectoration; causes dryness of throat.

❙❙Cough raises something from pit of throat, but it always gradually falls down again.

Loose, deep cough, without expectoration and without pain, especially in evening.

Loose cough at night.

❙❙Much hawking causing a short cough.

After coughing, is obliged to swallow, when irritation passes off; as soon as he swallows again is obliged to cough.

❙Epidemic cough among children, with coryza, inflammation of eyes and pain in ears.

❙Catarrh: with much phlegm and rheumatic pains; with rattling in chest.

Constantly obliged to expectorate.

When speaking, is obliged to spit out a frothy saliva.

Hawking; mucus yellowish and somewhat bloody.

Constant hawking, something is always loosening, but still something always remains adherent.

❝ **Neck and Back.** Pain deep in r. side of neck near œsophagus, a fine, sticking, cramplike, constant pain.

Pain in nape of neck which hinders turning.

Sticking pain in back as if something was sticking in spine, < by bending back.

Pain in back, which makes him bend back inward, with
heat in evening, disappearing in morning.

Sticking, burning, itching in a small spot on back, < after
scratching.

I I Pain in small of back and in calves.

I I Aching in sacrum and knees.

** Upper Limbs.** Skin recedes from thumb nail and suppurates.

** Lower Limbs.** Violent sticking, extending obliquely forward above l. crest of ilium, < when sitting erect, standing and bending toward l. side; > bending towards r.

Pain as if a band was drawn from crest of one ilium to
other; hip bones painful to pressure.

Pain in thighs and calves, he could hardly stand.

Paralytic pains in l. tibia and feet.

Cramps in soles of feet when moving at night.

Skin cracks between and about toes.

** Rest. Position. Motion.** Rising from lying down:
vertigo.

Sitting: whirling in head; sticking above l. crest of ilium
<; coldness as if he was naked.

Bending back: sticking pains <.

Bending inward: pain in back >.

Bending toward l. side: sticking above l. crest of ilium <.

Bending toward r. side: sticking above l. crest of ilium >.

Standing: sticking above l. crest of ilium <.

Could hardly stand: on account of pain in thighs and
calves.

Moving: cramps in soles of feet.

Walking: much exhaustive yawning; perspiration.

** Nerves.** Very much exhausted, but lively after drinking
coffee.

** Sleep.** Much exhaustive yawning when walking in open air.

Forgetting all his business he crept into a corner and said
he must sleep; he could not sleep, however, but still remained lying down.

After a sound midday sleep difficult waking, with much
thirst and bruised sensation.

Sound sleep undisturbed by any difficulties.

Stupid midday sleep with confused dream.

** Time.** Morning: seminal discharge; no erections.

All day: spits and hawks.

After midday nap: yellowish, bloody mucus in mouth;
violent erections.

Evening: dizzy and nauseated; headache lasts into night;
nausea, headache, vomiting; tears run out of eyes in
streams; unable to close eyes on account of burning;
violent internal itching in eyes and nose; cough more
frequent; heat in back.

Before midnight: heat.

Night: headache, burning in eyes, great thirst, much micturition; tears run out of eyes in streams; burning in eyes prevents sleep; violent thirst; heartburn; frequent urination; cough more frequent; cramps of soles of feet.

Temperature and Weather. Open air: much exhaustive yawning while walking, mornings.

Cold water: does not > burning in eyes; much thirst for.

Fever. Shiverings run over him after micturition.

Coldness, as if he was naked, while sitting.

||Hot hands.

Fever; heat before midnight, with little thirst and much perspiration, thereupon falling asleep; during fever and for several hours in morning, pain in back, > bending inward.

Perspiration and thirst after unsatisfactory coition.

Perspiration when walking.

|Catarrhal fever; thirst during chill; heat before midnight, with affection of trachea, throat, eyes; sweat when walking.

Attacks, Periodicity. During menstrual period: skin disease <.

Locality and Direction. Right: headache on side; whirling before eye; pain in eyeball above inner canthus; eye inflamed; pain in side near pit of stomach; pain deep in side of neck.

Left: neuralgia in forehead over eye; pain in corner of hyoid bone; pressure and sticking in side under ribs; violent sticking, extending obliquely forward above crest of ilium; paralytic pains in tibia.

Inward: as if stomach was drawn.

Backward: pressure in rectum.

Downward: labor like pressing in abdomen.

From above downward: stitching in abdomen.

Sensations. Internal pinching pains here and there.

Crawling, titillating pains.

Headache as if heavy board was lying on r. side; as from a sticking from all sides at once; as if everything was drawn together from within head; as if something was rolling in head; as if vision of r. eye would become dark; as though fire came out of eyes; biting as from pepper in eyes; as if stomach would be drawn inwards; as of cramp in orifice of stomach; as if a ten pound weight was hanging upon rectum; as if everything below rectum would fall out.

As if larynx was narrowed; as if something was sticking spine; pain as if a band was drawn from crest of one ilium to other; coldness as if he was naked.

Pain: in face some distance about pimples; on very small
spot in region of l. corner of hyoid bone; in r. side near
pit of stomach; in throat pit; in ears; deep in r. side
of neck near œsophagus; in nape of neck; in back; in
small of back; in calves; in thighs.

Violent sticking: above l. crest of ilium.

Fine, sticking, cramplike, constant pain: in side of neck.

Sticking, burning, itching: in a small spot on back.

Sticking: in pit of stomach; in l. side; under ribs; in back.

Slight stitching: in head.

Stitching: in abdomen.

Pressive, pinching pain; in small spot deep in forehead;
on vertex.

Contractive pinching pain: in eyeball; in small spot above
r. inner canthus.

Contractive pinching sensation: deep in stomach.

Pinching pains: in rectum.

Cramps: in soles of feet.

Colic, with labor like pressing downward in abdomen.

Neuralgia: in l. forehead over eye.

Paralytic pain: in l. tibia and feet.

Aching: in sacrum and knees.

Drawing: about navel as from a purge.

Twisting: in scrotum.

Pressure: in l. side under ribs; backwards during diarrhœa.

Burning: in head coming out at eyes; in eyes; in abdomen.

Biting: in eyes.

Whirling: in head; before r. eye.

Dryness: low down in throat.

Confused feeling: in upper abdomen like a coldness in it.

Violent internal itching: in eyes and nose.

Inward itching: in male sexual organs.

" **Tissues.** An old wound from a thrust became painful again.
ı ıRheumatic pain wanders from place to place, with
catarrh. ·

" **Touch. Passive Motion. Injuries.** Pressure: hip bones
painful to.

From a fall: inguinal hernia.

" **Skin.** ıComedones.

ıAcne, with pain extending for some distance around; the
skin disease is < during menstrual period.

ıı Pimples (sore acne) on face.

" **Relations.** Antidoted by *Coffea;* smoking tobacco antidotes
nausea.

Compare: *Lavroc.* and drugs containing hydrocyanic
acid; *Pulsat* (fugitive rheumatic pains).

JATROPHA.

Physic Nut. *Euphorbiaceæ.*

A shrub indigenous to the West Indies and South America. The alcoholic tincture is prepared from the powdered seeds.

Provings by Hering and provers; Jablancsy; Thorer and Lembke.

CLINICAL AUTHORITIES.—*Diarrhœa*, Stow, Raue's Rec., 1870, p. 209; Hencke, Raue's Rec., 1875, p. 146; A. H. Z., vol. 89, p. 63; B. J. H., vol. 33, p. 315; *Summer diarrhœa with vomiting*, Blake, Hom. Rev., vol. 20, p. 606; Times Retros., vol. 2, p. 14; *Cholera*, Hencke, A. H. Z., vol. 83, p. 119, and Raue's Rec., 1872, p. 148; Hencke, Brutger, Lembke, Riedel, N. A. J. H., vol. 1, p. 427; Jablancsy, Rummel, N. A. J. H., vol. 1, p. 433; *Lumbrici and ascarides*, Schulz, N. A. J. H., vol. 1, p. 434; *Vomiting of pregnancy*, Chase, N. A. J. H., vol. 1, p. 427.

[1] **Mind.** Apathy; indifference to pain.

Anxiety and anguish.

Anxiety, with burning in stomach and coldness of body.

[2] **Sensorium.** Giddiness, followed by unconsciousness and delirium.

Head hot, stupefaction, with yawning and nausea.

[3] **Inner Head.** Violent pressing pain in temples, > in open air, and reappearing when entering room.

Headache, with nausea and vomiturition, beginning in morning.

Heat and heaviness of head.

[4] **Outer Head.** Stiffness of muscles on forehead and neck.

[5] **Sight and Eyes.** [1]Quivering in l. upper lid.

[11]Itching and smarting of margins of lids.

[6] **Hearing and Ears.** Burning hot ears, with heat in back part of head.

[7] **Smell and Nose.** Itching of nose while eating.

Ulcers in nose and mouth.

[8] **Upper Face.** Pale face with blue margins around eyes.

[9] **Lower Face.** Painful cracked lips.

[11] **Taste and Tongue.** Metallic, bloody taste, with much spitting of saliva (in morning).

Long continued pain and burning of tongue.

Numbness of tongue, with heat and dryness of mouth.

[12] **Inner Mouth.** Increased accumulation of thin saliva.

Burning in mouth and throat, followed by dryness.

Dryness of mouth and tongue, without thirst (at night); mouth feels as if scalded.

Ulcers in nose and mouth.

¹³ **Throat.** ❚Dryness in fauces and throat.

Spasmodic constriction in throat, ascending from stomach.

¹⁴ **Appetite, Thirst. Desires, Aversions.** ❚Inextinguishable thirst, not satisfied by drinking cold water. *θ*Cholera.

¹⁵ **Eating and Drinking.** ❚Dreads to drink on account of nausea.

¹⁶ **Hiccough, Belching, Nausea and Vomiting.** Eructations.

❚Hiccough, followed by copious vomiting of bile. *θ*Cholera.

❚Vomiting: of large masses of dark green bile and mucus; of large quantities of watery, albuminous substances; water is almost immediately vomited.

❚Very easy vomiting of a great quantity of watery, glairy fluid, accompanied by watery diarrhœa; spasmodically contracting pains in stomach, burning in stomach, cramps in calves and coldness of body. *θ*Cholera.

❚Uninterrupted vomiting. *θ*Cholera.

¹⁷ **Scrobiculum and Stomach.** Sensation of sinking, with nausea in pit of stomach.

❚Crampy, constrictive pains in epigastrium.

❚Persistent dull pressure in stomach.

❚Heat and burning in stomach.

❚Spasmodically contracting pains in stomach.

¹⁹ **Abdomen.** ❚Much noise in abdomen, as if a full bottle was emptied, followed later by thin stool.

❚Rumbling in abdomen, with colic; > when walking in open air.

❚Abdomen: distended and soft; very much inflated, distended, tympanitic; swollen and sore to touch; contracted. *θ*Cholera.

❚Pain in region of navel, deep.

❚Burning in abdomen; seeks to cool himself by throwing off covering and lying on ground.

❚❚Lancinating, stinging pain with colic.

²⁰ **Stool and Rectum.** ❚Sudden desire for stool, and constant noises as of liquids in abdomen, especially in l. side.

❚❚Thin stool, preceded and followed by much rumbling, and at times a noise as if a bottle was being emptied.

❚Colic followed by discharge of large, watery, odorless stool.

❚Continued discharge of water by stool.

❚Stools painless, thin, watery, with loud, fluid rumbling, and gushing out of stool; < mornings.

❚❚Watery diarrhœa, as if it spurted from him.

❚Diarrhœa profuse; gushing out like a torrent.

❚Severe diarrhœa occurring suddenly in Summer, in connection with a sharp attack of vomiting.

❚After taking cold, sleepless; slight pain in bowels; after

midnight profuse watery discharge; a few hours later, again and again, weakening patient greatly; stools profuse, watery, without smell. θDiarrhœa.

▮Easy vomiting of large quantities of watery substance like albumen; diarrhœa, contents of rectum gush out like a torrent; anxiety, with burning at stomach; anguish, with coldness of body; viscid sweat; violent cramps in lower limbs; calves look like flat splints; abdomen flattened after many stools. θCholerine.

▮Vomiting, with cramp in abdomen; frequent, profuse, pale, watery, urgent stools; loud rumbling, as of water pouring from a bottle; abdomen flat; face pale, shrivelled; great thirst for water or lemonade.

▮During menstruation, which had ceased for thirty hours, uninterrupted vomiting of scentless, white, gelatinous fluid; cramps in calves and brachial muscles; body blue, cold as marble, and covered with cold, clammy sweat; pulse imperceptible; abdomen contracted; unquenchable thirst; drinks much cold water; burning in abdomen, which she seeks to relieve by lying on ground; mind placid, rather ecstatic, taking little notice of her cramps and other affections. θCholera morbus.

▮Fearful vomiting, coming up at once in quantity, of watery or glairy fluid, with crampy, constrictive pains in gastric region, or burning in stomach; continued discharge of water per anum; cramps in calves; general coldness of body. θCholera.

▮Sudden, violent vomiting of watery fluids, with cramps in stomach; cool skin; weak, soft, slow pulse; great debility; anxiety and fear, as though cramps in calves would set in; stool diarrhœic yesterday; to-day neither stool nor urine. θCholera.

▮▮First stage of cholera, before period of collapse.

▮Constipation.

▮Very abundant alvine evacuations, mushy, with a large number of lumbrici and ascarides.

▮Griping, sticking pains in abdomen, continuing a long time, accompanied by sensation as if balls were rolling together in abdomen; constipation; pains occasionally so severe that he shrieked and writhed about in bed; after five drops a copious evacuation with a quantity of lumbrici and ascarides; the same with the following evacuations.

▮▮Stitches in anus and rectum.

²¹ **Urinary Organs.** Frequent desire to urinate; urine pale yellow, frothy.

²⁴ **Pregnancy. Parturition. Lactation.** ▮Vomiting during pregnancy.

³⁰ Heart, Pulse and Circulation. ❚Pulse imperceptible. θCholera.

³² Upper Limbs. ❚Cramps in brachial muscles. θCholera.

³³ Lower Limbs. ❚Slight cramplike jerkings in both calves, with painless diarrhœa.

❚Cramps in calves. θCholera.

❚Violent, cramplike pain in lower legs, and cramps in calves, which become knotted.

❚Violent cramps in legs and feet.

Tingling in toes.

Itching between toes at night.

The heels are very sensitive when walking on them.

³⁵ Rest. Position. Motion. Walking: in open air, rumbling in abdomen; on heels, sensitive.

Writhed about in bed with pain.

³⁶ Time. Morning: headache begins; metallic, bloody taste, with much spitting of saliva; stools <.

Night: dryness of mouth and tongue, without thirst; itching between toes.

After midnight: profuse watery discharge; a few hours later again and again.

³⁹ Temperature and Weather. Open air: pressing pain in temples > ; rumbling in abdomen.

Entering room: pressing pain in temples returns.

Seeks to cool himself by throwing off covering and lying on ground.

⁴⁰ Fever. Chilliness in back, with heat in face and head.

Chilliness with cold hands and blue nails.

❚Coldness of body.

❚Body cold as marble and mottled blue. θCholera.

❚Cold hands, with heat in mouth and throat.

Heat in head, face and ears.

❚General cold, clammy perspiration.

❚Cold, clammy sweat on skin. ❚Cholera.

⁴¹ Attacks, Periodicity. Summer: severe diarrhœa occurring suddenly.

⁴² Locality and Direction. Left: quivering in upper eyelid; noise as of liquids in abdomen on side.

⁴³ Sensations. Mouth feels as if scalded; as if balls were rolling together in abdomen; rumbling as if a bottle was being emptied.

Pain: in region of navel.

Severe pain: in abdomen.

Lancinating stinging pain: in abdomen.

Violent cramplike pain: in lower legs.

Stitches: in anus and rectum.

Griping, sticking pains: in abdomen.

Violent cramps: in lower limbs.

Cramps: in calves; in abdomen; in bronchial muscles.
Violent pressing pain: in temples.
Contracting pains: in stomach.
Constrictive pains: in epigastrum, in gastric region.
Slight cramplike jerkings: in both calves.
Spasmodic constriction: in throat.
Persistent dull pressure: in stomach.
Smarting: of margin of lids.
Burning: in stomach; of tongue; in mouth and throat; in abdomen.
Burning hot ears.
Heat: of head; in back part of head; of mouth; in face; in ears.
Dryness: of mouth; of tongue; in fauces; in throat.
Numbness: of tongue.
Stiffness: of muscles on forehead and neck.
Sinking: in pit of stomach.
Heaviness: of head.
Tingling: in toes.
Quivering: in l. upper eyelid.
Itching: of margins of lids; of nose; between toes at night.

⁴⁶ Touch. Passive Motion. Injuries. Touch: abdomen sore; heels sore when walking on them.

⁴⁷ Stages of Life, Constitution. Woman, æt. 22; cholera. Woman, æt. 31; cholera.
Man, æt. 40; cholera.

⁴⁸ Relations. Effects cease by placing hands in cold water.
Compare: the Euphorbiaceæ, viz.: *Crot. tig.*, *Euphorb. coral.*, *Mancinella;* also *Veratr.* in cholera.

JUGLANS CINEREA.

Butternut.   *Juglandaceæ.*

Tincture of the bark of the root.
Provings by Paine, Clark, Cressor and Hale.   See Allen's Encyclopedia,
vol. 5, p. 193.

CLINICAL AUTHORITIES.—*Retrosternal pain*, Burnett, Hom. Rev., vol. 32, p.
205; *Scarlatina* (20 cases reported cured), Horton, A. H. O., vol. 8, p. 174; *Erysipelas*, Horton, A. H. O., vol. 4, p. 162; *Eczema*, Horton, A. H. O., vol. 3, p. 551, and
vol. 4, p. 161; *Herpes circinatus*, Horton, A. H. O., vol. 3, p. 551; *Impetiginous eruption*, Horton, A. H. O., vol. 3, p. 551; *Impetigo figurata*, Horton, A. H. O., vol. 3, p.
551; *Lichen lividus*, Horton, A. H. O., vol. 4, p. 162.

[1] **Mind.**   Depression of spirits.
[2] **Sensorium.**   Vertigo, with faintness.
[3] **Inner Head.**   ▮Aching pain in r. temple.
   Dull headache on rising, passing off on getting up.
   Fulness of head at night.
   ▮Sharp, shooting pains in occiput, often associated with
      liver disturbance.
[4] **Outer Head.**   ▮Eruptions on scalp.
[5] **Sight and Eyes.**   Inflammation, with pustules on lids and
      around eyes.
[6] **Hearing and Ears.**   Pain on swallowing, which is deep,
      drawing, tickling.
[7] **Smell and Nose.**   Coryza from l. nostril.
   Dryness of nose.
   ▮"Noli me tangere" on nose.
[8] **Upper Face.**   Erythema of face.
   ▮Erysipelas of entire face, < r. side, extending around to
      r. ear, which was swollen twice its natural size; eyelids
      turgid and infiltrated, nearly obscuring sight, < r. side.
[9] **Lower Face.**   Patch of herpes circinatus upon chin about
      size of dollar, steadily increasing in size.
[11] **Taste and Tongue.**   Tip of tongue sore, dryness of fauces.
[12] **Inner Mouth.**   ▮Swelling in submaxillary glands, < right.
[13] **Throat.**   ▮Pain in r. side of fauces.
   Sore throat, with dry lips and moist mouth.
   ▮Throat feels swollen, with pain on r. side.
   ▮Chronic inflammation of throat, with general debility.
[14] **Appetite, Thirst. Desires, Aversions.**   Loss of appetite,
      with coppery taste.

¹⁶ **Hiccough, Belching, Nausea and Vomiting.** Nausea in morning; vomiting, retching, with colic.

¹⁷ **Scrobiculum and Stomach.** Pain in epigastrium and boring in stomach.

Sinking sensation at stomach.

❙Indigestion, with gastric irritability; flatulence.

¹⁸ **Hypochondria.** ❙Pain in each hypochondriac region.

Stitching pains about liver and under r. scapula.

¹⁹ **Abdomen.** Flatulence and aching in abdomen after dinner.

Deep seated pain on l. side near kidneys.

Heat and pain in hypogastrium.

Irritation and inflammation of mucous membrane of bowels, followed by dysentery.

²⁰ **Stool and Rectum.** Loose stool which smells like onions.

Tenesmus and burning after stool.

❙Bilious, yellowish green stools with burning and tenesmus.

❙Constipation preceded by diarrhœa.

❙Colic, very severe and prostrating, with purging.

❙Diarrhœa of soldiers in camps.

²¹ **Urinary Organs.** ❙Diarrhœa with cutting in abdomen.

²⁵ **Voice and Larynx, Trachea and Bronchia.** Rattling in bronchia on coughing, without expectoration.

²⁷ **Cough.** Expectoration of very tenacious mucus and musty sputa.

²⁸ **Inner Chest and Lungs.** Great oppression in chest, with cutting pains in lungs.

❙Retrosternal pain, < or only felt when walking out of doors, after meals, or when hurried, or going up hill.

❙Suffocating pain in chest, especially when walking, so that he has to stand still. θAngina pectoris.

Pain in l. side, < on pressure.

Congestion of lungs.

❙Dropsy of chest of rheumatic origin, when there are bright red erythematous spots.

❙Scrofulous consumption, with great emaciation.

³¹ **Neck and Back.** ❙Stitchlike pain under r. scapula, when stooping.

Aching pain in small of back on stooping.

Aching or shooting pain in lumbar region.

³² **Upper Limbs.** ❙Aching in r., pain in l. shoulder.

Great pain in r. axilla, extending down arms along course of nerves.

Aching pains in arms and wrists, as if sprained.

³³ **Lower Limbs.** Heat on inner side of thigh, and in feet, with cramplike pain in l. hip at night.

³⁴ **Limbs in General.** ❙Rheumatic pain in r. shoulder, extending to pectoral muscles, producing inability to draw a deep inspiration; a single thickly set patch of impe-

tigo figurata upon inside of l. leg, between knee and in step which soon became crusted, discharging a purulent, ichorous secretion, irritating surrounding skin, producing a wide, inflammatory margin; painful and sore; difficulty in walking.

[35] Rest. Position. Motion. Rising: dull headache > when getting up.

Stooping: stitchlike pain under r. scapula; aching in small of back.

Could neither sit nor lie with any comfort on account of eruption.

Going up hill: retrosternal pain <.

Walking out of doors: retrosternal pain <; suffocating pain in chest so that he has to stand still; difficult on account of eruption on legs; pain from rectum to bladder >.

[36] Time. Morning: nausea.

Night: fulness of head; cramplike pain in l. hip.

Attacks come on first half of night: pain from rectum to bladder.

Latter half of night must walk his room.

[39] Temperature and Weather. When heated from overexertion: itching of whole body.

[40] Fever. ‖Scarlatina; anginose symptoms pretty well developed; no sequela.

[41] Attacks. Periodicity. One attack hardly subsides before a fresh crop appears: eczema.

[42] Locality and Direction. Right: aching pain in temple; erysipelas of face <, extending to ear; eyelid turgid and infiltrated; swelling in submaxillary glands <; pain in side of fauces; stitchlike pain under scapula; aching in shoulder; pain in axilla; rheumatic pain in shoulder.

Left: coryza from nostril; deep seated pain on side near kidneys; pain in side; pain in shoulder; cramplike pain in hip; a single thickly set patch of impetigo figurata upon inside of leg.

[43] Sensations. Arms and wrists as if sprained.

Pain: in r. side of fauces; in epigastrium; in each hypochondriac region; hypogastrium; retrosternal; in l. side; in l. shoulder; in eczema of hands.

Great pain: in r. axilla, extending down arms along nerves.

Cutting: in abdomen; in lungs.

Sharp pain: in occiput.

Shooting pain: in lumbar region.

Stitchlike pain: under r. scapula; in occiput; about liver.

Suffocating pain: in chest.

Severe pressing pain: extending from rectum to neck of bladder.

Very severe and prostrating colic.

Cramplike pain in l. hip.

Boring: in stomach.

Deep seated pain: on l. side near kidneys.

Deep, drawing, tickling pain: in ears.

Aching: in r. temple; in abdomen; in small of back; in r. shoulder; in arms and wrists.

Rheumatic pain: in l. shoulder; extending to pectoral muscles.

Dull pain: in head.

Heat: in hypogastrium; on inner side of thigh; in feet.

Soreness: of tip of tongue.

Unbearable smarting pains: eczema of hands.

Dryness: of nose; of fauces; of lips.

Fulness: of head.

Oppression: in chest.

Sinking sensation: at stomach.

Tension: eczema of hands.

Painful itching: of eruption upon body, face and arms.

Intolerable itching and soreness of eczema of hands

Violent itching: over whole body in spots.

" **Tissues.** *Scrofulous swelling of glands.

" **Touch. Passive Motion. Injuries.** "Noli me tangere": on nose.

Pressure: pain in l. side <.

" **Skin.** *Redness of skin, resembling flush of scarlatina; violent itching over whole body, in spots, changing about, first one place then another; < when being heated from overexertion.

*Erysipelatous inflammation of skin of body and extremities.

*Numerous and extensive patches of eruption on body and extremities, varying in size from a dollar to a man's hand. θErythema nodosum.

*Eruption upon body, face and arms; painful itching causing an irresistible inclination to tear off the crusts. θEcthyma.

*Eruption resembling eczema simplex.

*Eruption general and almost confluent; pustules large and thickly set; those upon face seemed to be drying, with steady increase and aggravation of those upon body and extremities; could neither sit nor lie with any comfort; worried; slept but little; appetite poor; diarrhœa. θEcthyma.

*Impetiginous eruption upon chin, which had been torn and broken, producing hard crusts, which nearly covered entire surface; some scattering crusts of same upon hands and arms; several large aphthous sores upon in-

side of lips and upon tongue; constipation; child fretful and feverish; ichorous secretion of sores had inocu-
lated mother's breast, producing similar sores around
nipples.

Pemphigus.

❚Pustular eruptions.

❚Various forms of eruptions emanating from a psoric or
sycotic taint.

❚Entire circumference of leg, from knee to ankle, covered
with lichen lividus; the livid character of papulæ, and
ecchymosed streaks running from pimple to pimple,
appeared almost like a coarse purple net drawn around
limb; severe pressing pain extending from rectum to
neck of bladder, thence radiating up spermatic cords;
attacks come on first half of night during sleep; >
walking; must walk his room the entire latter half of
night.

❚Chronic eczema of hands, one attack hardly subsiding
before a fresh crop made its appearance, often passing
from simple to impetiginous variety; the ichorous and
semi-purulent secretion oozing upon exercising the
hands, would crust over again, causing most intolerable
itching and soreness; is awakened at times from sound
sleep and finds himself scratching the skin off hands:
dyspepsia, with bronchial irritation and cough.

❚Simple eczema of hands and wrists, assuming finally all
characteristics of a fully developed impetigo figurata, in
its pustular stage; the patches had coalesced and eruption had become confluent generally; pustules were discharging and crusting over, and there was an unbearable degree of tension and pain about them.

❚Eczema of hands, disease having reached impetiginoid
degree, extending over entire back of both hands, and
around ball of thumbs nearly to middle of palms; upon
removing bread poultices which patient had applied
the softened crusts and intervening epidermis adhered
to them, leaving a raw surface, and this was followed
by a copious discharge of blood; unbearable smarting
pains.

" Stages of Life, Constitution. Girl, æt. 18 mos., impetiginous eruption.

Boy, æt. 2, suffering three months; ecthyma.

Girl, æt. 4; herpes circinatus.

Girl, æt. 8; ecthyma.

Boy, æt. 14; impetigo figurata.

Man, had ill health for some time; complained of languor;
slight nausea at times, and occasional wandering pains
about limbs; was seized quite suddenly during night

JUGLANS CINEREA.

Very severe and prostrating
Cramplike pain in l. hip.
Boring: in stomach.
Deep seated pain: on l. sid
Deep, drawing, tickling p
Aching: in r. temple; in
r. shoulder; in arms a
Rheumatic pain: in l.
muscles.
Dull pain: in head.
Heat: in hypogastriu
Soreness: of tip of to
Unbearable smartin
Dryness: of nose;
Fulness: of head.
Oppression: in cl
Sinking sensatio
Tension: eczem
Painful itchin
Intolerable it
Violent itchi
" **Tissues.** Se
" **Touch. Pas**
on nose.
Pressure:
" **Skin.** R
violen
abou
fro
Ery
ti
N

Protrusion of eyeballs.

Conjunctiva glassy.

Dyspnœa; injected conjunctivæ, and eyeballs fixed.

Right eye weaker; watery, as after weeping.

Upper Face. :Nodular eruption on face; boils.

Furfuraceous eruption in beard.

Taste and Tongue. ١١Tongue coated on edges only with mucous stripes. θNeuropathia.

ıIn middle towards tip of tongue smooth red spot with troublesome burning and numbness. θNeuralgia of tongue.

πTongue swollen, felt too large in mouth.

Throat. πSensation in throat and larynx as if forced asunder.

Hiccough, Belching, Nausea and Vomiting. ١١For one or two hours, repeated every five or ten minutes, sensation as of a ball rising from pit of stomach to larynx threatening suffocation, > by loud belching. θNeuropathia.

[17] **Scrobiculum and Stomach.** ١١From pit of stomach to spine an anxious feeling, accompanied by palpitation, not perceptible objectively. θNeuropathia.

١١Empty feeling in stomach. θNeuropathia.

[20] **Stool and Rectum.** ١١Violent diarrhœa.

[23] **Female Sexual Organs.** ıCauliflower excrescence of os uteri, with flying pains, pressure below os pubis, and stinking discharge.

[29] **Heart, Pulse and Circulation.** ıPulse weak and contracted. θMelancholy and jealousy.

١١Pulse small, scarcely perceptible, rapid. θNeuropathia.

[33] **Lower Limbs.** ıVaricose veins of legs.

ıUlcers on legs with general psoriasis.

[34] **Rest. Position. Motion.** Cannot sit up in bed: on account of weakness.

Walking: causes perspiration.

[36] **Nerves.** ١١Such weakness she cannot sit up in bed; a loud noise or sudden, unexpected motion throws her whole body into a tremor. θNeuropathia.

[38] **Time.** Night: intolerable itching of eruption.

[39] **Temperature and Weather.** Warmth: < dry chronic eczema.

Undressing: at night, itching of eruption <.

[40] **Fever.** ıTemperature of surface diminished. θMelancholy and jealousy.

Lassitude with febrile heat.

Perspiration when walking.

[41] **Attacks, Periodicity.** ١١Worse every other day in the morning. θNeuropathia.

with acute pain through r. hypochondriac region, darting upward into chest; difficult respiration and cough,
nausea and fever; *Acon.* relieved, and three days after
there appeared erythema nodosum.

Man, after feeling indisposed a week or two; impetigo
figurata.

Woman, æt. 35, afflicted occasionally, for years; eczema.

Man, æt. 65, formerly farmer, debilitated, broken down
constitution; lichen lividus.

Woman, æt. 80; erysipelas.

⁴⁸ **Relations.** Compare: *Bryon.* in rheumatic pains, dropsy of
chest, stitching in liver, occipital headache; *Chelid.* in
liver pain, especially under r. scapula, bilious stools;
Nux vom. in jaundice, liver pains, occipital headache;
Gelsem., Coccul. and *Carbo veg.* in occipital headaches.

KALI ARSENICOSUM.

Potassium Arsenite (Fowler's Solution). $As_2O_3K_2O.$

A short proving, Med. and Surg. Journ., 1848, p. 459; physiological and pathogenetic effects by Berndt and Cattell; see Allen's Encyclopedia, vol. 5, p. 212;
pathogenetic effects observed by Hering, MSS.

CLINICAL AUTHORITIES.—*Melancholy and jealousy*, N. N.; *Affection of uterus*,
Cattell, B. J. H., vol. 11, p. 350; *Neuropathia*, Gradowicz, Med. Ztg., vol. 3, p. 180,
1846; *Psoriasis*, Cattell, B. J. H., vol. 11, p. 350.

¹ **Mind.** ▮Scolding, morose, retired, quarrelsome and discontented, jealous, indifferent to everything, scarcely an-
swered questions addressed to her, or replied to them in
a peevish tone; eyes had a fixed look, face looked
· frightened and anxious; < every third day. θMelancholy.

πThought her head felt larger.

πHeadache in l. parietal bone, as if it was sore and pressed
upon by a hand; behaves like a crazy person.

ⅠⅠConstricted feeling in head, as if there was a wound on
parietal bone which was being scratched; the place feels
hot; pressure does not relieve. θNeuropathia.

⁴ **Outer Head.** :Crusta lactea.

⁵ **Sight and Eyes.** ⅠⅠStartled look, with protruding, brilliant
eyes, pale face and sunken cheeks. θNeuropathia.

πProtrusion of eyeballs.

Conjunctiva glassy.

πDyspnœa; injected conjunctivæ, and eyeballs fixed.

πRight eye weaker; watery, as after weeping.

⁸ Upper Face. : Nodular eruption on face; boils.

: Furfuraceous eruption in beard.

¹¹ Taste and Tongue. I I Tongue coated on edges only with mucous stripes. θNeuropathia.

I In middle towards tip of tongue smooth red spot with troublesome burning and numbness. θNeuralgia of tongue.

πTongue swollen, felt too large in mouth.

¹³ Throat. πSensation in throat and larynx as if forced asunder.

¹⁶ Hiccough, Belching, Nausea and Vomiting. I I For one or two hours, repeated every five or ten minutes, sensation as of a ball rising from pit of stomach to larynx threatening suffocation, > by loud belching. θNeuropathia.

¹⁷ Scrobiculum and Stomach. I I From pit of stomach to spine an anxious feeling, accompanied by palpitation, not perceptible objectively. θNeuropathia.

I I Empty feeling in stomach. θNeuropathia.

²⁰ Stool and Rectum. I I Violent diarrhœa.

²³ Female Sexual Organs. I Cauliflower excrescence of os uteri, with flying pains, pressure below os pubis, and stinking discharge.

²⁹ Heart, Pulse and Circulation. I Pulse weak and contracted. θMelancholy and jealousy.

I I Pulse small, scarcely perceptible, rapid. θNeuropathia.

³³ Lower Limbs. I Varicose veins of legs.

I Ulcers on legs with general psoriasis.

³⁴ Rest. Position. Motion. Cannot sit up in bed: on account of weakness.

Walking: causes perspiration.

³⁵ Nerves. I I Such weakness she cannot sit up in bed; a loud noise or sudden, unexpected motion throws her whole body into a tremor. θNeuropathia.

³⁸ Time. Night: intolerable itching of eruption.

³⁹ Temperature and Weather. Warmth: < dry chronic eczema.

Undressing: at night, itching of eruption <.

⁴⁰ Fever. I Temperature of surface diminished. θMelancholy and jealousy.

Lassitude with febrile heat.

Perspiration when walking.

⁴¹ Attacks, Periodicity. I I Worse every other day in the morning. θNeuropathia.

For one or two hours, repeated every five or ten minutes: sensation of ball rising from pit of stomach to larynx.

Every third day: mind symptoms $<$.

⁴² **Locality and Direction.** Left: headache in parietal bone.

⁴³ **Sensations.** Head felt larger; as if l. parietal bone was sore and pressed upon by a hand; as if there was a wound on parietal bone which was being scratched; tongue felt too large; sensation in throat and larynx as if forced asunder; as if a ball was rising from pit of stomach to larynx.

Pain: in l. parietal bone.

Flying pain: in uterus.

Troublesome burning: in middle towards tip of tongue; of eruption on trunk, legs and forearms.

Anxious feeling: from pit of stomach to spine, accompanied by palpitation.

Constricted feeling: in head.

Pressure: below os pubis.

Lassitude: with febrile heat.

Numbness: of middle towards tip of tongue.

Intolerable itching, stinging: of eruption on trunk, legs and forehead.

⁴⁴ **Tissues.** ▮ Phagedenic ulcers, deep base and turned up edges.

Eruptions; lichen, psoriasis, icthyosis.

: Rheumatic, gouty and syphilitic pains.

: Gouty nodosities.

⁴⁵ **Touch. Passive Motion. Injuries.** Pressure: does not relieve constricted feeling in head.

⁴⁶ **Skin.** ▮▮Dry, wilted skin; emaciated to a skeleton. θNeuropathia.

▮ Acne, appearance like that in early stage of variola.

▮ Eruption covering entire body except scalp, comes out in red papulæ, varying in diameter from size of pin's head to that of a three cent piece; vesicles form on summit, suppurate, crusts form and fall off, leaving a sore which heals; the places occupied by these sores are marked by a dark colored cicatrix, and the skin generally has a dusky look; intolerable itching, stinging and burning, especially on undressing at night; it is worst on trunk, legs and forearms; mind much depressed.

▮▮Lichen confluens over whole body, except face, palms and soles, and part of chest; the rest studded with papulæ, particularly distinct about outer sides of thighs, arms and back; they are covered with very minute, flimsy, whitish scabs, causing a powdery appearance of skin; head very scurfy; hair crisp and dry; often irritation in skin, which becomes reddened and cracked, particularly about bend of arms and knees.

ı ı Dry chronic eczema; skin of arms thicker and rougher than natural, covered with flimsy exfoliations of epidermis; very irritable, itching and tingling when she gets warm; intensely fissured about bends of elbows and wrists; occasional exacerbation, with eruption of distinct vesicles; languor and lassitude; pale, sallow complexion; catamenia irregular.

ı ı Patches of psoriasis on back, arms and spreading from elbows, and anteriorly on legs, size of a crown piece, and indolent.

ı ı Lepra.

ı ı Psoriasis: scaly itchings, causing him to scratch till an ichorous fluid discharges, forming a hard cake.

ı ı Discoloration of skin after psoriasis and lepra.

ı ı Psoriasis in numerous patches, with great itching; the patches becoming more active, scale off, and are replaced by smaller, they leave beneath them a red skin.

⁴⁸ Relations. Compare *Arsen.* which it greatly resembles; *Cinchon.* in periodicity; *Cicuta* in fixed eyeballs; *Iodum, Kali bich., Merc. cor.*

For one or two hours, repeated every five or ten minutes: sensation of ball rising from pit of stomach to larynx.

Every third day: mind symptoms <.

⁴² Locality and Direction. Left: headache in parietal bone.

⁴³ Sensations. Head felt larger; as if l. parietal bone was sore and pressed upon by a hand; as if there was a wound on parietal bone which was being scratched; tongue felt too large; sensation in throat and larynx as if forced asunder; as if a ball was rising from pit of stomach to larynx.

Pain: in l. parietal bone.

Flying pain: in uterus.

Troublesome burning: in middle towards tip of tongue; of eruption on trunk, legs and forearms.

Anxious feeling: from pit of stomach to spine, accompanied by palpitation.

Constricted feeling: in head.

Pressure: below os pubis.

Lassitude: with febrile heat.

Numbness: of middle towards tip of tongue.

Intolerable itching, stinging: of eruption on trunk, legs and forehead.

⁴⁴ Tissues. ▮Phagedenic ulcers, deep base and turned up edges.

Eruptions; lichen, psoriasis, icthyosis.

: Rheumatic, gouty and syphilitic pains.

: Gouty nodosities.

⁴⁵ Touch. Passive Motion. Injuries. Pressure: does not relieve constricted feeling in head.

⁴⁶ Skin. ❙❙Dry, wilted skin; emaciated to a skeleton. θNeuropathia.

▮Acne, appearance like that in early stage of variola.

▮Eruption covering entire body except scalp, comes out in red papulæ, varying in diameter from size of pin's head to that of a three cent piece; vesicles form on summit, suppurate, crusts form and fall off, leaving a sore which heals; the places occupied by these sores are marked by a dark colored cicatrix, and the skin generally has a dusky look; intolerable itching, stinging and burning, especially on undressing at night; it is worst on trunk, legs and forearms; mind much depressed.

❙❙Lichen confluens over whole body, except face, palms and soles, and part of chest; the rest studded with papulæ, particularly distinct about outer sides of thighs, arms and back; they are covered with very minute, flimsy, whitish scabs, causing a powdery appearance of skin; head very scurfy; hair crisp and dry; often irritation in skin, which becomes reddened and cracked, particularly about bend of arms and knees.

ı ı Dry chronic eczema; skin of arms thicker and rougher than natural, covered with flimsy exfoliations of epidermis; very irritable, itching and tingling when she gets warm; intensely fissured about bends of elbows and wrists; occasional exacerbation, with eruption of distinct vesicles; languor and lassitude; pale, sallow complexion; catamenia irregular.

ı ı Patches of psoriasis on back, arms and spreading from elbows, and anteriorly on legs, size of a crown piece, and indolent.

ı ı Lepra.

ı ı Psoriasis: scaly itchings, causing him to scratch till an ichorous fluid discharges, forming a hard cake.

ı ı Discoloration of skin after psoriasis and lepra.

ı ı Psoriasis in numerous patches, with great itching; the patches becoming more active, scale off, and are replaced by smaller, they leave beneath them a red skin.

⁴⁵ Relations. Compare *Arsen.* which it greatly resembles; *Cinchon.* in periodicity; *Cicuta* in fixed eyeballs; *Iodum*, *Kali bich.*, *Merc. cor.*

ing ten hours, leaving soreness of scalp. *θ*Supraorbital
neuralgia.

▮Pain in l. temple, stretching across forehead to r. temple,
and round eye and malar bone of r. side; complete loss
of sight in r. eye, and puffy swelling on malar bone
during pain; attack begins 9 A.M. and goes off in afternoon. *θ*Supraorbital neuralgia.

▮Shooting pains over eyebrow.

▮Acute throbbing pain in centre of r. eyebrow, commencing in morning, lasting all day, and accompanied by
persistent retching and vomiting of food and bile, without relief. *θ*Migraine.

▮Pain in l. side of head and over l. eye; < at night; pain
in r. side of chest, from scapula round to anterior part;
gnawing at epigastrium after meals; catamenia scanty;
leucorrhœa. *θ*Headache.

▮Sudden violent pain in temples; a shooting outward, in
temples and over eyes, continuing day and night, but
less severe during night; < stooping, which also brings
on vertigo; no coryza. *θ*Headache.

Stinging headache in one temple.

▮Blindness, followed by violent headache, must lie down;
aversion to light and noise; sight returns with increasing headache.

Headache which involves optic nerve; comes in morning,
sight is blurred; as pain increases, dimness of sight de-
creases; comes and goes with sun and is accompanied
by nausea.

Burning headache with vertigo, during which all objects
seemed to be enveloped in a yellow mist; > by warm
soup.

▮Violent pain in l. side of head, at zygomatic process; <
when lying on it; shooting inwards and towards throat;
throat a little reddened but not swelled; gastric symptoms present. *θ*Headache.

Periodical attacks of semilateral headaches on small spots
that could be covered with point of finger; nausea, eructation, vomiting.

▮Periodic headache with vertigo and nausea, morning
awaking, also in evening; often > by pressure, in open
air, or by eating.

▮Pain in head, at a point.

▮In morning, on awaking, pain in forehead and vertex;
later extends to back of head.

▮Headache from suppression of discharge from nose.

⁴ **Outer Head.** ⅠⅠViolent shooting pains from root of nose
along l. orbital arch to external angle of eye, with dim
sight, like a scale on eye; begins in morning, increases
till noon, and ceases towards evening.

| | Frontal headache: usually over one eye; shooting at intervals in r. temple.

| Semilateral headache in small spots, or along course of a few nerves.

| Darting or aching pains on one side; flying pains.

| | Pressure on vertex, as from a weight.

| | Bones of head feel sore; sharp stitches in bones. θRheumatic headache.

| Eczema of scalp, which all over and down to eyebrows was red, raw and oozing a thin moisture, which dries into yellow scabs here and there; hair thin and scattered, and nearly all fallen off; much creeping, itching and smarting of affected parts.

| Circumscribed patches of eruption, varying greatly in size, commencing at supraorbital regions, and covering nearly entire scalp; eruption consists of a number of minute vesicles closely crowded together, and filled with a transparent, viscid fluid, which burst and form thick, laminated crusts, of a dirty grey color; no inflammation or swelling of skin between patches of eruption; much itching; agglutination of lids, and discharge of purulent matter from inner canthus; patches of eruption on face, and thick crusts around nostrils; external ears greatly swollen, red and glazed, behind ears excoriated with profuse discharge of serous fluid; patches of eruption about 1½ inches in length, deeply fissured, in folds of skin of neck, with sero-purulent discharge; fretful, rests badly; sucks with difficulty, from stuffing up of nostrils; emaciation; green, slimy diarrhœa.

| Eruption began on ear and spread over half the head; greenish crusts, with oozing of whitish, thick matter.

| Eruption of painful small boils on back of head.

⁵ **Sight and Eyes.** | Photophobia only by daylight; when opening lids they twitch.

| Various colors and bright sparks before eyes.

| | Burning headache with giddiness, during which objects seem to be covered with a yellow veil.

| | Eyeball tender when rubbed, especially the left; sees point of pen double.

| Sight dim, confused: before headache; with vertigo; with yellow sight.

Indistinct outline; figures vanish on looking at them.

| Granular lids, complete pannus of r. eye so could barely count fingers, and partial pannus of l. eye; considerable discharge; everything appeared slightly red to him; > when lying on face. θTrachoma with pannus.

| Rheumatic sclero-iritis, with excessive pain and photophobia. θSyphilis.

∎Sequelæ of iritis; pains pricking, stinging, wandering; mostly l. eye; lymph and pigment deposited upon anterior capsule of lens, or posterior wall of cornea; photophobia not commensurate with degree of inflammation; œdema of lids; great desire to rub lids; conjunctival chemosis with small spots here and there like ecchymoses.

∎Indolent ulcers of cornea; pale ring around cornea.

❘Right eye inflamed; lids ulcerated; ulcer on cornea; slight blepharospasm.

∎Ulcers and pustules of cornea with no photophobia, no redness.

∎Ulcer with slight photophobia in morning and agglutination; smarting < after rubbing; stringy discharge from eye. θUlceration of cornea.

∎Corneal ulcers which have a tendency to bore in without spreading laterally.

❘❘Small, white, granular pustules on l. cornea, with pricking pain.

∎Cornea affected with a large opaque spot, to which large red vessels ran from injected conjunctiva across clear margin; a zone of fine injection of bulb round cornea. θCatarrho-strumous ophthalmia.

∎Much injection of conjunctiva, both of the bulb and eyelids of both eyes; very red at edges of cornea, and phlyctenulæ on edge; several deep ulcers on the cornea; great photophobia and flow of tears; no pain. θScrofulous ophthalmia

∎Long lasting dense opacities of cornea.

∎Pustule on l. cornea, with surrounding indolent inflammation.

∎Left eye greatly injected; cornea dim; much photophobia in both eyes; upon r. eye an old cicatrix; eczema squamosum over whole body. θConjunctivitis scrofulosa.

∎Mild cases of croupous conjunctivitis (a condition midway between purulent and genuine croupous inflammation), in which the false membrane is loosely adherent, easily detached, and has a tendency to roll up and separate in shreds, which come away in discharges, giving them a stringy appearance; conjunctiva very much inflamed, even chemosis; lids swollen and cornea may be hazy.

∎True descemititis; fine punctate opacities in membrane of Descemet, especially over pupil, with only moderate irritation of eye.

∎Iris muddy and sluggish; cornea looked projecting; fine sclerotic injection round it, and some conjunctival injection; sight very dim, like a gauze; lachrymation on exposure; stiffness at outer canthus; burning pain on upper eyelid on touching it. θRheumatic inflammation.

▌Small white pustules in conjunctiva.

▌On opening eyes, lachrymation and burning.

▌Itching and burning in both eyes, lachrymation and photophobia.

▌Burning in eyes.

▌Heat and pressure in eyes.

▌Heat and redness in eyes, with desire to rub them.

▌Conjunctiva red, traversed by large vessels; or chemosis,
with small spots here and there, like ecchymoses.

▌Inflammation of eyes; conjunctiva reddened, injected
and chemosed; much flow of tears; eyelids reddened
and agglutinated, with thick matter at edges.

▌Conjunctivitis, congestion of lids and globe; no photophobia; soreness in eyes < by reading or using eyes,
with smarting lachrymation upon using.

▌Catarrhal inflammation, stringy discharge, or scanty secretion, < morning on awaking.

▌Inflammation of eyes, with yellow discharge and agglutination, in morning.

▌White of eye dirty yellow, puffy, and covered with yellow brown points.

▌Lids agglutinated in morning; yellow matter in canthi.

▌Œdema of lids; great desire to rub them.

▌Heaviness of upper lids on waking; requires an effort to
open them.

▌Lids red, itching, tender; tarsi seem rough, causing a
sensation as from sand in eyes; granular lids.

▌Margin of lids very red.

▌Eyelids burning, inflamed, much swollen; granular.

▌Large acute granulations of lids

▌Large polypus springing from conjunctiva of upper lid.

' Hearing and Ears. ▌Stitches in l. ear and l. parotid gland,
with headache.

▌Violent stitches in l. ear, extending into roof of mouth,
side of head and neck; glands swollen, neck painful to
touch.

▌▌Stinging from external meatus into internal ear.

▌Pulsating pain at night, purulent otorrhœa; stitches extending into mouth, or down neck, enlarged parotid.

▌Pulsating pains in ears at night, also stinging; external
meatus swollen and inflamed.

▌Thick, yellow, fetid discharge from both ears. θAfter
scarlatina.

▌▌Chronic suppuration; membrana tympani perforated;
cicatrization of edges of perforation complete; tissues
appear as if changed to mucous membrane, and secretion is often more mucus than pus; discharge yellow,
thick, tenacious, so that it may be drawn through per-

foration in strings; lancinations, sticking sensations that cannot be located with any degree of positiveness.

∎Ulcers upon tympanum, dry but not painful, excepting sharp stitches.

∎Violent tickling and itching in ears.

∎∎External meatus of l. ear swelled and inflamed.

∎Redness; heat and itching of external ears.

∎Eruption covering both ears, and considerable portion of surrounding skin; hot and itching, and constant oozing of watery discharge. θEczema.

∎Itching of r. ear lobe, waking him.

∎Mumps on r. side lip.

⁷ **Smell and Nose.** ∎Loss of smell.

∎∎Fetid smell from nose.

∎∎Dryness of nose.

∎∎Nose very dry, with feeling of pressure in nasal bones.

∎Nose painfully dry; air passes with great ease through it.

∎Dryness of nose; constant feeling of being stopped up; disagreeable feeling of burning and swelling, and at times actual swelling; tensive feeling as if it must burst; hot upper lip; eyes affected; < in warm, > in cool temperature. θChronic inflammation of mucous membrane of nose.

∎∎Dryness of nose with pressive sensation at root as in commencement of stopped catarrh; pressive pain extended to temples and affected head.

∎Disagreeable sensation in nose, as if it were swollen, mucous membrane dry; walls of nose feel stiff and velvety.

∎Sensation of a hard substance compelling one to blow nose, but there is no discharge.

∎Sensation as if nose was swollen and stiff; must blow out a thick substance, but no discharge; feels as if a heavy weight was hanging from it.

∎Sensation as if nostrils were made of parchment.

∎Burning and beating inside of root of nose; externally heat and distinct throbbing rhythmical with pulse; nose swollen at root and hot without being red; nose seemed thick and full, "spoke through it;" frequently inclined to blow nose on account of sensation of thick substance in it, but nothing was expelled; nose dry; sensation as of a heavy weight hanging from it.

∎Violent shooting pains from root of nose along l. orbital arch to external angle of eye, with dimness of sight like a scale on eye; beginning in morning, it increases till noon, and gives way towards evening θOzæna.

∎∎Pressure and pressive pain in root of nose.

∎Aching pain at root of nose, with acrid discharge.

‖Soreness in nose; yellow scab at lower (outer) surface of septum; dorsum of nose painful to touch.

‖On blowing nose violent stitches in r. side of nose, as though two loose bones were rubbed against each other.

‖The nose feels too heavy.

‖‖Expired air feels hot in nose.

‖Tickling, as from a hair, high up in l. nostril.

‖Frequent sneezing: in morning; on going into open air.

‖Constant snuffling in warm, damp weather.

‖Watery secretion, great soreness and tenderness of nose.

‖Burning, excoriating, watery discharge from r. nostril; whitish scabs in nostril; sensation of pressure at root of nose; eyes watery, < in wind; dizzy on stooping and on going up stairs; easily takes cold. θNasal catarrh.

‖Watery discharge with redness of nose and putrid smell.

‖Scanty, acrid, mucous discharge from nose, causing burning of septum.

‖Coryza fluent, excoriating nose and lip; nostrils sensitive, ulcerated; round ulcer or scabs on septum.

‖Small perforating ulcer on septum.

‖Distress and fulness from inflammation in frontal sinuses.

‖Coryza, with pressure and tightness at root of nose; < evenings and in open air; in morning obstruction and bleeding from r. nostril.

‖Troublesome coryza and loss of sense of smell and taste; after syphilis and large doses of mercury.

‖Constant running from eyes and nose, severe pain in frontal sinuses, some fever and great weakness; cough prevents sleeping; always < at night.

‖Sneezing, redness of Schneiderian membrane and alæ of nose, suffused eyes, lachrymation, rawness of throat and great languor. θHay fever.

‖‖Nose stuffed up; especially upper part, with a difficulty of detaching thick mucus which more readily passes by posterior nares.

‖‖Formation of plugs in nostrils.

‖Nose constantly full of thick mucus.

‖‖Clinkers in nose; if allowed to remain a few days can be easily detached; but if pulled away too soon, it causes soreness at root of nose, and intolerance to light.

‖Discharge of large masses of thick, clean mucus from nose; if that ceases he has violent headache; pain from occiput to forehead.

‖Pinching pain in bridge of nose, > by hard pressing; small, lumpy, nasal discharge; greater portion, which is tough and ropy, passes down from posterior nares into throat, and is hawked up with difficulty and disgust. θNasal catarrh.

∎Ropy, tough discharge, often from posterior nares; offensive or not.

∎Nasal catarrh, with acrid or thick yellow, ropy discharge
from posterior nares.

∎Constant discharge of thick yellow matter from l. nostril,
mostly early in morning, and fetid smell, after any
fresh cold; severe pain up muscles of l. side of neck to
one small spot in side of head, brought on and aggravated by blowing nose; in l. nostril, half way up, severe
smarting pain, extending to malar bone below eye; constipation; tongue white. θChronic inflammation of
Schneiderian membrane.

∎∎Discharge of tough, green masses, or hard plugs.

∎On blowing nose, violent sticking in r. side of nose, as
though two loose bones rubbed against each other; frequent discharge of greenish colored masses of offensive
odor, that, passing through posterior nares, have very
disagreeable taste; r. nostril filled with hard masses;
small ulcers on external borders of nostrils.

∎∎Mucus tough, ropy, green, bloody; in clear masses, and
has violent pain from occiput to forehead if discharge
ceases.

∎Nostrils filled with a dry, hard crust, bloody at edges when
discharged; itching pains in ethmoid bone; crista na-
salis, or septum narium, which irritation often affects
periosteum of superior maxilla. θCatarrh.

∎Discharge of crusts slightly tinged with blood.

∎Internal ulceration, with thin, watery discharge or collection of elastic plugs, which cause great pain in removal,
and leave nose very sore.

∎Membrane of septum dotted with minute ulcerations.

∎Ulceration of septum narium; purulent inflammation of
whole nasal mucous membrane.

∎∎Entire cartilaginous septum destroyed, and whole nasal
mucous membrane in a state of purulent inflammation;
disease mistaken for syphilis.

∎∎Septum narium completely ulcerated away.

∎Swelling of a highly vascular spongy texture in r. nostril,
distending it and apparently growing upwards, finally
also traveling downward and protruding externally; l.
nostril also became affected in same way; soft parts of
alæ nasi involved, but bony structure unaffected; very
slight and occasional muco-purulent discharge; fetor;
occasionally, severe paroxysms of lancinating pain in
affected parts, making him cry out; by the continued
growth and pressure of the tumors neighboring soft
parts were absorbed, causing much disfigurement; voice
hoarse. θMalignant ulceration of nose.

∎Syphilitic caries of septum narium.

Small ulcers on edge of r. nostril, violent burning when touched.

∎Spot in r. lachrymal bone is swollen and throbbing; profuse secretion from nostril.

∎ Ulceration of frontal sinuses, with violent headache at root of nose, and in frontal prominences, if discharge stops.

∎Nasal polypi, recent or of long standing.

∎Thick, dark red blood from nose; irregular, small, contracted pulse.

׀׀Nasal lupus.

⁸ **Upper Face.** Face: pale, yellowish; red, in blotches; flushed; expression anxious.

∎Sensitiveness of bones of upper jaw, beneath orbit.

∎Shooting pain in l. upper maxillary bone, towards ear.

∎Shooting inward in l. malar bone, with pressure; also same across bridge of nose; hot and cold alternately; cough < in morning; sputa greenish yellow, bitter; inclined to cry; shooting sometimes in bone over the eye; cough hurts painful part of cheek.

∎Thick brown scabs, under which yellow matter formed; much itching; eruption extended from root of nose to upper lip. θSyphilitic eruption.

∎Twenty years previously small tubercle appeared on r. side of nose; this gradually melted away and formed an ulcer, which has ever since slowly traveled in furrows, healing behind; there is now present an irregular sulcus one inch and a half long; besides this there are scabs on nose, and scars indicating the sites of former sores; troublesome itching. θLupus.

⁹ **Lower Face.** Twanging like wires in l. face and neck, followed by burning sensation, as if losing her reason.

∎Sore on l. cheek about size of large almond; base clear and raw; profuse discharge of clear, watery fluid, very hot and scalding. θHerpes exedens or lupus.

∎Pustules on cheeks, forehead and chin, becoming covered with brownish scab, without oozing of matter; itching after washing.

∎Impetiginous eruption on face; pustules form frequently, discharge a watery pus and leave a brownish scab, and are accompanied with much itching.

׀׀Perspiration on upper lip.

∎Lower lip swelled, chapped.

∎Ulcerations with indurated edges and smarting pain on mucous surface of both lips.

∎Digging in rami of lower jaw.

∎Mumps on right side.

∎Parotids swollen; pains from ears into glands.

¹⁰ **Teeth and Gums.** ∎Gum of r. lower jaw very much swollen, of a dirty white color, and extremely tender to touch; teeth on that side quite loose, and will not bear slightest pressure; profuse ptyalism; gums of both sides of mouth unusually sensitive; cannot masticate any food; liquid food causes gums to feel very sore, and tongue rough; tongue furred, dirty brown at sides, in centre red and irritable looking; throat swollen and painful; sour taste in mouth; constant eructation for some time after taking food; after meals aching pain in forehead and occiput, and a feeling of giddiness and faintness; light pain across lower part of chest, extending to between scapulæ, particularly when eating; is very weak and has become thin. *θ*Stomacace.

¹¹ **Taste and Tongue.** Taste: coppery; sweetish; sour; bitter, in morning.

∎Tongue dry, smooth, red, cracked; dry and red.

∎Tongue broad and flat, with raised, almost scollop shaped edges, surface rough and yellowish, dry or moist, while underlying this yellow roughness tongue is very red, fur being thin, and lying on a red ground. *θ*Dyspepsia.

∎Tongue coated: yellowish white; thick yellow mucus, edges red and full of small painful ulcers.

∎Thick yellow fur toward base of tongue. *θ*Catarrh of stomach.

∎Papillæ of tongue very long on dorsum; with a brown colored patch.

∎Tongue coated, thick brown, as with thick yellow felt, at the root; papillæ elevated.

∎Syphilitic ulcers on tongue; deep; stinging; yellow base.

∎Deep ulcer on edge of tongue.

∎Stinging and pricking pains in tongue.

∎Sensation of a hair on back part of tongue and velum; not > by eating or drinking.

¹² **Inner Mouth.** ∎∎Dryness in mouth.

∎Dryness of mouth and lips, > by drinking cold water.

∎Sticky saliva in mouth and upper part of throat about uvula.

Saliva: increased, bitter, viscid, frothy, tasting salt.

In forepart of palate single circumscribed spots, of size of barley corn, colored red, as if little ulcers were about to form.

∎Ulcer on roof of mouth, with sloughing. *θ*Syphilis.

∎Ulcers with hard edges, smarting, at mucous surface of lips.

∎Aphthous ulcers, deeply corroding.

∎∎Syphilitic affections of mouth and fauces.

¹³ **Throat.** ∎Soft palate slightly reddened; uvula relaxed, with sensation of a plug in throat, not > by swallowing.

▪Sensation as if an acid acrid fluid was running through posterior nares over palate, causing cough.

▪Œdematous uvula.

▪Deep, excavated sore, with a reddish areola, and containing a yellow, tenacious matter, at root of uvula; fauces and palate erythematous, bright or dark red, or coppery.

▪Uvula and tonsils red, swollen and painful, finally becoming ulcerated.

▪Swollen tonsils with deafness of children.

▪Tonsils swollen; neck thick outwardly below angle of jaw; Eustachian tubes seem blocked up; is very deaf; could not hear watch, except when very close to ear.

▪Sharp, shooting pains in l. tonsil, extending toward ear > by swallowing; suppuration of tonsils.

▪Indolent enlargement of tonsils, where there is little perceptible inflammation; patient flabby; leuco-phlegmatic habit of body; foul tongue; thickening of nasal mucous membrane, and disposition to scabby nostrils.

▪Subacute inflammation of tonsils, with little fever, but tendency to formation of small ulcers on tonsils and velum.

▪Swelling of amygdalæ with dirty redness, violent pain on swallowing; no suppuration; very little fever.

▪Ulcers on tonsils and throat, surface of which seemed covered with an ashy slough; surrounding mucous membrane dark, livid and swollen.

▪Congestion of all vessels, ulcers on tonsils, pimples on uvula, uvula swollen and red.

▪Sensation of hair in fauces.

▪Dryness in mouth and throat.

▪Dryness and burning in throat, morning; often coincident with inability to breathe through nose.

▪Throat pains more when putting tongue out.

▪▪Much tenacious mucus, sometimes thick, gelatinous, hawked in morning.

▪Mucus so viscid that it draws out like a long thread from gullet and throat; continually a troublesome retching and cough.

▪Very sore throat, pain much < by swallowing; throat full of tough mucus which she could neither swallow nor hawk up; pains < putting tongue out; pain in side of head; shooting pain in l. ear; l. side of neck painful to touch and much swollen; tonsils, especially l., much swollen and inflamed.

▪Burning in pharynx, extending to stomach; solids cause pain when swallowed, and leave a sensation as of something remaining there.

▪Posterior wall of pharynx dark red, glossy, puffed, showing ramifications of pale red vessels; to l. of middle a small crack, exuding blood.

▮Two ulcers in back part of throat, over one half inch in diameter, deep, filled with cheesy looking matter, edges elevated, with well defined borders; also one ulcer which had eaten through velum palati, and from which continually oozed matter like that of the others; pale; emaciated; loss of appetite; very weak; "miserable all over." θUlcerated sore throat.

▮Follicular enlargement of mucous membrane of pharynx, with chronic coryza, that forms hardened yellow pieces of mucus.

▮Ulcers in fauces, also in pharynx, discharging cheesy lumps of offensive smell.

▮▮Deep-eating ulcers in fauces, often syphilitic.

▮Chronic ulcer of pharynx.

▮Tonsils red, ulcerated; uvula nearly destroyed, only a very small portion remaining; large ulcer on gums gradually increasing in size, with dirty edges and foul discharge; destruction of nasal septum, foul smelling ozæna, thick, puslike discharge from nose; upon drinking water it escapes through nose; glands of neck and lower jaw enlarged; severe pain on swallowing; voice hoarse, nasal; excruciating pains in small of back. θSyphilis.

▮Ulceration of fauces to a great extent, with much redness of tissue surrounding ulcerated parts; at one part ulcer has perforated velum palati, forming a clean oval hole; much pain on swallowing; cough and thick, blackish mucus in morning; frequent tickling cough; swelling and feeling of fulness in nose and sensation of a fetid smell. θSyphilis.

▮Syphilitic mercurial sore throat, full of pockets.

▮Increased redness of sound places of mucous membrane of mouth and fauces, with heightened sensitiveness. θDiphtheritis.

▮Pharynx red and swollen; thick, tenacious, ashy grey membrane, tough and glutinous, on tonsils and between them; thick, gurgling sound, with a flapping noise as of a piece of loose membrane, heard over larynx; face and especially forehead, of a bluish tinge; nose pinched; mouth drawn; low fever; unable to swallow. θDiphtheria.

▮Entire throat much swollen; thick, tenacious membrane covering both tonsils and extending down pharynx, and also to nostrils and eyes; fetid discharge from nose; shivering chills followed by dry heat; prostration extreme. θDiphtheria.

¦¦Diphtheria; pseudo-membranous deposit, firm, pearly, fibrinous, prone to extend downwards to larynx and trachea; bladder-like appearance of uvula, much swelling, but little redness.

¦Entire pharynx coated with tenacious, greyish, pseudo-membrane of offensive odor; harsh and stridulous breathing; voice partially suppressed; harsh cough. θDiphtheria.

¦During course of diphtheria, croupy cough; epiglottis covered on apex and sides with membrane; breathing labored; could not lie down; cough hard, expectoration consisting of long, tenacious mucus; paroxysms of suffocation at night; great drowsiness. θDiphtheritic croup.

¦Patch on r. tonsil, croupy cough, bad odor from mouth, no appetite; temperature 101°; pulse 100. θDiphtheritic croup. (*Kali bich.* during day and *Spongia* at night.)

¦Shrill, croupy cough, occasionally whistling and wheezing; rough, hoarse sound of voice with difficult breathing, as though lungs were stuffed with cotton; throat purple, with numerous isolated patches of greenish yellow exudation all over fauces; tongue, cheeks, gums smelling like decayed meat; pains extending to r. ear, when swallowing: expectoration frequently streaked with blood; exudation tough and firmly adhering, spreading upwards into nostrils and down into larynx; tendency to diphtheritic deposits upon remote mucous membranes; great weakness; cachectic look; swollen glands. θDiphtheria.

¦Almost unconscious condition; when aroused from it or when awaking from apparent sleep, complains most, or feels worse; awakes often with desire to cough, or to hawk up detached portions of diphtheritic deposit; while making this attempt throws off tough, ropy, yellow, discolored mucus; very great fetor; deposit covers throat, uvula, tonsils and even roof of mouth, and is of a yellow greyish color; becomes hoarse; tongue either quite red, or covered with a thick, yellow substance; the (r.) parotid gland is much smaller and, upon deglutition, pain shoots up to ear and down neck of affected side. θDiphtheria.

¦Diphtheria: pain in ear extending to swollen parotid glands and to head; tongue coated yellow, especially at root; pricking in tonsils and scraping with stitches in throat; burning in throat; after abuse of Iod. of Mercury.

¦Violent stitches in l. ear extending into roof of mouth, into corresponding side of head and same side of neck,

which was painful to touch and glands swollen.   θDiphtheria.

∎Diphtheria on a wounded palate; much prostration;
exudation looked like mould on bread; discharge from
nostrils.

∎Extensive, well organized deposit, exciting much cough.

∎Corresponds to form of disease in which vegetable parasite
found in diphtheritic deposit resembles the spirobacteria.

¹⁴ **Appetite, Thirst. Desires, Aversions.** ∎Appetite lost;
thirst increased; foul tongue; languor.

∎Longing for beer; for acid drinks, which increases.

∎Dislike to meat.

¹⁵ **Eating and Drinking.** ∎Food lies like a load; sensation
after a full meal as if digestion was suspended.   θDyspepsia.

∎Pressure and heaviness in stomach, immediately after
eating.   θDyspepsia.

∎After dinner external stitches in epigastrium and breast
into nipple (male), and in r. hypochondrium.

∎Secondary bad effects from malt liquors; especially from
lager beer.

¹⁶ **Hiccough, Belching, Nausea and Vomiting.** ∎Fetid
eructations.

∎∎Eructations of air, relieving an uneasiness of stomach,
like from pent up wind at great curvature.

∎Sudden nausea.

∎Nausea: feeling of heat over body, with giddiness, rush
of blood to head; < on moving about, in morning, at
sight of food, after meals, and after stool; excited by
drinking and smoking; > by eating and in open air.

Nausea, with burning pain in anus, and erections lasting
half an hour.

∎Giddiness, followed by vomiting of an acid, white, mucous
fluid, with pressure and burning in stomach.   θUlcer of
stomach.

∎Almost immediately after eating, vomits all her food,
sour; appetite good; tongue red in middle; bitter taste;
constipation.

∎Vomiting: sour, undigested; of bile, bitter; pinkish,
glairy fluid; of mucus and blood; of blood, with cold
sweat on hands, face hot; of yellow, purulent mucus.

∎∎Nausea and vomiting of drunkards.

¹⁷ **Scrobiculum and Stomach.** ∎Swelling of stomach (evening), with fulness and pressure; cannot bear tight
clothing; tongue yellow.

∎Pressure and heaviness in stomach; immediately after
eating.

∎Food lies on stomach like a load; digestion suspended.

ǁAwakens with a start; heat in pit of stomach and spitting of blood; 2 A.M.

▮Awoke with uneasiness, soreness and tenderness, especially in a small spot towards l. of ensiform cartilage; headache in a small spot.

▮Feeling of coldness in stomach and bowels.

▮Pains and uneasiness in stomach, alternate with pains in limbs.

Gastric pains > after eating and rheumatic pains reappear; when gastric symptoms reach to any height rheumatic pains subside.

▮Organic cardialgia; eructations; nausea like sea sickness; sensation of fulness, heaviness; malaise after a meal; chilliness; inflation; gnawing, burning, constricting pain in stomach and hypochondria, < in morning and during motion, > by eating.

▮After food, choking, as if there was something hard all down œsophagus, then a hiccup, and a jumping and shaking as if stomach jerked up, not painful; then a curious feeling as of something eating in bowels; gulping up of food unchanged and not sour, with pain across middle of back; constipation. θGastric affections.

▮Constant nausea and at times vomiting; choking feeling, like a hair in back of throat, comes suddenly and causes sickness; constant tearing pain at epigastrium; smarting between scapulæ; bad taste; tongue white; vertigo on rising. θGastric disorder.

▮Want of appetite; fulness at chest, much flatulence; taste of rotten eggs coming into mouth, with constant nausea; great dislike to fat meat; tongue reddish and rough; sharp, shooting, stabbing pains all over head, < afternoon and evening; constipation; heat of whole body when walking; eyes weak; pain in eyeballs; drowsiness and languor in daytime, sleeplessness at night; frequently sharp, shooting, aching pains in sides and back.

▮Nausea on moving about or taking a short walk; frequent sensation of nausea rising from stomach to pit of throat; paleness of face; flow of water in mouth; coppery taste; faintness and general coldness, and desire to lie down; frequent pain at epigastrium, pricking through to back, lasting about half an hour; thirst; brown tongue in morning; bowels very constipated; abdomen distended; constant hunger and craving; milk disagrees; almost daily headache, shooting from back to front; pains in both hypochondria on walking; excessive languor and indisposition to bodily and mental exertion; sleep unrefreshing. θAffection of stomach.

▮Pain in r. hypochondriac region, towards epigastrium, <

by touch and walking; vomiting of greenish, watery mucus in morning; thick yellow fur on tongue; no appetite. *θ*Gastric derangement.

▮Appetite poor, but must eat often; as otherwise she felt faint; nausea, > after a meal; heartburn; not much flatulence; risings after food; metallic taste in mouth; pain or weight at stomach immediately after taking food, especially after meat; headache and giddiness; constipation; urine high colored; abdomen bloated; tongue too red and dry, but with a yellowish or brownish fur on it; arches of palate red; catamenia irregular and excessive; great weakness; rheumatism even when well. *θ*Dyspepsia.

▮▮Bad effects of overindulgence in beer or other malt liquors; great weight in pit of stomach; flatulency; loss of appetite; oppression of food immediately after eating; nausea, confused feeling, especially in morning, and vomiting of mucus; bad humor.

▮Dines at 6 P.M., and in about three hours has waterbrash, raises phlegm continually, vomits whatever food remains in stomach, and rarely sleeps before midnight, as phlegm chokes him; cough; constipation, stools hard and passed with some exertion. *θ*Affection of stomach.

▮Vomiting of food, sour, with nausea, coming on an hour after eating; pain at pit of stomach, like a stone; tongue white and flabby; bowels costive; meat, tea or coffee vomited immediately. *θ*Dyspepsia.

▮Stomach complaint when there is pain in region of liver and sodden looking tongue, without much acidity or other symptoms, except general discomfort and sometimes white stools.

▮Gastric catarrh with acid vomiting; sudden dyspepsia while eating.

▮Dyspepsia and vomiting from chronic gastric catarrh; tongue coated thick, yellowish.

▮Chronic catarrh of stomach.

▮Ulceration of stomach and duodenum.

▮Round ulcer of stomach.

[18] **Hypochondria.** ▮Dull pain or stitches in r. hypochondrium, especially when limited to a small spot; clay colored stools; metallic taste; confusion in head.

▮In evening is seized with a violent aching continued pain, drawing her downwards, in r. hypochondrium, stretching from epigastrium round to shoulder; must undress immediately, though not perceptibly swelled; great oppression of breathing; pain lasts several hours and subsides gradually, without any evacuation or passing of wind; at times it is accompanied with nausea and some little vomiting; tongue flat and furred; bowels regular; complexion not yellow.

∎Pain in a small spot in r. hypochondrium; pretty constant, but < to a sharp stitch on sudden motion after sitting; appetite good and health not much affected.

∎Pain in l. hypochondrium, under ribs, unaffected by eating or pressure, or respiration, < by a chill, or great bodily exertion.

∎Constant dull aching in r. hypochondriac region.

∎Spasmodic attacks resembling those accompanying gall stones.

∎Dull, heavy pressure or stitches in region of liver.

∎Stitches in region of spleen, extending into lumbar region, < from motion or pressure.

¹⁹ **Abdomen.** ∎Tympanitis; abdomen feels bloated, followed by eructations.

ι ιSensitiveness of abdomen to least pressure.

∎Stitches through abdomen, extending to spinal column.

∎Cutting, as from knives, soon after eating; colic, alternating with cutting at navel, during night.

∎Cutting pains in lower intestines, and rumbling of gas in upper.

ι ιDull, colicky pain round navel, coming on after any exposure to cold wind.

∎Almost immediately after eating complains of coldness and nausea, looks pale, and has pain in abdomen; then vomiting of food, unchanged, sometimes sour or tinged with bile; vomiting gives relief; during rest of day languid, drowsy, and complains of cold, though body is hot; frequent colicky pains in abdomen; tongue white, furred; thirst; bowels moved several times a day; stools pale and liquid. θGastro-intestinal irritation.

∎Attacks of periodical spasmodic constriction of intestines, with nausea, followed by a papescent stool and burning in anus, with tenesmus.

∎Pain as in enteritis; vomits in rapid succession bilious, bloody matter; blood bright and clotted; listless, indifferent, languid mood. θIntussusception.

∎Gastro-intestinal inflammation, cramps here and there, < in calves and inner parts of thighs.

ι ιChronic ulceration of mucous membrane attended with vomiting of ingesta, hectic and emaciation.

²⁰ **Stool and Rectum.** ∎Watery, gushing diarrhœa in morning; awakes from urgent desire; followed by violent tenesmus, which prevents her rising; later, burning in abdomen, nausea and violent straining to vomit.

∎∎Diarrhœic stool, of brown, frothy water, with excessively painful pressure, urging and tenesmus in anus.

■Stools frequent, clay colored, thin, with lumps, blood streaks, much straining; little appetite, no thirst, no fever; insular large patches on tongue.

■Clay colored stools. *θ*Chronic diarrhœa.

■Chronic morning diarrhœa; cough; early in morning, pains darting through r. lung, from below mamma to back below r. scapula; very acute pains darting from behind l. hip down on outside of l. thigh, and sometimes to calf of leg; severe acute pains about l. eye and l. side of forehead.

■Chronic whitish diarrhœa with hepatic derangement of children.

■Diarrhœa < from lager beer.

■Stools: blackish, watery; yellowish, watery; clay colored, watery and lumpy; jellylike; involuntary and often painless and odorless; bloody and extremely painful.

■Dysentery: brownish, frothy, watery, or frequent bloody evacuations, gnawing about navel, tenesmus; tongue smooth, red, cracked; after a burn.

■Diarrhœa, or dysentery after rheumatism.

■Periodical dysentery every year; early part of Summer.

■After *Canthar.* has removed stools like scrapings, jellylike stools will sometimes appear; *Kali bich.* will then complete cure. *θ*Dysentery.

Before stool: abdominal pains; erections.

During stool: painful urging; burning and straining in anus; succus prostaticus; gnawing about navel; pain in region of spleen; metallic taste in mouth; offensive breath; confusion in head.

After stool: remission of complaints; tenesmus; burning soreness or drawing in anus with nausea.

Papescent evacuations, with much rumbling in intestines.

■Constipation, debility, coated tongue, headache, cold extremities; stools dry, knotty.

■Great constipation; stools too large in size, and very painful to expel; insular large patches on tongue.

■Stool in one mass, of excessive hardness.

■Hard, dry, knotty, difficult stools.

■Hard evacuation, followed by burning and pressure in anus.

■Scanty, lumpy stool, followed by burning in anus.

■Habitual constipation; stools scanty, knotty, followed by painful retraction of anus.

■Stools dry, with burning at anus.

■Tendency to constipation, especially when there exists an aggravation of general symptoms in consequence of its presence.

■Periodic constipation every three or six months.

During an emission of wind per anum, sweat all over body, but especially on face, from which it runs in streams.

❚Falling of rectum.

Pressing and straining in anus, with tenesmus.

❚Burning in anus after dry and knotty stool.

❚Sensation of plug in anus, can scarcely sit down.

❚Soreness at anus, making it very painful to walk.

❚Fulness in hemorrhoidal vessels.

❚Painful dry piles, protruding after stool.

❚Hemorrhage from bowels; strength much impaired; lips completely blanched; palpitation on slightest exertion; tenderness over cæcum; stools sometimes natural, sometimes mucus streaked with blood, sometimes almost pure blood; somewhat distended abdomen; stools never caused pain when they were solid, but when there was mucus or blood there was some tenesmus.

²¹ **Urinary Organs.** ❚Pain across back, with red urine.

❚Shooting in renal region, small pulse, prostration; suppressed urine.

Constant aching in region of kidneys, < in r. side, where pain was frequently shooting through to bowels; soreness at stomach and acidity; urine high colored and scanty.

❚Continuous desire to urinate during day.

❚Frequent discharge of watery urine, of strong smell, awaking him at night.

Suppression of urine, with much pain in renal region.

❚Suppression of urine following cholera.

❚❚Scanty, reddish urine.

❚Scanty, high colored urine, with copious, whitish sediment and pain in back.

❚Scanty urine, with a white film and whitish deposit; mucous sediment.

❚Urine alkaline and ropy.

❚Painful drawing from perineum into urethra.

❚Before urination: pain in coccyx, extending into urethra.

❚During urination: heat in urethra; burning in glandular part of urethra, continuing long after; burning in fossa navicularis or in bulbus of urethra; backache.

❚After urination: burning in back part of urethra, with sensation as if one drop had remained behind, with unsuccessful effort to void it; stitches in urethra.

²² **Male Sexual Organs.** ❚❚Sexual desire absent, in fleshy people.

❚Constrictive pain at root of penis; morning on awaking.

❚Itching in hairy parts, skin inflames, small pustules form, of size of a pin's head.

∎Chancres ulcerating deeply.
❘❘Indurated chancre.
▪Pricking and itching at glans penis; ulcers.
∎Stitches in prostate when walking, must stand still; prostatic fluid escapes at stool. θChronic prostatitis.
∎Gleet, with stringy or jellylike, profuse discharge.

²³ Female Sexual Organs. ❙❙Prolapsus uteri, seemingly from hot weather.
∎Subinvolution of uterus.
▪Membranous dysmenorrhœa.
∎Menses: too soon, with vertigo, headache, nausea and feverishness; obstinate suppression of urine or red urine.
∎Soreness and rawness in vagina.
❘❘Swelling of genitals.
∎Itching, burning and excitement about vulva; genuine pruritus.
∎Leucorrhœa yellow, ropy; pain and weakness across small of back, and dull, heavy pains in hypogastrium.
∎Leucorrhœa that can be drawn out in long strings; yellow, ropy, stiffening the linen.
▪Accumulation of thick, tenacious mucus.
∎Flushes in face, during climacteric period.

²⁴ Pregnancy. Parturition. Lactation. Sudden nausea; yellow coated tongue; inward coldness and heat of face; constipation; violent abdominal pains; faintness. θVomiting of pregnancy.
∎Long and continued vomiting during pregnancy; can retain no food in stomach; great emaciation and debility.
∎Milk, as it flows from breast, has appearance of being composed of stringy masses and water.

²⁵ Voice and Larynx. Trachea and Bronchia. ❙❙Rough, hoarse or nasal voice.
❘Hoarseness and accumulation of mucus in larynx, in morning.
❘❘Hoarseness in evening.
∎Chronic hoarseness with laryngitis.
∎Throat dry and rough, with great hoarseness or aphonia.
∎Tickling in throat, causes cough.
▪Accumulation of tough mucus in larynx, causes hawking.
∎Hawks copious, thick blue mucus, in morning.
∎Sensation as from ulceration in larynx.
∎Frequent attacks of hoarseness, cough and difficulty of swallowing; sore throat and sensation of a lump, partially > by swallowing; hoarseness and loss of voice; cough with blackish sputa, most in morning, with pain at sternum "like pins and needles."
∎Pain in throat, and feeling of swelling in larynx; hoarse, husky voice; cough with sputa difficult to detach;

cough and dyspnœa in morning; pain across epigastrium and abdomen; constipation. θAffection of larynx.

∎After catching cold, sensation of dryness in throat sometimes becoming a burning, which extended to larynx; voice rough, hoarse; at times, short, dry cough; greyish white coating on posterior wall of pharynx; debility and lassitude. θLaryngitis.

∎Oppression of chest; without cough, expectoration of blood mixed with phlegm, brought on by any exertion, or by reading or talking loud or laughing; < morning; cannot bear clothes tight over chest or throat, otherwise a sensation of faintness comes on; sore, smarting feeling in l. side of throat, somewhat > by swallowing; feeling of throat as if lined with wash leather; > dry, warm air; < in damp weather, whether hot or cold. θAffection of fauces and larynx.

∎Catarrhal laryngitis and catarrhal aphonia; < in evening and when weather is going to change, and after long talking.

∎Attacks of dyspnœa, and more or less difficulty in taking an inspiration at all times; tough, offensive expectoration; constant hoarseness; appetite poor; emaciation. θChronic inflammation of larynx and trachea.

∎Pharynx bluish with varicose veins; vocal cords and posterior parts of larynx red and puffy and covered with greyish mucus; sensation of dryness; tickling in larynx when speaking; voice rough and hollow; cough with scanty, stringy expectoration, provoked by speaking and laughing; chronic laryngitis.

∎Chronic laryngitis, with congestion; swelling of tissues and increased secretion of a glutinous fluid; < towards morning, when tough mucus nearly strangles him. θFollicular laryngitis.

∎Gradual and insidious onset; at first only slight difficulty of breathing, when mouth is closed; as disease progresses there is fever, increased difficulty of breathing, hoarse voice, constant cough at intervals; cough hoarse, dry, barking, metallic; deglutition painful; tonsils and larnyx red, swollen, covered with false membrane, difficult to detach, with expectoration of tough, stringy mucus; finally breathing performed only by abdominal muscles, and those of neck and shoulders; head bent backwards, breath offensive; diminished temperature, prostration, stupor and death from asphyxia, if not relieved. θMembranous croup.

∎Croupy cough; labored and quick breathing; epiglottis slightly covered with a pale, pearly coating; cough dry and severe; pain and soreness in larynx; expectoration gelatinous. θMembranous croup.

∎Fever, fluent coryza, croupy cough, < in morning; membrane throughout fauces, tending to spread downwards to larynx; epiglottis faintly covered; coughed up tough, chunky mucus. θMembranous croup.

∎On fourth day of slight attack of diphtheria, sudden croupy cough; breathing labored; could not lie down; cough hard; expectoration of long, tenacious mucus; very drowsy; epiglottis covered on apex and sides with membrane. θDiphtheritic croup.

∎Croupy cough and difficult breathing, with wheezing; expectoration of yellow, somewhat stringy mucus, which had to be removed with finger; tonsils and fauces lined with a white, pearly coating, extending down to larynx; < on r. side. θMembranous croup.

∎After riding against a cold west wind, cold in head and throat, followed by croupy cough; increased dryness of throat at night, breathing could be heard distinctly through house; cough in paroxysms, fearfully increased after sleep. θCroup.

∎∎Membranous or diphtheritic croup invading larynx, trachea and even bronchi; voice hoarse, uncertain, cough hoarse, metallic; deglutition painful, tonsils red, swollen, or covered with false membrane difficult to detach, with expectoration of tough, stringy mucus; coughs up casts of elastic, fibrinous nature; loud mucous râles; wheezing rattling in sleep; insidious approach; fat, chubby, light haired children.

∎Early, formative stage of croup; < 2 to 3 A.M.; tough mucus strangles him.

∎Sensation of lump in upper part of trachea, and of hairs across base of tongue, which neither hawking, swallowing nor eating relieves.

∎Catarrh of fauces and trachea; great accumulation of ropy mucus; hoarseness; cough; suppressed voice; burning of mucous membrane, extending up into nostrils; tonsils enlarged, causing dulness of hearing; ulceration of pharynx and larynx; oppressed breathing.

∎Burning sensation in trachea and bronchi.

∎∎Sensation of dryness in bronchi in morning.

∎Violent ringing cough; difficult, yellowish white expectoration; burning, raw pain down throat and along sternum; dyspnœa and wheezing, must sit partially up in bed; pulse quick and small; no sleep throughout whole night. θAcute bronchial catarrh.

∎Constant cough, keeping him awake whole night, and causing much distress from pain in chest, which he described as a tearing and burning; constant running from nose; pain in frontal sinuses; general feeling of lassitude and languor. θCatarrh of chest.

∎Frequent severe paroxysms of cough, loose, wheezing sound, no sputa; perspiration < at night; loud wheezing and rattling; dyspnœa on lying down. θBronchial catarrh.

∎Violent paroxysms of cough, with little expectoration, and that of stringy mucus, leaving patient excessively exhausted, sometimes attended with dry retching. θBronchitis.

∎Acute capillary bronchitis.

∎Every two or three weeks, after any slight exposure, is seized with chilliness and languor, with flushed face, headache and hot hands for half a day; then heat of whole body; disturbed sleep and screaming at night, followed by paroxysms of coughing, with vomiting of tough mucus like white of egg and yellow, acid fluid; then for several days cough; want of appetite; foul tongue; constipation. θBronchial attacks after whooping cough.

∎Common bronchitis, vacillating between acute and torpid inveterate character of disease, and especially if attended by periosteal or rheumatic pains of chronic character.

∎Violent, tight, dry cough, < during day, and always excited by any exposure to smoke; wheezing at night in bed. θChronic bronchitis.

∎Rattling in chest, dyspnœa on lying down. θChronic bronchitis.

∎Chronic bronchitis for many months; cough slight, but much viscid expectoration, in grey lumps; slight sore throat; pain at epigastrium; flatulence.

∎After catching cold, one year ago, cough, with great oppression of chest and swelling of veins of neck; sputa in tough, black lumps; cough < after eating or drinking; dyspnœa on exertion. θChronic bronchitis.

∎Stringy expectoration; sensation of choking on lying down. θChronic bronchitis.

∎Chronic bronchitis caused by inhalation of vapor of arsenic.

∎Subacute and chronic inflammatory processes in larynx or bronchial tubes, with congestion and swelling of tubes and increased secretion of glutinous mucus, which veils and alters voice.

∎Bronchial dilatation with fetid breath and expectoration.

²⁶ **Respiration.** Oppressed breathing, awakens at 2 A.M.; palpitation; orthopnœa, sits bent forward; caused by mucus, croup, croupous diphtheria, chronic bronchitis, membranous bronchitis, or from disturbed circulation; cold sensation and tightness about heart, lower portions of lungs oppressed.

Pressure and heaviness on cnest, as from a weight; wakens
with this sensation at night and is relieved after rising.
Like a heavy load on chest when awaking from sleep.
I Wheezing, panting on awaking; then cough which forces
him to sit up, bent forward.
I Wheezing at night after whooping cough.
I Dyspnœa.
I Slight dyspnœa, as if mucous membrane of bronchi was
thickened, on rising in morning.
I Tightness at bifurcation of bronchi.
I Sensation of choking on lying down.
²⁷ **Cough.**   I Cough excited by: tickling in larynx, or at bron-
chial bifurcation; by oppression at epigastrium, or accu-
mulation of mucus in larynx.
I Dry, short, continual tickling cough and pain in larynx,
as if from an ulcer.
I Cough accompanied by inward soreness in chest, especially in one point, as if an ulcer was there.
I I Cough, with pain, from mid-sternum through to back;
severe stitching, or weight and soreness in chest.
I Dry cough, with stitches in chest, pain in loins, vertigo,
dyspnœa, shootings in chest.
I During cough: bloody taste in mouth; nausea; ulcerative pain in throat; pressure in sternum and larynx, extending into os hyoides; burning pain in sternum, extending into shoulders; heaviness, sensitiveness and
pains in chest; palpitation with rattling in throat; pains
in sides and loins > by pressure.
I Loud, harsh cough, in single coughs, at different times,
for an hour or two, and then not for some hours, most
in morning on waking.
I I Cough in morning on awakening, with dyspnœa, >
by lying down.
I I Cough, especially in morning, with expectoration of
white mucus, "tough as pitch," can be drawn out into
strings.
I Constant hacking cough, sometimes with expectoration
of blood; nocturnal perspiration; night disturbed by
cough; tickling irritation in larynx; no appetite; pale;
phthisical habitus.
I Continuing cough, with expectoration of blood; irritation
to cough coming from larynx; sweating in sleep nights.
Cough <: undressing; morning on awaking; after eating; deep inspiration; > after getting warm in bed.
I Wheezing and panting, then violent cough, with retching
and difficult expectoration of mucus, so viscid that it
can be drawn in strings down to feet.
I Cough caused by eating; dry cough after dinner.

*Cough with smooth or follicular inflammatory redness of pharynx and fauces.

*Dyspnœa and dry cough for six weeks, followed by expectoration of dark grey mucus of consistence of white of egg, with soreness and oppression of chest.

*Cough resonant, whistling, with nausea and expectoration of thick mucus; whistling, loud rattling in chest.

*Choking cough, with tough, stringy mucus, which sticks to throat, mouth and lips.

**Cough hoarse, metallic, in croup (membranous or diphtheritic), with expectoration of tough mucus or fibroelastic casts.

*Stuffing cough with pain at chest, and expectoration of yellowish, heavy, tough matter.

*Cough with expectoration of yellowish green tough matter.

*Cough with thick, heavy expectoration, bluish lumps of mucus.

*Cough with transparent, dirty, slate colored sputa.

*After whooping cough, six months previously, cough still continued, loose and rattling and tickling in fits at night; wheezing during day without cough; occasional pituitous vomiting.

*Whooping cough; mucus so viscid that it stretched in long strings from mouth to ground.

**Expectoration is very glutinous and sticky; adhering to fauces, teeth, tongue and lips, finally leaving mouth in long, stringy and very tenacious mass.

*Expectoration with traces of blood.

Inner Chest and Lungs. *Pains from back to sternum; or, from mid-sternum darting to between shoulders.

*Itching behind sternum, causing violent, racking, paroxysmal cough.

*Face slightly flushed; nasal mucous membrane irritable, either dry or secretes copiously a yellow mucus; eyes now healthy, often catarrh in corners; teeth all destroyed (mercurial sequela); tongue clear at tip, which is covered with red points, root thickly coated yellow; great dryness of mouth, alternating with salivation; gums livid; fauces and pharynx covered with red granulations, interlaced with white streaks and reaching down to œsophagus; constant irritation, as from a foreign body in throat, sometimes severe burning and scratching; taste sour, often metallic; great thirst; stomach bloated, with sensitiveness, fulness and pressure; vomits sometimes; region of rectum sensitive to pressure; urine very acid; stool hard and defecation difficult; dysmenorrhœa; dull percussion sound over r. upper anterior and posterior part of chest; weak, rattling murmur in apex of

r. lung; same symptoms on l. side, only weaker;
cough mostly dry, but troublesome, especially in morning after dressing and late in evening; thick, tough,
white sputa; heat and titillation in larynx before coughing, causing restlessness and impatience. θConsumption.

∎Cough, with profuse, yellow, stringy expectoration, and
much sweating; pain, as of ulceration of larynx, causing
cough at almost every inspiration; feeling of stiffness in
larynx. θPhthisis pulmonalis.

❘❘Scirrhous degeneration of both lungs, expectoration so
viscid that it could be drawn a yard from mouth; cough
very violent, preventing sleep and rest.

∎Hæmoptysis; pneumonia.

²⁹ Heart, Pulse and Circulation. ∎Cold sensation about heart;
tightness of chest; dyspnœa.

∎Pressure on heart after eating.

∎Pricking pain in region of heart.

∎Palpitation, dyspnœa, accelerated pulse, heat; awakens
suddenly with a start, 2 A.M.

∎Hypertrophy of heart; insufficiency of aortic valves.

∎Pulse: irregular, small, contracted, with nosebleed; accelerated, often soft, weak, even fluttering.

∎Pulsation felt in all the arteries.

³⁰ Outer Chest. Dull pain in r. side over a circumscribed spot,
< on inspiration.

³¹ Neck and Back. ∎Stiffness of nape of neck on bending
head.

Brown spots on throat like freckles.

∎Stabbing from third cervical to fifth dorsal vertebra,
striking forward through chest to sternum, < on motion;
inability to straighten spine after stooping.

∎Pain in back striking through to sternum with cough and
expectoration of tough, black mucus.

❘❘Pain in small of back.

∎Sharp, shooting pains, first l. then r. renal region, extending down thighs, < on motion.

∎∎Sharp, stinging pain in region of kidneys.

∎Aching in back and down l. side into hip.

❘❘Pain: as from a knife, through loins; cannot walk.

❘❘Pains across loins with coldness of extremities.

∎Rheumatic pains in back, while stooping felt as if
something cracked across sacrum, cannot stoop or move
for pain, which remains constant even while at rest, but
< on least movement of trunk or legs.

∎A violent aching pain, "like a gathering," in a small spot
in sacrum, a steady, throbbing pain, most felt at night
and hinders sleep; > in day, when up and walking
about, but unable to lift anything.

▮Pain in sacrum ; cannot straighten himself.
▯ ▯Cutting pain in outer l. side of sacrum, shooting up and
down.
▮Pains in os coccygis, < from walking, or touch, and after
rising after long sitting.
▮▮Pain in coccyx, while sitting.

꒪ **Upper Limbs.**   ▮Rheumatic pains in both shoulders, < at
night.
▯ ▯Stitches at lower angle of l. shoulder blade.
▯ ▯Stiffness of shoulder joint.
Painful stiffness of r. arm.
Sensation of lameness in r. arm, as if it had gone to sleep.
▮Burning pain in middle of forearm, extending to wrist.
Swelling of arm, followed by a boil-like elevation, which
turned into a large ulcer with overhanging edges.
Pustules on arms size of split pea, with a hair in centre.
Itching of forearms and hands, then intolerable pain and
formation of numerous ulcers, from which above a dozen
nearly solid masses of matter fell on striking the arm
firmly, leaving ulcers clean, dry cavities, which slowly
filled up and healed.
▮Rheumatic pains in elbows and wrist joints; stinging in
l. elbow.
▮Papular eruption on forearms, lasting a few days, and frequently recurring. .
▯ ▯Redness, swelling and itching in a spot on wrist; then
great pain; after some time matter formed and broke
the skin, and continued to ooze out for two or three
months, then healed, leaving a cicatrix depressed as if
scooped out.
▮Great weakness of hands.
▮Spasmodic contraction of hands.
▯ ▯Psoriasis diffusa of hands, after some time degenerating
into impetigo.
▮Hands completely covered with depressed cicatrices which
look as if they had been punched out with a wadding
cutter.
Hands become covered with deep, stinging cicatrices.
▮Bones of hands as if bruised, when pressed; ulcers on
fingers, with caries.
▮Rheumatic pains in finger joints.
After redness and swelling of finger, with some throbbing
pain, an ulcer formed over joint of forefinger, with white
overhanging edges and dark, gangrenous central points,
skin and cellular tissue movable as if separated from
their attachments.
▮Small pustules on roots of nails, spreading over hands to
wrists; arm became red and axillary glands suppurated;

small pustules on hands secreted a watery fluid when broken; if not touched fluid became thickened to a yellow, tough mass.

Painful ulcer under thumb nail.

³³ **Lower Limbs.** ∎Rheumatic pains in hip joints and knees, on walking or moving, also with restlessness, in diphtheria.

∎Pain in course of l. sciatic nerve, from behind great trochanter to calf; > in motion.

Stitches in r. side of chest and in l. sciatic nerve.

Sciatica: in males; l. side, pain running from hip to knee; wandering, erratic pains, sharp pain in knee and hip joint, aching in leg, with trembling; pains come on quickly and subside soon; jerking aching pain in hip; pain > by walking and flexing leg; < in hot weather, by standing, sitting, or lying in bed; pressure causes pain to shoot along entire length of nerve. θSciatica.

∎Severe pains in hip and down outside of thigh; < in afternoon and evening, > in bed; < on any change in weather. θSciatica.

∎Pain aggravated by standing, sitting, or lying in bed; > by walking and flexing leg; pressure caused pain to shoot along entire length of nerve; l. leg affected. θSciatica.

∎Sciatica from getting her clothes damp; pain in l. hip, > from motion.

∎Pain in r. hip, extending to knee.

∎Heaviness of legs; aching and weakness in calves on walking or going up stairs.

Eruption on legs and thighs of reddish, hard knots, from size of a pin's head to that of a split pea, with a depressed, dark scurf in centre, with an inflamed base.

∎Violent pains in shin bones and burning, extending up legs; aching and shooting in front of thighs and knees; < at night, without swelling.

∎Pain in tendons of muscles of calf, as if stretched, causing lameness.

∎Tearing in r. tibia.

∎Tearing pains in tibia, from tertiary syphilis.

Pain in middle of tibia.

∎Periostitis from a blow on shin, leaving an ulcer on spot about size of a shilling, skin and cellular tissue around it much inflamed; great pain in leg when he stands; violent pain shooting up to knee; stiffness of flexor muscles of knee.

∎Red, painful, doughy swelling on r. shin; tender to touch and after standing, but especially painful at night, when gnawing and scraping pains keep her awake; leucorrhœa and itching of vulva. θSyphilitic periostitis.

▮A number of small, irregular ulcers on leg, which leave a depressed cicatrix on healing. θSyphilis.

Small pimples on legs, which spread into large scarlet blotches, discharging yellow matter.

Sensation of dislocation in l. ankle.

▮Violent burning heat around ankle and heel, deep seated, and hindering sleep; three small, irregular, shallow ulcers; costive bowels; fluttering at heart.

▮Soreness·in heels when walking.

Blister, full of serum, on sole of r. foot.

▮Ulcers on previously inflamed feet.

³⁴ **Limbs in General.** ▮Shooting pricking pains, < in morning.

▮Frequent and severe pain in limbs, especially arms, attended with cramping of hands; when free from pain in limbs had pain and uneasiness in stomach and pain in malar bones.

▮Periodical, wandering pains, also along bones; generally without localized inflammatory processes.

▮Pain in limbs shifting from place to place.

Bones feel bruised; cracking in joints from motion.

▮Stiff all over, could hardly move in morning.

All the limbs stiff, with shooting pains, < in morning.

▮Rheumatism of limbs, especially in joints.

Rheumatic pains: in limbs; in hips and fingers, < during day.

Chronic rheumatism of a cold variety; bones feel sore and bruised.

Periosteal and syphilitic rheumatism.

Audible cracking in joints on slight motion of wrists, ankles and spine, < by motion.

³⁵ **Rest. Position. Motion.** Lying: throbbing over eyes >; on painful side <; dyspnœa; sensation of choking; cough >; sciatica <; pains from patella to foot <.

Lying on face: pannus of eyes >.

Bending head: stiffness of nape of neck.

Head bent backward: membranous croup.

Twisting head: during epileptic attack.

Must lie down: on account of violent headache.

Inclination to lie down.

Could not lie down: during diphtheria.

Stooping: lightness in head; throbbing over eyes <; shooting in temples and over eyes <; dizziness; felt as though something cracked across sacrum.

After stooping: cannot straighten spine.

Rising after sleep: sensation of weight on chest >.

Rising from a seat: vertigo.

Sitting: pain in coccyx; sciatica <; profuse sweat on back.

After rising after long sitting: pains in os coccygis <.

Could hardly sit down: sensation of plug in anus.

Must sit up partially in bed: on account of dyspnœa.

Sits bent forward: orthopnœa; on account of wheezing.

Standing: sciatica <; great pain in leg.

After standing: doughy swelling on r. shin.

Motion: aversion to; organic cardialgia <; sudden, after sitting, sharp stitch in r. hypochondrium; pain through chest to sternum <; shooting pain in renal region <; rheumatic pain < on movement of trunk and limbs; rheumatic pains in hip joints and knees; pain in course of sciatic nerve >; cracking of joints.

Slightest motion: pain in blood boil on r. side of spine.

Slightest exertion: causes palpitation; expectoration of blood mixed with phlegm; dyspnœa.

Moving about: throbbing over eyes <; nausea <.

Cannot stoop or move: with pain across sacrum which remains constant even while at rest.

Putting tongue out: pain in throat <.

Going up stairs: dizziness; aching in calves.

Flexing leg: > pain in hip.

Walking: heat of whole body; pains in both hypochondria; in r. hypochondriac region; painful on account of soreness at anus; stitches in prostate, must stand still; pain in sacrum >; pain in os coccygis <; rheumatic pains in hip joints and knees; jerking aching pain in hip >; aching in calves; soreness in heels.

Must walk up and down room whole night on account of burning itching of papular itching.

Cannot walk: on account of pain through loins.

Tossing arms: during sleep.

⁵⁶ **Nerves.** ‖Great wearines, and general discomfort; debility, with desire to lie down.

‖Weariness in limbs as the pains subside.

‖Prostration; face pale, cold sweat on face and body.

‖‖Neuralgia every day at same hour.

‖Epileptic attacks; hands get lame; nausea followed by chill, gaping, fainty feeling and headache; loses consciousness with the headache; winking with eyelids during attack; twisting the head; loud screaming; face changing, now pale, now red; froth at mouth; tough, stringy fluid runs from mouth, could be drawn out in a thread six yards long.

⁵⁷ **Sleep.** Great inclination to yawn and stretch.

Drowsy in open air.

‖Unrefreshing sleep; feels debilitated, especially in extremities.

‖During sleep frequent starts, incoherent talk, tossing arms.

■Awakened: with desire to urinate; by dyspnœa; palpitation; heat; headache.
■Worse on awaking: head and chest symptoms especially.
** Time.** Most symptoms appear in morning, or are then
most severe.

2 A.M.: heat in pit of stomach and spitting of blood; oppressed breathing awakens; awakens with a start.

2 to 3 A.M.: croup <.

Mornings: lightness in head <; pain in one side of head
comes on; acute throbbing in eyebrows, lasting all day;
sight is blurred; on awakening, headache; pain in forehead and vertex; slight photophobia; catarrhal inflammation < on awaking; inflammation of eyes with agglutination; frequent sneezing, obstruction and bleeding
from r. nostril; thick, yellow discharge from l. nostril;
cough <; taste coppery, sweetish, sour, bitter; dryness and burning of throat; much tenacious mucus
hawked; black mucus from throat; nausea <; organic
cardialgia <; brown tongue; confused feeling; watery,
gushing diarrhœa; chronic diarrhœa; pains darting
through r. lung; on awaking, constrictive pain at root
of penis; hoarseness and accumulation of mucus in
larynx; hawks copious, thick, blue mucus; cough with
blackish sputa; cough and dyspnœa; expectoration of
blood mixed with phlegm <; chronic laryngitis <
towards morning, when tough mucus nearly strangles
him; fever and croupy cough <; dryness of bronchi;
when rising, slight dyspnœa; loud, harsh cough <;
cough with dyspnœa; cough <; limbs stiff with shooting pains <; great thirst.

9 A.M.: attack of pain in head begins, goes off in afternoon.

Begins morning, increases till noon, ceases towards evening: violent shooting from root of nose to external angle
of eye.

Day: shooting in temples and over eyes; drowsiness and
languor; continuous desire to urinate; violent, tight
cough <; wheezing without cough; aching in sacrum
>; rheumatism of hips and fingers <.

Afternoon: sharp pains all over head; sciatica <.

Evening: headache; coryza <; swelling of stomach;
sharp pains all over head; violent aching pains in r.
hypochondrium; hoarseness; catarrhal laryngitis; catarrhal aphonia <; cough <; sciatica <.

Night: pain in l. side of head <; shooting in temples and
over eyes; pulsating pain in ears; running from nose
and eyes, always <; paroxysms of suffocation; sleeplessness-
ness; cutting at navel; frequent discharge of watery
urine of strong smell awakening him; dryness of throat

<; no sleep on account of cough; perspiration <; dis-
turbed sleep and screaming; wheezing in bed; sensation
of weight on chest; sweats; cough; tickling cough;
aching in small spot in sacrum <; rheumatic pain in
shoulders; aching in front of thighs and knees <;
doughy swelling on r. shin; heat and itching of skin;
burning itching of papular eruption; throat sore on
swallowing.

³⁹ **Temperature and Weather.**   ǁComplaints in hot weather.
ǀLiability to take cold in open air.
ǀǀEruptions begin in warm weather. (*Rhus* in cold.)
ǀModerately cold air is felt very unpleasantly.
ǀǀGeneral feeling better outdoors, particularly vertigo >
while walking in open air; chilliness and complaints of
stomach < in open air.
ǀǀUncovering <; wrapping up >.
Open air: throbbing over eyes >; headache >; frequent
sneezing and coryza <; nausea >; drowsy.
In bed: sciatica >; pain from patella to foot <.
Seeks a warm place: on account of chilliness in back.
Dry, warm air: throat >.
Warm temperature: dryness of nose <; cough >; itching
of skin.
Warm, damp weather: constant snuffling; throat <.
Warm soup: burning headache >.
Hot weather: prolapsus uteri, seemingly from; sciatica <;
violent itching of eruption <; eruption begins.
Wind: watery discharge from r. nostril <.
Cool temperature: dryness of nose >.
Cold weather: itching of eruption >; ulcers painful.
Cold, west wind: riding against caused cold in head fol-
lowed by croup.
Cold winds: cause dull, colicky pains around navel.
Cold, damp weather: throat <.
Drinking cold water: does not > dry mouth and lips.
Change of weather: sciatica <.
When weather is going to change: catarrhal laryngitis <.
Undressing: cough <.
After catching cold: cough.
⁴⁰ **Fever.**   ǀChilliness in back, sleepiness; seeks a warm place.
ǀChilliness alternating with flushes of heat.
ǀChilliness with giddiness and nausea, followed by heat,
with sensation of coldness and trembling; periodical
stinging pains in temples; without thirst.
ǀAttacks of chilliness from feet upwards, and sensation as
if skull at vertex became contracted, in frequently returning paroxysms.
ǀChill, followed in an hour by heat, with dryness of mouth

and lips, which have to be moistened all the time; followed in morning by great thirst but no sweat; ill
humor.

▮Chilliness, especially on extremities, and flushes of heat
alternating with general sweat.

▮Burning heat of upper part of body and face, with internal chilliness and violent thirst.

ⅠⅠGiddiness; violent, painful vomiting followed by pain
in forehead, burning of eyes, great burning heat of
upper part of body and face, with internal chilliness and
violent thirst.

▮Flushes of heat; in face. θClimaxis.

▮Heat of hands and feet; nausea; pain in upper part of
abdomen; dryness of mouth; sleeplessness; followed by
sweat of hands, feet and thighs.

ⅠⅠFlushes of heat alternating with general sweat.

ⅠⅠHands cold and bathed in cold sweat.

ⅠⅠSweat on forehead; rest of face dry.

▮Sweat: on back, during effort at stool; profuse while sitting quietly; cold on forehead and hands; on hands,
feet and thighs.

⁴¹ **Attacks, Periodicity.** Pains fly rapidly from one place to
another, not continuing long at any place, and intermit.

▮Symptoms alternate.

▮Gastric symptoms supersede rheumatic.

ⅠⅠPains appear rapidly, disappear suddenly.

Frequently returning paroxysms: sensation as if skull or
vertex became contracted.

Periodical attacks : of semilateral headaches ; spasmodic
constriction of intestines; of stinging pains in temples.

Periodic: headaches; constipation.

At intervals: shooting in r. temple.

An hour after eating: vomiting of food with nausea.

One hour after chill: heat.

Several times a day: bowels moved.

Comes and goes with sun: headache.

Every day at same hour: neuralgia.

Almost daily: headache.

On fourth day of diphtheria: sudden croupy cough.

For several days, after exposure: cough, want of appetite.

Every two or three weeks: after slight exposure is seized
with chilliness and languor, flushed face, headache, hot
hands for half a day.

For six weeks: dyspnœa and dry cough.

Every three or six months: constipation.

Fall and Spring: alternately gastric symptoms and rheumatism.

For many months: chronic bronchitis.

Every year: periodical dysentery.

One year ago: after catching cold, cough.

Dines at 6 P.M., and in about three hours has waterbrash.

Lasting half an hour: erections; pricking through back.

Lasts ten hours: pain in head.

Lasting a few days: papular eruptions on forearms.

" **Locality and Direction.** Right: pain beginning in supra-orbital ridge, spreading over one side of head; pain round eye and malar bone; loss of sight of eye; acute throbbing in centre of eyebrow; pain in side of chest; shooting in temple; complete pannus of eye; eye inflamed; an old cicatrix upon eye; itching of ear lobe; mumps on side of lip; on blowing nose violent stitches in side of nose; watery discharge from nostril; obstruction and bleeding from nostril; violent sticking in side of nose on blowing it; nostril filled with hard masses; swelling of a highly vascular, spongy texture in nostril; small ulcer on edge of nostril; spot in lachrymal bone swollen and throbbing; small tubercle on side of nose; mumps; gum of lower jaw very much swollen; patch on tonsil; pains extending to ear; stitches in hypochondrium; pain in hypochondriac region; aching in hypochondrium; pains in a small spot in hypochondrium; constant dull aching in hypochondriac region; pains dart through lung from below mamma to back below scapula; aching in region of kidney; dull percussion sound over upper anterior and posterior part of chest; weak, rattling murmur in apex of lung; dull pain in side over a circumscribed spot; painful stiffness of arm; stitches in side of chest; pain in hip to knee; tearing in tibia; red, painful, doughy swelling on shin; blister full of serum on sole of foot; blood boil on thigh; blood boil on side of spine; blisters full of serum on sole of foot.

Left: pain in temple stretching to r. temple; pain in side of head and over eye; violent pain in side of head, zygomatic process; shooting pain along orbital arch; eyeball tender when rubbed; partial pannus of eye; pricking, stinging pains in eye; small, white, granular pustules on cornea; eye greatly injected; shooting pains in ear; stitches in ear and parotid gland; violent stitches in ear extending to roof of mouth, side of head and neck; external meatus of ear swelled and inflamed; tickling high up in nostril; constant discharge of thick, yellow matter from nostril; severe pain up muscle of side of neck; half way up nostril severe smarting pain; spongy swelling in nostril; shooting pain in upper maxillary bone towards ear; shooting inward in malar bone;

twanging like wires in face and neck; sore on chest;
shooting pain in tonsil; uneasiness, soreness and tenderness in a small spot towards l. of ensiform cartilage;
pain in hypochondrium; acute pains darting from behind hip, down on outside of thigh; acute pains about
eye and side of forehead; smarting feeling in side of
throat; weak, rattling murmur in apex of lung; aching
down side into hip; pain in outer side of sacrum;
stitches at lower angle of shoulder blade; stinging at
elbow; pain in course of sciatic nerve; stitches in sciatic
nerve; pains running from hip to knee; sensation of
dislocations in ankle.

First l. then r. renal region: sharp, shooting pains.

Outward: a shooting in temples and over eyes.

⁴³ **Sensations.** ❚❚Pains in small spots, which can be covered
with point of finger.

❚❚Pains attack first one part, then reappear in another.

❚Heavy feeling in many parts.

As if head would burst; pressure on vertex as from a
weight; sensation as from sand in eyes; as if nose must
burst; as if nose was swollen; a stiff sensation of a hard
substance in nose; as if a heavy weight was hanging
from nose; as if nostrils were made of parchment; as if
two loose bones were rubbed against each other; nose
feels too heavy; tickling as from a hair high up in l.
nostril; as if losing her reason from burning sensation
in face; sensation of a hair on back part of tongue;
sensation of a plug in throat; as if acid fluid was
running through posterior nares over palate; as if something remained in throat after swallowing; as though
lungs were stuffed with cotton; as if digestion was
suspended; as if there was something hard all down
œsophagus; as if stomach jerked up; as if something
was eating in bowels; sensation of plug in anus; as
from ulceration in larynx; as from a lump in
throat; feeling of swelling in larynx; throat as if
lined with wash leather; cutting as from knives in
abdomen; sensation as if one drop of urine had remained behind; pain at sternum "like pins and
needles;" as if a lump was in upper part of trachea,
and of hairs across base of tongue; like a heavy load on
chest; as if mucous membrane of bronchi was thickened; pain in larynx as if from ulcer; as if an ulcer
was in chest; irritation as from foreign body in throat;
as from a knife through loins; as if something cracked
across sacrum when stooping; as if r. arm had gone to
sleep; cicatrices on hands look as if they had been
punched out with a wadding cutter; bones of hands as

Rheumatic pains: in stomach; in back; in both shoulders; in elbows and wrist joints; in finger joints; in hip joints and knees; in limbs.

Raw pain: down throat and along sternum.

Pressive pain: in root of nose.

Colicky pains: in·abdomen.

Gnawing: at epigastrium; in stomach; in hypochondria; about navel; in r. chin.

Cramps: in hands; in calves and inner side of thigh.

Dull aching: in r. hypochondriac region.

Throbbing, dull, heavy: above eyes; distinct and rhythmical with pulse; in r. lachrymal bone.

Beating: inside of root of nose.

Light pain: across lower part of chest.

Semilateral headache: in small spots.

Gastric pains: in stomach.

Dull pain: in hypochondrium; around navel; in r. side.

Dull, heavy pain: in hypogastrium.

Painful pressure: in anus.

Drawing: in anus; painful, from perineum into urethra.

Twanging like wires: in l. face and neck.

Bruised feeling: in bones.

Scratching: in throat.

Smarting: of affected parts; between scapula; in l. side of throat; scabs of pustules on arms and legs; on mucous surface of lips.

Sticking sensations: in ear.

Soreness: of bones of head; in eyes; in nose; of gums; in small spot towards l. of ensiform; in anus; at stomach; in vagina; of throat; of larynx; of chest; in heels.

Rawness: in vagina.

Violent burning: in small ulcer on r. nostril; in throat; around ankle.

Great burning heat: of upper part of body.

Burning: in both eyes; in eyelids; of nose; inside of root of nose; of septum; in face; in throat; in pharynx; in stomach; in hypochondria; in anus; in abdomen; in glandular part of urethra; in fossa navicularis; in bulbous portion of urethra; about vulva; of mucous membrane extending up into nostrils; in trachea and bronchi; in shin bones and up legs; in skin.

Heat: in eyes; of external ears; in external nose; in pit of stomach; in urethra.

Painful stiffness: of r. arm.

Dull, heavy pressure: in region of liver.

Constriction: of intestines.

Tightness: about heart; at bifurcation of the bronchi; of chest.

Pressive sensation: at root of nose; in temples.
Stiffness: of larynx; of nape of neck; of shoulder joint.
Stiff sensation: in walls of nose.
Lameness: in r. arm; of hands.
Fulness: in stomach; at chest.
Great weight: in pit of stomach; in chest.
Pressure: on vertex; in eyes; at root of nose; in stomach;
  in anus; on chest; in sternum; on heart.
Heaviness: of head; of upper eyelids; in stomach; on
  chest; of legs.
Oppression: of chest.
Lightness: in head; across forehead.
Confusion: of head.
Sensation of choking: on lying down.
Dryness: of nose, of mouth and lips; in throat; in bronchi.
Velvety feeling: on walls of nose.
Gaping, fainty feeling: with headache.
Uneasiness: in stomach.
Sensation of dislocation: in l. ankle.
Tickling: high up in l. nostril; in throat; in larynx; in
  bronchial bifurcation.
Violent tickling and itching: in ears.
Intense burning itching like fire: of eruption over body.
Violent itching: over whole surface of body.
Itching pain: in ethmoid bone.
Itching: of affected parts; of eruptions on scalp; of lids;
  of external ears; of eruption on ears; of r. ear lobe; of
  scabs on face; of pustules on face; in hairy parts of
  male sexual organs; at glans penis; about vulva; be-
  hind sternum; of forearms and hands; in a spot over
  wrist; of chin.
Creeping: of affected parts.
Inward coldness and heat: of face.
Feeling of coldness: in stomach and bowels.
Cold sensation: about heart.

" **Tissues.** Emaciation; anæmia; general cachexia.
  ❙Diphtheritic formations in nose, mouth, fauces, pharynx,
    larynx, trachea, bronchi, and even uterus and vagina.
  ❙Plastic exudations.
  ❙❙Affections of any mucous membranes, with discharges
    of tough, stringy, adherent mucus, or can be drawn out
    into long strings.
  ❙Catarrh alternating with rheumatic pains.
  ❙Rheumatism alternating with gastric symptoms, one ap-
    pearing in the Fall, the other in Spring.
  ❙Bones feel bruised; caries.
  ❙Cracking in all joints from least motion.
  ❙Rheumatic pains in nearly all joints.

Rheumatic pains: in stomach; in back; in both shoulders; in elbows and wrist joints; in finger joints; in hip joints and knees; in limbs.

Raw pain: down throat and along sternum.

Pressive pain: in root of nose.

Colicky pains: in·abdomen.

Gnawing: at epigastrium; in stomach; in hypochondria; about navel; in r. chin.

Cramps: in hands; in calves and inner side of thigh.

Dull aching: in r. hypochondriac region.

Throbbing, dull, heavy: above eyes; distinct and rhythmical with pulse; in r. lachrymal bone.

Beating: inside of root of nose.

Light pain: across lower part of chest.

Semilateral headache: in small spots.

Gastric pains: in stomach.

Dull pain: in hypochondrium; around navel; in r. side.

Dull, heavy pain: in hypogastrium.

Painful pressure: in anus.

Drawing: in anus; painful, from perineum into urethra.

Twanging like wires: in l. face and neck.

Bruised feeling: in bones.

Scratching: in throat.

Smarting: of affected parts; between scapula; in l. side of throat; scabs of pustules on arms and legs; on mucous surface of lips.

Sticking sensations: in ear.

Soreness: of bones of head; in eyes; in nose; of gums; in small spot towards l. of ensiform; in anus; at stomach; in vagina; of throat; of larynx; of chest; in heels.

Rawness: in vagina.

Violent burning: in small ulcer on r. nostril; in throat; around ankle.

Great burning heat: of upper part of body.

Burning: in both eyes; in eyelids; of nose; inside of root of nose; of septum; in face; in throat; in pharynx; in stomach; in hypochondria; in anus; in abdomen; in glandular part of urethra; in fossa navicularis; in bulbous portion of urethra; about vulva; of mucous membrane extending up into nostrils; in trachea and bronchi; in shin bones and up legs; in skin.

Heat: in eyes; of external ears; in external nose; in pit of stomach; in urethra.

Painful stiffness: of r. arm.

Dull, heavy pressure: in region of liver.

Constriction: of intestines.

Tightness: about heart; at bifurcation of the bronchi; of chest.

Pressive sensation: at root of nose; in temples.
Stiffness: of larynx; of nape of neck; of shoulder joint.
Stiff sensation: in walls of nose.
Lameness: in r. arm; of hands.
Fulness: in stomach; at chest.
Great weight: in pit of stomach; in chest.
Pressure: on vertex; in eyes; at root of nose; in stomach; in anus; on chest; in sternum; on heart.
Heaviness: of head; of upper eyelids; in stomach; on chest; of legs.
Oppression: of chest.
Lightness: in head; across forehead.
Confusion: of head.
Sensation of choking: on lying down.
Dryness: of nose, of mouth and lips; in throat; in bronchi.
Velvety feeling: on walls of nose.
Gaping, fainty feeling: with headache.
Uneasiness: in stomach.
Sensation of dislocation: in l. ankle.
Tickling: high up in l. nostril; in throat; in larynx; in bronchial bifurcation.
Violent tickling and itching: in ears.
Intense burning itching like fire: of eruption over body.
Violent itching: over whole surface of body.
Itching pain: in ethmoid bone.
Itching: of affected parts; of eruptions on scalp; of lids; of external ears; of eruption on ears; of r. ear lobe; of scabs on face; of pustules on face; in hairy parts of male sexual organs; at glans penis; about vulva; behind sternum; of forearms and hands; in a spot over wrist; of chin.
Creeping: of affected parts.
Inward coldness and heat: of face.
Feeling of coldness: in stomach and bowels.
Cold sensation: about heart.
" **Tissues.**   Emaciation; anæmia; general cachexia.
  ▮Diphtheritic formations in nose, mouth, fauces, pharynx, larynx, trachea, bronchi, and even uterus and vagina.
  ▮Plastic exudations.
  ▮▮Affections of any mucous membranes, with discharges of tough, stringy, adherent mucus, or can be drawn out into long strings.
  ▮Catarrh alternating with rheumatic pains.
  ▮Rheumatism alternating with gastric symptoms, one appearing in the Fall, the other in Spring.
  ▮Bones feel bruised; caries.
  ▮Cracking in all joints from least motion.
  ▮Rheumatic pains in nearly all joints.

ı ı Bone pains with stitches as if from sharp needles.
ıSyphilis.

" Touch. Passive Motion. Injuries. Touch: burning
pain on upper eyelid; neck painful; dorsum of nose
painful; violent burning in ulcer on nostril; gum on
r. lower jaw tender; l. ear and neck painful; pain in
hypochondriac region <; pain in os coccygis <; swelling like a knot painful.

Pressure: hard, > throbbing over eyes; headache >;
pinching pain in bridge of nose >; teeth will not bear
slightest pressure; stitches in region of spleen <; abdomen sensitive; pains in sides and loins >; region
of rectum sensitive; causes pain to shoot along length
of sciatic nerve.

Cannot bear clothes tight over chest or throat.

Must undress immediately on account of pain in r. hypochondrium.

Desire to rub eyes.

Rubbing: smarting of eyes <.

After an abrasion: swelling like a hurt.

From a blow on chin: periostitis.

" Skin. ıBurning stinging in skin.
ıSkin hot, dry and red.

ıWhole of lower part of body, from a little below navel
in front and from top of nates behind, down thighs and
legs, covered with a smooth, shining, elevated, bright
red eruption, giving those parts appearance of boiled
lobster shell; skin has an appearance of thickening and
induration; not much irritation or heat.

ıHeat and itching of skin at night, when warm in bed,
followed by reddish, hard knots, from size of pin's head
to that of a split pea; centre depressed, with a dark
scurf, surrounded by an inflamed base.

ıDry eruption like measles.

ıUpon development of eruption, hoarse, croupy, distressing cough; nose sore, small ulcers in nostrils, and discharge tough, thick, viscid, stiff; expectoration stringy
and tough, and detached with great difficulty.
θMeasles.

ıPapular eruption, began as a spot on calf of leg and spread
all over body; large papular elevations, red and irregular, like measles, but more raised, with intense and excessive burning itching like fire, especially at night,
compelling her to walk about room whole night; general debility; gnawing and pain at epigastrium, and
sensation of internal itching there, > taking food;
bowels open; urine hot and high colored, and at times
scanty; catamenia regular.

▮Violent itching of whole surface; then small pustules form, mostly on arms and legs; scabs smart, pain and burn; < in hot, > in cold weather.

▮Small pustules over body like small pox; they disappear without bursting; mostly on face and arms.

Pustules over whole body, appearing on inflamed parts of skin, as large as a pea, with a small black scab in middle.

▮Eruption all over body, beginning as a small lump on skin, which inflames and gets red, and finally discharges a bloody fluid, and leaves a small, depressed, ulcerative surface with an inflamed base, which heals and breaks out again; wherever discharge touhes it causes a fresh spot; violent itching at night. *θ*Pustular eruption.

▮Small pustules on roots of nails, spreading over hands to wrists; arm red, axillary glands suppurate; small pustules on hands secrete a watery fluid when broken; if not touched, fluid thickens into a yellow, tough mass.

▮Boil-like elevation which turned into a large ulcer, with hard centre and overhanging edges.

▮Blood boil on r. thigh; r. side of spine, near last rib; painful on least motion.

Vesicular eruptions.

▮Blisters full of serum on sole of r. foot.

Herpes after taking cold, with fluent coryza and bronchial irritation.

▮Scabs on fingers, or corona glandis; deep, stinging cicatrices on hands.

▮Brown spots like freckles on throat.

▮Suppurating tetter (ecthyma.)

▮Pustular syphiloderma.

▮Impetigo, pustules.

▮Zona.

▮Lupus, chronic form, with burning and itching.

▮The eruption begins in hot weather.

After an abrasion, swelling like a knot, forming an irregular ulcer, covered with a dry scab and painful to touch; under skin, hard, movable knot, like a corn, with small, ulcerated spot in middle, where it touches the cuticle; the hard, knotty feel remains after the healed ulcer is covered with white skin.

▮▮Ulcers: deep yellow, dry, oval; edges overhanging, bright red areola; base hard, corroding; becoming deeper; blackish spot in centre; cicatrix remains depressed; deep as if cut out with a punch, edges regular.

▮Syphilitic ulcers, deep with hard edges, on genitals, in throat, uvula, septum of nose, etc.

▮▮Ulcers painful in cold weather.

■Suppurating, solitary skin tubercles, forming deep holes.

■Head and scalp covered with dry, red, scaly patches at roots of hair, and bringing out hair; much itching at night, but no moisture or pain; on face and body brown flat spots and papulæ; cervical glands behind ears swollen and painful; violent pains from patella to foot, of a "linking" character, and as if in the bone; pains < in bed and on lying down; at night must get up and walk about most of the time; at times much swelling along tibia; leg feels swelled and doughy along the bones; throat sore on swallowing, especially at night, and is red but not ulcerated; several flat, elevated ulcerations on tongue, and one large patch in centre; voice hoarse; constipation; nausea after meals; flushes of heat and perspiration; catamenia regular but painful.

θEruption and periostitis, probably syphilitic.

" **Stages of Life, Constitution.** ■■Fat, light haired persons, who suffer from catarrhal, syphilitic, or scrofulous affections.

■■Fat, chubby, short necked children, disposed to croupous inflammations.

Persons of florid complexion, of a blotchy, red appearance and thick skin.

■Dyspeptic beer drinkers.

■Suited to persons subject to catarrhs of mucous surfaces.

Boy, æt. 5 months; constipation.

Child, æt. 5 months, strumous constitution, ailing three months; eruption on head.

Boy, æt. 10 months, bright, vivacious, light complexioned; membranous croup.

Child, æt. 11 months; diphtheria.

Girl, æt. 18 months; eruption on body.

Child, æt. 1½; six months ago had whooping cough, since then suffering; cough.

Boy, æt. 2; scrofulous conjunctivitis.

Boy, æt. 2½, suffering nine months; hoarseness.

Boy, æt. 3, good constitution; bronchitis.

Girl, æt. 3; membranous croup.

Child, æt. 3; diarrhœa.

Boy, æt. 4; scrofulous conjunctivitis.

Child, æt. 4; diphtheria.

Girl, æt. 4, fair complexion; diphtheritic croup.

Girl, æt. 4, light complexion, flaxen hair; membranous croup.

Boy, æt. 4, sanguine temperament; chronic diarrhœa.

Boy, æt. 5; diphtheritic croup.

Girl, æt. 5, fair haired, had whooping cough, after which she caught cold; gastro-intestinal irritation.

Girl, æt. 5; pustular eruption.

Boy, æt. 6, suffering two days; catarrhal ophthalmia.

Boy, æt. 6; scrofulous conjunctivitis.

Child, æt. 6; diphtheria.

Girl, æt. 7, affected most of her life; scrofulous ophthalmia.

Boy, æt. 7, lymphatic, pale complexion, sanguine temperament; eruption.

Girl, æt. 8, had whooping cough four years ago, since then ill; recurring bronchial attacks.

Boy, æt. 8, stout, large head, after a burn; dysentery.

Girl, æt. 8½; scrofulous conjunctivitis.

Boy, æt. 9; scrofulous conjunctivitis.

Child, æt. 10; diphtheria.

Girl, æt. 10, ill six weeks; eczema.

Girl, æt. 11, ill two months; vomiting.

Girl, æt. 12, had croup six years ago, since which she has been suffering; hoarseness; cough.

Girl, æt. 13, suffering a month; scrofulous ophthalmia and ulceration of cornea.

Girl, æt. 13; sore throat.

Girl, æt. 13; croup.

Girl, æt. 14, not yet menstruated; affection of stomach.

Boy, æt. 14, lymphatic, nervous temperament, fair hair, light eyes; pustular eruption.

Girl, æt. 15, suffering for a year; catarrh of nose.

Young lady, æt. 17, just returned from India; pain in r. hypochondrium.

Girl, æt. 17, caught cold one year ago, since which she has been suffering; bronchitis.

Young girl, suffering several months, operation unsuccessful; nasal polypus

Girl, sanguine, lymphatic temperament, for six years after diphtheritis; pains in limbs.

Lady, æt. 22; pain in hypochondriac region.

Man, æt. 22, had syphilis two years ago; ulcers on leg.

Woman, æt. 22; syphilis.

Man, æt. 24, has gastric and rheumatic troubles; pain in back.

Young man, blonde; gastric derangement.

Young tenor singer, after catching cold; laryngitis.

Man, æt. 24, healthy, suddenly seized with violent pain in temples a month ago, since which he has suffered; headache.

Officer, æt. 24, strong, plethoric constitution, choleric temperament, 15 months ago had chancre; syphilis.

Young woman, mother of two children; ulcerated sore throat.

Woman delicate, married five years; eruption and periostitis.

Woman, æt. 25, unmarried, suffering for three months; stomacace.

Lady, æt. 25, strumous constitution, suffering many years; lung fever.

Man, æt, 26; chronic bronchitis.

Woman, æt. 26, blonde, small figure, steel grey eyes, oxygenoid constitution; gracile, but not phthisicky habit; excessively nervous, anxiety at least ailment; irritability and tendency to spasm, and of tearful disposition; catches cold easily and then coryza and cough are troublesome for a long time; suffered from acute gastric and intestinal catarrh, for which she took very large doses of nitrate of silver; consumption.

Woman, æt. 27, married; migraine.

Man, æt. 27; trachoma with pannus.

Woman, æt. 28; ulcer.

Man, æt. 28; pustular eruption.

Woman, æt. 30, had syphilis eleven years ago, and was treated with mercury, had one stillborn child; syphilitic sore throat.

Irishman, æt. 30, strong and hearty, during day is able to work and enjoys his breakfast and lunch; affection of stomach.

Man, æt. 30, after being exposed to cold some months before; affection of kidneys.

Lady, æt. 30, unmarried, suffering for years; affection of fauces and larynx.

Woman, æt. 30, since confinement three months ago; cough.

Mrs. ——, æt. 30, delicate, subject to perspirations; papular eruption.

Man, æt. 32; supraorbital neuralgia.

Man, æt. 32, suffering three years; pain in r. side.

Mrs. D., æt. 32, phthisical habit, lymphatic temperament; convalescent from mild attack of gastric fever; pain in tibia.

Woman, æt. 33, had syphilis several years ago; affection of nose and throat.

Woman, æt. 35, married, fair hair, stout; suffering daily for about ten days; pain in r. hypochondrium.

Policeman, æt. 35, suffering for one month; sciatica.

Maid servant, æt. 36, suffering three years; eczema of scalp.

Woman, æt. 36, suffering two months; affection of larynx.

Woman, æt. 37, ill seven weeks; gastric disorder.

Woman, æt. 38, suffering six months, headache.

Man, æt. 38, spare, blonde, father of four healthy children, four years ago had syphilis and was subjected to severe mercurial treatment; coryza with loss of taste and smell.

Man, æt. 39, suffering 18 months; dyspepsia.

Woman, æt. 39, general health impaired, feeble frame; ulcer on leg.

Man, æt. 40; boils on head.

Man, æt. 40, in bad health for two years, has had rheumatic gout and rheumatic iritis; inflammation of eyes.

Lady, æt. 40, fat, fair, of florid complexion, uses beer at meals, and whiskey in evening, suffers from enlarged liver and jaundice; dyspepsia.

Middle aged woman, suffering for four years; gastric affection.

Man, tall, spare frame, suffering for eight years; sciatica.

Florid, red haired woman, husband had syphilis before marriage; five years ago, had sore throat and ulcer on lips, first two children premature and stillborn, remaining two delicate, now nursing for last six months; syphilitic periostitis.

Woman, æt. 44, suffering for a fortnight; supraorbital neuralgia.

Lady, æt. 44, stout, florid countenance, subject to chronic coughs; acute bronchial catarrh.

Man, æt. 45; laryngitis.

Mrs. ——, æt. 45, nervous temperament; chronic inflammation of larynx and trachea.

Man, æt. 45; chronic bronchitis.

Man, æt. 45; cough.

Woman, æt. 46, suffering one month; headache.

Man, æt. 46, suffering seven years; pustular eruptions.

Man, æt. 48; chronic bronchitis.

Man, æt. 48; pustular eruption.

Man, æt. 50, operated upon three times within last 23 years; nasal polypus.

Mrs. H., æt. 50, subject to colds in head, and determination of blood to head, catamenia ceased about two years ago, after influenza two years previously; chronic catarrh of nose.

Man, æt. 50, stout, red faced, suffering many months, had been treated with caustics and counter irritants; enlarged tonsils with deafness.

Woman, æt. 50, delicate; laryngitis.

Man, æt. 50, rheumatic; general pains.

Man, æt. 50, after a blow; periostitis.

Man, æt. 50; affection of kidneys.

Lady, æt. 52; polypus of conjunctiva

Man, æt. 55, major; chronic inflammation of larynx and trachea.

Man, æt. 55; chronic bronchitis.

Woman, æt. 60, weak, rheumatic, for several weeks has

been suffering from sudden and profuse discharges of clear, watery fluid from nose which suddenly ceased; affection of œsophagus.

Man, æt. 60, fell and hurt leg 16 years ago; periostitis.

Mrs. ——, æt. 60, subject to attacks of dyspepsia and sick headache; lupus.

Man, æt. 62; chronic rheumatism.

Man, æt. 64, had syphilis 40 years ago, but no symptoms of it during intermediate time, for last ten years; sore on cheek.

Woman, æt. 65; cough.

Man, æt. 67; bronchitis.

Man, æt. 69; chronic bronchitis.

Man, æt. 82, lived for thirty years in India, had fever, dysentery, bronchitis; bowels generally loose, habitual snuff taker; malignant ulceration of nose.

[45] **Relations.** Antidoted by: *Arsen.*, *Laches.* (croup, diphtheria, etc.), *Pulsat.* (wandering pains).

It antidotes: effects of beer; effects of arsenical vapors; *Mercur.*, *Merc. jod.*

Compatible: after *Canthar.* in dysentery; after *Iodum* in croup, when hoarse cough, with tough membrane, general weakness and coldness are present; *Ant. tart.* follows well in catarrhal affections and skin diseases.

Compare: *Bromium* in croup; *Cannab.* in orbital pains; *Hepar* in croup, ulcers, etc.; *Kali jod.* in syphilitic affections after mercury; *Mezer.* in bone diseases; *Nitr. ac.* in syphilis; *Phytol.* in syphilitic bone affections; *Spongia* in croup; *Silica* in bone affections.

KALI BROMATUM.

Potassium Bromide.   *K. Br.*

For general effects and experiments with the crude drug, see Allen's Encyclopedia, vol. 5, p. 264.

We need provings, particularly with the higher potencies, to bring out the finer characteristics of the drug.

CLINICAL AUTHORITIES.—*Melancholy and loss of memory; Affection of mind at climacteric period*, Wesselhœft, N. E. M. G., vol. 8, p. 520; *Incipient basilar meningitis*, Hale's Sympt., p. 117; *Diphtheria*, Noack, Œhme's Therap., p. 44; *Diabetes mellitus* (2 cases), Begbie, Hale's Therap., *Cholera infantum* (157 cases reported cured), Caro., Hale's Therap.; *Polypus of rectum*, Helmuth, B. J. H., vol. 29, p. 745; *Nymphomania*, Hale, N. A. J. H., vol. 13, p. 212; *Ovarian enlargement*, Hughes, B. J. H., vol. 28, p. 793; *Ovarian cyst*, Black, Trans. World's Hom. Con., 1876, p. 763; Raue's Rec., 1870, p. 244; *Menstrual disorders*, Cowley, Trans. H. M. S. Pa., 1876, p. 439; *Puerperal eclampsia*, Woodbury, Raue's Rec., 1872, p. 193; *Capillary bronchitis*, Blakelock, Raue's Rec., 1872, p. 11; *Epilepsy, menstrual or hysterical* (15 cases), Locock, N. A. J. H., vol. 13, p. 210; *Epilepsy*, Cook, B. J. H., vol. 24, p. 330; (3 cases), Hubbell, N. E. M. G., vol. 3, p. 94; (3 cases), Neidhard, Trans. Hom. Med. Soc. Pa., 1881, p. 354.

[1] **Mind.** Unconscious of what is occurring around them; cannot recognize, nor be comforted by their friends.

Loss of memory.

Memory absolutely destroyed; anæmia; emaciation.

Loss of memory, despondency, inability to concentrate mind on any object; constant worry, fears to see people or to be spoken to; vertigo, with falling, < from stooping; failure of mental and bodily strength; pricking sensation all over body, palpitation; constantly busy, tying his shoes, fumbling in his pockets, picking threads, etc. θMental derangement.

Loss of memory, forgets how to talk, absentmindedness.

Loss of memory; had to be told the word before he could speak it. θAmnesic aphasia.

Single words forgotten; syllables are dropped.

Inability to express oneself.

Mentally dull, torpid; perception slow, answers slowly.

Imagines he is singled out as an object of divine wrath; extreme drowsiness.

Imagines she is a devil; cannot sleep; fears to be alone.

Positive delusions of various kinds.

Delusions during and after delirium tremens.

∎In first stage with horrid illusions, flushed face, red eyes, and hard and quick pulse. θDelirium tremens.

∥Frightful imaginings at night (in pregnant women during latter months), they are under impression that they have committed, or about to commit, some great crime and cruelty, such as murdering their children or husbands.

Hallucinations of sight and sound, with or without mania, precede brain and paralytic symptoms.

∎Delirium, with delusions; thinks he is pursued; will be poisoned; is selected for divine vengeance; that her child is dead, etc.

∎Delirium tremens, in first or irritative stage; face flushed; eyes red; delirium active; horrid illusions; hard, quick pulse.

∎Puerperal mania.

∥Acute mania, with fulness of bloodvessels of brain.

∎Insanity; manner excited, rambling.

∎Feels as if he would go out of his mind.

∎She is very fretful, crying at trifles, constantly brooding over loss of a daughter; almost crazy; from fretting, loss of rest and want of nourishment, is seized with nervous dysentery.

∥Hands constantly busy; all sorts of fearful delusions; walks the room groaning, bemoaning his fate; full of fear; unsteady.

∥Fits of uncontrollable weeping and profound melancholic delusions.

∎Feeling of lightness and exhilaration in place of heaviness and depression.

∥Depressed; lowspirited; has nervous anxiety.

∎Remarkably depressed, well marked amnesic aphasia.

∎Deep depression, with painful delusions, with persistent sleeplessness, and dread of impending destruction of all near to her.

∥Great despondency; "feel as if they should go out of their minds."

∎Profound melancholic depression, with religious delusions and feeling of moral deficiency; frequent shedding of tears, lowspirited and childish, giving way to her feelings; profound indifference and almost disgust for life. θMelancholia.

∎Profound melancholy, from anæmia.

∥Great despondency, with insanity, a feeling of moral deficiency, or a religious delusion, from anæmia.

∎Melancholy, with delusions; often childish; fits of uncontrollable weeping.

∥Night terrors of children (not from indigestion), with

screaming, unconsciousness of what is occurring around them; cannot recognize, nor be comforted by their friends; sometimes followed by squinting.

∎Apathetic, indifferent.

ı ıTimid, suspicious, full of fear.

∎Much concerned about health; complains without cause; ⌣ restless and trembling in evening; lowspirited, with great and uncontrollable sensation of fear and anxiety; thinks she is becoming deranged; change of life.

∎So sensitive and irritable of mind she cannot give her music lessons; very thought of piano breaks her down, makes her shake all over, and then cry with fear and apprehension that she is losing her mind; cries easily; so easily confused that she cannot say what she wishes to; least thing worries her; makes her utterly miserable to be looked at or spoken to; fears to see people; always depressed and lowspirited; memory weak and unreliable. θMelancholia.

∎Overtaxed brain.

² **Sensorium.** ∎Congestive paralysis approaching apoplexy; lay unconscious for twenty-four hours; flushed face; feeble pulse, contracted and non-reacting pupils; followed by vertigo and mental weakness.

ı ıHeaviness, confusion; slow speech, staggers as if drunk.

ı ıDizziness, noises in ear; nervous excitement; sleepless.·

∎Vertigo: palpitation, nausea, even unconsciousness; memory growing weak; as if ground gave away; staggering gait; confusion and heat of head, drowsiness, stupor; fainting and nausea followed by sound sleep.

∎Confusion of head.

³ **Inner Head.** ∎Migraine, with flushed face, throbbing temples, injected conjunctiva, photophobia and much congestion of brain.

∎Constrictive sensation in brain as if too tight, with a feeling of anæsthesia of brain.

ı ıHeadache in r. frontal protuberance; sleepy.

∎Severe, throbbing aching pains in occipital region, extending down as far as dorsal region; cannot sit up or walk, or shake head without feeling <; great weakness and depression of mind.

∎Violent headache, particularly in occiput.

∎Brain irritated, face flushed, pupils dilated, eyes sunken; rolls head; awakes now and then screaming; extremities cold. θCholera infantum.

∎Reflex cerebral irritation, with active congestion in children during teething, cholera infantum, or scarlet fever; first stage of hydrocephaloid from cholera infantum.

ı ıFlushed face, throbbing of carotids and temporals, suffusion of eyes; feeling of fulness of head.

∎Headache, with dizziness; staggering as if intoxicated; stupefaction; sopor; muscular weakness; anæsthesia of pharynx and velum palati and external skin; sight weakened and hearing impaired; gastralgia; vomiting; colic; constipation. θAlcoholism.

∎Active congestion, or first stage of inflammation, before effusion has occurred.

∎Acute congestions or inflammatory diseases of brain.

∎Incipient basilar meningitis; severe headache, nearly all the time, < at night; would play a few minutes, then lay head down on chair or other support and cry with headache; weak, emaciated, dull, heavy eyed; no appetite; sleep disturbed by groans, grinding of teeth, starting up frightened; terrible headache; tongue clean; pulse 90 to 100, quick and wiry; constipation; scanty urine; too much heat about head.

∣∣Anæmia of brain from loss of fluids; constant drowsiness; coma; pupils dilated, eyes sunken, eyeballs moving in every direction without taking any notice; feet and hands blue and cold; pulse imperceptible. θHydrocephalus.

∣∣Bad results from overtaxing brain; especially with grief or anxiety; nervousness.

∣∣Violent headache, from concussion of brain.

∣∣Mercurial headache.

⁴ Outer Head. Drooping of head; cannot hold it erect.
∣∣Scalp feels tight, brain numb, confused; difficult walking.

⁵ Sight and Eyes. ∎Vision dim, pupils dilated; with heavy lids and invincible drowsiness.

∎Eyes sunken, lustreless; gaze fixed.

∣∣Eyeballs moving in every direction.

∣∣Dilated pupils and sunken eyes. θCholera infantum.

∣∣Pupils dilated, contract sluggishly, vertigo and confusion of head; pupils contracted.

∎Vessels of fundus enlarged; conjunctivæ congested.

∎Eyes suffused.

∎Squinting; after night terrors of children.

⁶ Hearing and Ears. ∣∣Ringing in ears.

∎Roaring in ears at night synchronous with pulse.

∎Sounds echo in ears; headache.

∎Hardness of hearing.

⁷ Smell and Nose. ∎Smell impaired.

∎Thick mucus and yellow scabs in nostrils.

∣∣Erythematous swelling of nose.

⁸ Upper Face. Expression: pale, but otherwise appeared as one drunk, with hallucinations, etc.; wearied, anxious; dull, stupefied; imbecile.

∎Expressionless face; incipient softening of brain.

ıComplexion yellow, cachectic.

ıFace flushed.

ıAcne on face in young fleshy people of gross habits.

ı ıPapular rash.

¹⁰ **Teeth and Gums.** ı ıOdontitis in children.

ı ıDifficult dentition of children.

ıVomiting and diarrhœa of teething children.

¹¹ **Taste and Tongue.** Taste: foul; salty; lost.

ıDifficult speech; action of tongue disordered; slow and difficult after waking; stammering.

Tongue: red, dry, enlarged; red, later dry and brown; white, with languor and sleepiness; pale and cold.

ı ıWhite tongue. θDyspepsia.

ı ıTongue red and tender; gums spongy. θDiabetes.

¹² **Inner Mouth.** ıFetid breath; a peculiar sickening odor; tongue white.

ıSaliva profuse, with fetid breath.

ı ıSuppressed salivation in teething children.

¹³ **Throat.** ıAnæsthesia of mouth, throat and pharynx; chronic alcoholism.

ıDysphagia of liquids (in infants); can swallow only solids.

ıUvula and fauces congested, then œdematous.

ıDryness of throat.

ıFace very red, throat swollen; pulse 150; impossible to move head; submaxillary glands swollen and painful, especially on r. side; tonsils swollen and purple; very thick exudate, covering tonsils and uvula; distinct, crooked line of demarcation between healthy and affected part; mouth dry, hot; anxiety; excitement alternating with comatose somnolence. θDiphtheria.

ıDiphtheritis with quick pulse; fever; dry tongue; offensive breath; highly injected and dusky red fauces; patches of wash leather exudation on tonsils or pharynx.

¹⁴ **Appetite, Thirst. Desires, Aversions.** ıLoss of appetite; tongue white; languor.

ıThirst intense with dry mouth.

¹⁵ **Eating and Drinking.** ı ıChildren, from time of birth, can swallow solids with ease, yet choke every time they try to drink.

ı ıTroublesome pressure at stomach after dinner; lassitude.

¹⁶ **Hiccough, Belching, Nausea and Vomiting.** ı ıRepeated retching and emesis; sick and giddy.

ıHysterical women who vomit their food after each meal, especially if subjected to exciting emotions.

ıVomiting: with intense thirst; when ganglionic system is affected; of drunkards after a debauch; in whooping cough; of meconium.

ıChronic morning vomiting of drunkards.

∎Headache, with dizziness; staggering as if intoxicated; stupefaction; sopor; muscular weakness; anæsthesia of pharynx and velum palati and external skin; sight weakened and hearing impaired; gastralgia; vomiting; colic; constipation. θAlcoholism.

∎Active congestion, or first stage of inflammation, before effusion has occurred.

∎Acute congestions or inflammatory diseases of brain.

∎Incipient basilar meningitis; severe headache, nearly all the time, < at night; would play a few minutes, then lay head down on chair or other support and cry with headache; weak, emaciated, dull, heavy eyed; no appetite; sleep disturbed by groans, grinding of teeth, starting up frightened; terrible headache; tongue clean; pulse 90 to 100, quick and wiry; constipation; scanty urine; too much heat about head.

❘❘Anæmia of brain from loss of fluids; constant drowsiness; coma; pupils dilated, eyes sunken, eyeballs moving in every direction without taking any notice; feet and hands blue and cold; pulse imperceptible. θHydrocephalus.

❘❘Bad results from overtaxing brain; especially with grief or anxiety; nervousness.

❘❘Violent headache, from concussion of brain.

❘❘Mercurial headache.

⁴ Outer Head. Drooping of head; cannot hold it erect.

❘❘Scalp feels tight, brain numb, confused; difficult walking.

⁵ Sight and Eyes. ∎Vision dim, pupils dilated; with heavy lids and invincible drowsiness.

∎Eyes sunken, lustreless; gaze fixed.

❘❘Eyeballs moving in every direction.

❘❘Dilated pupils and sunken eyes. θCholera infantum.

❘❘Pupils dilated, contract sluggishly, vertigo and confusion of head; pupils contracted.

∎Vessels of fundus enlarged; conjunctivæ congested.

∎Eyes suffused.

∎Squinting; after night terrors of children.

⁶ Hearing and Ears. ❘❘Ringing in ears.

∎Roaring in ears at night synchronous with

∎Sounds echo in ears; headache.

∎Hardness of hearing.

⁷ Smell and Nose. ∎Smell impaired.

∎Thick mucus and yellow scabs in

❘❘Erythematous swelling of nose

⁸ Upper Face. Expression: pale, one drunk, with hallucinat dull, stupefied; imbecile.

∎Expressionless face; inci

ι Complexion yellow, cachectic.
ι Face flushed.
ι Acne on face in young fleshy people of gross habits.
ι ι Papular rash.

10 Teeth and Gums.   ι ι Odontitis in children.
   ι ι Difficult dentition of children.
   ι Vomiting and diarrhœa of teething children.

11 Taste and Tongue.   Taste: foul; salty; lost.
   ι Difficult speech; action of tongue disordered; slow or
      difficult after waking; stammering.
   Tongue: red, dry, enlarged; red, later dry and brown,
      white, with languor and sleepiness; pale and co..
   ι ι White tongue. θ Dyspepsia.
   ι ι Tongue red and tender; gums spongy. θ Diabetes

12 Inner Mouth.   ι Fetid breath; a peculiar moisture..
      tongue white.
   ι Saliva profuse, with fetid breath.
   ι ι Suppressed salivation in teething children.

13 Throat.   ι Anæsthesia of mouth, throat and ....
      alcoholism.
   ι Dysphagia of liquids (in infants): can swallow ... .
   ι Uvula and fauces congested, then ... . dis-
   ι Dryness of throat.   ...owels;
   ι Face very red, throat swollen: ... ... rectum.
      move head; submaxillary glands ... ...ls.
      especially on r. side; tonsils swollen ... and painful
      thick exudate, covering ...
      crooked line of ... ... extending in
      part; mouth dry, but ... ...s copious urine.
      with comatose ... r.
   ι Diphtheritis with gu...
      sive breath; hi... ...ssages.
      patches of w... ...ra.

14 Appetite, Thirst.   ...th abundance of phos-
      tongue w... ...even suppressed in col-
   ι Thirst ... ...w drops at beginning of

15 Eating
                           ...missions of urine.
                           θ Cholera infantum.
                    ...: skin cold and dry; pulse rapid
               ...e red and tender; gums spongy and
         ...excessive; appetite voracious; bowels
      urine pale, frequent, large quantity, of
   ...and loaded with sugar; liver tumid and
      θ Diabetes mellitus.
   ...al Organs.   ι Sensual and lascivious fancies and

[17] **Scrobiculum and Stomach.** I I Weakness of stomach; dyspepsia.

I Anorexia, foul breath, white tongue, involving edges as well as dorsum, and not necessarily furred; great languor; violent headache; loathing; vomiturition or vomiting of mucus; saltish taste in mouth; vomiting of drunkards after debauch; troublesome pressure at stomach after dinner.

[18] **Hypochondria.** I I Enlargement of liver and spleen.
I I Small tumor in region of spleen.

[19] **Abdomen.** I Sensation as if bowels were falling out.
I Internal coldness of abdomen.
I I Abdomen sunken, almost stuck to vertebral column. θCholera infantum.
I Abdominal spasms, walls retracted, convulsive motions of eyes and limbs; frequent, green, watery stools. θSummer complaint.
I I Colic in young children; walls of belly are retracted and hard, while intestines can be seen at one spot contracted into a hard lump, of size of a small orange, and contraction can be seen through abdominal wall to travel from one part of intestines to another; attacks frequent and excruciating, unconnected with diarrhœa or constipation, but often associated with an aphthous condition of mouth.
I Periodic colic in infants, occurring about 5 P.M.
I Flatulent colic in children and hysterical women.
I I Ascites of hepatic or splenic origin.

[20] **Stool and Rectum.** I I Painless diarrhœa, with great chilliness, even in a hot room; fifteen or twenty passages in twenty-four hours; burning in chest; internal coldness of abdomen; pulse frequent and weak; urine scanty, dribbling of a few drops in beginning; at every stool, sensation as if bowels were falling out; restless and shaky as if from palsy.
I Stools: watery (like rice water); painless.
I Frequent, green, watery discharges, with violent abdominal spasms, during which abdomen gets hard; thrush in mouth; convulsive motions of eyes and limbs.
I I Bloody muco-purulent diarrhœa, with intense thirst, vomiting, eyes sunken, pupils dilated, skin corrugated and spotted blue, body cold, tongue red and dry, pulse imperceptible, urine suppressed.
I Cerebral irritation during cholera infantum; pupils dilated, eyes sunken, eyeballs moving in every direction without taking any notice; feet and hands blue and cold; pulse imperceptible.
I Cholera infantum, with reflex cerebral irritation of brain, before effusion.

∎Cholera infantum, sudden in onset, attended by great prostration, cold hands and feet, hot head, dilated pupils, rolling of eyes and head, starts, jactitation, spasms, watery, very offensive stools, vomiting of all drinks and intense thirst; nervous and vascular excitement.

ı ıGreat prostration, coldness of surface and symptoms of hydrocephaloid. *θ*Cholera infantum.

ı ıAsiatic cholera, first stage, vomiting, cramps, rice water discharges; restores secretion of urine.

ı ıConstipation; stools very dry, hard and infrequent.

ı ıRetention of meconium, with vomiting of all food and obstinate constipation.

∎During stool: sensation as if bowels were falling out; dribbling of urine.

∎Spasmodic stricture of sphincter ani.

∎Constant diarrhœa and more or less tenesmus, and passage of much blood; on making efforts to expel, protrusion of several elongated bodies, resembling earthworms in shape, but of much more brilliant red color; they presented a soft, vascular, shreddy appearance, bearing some resemblance to sarcomatous growths; with this expulsion there was always a yellow, very fetid discharge; feces flattened; flatulent distension of bowels; patient pale and sickly looking. *θ*Polypus of rectum.

∎Blind, intensely painful varices with black stools.

: Pain in hemorrhoids, fissure of rectum, and painful growths.

ⁿ Urinary Organs. Pain in region of kidneys extending in direction of ascending colon ; afterwards copious urine.

ı ıSpasmodic affection of neck of bladder.

ı ıNeuralgia of neck of bladder.

ı ıAbnormal irritability of urinary passages.

∎Diminution of sensibility of urethra.

∎Urine: profuse with thirst; with abundance of phosphates; copious, pale; scanty, even suppressed in collapse; scanty, dribbling a few drops at beginning of every stool.

∎Incontinence of urine.

ı ıNocturnal involuntary emissions of urine.

ı ıSuppression of urine. *θ*Cholera infantum.

ı ıEmaciation; paleness; skin cold and dry ; pulse rapid and feeble; tongue red and tender; gums spongy and bleeding; thirst excessive; appetite voracious; bowels constipated; urine pale, frequent, large quantity, of high density, and loaded with sugar; liver tumid and tender. *θ*Diabetes mellitus.

ⁿ Male Sexual Organs. ∎Sensual and lascivious fancies and dreams.

▮Excessive sexual desire, with constant erections at night.
▮Satyriasis.
▮Diminution of sexual desire; lessened even to impotence.
▮▮Erections at night; backache; uncontrollable fidgetiness.
▮▮Impotence with melancholy, loss of memory; nervous prostration; epilepsy.
▮Effects of sexual excesses, such as impotency, paralysis and spasms from exhaustion of spinal cord.
▮Frequent pollutions from ardent imagination.
▮▮Seminal emissions, with depressed spirits, dull thought, backache, staggering gait and great weakness.
▮Nocturnal emissions, with amorous dreams and erections.
▮Spermatorrhœa, before paralytic symptoms have set in; erections normal but teasing and persistent, with nocturnal emissions and nervous disturbances growing out of unsatisfied sexual desire.
▮Chordee, during gonorrhœa.
² Female Sexual Organs. ▮Nymphomania.
▮Sterility from excessive sexual indulgence.
▮▮Abolition of all sexual feeling during coition.
▮Aversion to coition; menses scanty.
▮Enlargement of uterus after parturition, with abnormal discharges.
▮▮Subinvolution of uterus.
▮Induration of uterus; enlargement of uterus (after parturition), with abnormal discharges.
▮▮Uterine fibroids.
▮Ovarian neuralgia from ungratified sexual desire; nervous unrest.
▮Neuralgia of ovaries; pain, swelling, tenderness of l. ovary; diminution of sexual desire.
▮Epilepsy from ovarian irritation.
▮Large tumor, smooth and tense in hypogastric and r. iliac region; tumor slightly tender when pressed, and there is indistinct fluctuation; measurement of abdomen taken in a line with crests of ilium shows an increase in size of ten inches; urine scanty and frequent calls to pass it. θOvarian cystic tumor.
▮Abdomen large but not tense; on palpation, well defined, elastic tumor, yielding indistinct fluctuation, in l. iliac region, here also movements are felt as in quickening. θOvarian enlargement.
▮Ovarian cystic tumor, after tapping.
▮Metrorrhagia from reflex irritation, or of nervous origin.
▮Menorrhagia, metrorrhagia, nymphomania and menstrual epilepsy; nervous symptoms led to its use.
▮Menorrhagia from ovarian irritation caused by strong sexual desire.

: Flooding, especially in young women.

❙Erotomania, a few days after menses.

❙Before menses: headache.

During menses: epileptic spasms, nymphomania, itching.
burning and excitement in vulva, pudenda and clitoris.

After menses: headache, insomnia and heat in genitals.

❙Epileptic attacks at or near menstrual periods.

❙❙Scanty menstruation, in fleshy women.

❙Change of life: restless, must be on the move; sleepless;
trembling; flushings of face and much congestion of
blood to head; palpitation of heart; menorrhagia.

❙❙Vaginismus.

❙Voluptuous itching, tingling and irritation in external
genital organs.

❙Pruritus of genitals, arising from irritation of uterus, or
ovaries, or any hyperæsthesia of veins of that location;
sexual excitement intense, often actual nymphomania.

²⁴ **Pregnancy. Parturition. Lactation.** ❙Nymphomania
during puerperal state.

❙Puerperal mania, attended by ferocious or erotic delirium.

❙Frightful imaginings in pregnant women, usually caused
by engorged condition of brain.

: Frightful imaginings at night, labors under impression
that she has committed, or is about to commit, some
great crime or cruelty, as the murder of her children
or husband. θPregnancy.

❙Morning sickness and vomiting during pregnancy.

❙Constant hacking cough during pregnancy; irresistible
desire to urinate, but no flow except with urging and
difficulty.

❙Nervous cough during pregnancy, threatening abortion;
the cough dry, hard and almost incessant.

❙Convulsions during labor.

❙Enlarged uterus.

²⁵ **Voice and Larynx. Trachea and Bronchia.** ❙❙After
parturition voice changed, whispering.

❙❙Hoarseness, extremely painful and disagreeable.

❙Aphasia, from embolism of middle cerebral artery.

❙❙Hyperæsthesia of laryngeal nerves.

❙Loss of sensibility.

❙Chronic catarrh with purulent slate colored sputa.

❙Follicular and catarrhal laryngitis.

❙❙Laryngismus stridulus, uncomplicated, from neurosis or
reflex irritation.

❙❙Spasmodic, dry croup, occurring suddenly in night;
from reflex irritation, teething, worms, not catarrhal.

❙Spasmodic croup; in earlier stages when child appears
well in daytime; at night is agitated, face flushed, suf-

fused and bloodshot eyes; after several hours he sleeps, breathing easily and naturally, but soon awakens in a paroxysm; hyperæsthesia of laryngeal nerves followed at later stage by natural reaction; loss of sensibility in larynx; exudation of whitish, firm texture, affecting trachea and bronchi; harsh, painful voice, with hoarseness; hacking cough with dulness and confusion of head; wakes suddenly from sound sleep with sensation of suffocation, with peculiar ringing, dry, brassy cough and hurried breathing. *θ*Croup.

▮Membranous croup, with whitish exudation.

▮Torpid cases with copious purulent expectoration. *θ*Bronchitis.

▮Infantile capillary bronchitis with severe dyspnœa, throwing arms wildly about; spasmodic action of muscles, opisthotonos.

²⁶ **Respiration.** ▯▯Breath hot and hurried.

▯▯Breathlessness, nervous headache and want of sleep.

▯▯Asthma of nervous origin.

▮Spasmodic asthma, with dry, nervous, spasmodic cough, great tightness of breathing.

▯▯Spasmodic asthma of children; great dyspnœa, lividity of face; no sleep, urine suppressed, general œdema.

▮Severe dyspnœa, tossing arms about wildly; spasmodic action of muscles, throwing child into a state of opisthotonos. *θ*Capillary bronchitis.

²⁷ **Cough.** ▯▯Paroxysmal, dry cough.

▮Dry, fatiguing cough at intervals of two or three hours, with difficult respiration, followed by vomiting of mucus and food, < at night and when lying down; tightness of chest when breathing.

▮Weak, nervous children, arouse with a dry, spasmodic cough, which greatly frightens them, causing them to cry out in terror.

▮Hacking cough with dulness and confusion of head.

▮Dry cough, due to reflex action from stomach, intestines, or uterus.

▮Nervous, dry, hysterical cough of women, especially if pregnant.

▯▯Whooping cough, with spasmodic, dry cough; spasm of glottis; with convulsions.

²⁸ **Inner Chest and Lungs.** ▯▯Burning in chest.

▮Pneumonia in drunkards.

²⁹ **Heart, Pulse and Circulation.** ▮Feeble, intermitting action of heart; so nervous she must be busy and walk; slow and small pulse; heart's beats wanting in energy, and its sounds distant and feeble; action of heart slow and fluttering.

■Cardiac neuroses from spinal or uterine irritation.

Pulse: accelerated, later slower; slow, small, weak; rapid and weak; 100, weak; 50, small and feeble; 40, skin cold, clammy; imperceptible with coldness and collapse.

ı ı Vascular bruit de souffle.

³¹ **Neck and Back.** ■Tabes dorsalis from sexual excesses.

■Backache; tired lameness of legs. θSeminal emissions.

³² **Upper Limbs.** ■Trembling of hands during voluntary motion; or, as in delirium tremens.

■Hands and fingers in constant action; busy twitching of fingers.

³³ **Lower Limbs.** ■Cannot stand erect; legs weak.

. ■Unsteady gait; frequently taken for a drunken man.

■Gait staggering, uncertain; looks to see if legs are really moving; feels as if his legs were all over sidewalk. θLocomotor ataxia.

■Loss of sensibility; pinching or burning causes no pain. θLocomotor ataxia.

ı ı Legs and feet cold and blue; on being touched leave white impress of fingers for more than twenty-five seconds. θCholera infantum.

³⁴ **Rest. Position. Motion.** Difficulty of holding head erect.

Stooping: vertigo <.

Lying down: cough <.

Cannot sit, or walk, or shake head without feeling < of headache.

Cannot stand erect.

Straightening out in bed during spasm.

Restless, must be on the move.

Impossible to move head on account of swollen throat.

Difficult walking.

³⁵ **Nerves.** ■The thought of something to be done makes her shake all over.

■■Nervous, restless; cannot sit still, but must move about or otherwise occupy oneself; often suits nervous women.

■Restlessness, fitfulness of motion, with giddiness.

■Almost constant twitching of fingers and a busy occupation of them in matters of no importance.

■Nervous irritability caused by severe illness or death of some dear friend, or loss of property or reputation; constant fretting; will not eat, cannot sleep, is very irritable; pulse quick, tongue coated; fetid breath.

■Restlessness and sleeplessness due to worry and grief.

■Nervous excitement, irritation and congestion of cerebral meninges, with mania.

■Hysterical spinal irritation.

■Reflex excitability.

▌Languor, disinclined to talk, or use mind or work, indifferent, sleepy; by strong effort of will can act as usual.

▌▌Trembling sensation through body.

▌Mercurial trembling.

▌Symptoms from affection of vasomotor nerves: occasional sudden paroxysmal feeling of numbness; pins and needles; deadness and weakness; indescribable feeling of something wrong; feeling of largeness, or as if limbs were swollen; aching, uneasiness or actual pain not very severe; feeling of coldness, occasionally obvious fact of coldness; sudden weakness; paralyzed feeling; unable to retain grasp of an object, hastily putting it down, or allowing it to fall; muscles do not respond readily to will; co-ordination of movement defective; writing or needlework have to be discontinued; rubs the limbs by, as it would seem, an almost instinctive impulse; sensations allied to cramp, or actual cramp, with varying amounts of pain.

▌General delirium, hallucinations, fancies about being persecuted; ataxia; as in general paralysis.

▌Gait: unsteady, reeling, as if drunk; staggering; false steps frequent; with rolling and staggering; as one walks with locomotor ataxia; looks too see if legs are really moving.

▌Weakness of extensors of legs and feet.

▌▌Weakness of muscles of arms.

▌Inco-ordination of muscles; nervous weakness, even paralysis of motion and numbness.

▌▌Great difficulty in getting and keeping right word, although right idea is present to mind. θAnæmia of frontal lobe of brain.

▌Amnesic aphasia.

▌Anæsthesia, particularly of gums, pharynx and genitalia.

▌▌Spasms: from fright, anger and other emotional causes, occurring in plethoric, nervous persons, or in women at time of menses; during parturition; from sexual excitement or excessive venery; too great reflex excitability, sleeplessness; during teething, whooping cough, or laryngismus stridulus; from Bright's disease.

▌Neuroses involving brain, accompanied by convulsions.

▌At intervals of seven, ten and fifteen days, is attacked, usually at 4 A.M., with spasms; straightens out in bed and makes the noise peculiar to this disease; face almost immediately becomes livid, and unless temples and face are rubbed during fit, dark purple spots remain for two or three days; livid ring about eyes; after from one to three minutes, muscles relax and she goes into a comatose sleep, in which she remains several hours; feels languid on awaking; head aches, and has a severe pain always at pit of stomach, and sometimes nausea, eats nothing for twenty-four hours, and then feels nearly as well as usual. *θ*Epilepsy.

▮Mental hebetude, slowness of expression, failure of memory; confusion and heat of head, great vertigo; dull, stupefied expression; languor in extremities, whole mind and body given up to lassitude. *θ*Epilepsy.

▮At each menstrual period one severe convulsion; falling while at work; stupid and prostrated remainder of day.

▮Attacks at new moon, regularly at 2 A.M.; nausea, trembling in bowels; eyes staring and wide open; jerking of l. foot and then of arms; then deep sleep; complete unconsciousness, but no foaming at mouth; urine involuntary. *θ*Epilepsy.

▮No foaming at mouth; headache after attacks; menses deficient, with prolapsus uteri; undoubted heredity. *θ*Epilepsy.

▮Fits as often as once a fortnight, and at times twice a week. *θ*Epilepsy.

▮Fit each month, usually a day or two before menses.

▮Frequent and violent convulsive seizures; epileptiform attacks, dependent on presence of a tumor or other coarse organic lesion of brain, are usually suspended; attacks especially occurring during daytime; grand mal rather than petit mal.

▮Epilepsy when attacks are attended or caused by unmistakable congestion of brain; epilepsy of recent character, and not dependent on constitutional causes; congenital and syphilitic epilepsy greatly modified.

▮Epilepsy from cerebral congestion, with vascular fulness of retina.

▮Epilepsy from tuberculosis.

▮Acts like a crazy person; enfeebling of mental power; trembling of hands; gait unsteady, irregular, staggering, as if drunk; eruption on lower extremities, generally on calves of legs, spotted yellow, indurated base, thick, yellow scabs. *θ*Chorea.

ı ı Tongue protruded with a jerk; muscles of face, r. arm and legs in constant jactitation, quite violent. *θ*Chorea.

ı ı Unable to dress herself or work, could hardly speak; face, arm and leg of r. side affected. *θ*Chorea.

▮Very violent chorea from fright.

▮Tetanus.

▮Paralysis agitans.

³⁷ **Sleep.** ▮Sleepiness; deep sleep, often broken by a start, though waking is very difficult; confused dreams.

▮Sleepy; drops asleep in his chair; if aroused falls right asleep again; during day.

‖Sleepless; restless; can only calm herself by incessant occupation.

∎Sleeplessness: especially in anæmic patients, or nervous persons who are exhausted but irritated; from overfulness of cerebral bloodvessels; during convalescence from acute diseases; in case of mercurial poisoning; accompanying mental anxiety, hysteria, pregnancy and general nervous irritability.

∎Deep, profound and quiet slumber.

Profound and yet disturbed sleep, always awakens with a mental struggle, not knowing at first where he was or what had become of him.

∎Grinding of teeth during sleep, with moans and cries.

‖Night terrors of children; grinding teeth in sleep, moans, cries; horrible dreams.

‖Somnambulism in children.

∎Awakes from a profound sleep, not knowing where he is.

∎Waking with severe headache in a child.

³⁸ Time. During day: sleepy.

Evening: restless and trembling.

Night: frightful imaginings; headache <; roaring in ears; involuntary emission of urine; suddenly at night, spasmodic croup; child with croup is agitated; face flushed; cough <; itching.

³⁹ Temperature and Weather. Hot room: chilliness.

High temperature: itching.

⁴⁰ Fever. Body cold; skin corrugated and mottled.

∎Shivering with cold and cold skin, although child was covered with mustard plasters.

‖Chilliness and general feeling of coldness, more pronounced about extremities. θAgue.

‖Heat, like cold stage, not very strongly marked.

‖Heat in face and fugitive flushings here and there.

∎Head hot, feels as if in a furnace, with coldness and chills.

‖Sweat abundant and viscid, all over body; unusually long lasting and exhausting. θAgue.

∎Quotidian ague.

⁴¹ Attacks, Periodicity. Symptoms recur paroxysmally.

5 P.M.: periodic colic in infants.

At intervals of two or three hours: dry, fatiguing cough.

For several hours: comatose sleep.

At every stool: sensation as if bowels would fall out.

In 24 hours, fifteen or twenty passages.

At times: fits twice a week.

At intervals of seven, ten and fifteen days, is attacked, usually at 4 A.M., with spasms.

Every fortnight: fits.

Attacks at new moon: regularly at 2 A.M.

Before menses: headache. '

During menses: epileptic spasms.

After menses: headache; insomnia; heat in genitals.

At each menstrual attack: one severe convulsion.

In winter: slightly elevated, smooth, red patches like urticaria.

⁴² **Locality and Direction.** Right: headache in frontal protuberance; submaxillary glands swollen and painful;
large tumor in iliac region; muscles of arm in constant
jactitation; chorea affecting arm and leg.

Left: tenderness of ovary; jerking in foot.

⁴³ **Sensations.** Paroxysms of numbness; feels as if needles
were pricking him.

Parts feel as if growing large, swollen.

▮▮Loss of sensibility; body generally, also fauces, larynx,
urethra, etc.

Feels as if he would go out of his mind; staggers as if
drunk; as if ground gave way; brain, as if too tight;
as if bowels were falling out; restless and shaky as if
from palsy; feels as if legs were all over sidewalk; as if
limbs were swollen; as if in a furnace.

Pain: in r. frontal protuberance; in hemorrhoids; in
region of kidneys, extending in direction of descending
colon; in l. ovary.

Excruciating colic.

Violent pain: in head, particularly in occiput.

Terrible headache.

Intensely painful varices with black stools.

Neuralgia: of neck of bladder.

Severe, throbbing, aching pains: in occipital region.

Throbbing: in temples; in carotids and temporals.

Colic: in children.

Pricking sensation: all over body.

Hoarseness: extremely painful.

Tingling: in external genital organs.

Burning: in chest; in vulva.

Heat: in genitals.

Confusion: of head.

Fulness: of head.

Pressure: at stomach.

Tight feeling: in scalp.

Tightness: of chest when breathing.

Constrictive sensation: in brain.

Sensation of suffocation.

Dryness: of throat.

Lameness: of legs.

Jerking: in l. foot and then of arms.

Trembling sensation: through body; in bowels.

Itching : in external genital organs.

Internal coldness : of abdomen.

" Tissues. Diminishes reflex excitability of nervous centres; the functions of organic life are not disturbed.

Great weakness of muscles.

❙Muscles irritated, rendered inco-ordinate and then paralyzed.

It is supposed to cause contraction of capillaries.

❙Sedative effect upon action of heart.

Septicæmia, lethargy, brain and spinal symptoms; multiple abscesses.

Swelling of lymphatic glands.

Sebaceous cysts.

❙Ascites.

Diseased organs are in hypertrophic condition.

: It removes pathological deposits of fatty matter only, while the iodide removes normal adipose matter.

Emaciation; decrease of temperature; pallor.

Lowers temperature, with coldness of extremities, hands and wrists icy cold and wet, cerebral irritation, in cholera infantum.

" Touch. Passive Motion. Injuries. Touch : leaves white impress of fingers.

Pressure: tumor slightly tender.

Pinching: causes no pain.

" Skin. ❙Skin cold, blue, spotted, corrugated. *θ*Cholera infantum.

❙Moist eczema of legs with pityriasis of scalp.

❙Moist eruptions.

❙Slightly elevated, smooth, red patches, like urticaria, but with hardened bases, like erythema nodosum; itching at night in bed and in a high temperature; appear in winter.

❙Acne simplex and indurata; bluish red, pustular, < on face and chest; especially in lymphatic constitutions.

❙Acne on face and shoulders; centre becomes depressed; leave scars.

❙Rose colored mammilated eruption on lower extremities; sometimes pustules in centre of patches that become umbilicated, exuding a creamy moisture and forming thick, yellow scabs.

❙Eruption of small boils in successive crops, mostly on face and trunk, with troublesome itching.

❙Large, indolent, painful pustules; boils.

❙Long lasting scrofulous ulcerations.

❙Syphilitic psoriasis.

" Stages of Life, Constitution. Acts more satisfactorily in children than in adults.

Especially adapted to large persons inclined to obesity.

Child, æt. 3; threatened inflammation of brain.

Girl, æt. 5, delicate, thin, complaining for several weeks; incipient basilar meningitis.

Child, æt. 8, lymphatic temperament, disposed to frequent sore throats; diphtheria.

Girl, æt. 16, menses appeared at 13 without any influence upon the disease, animal magnetism and electricity benefited for a short time; epilepsy.

Young lady, of robust habit and sanguine temperament, usually modest and retiring; nymphomania.

Young woman, single, seamstress; epilepsy.

Woman, æt. 19, stout, healthy looking, began to menstruate at 14 years of age; epilepsy.

Woman, æt. 20, dwarfish appearance, suffering eight years; polypus of rectum.

Woman, æt. 25, single, teacher of music; melancholia.

Woman, æt. 30; threatened inflammation of brain.

Lady, æt. 32, unmarried, dark hair, healthy appearance, subject to severe cutting pains in hypogastrium and headaches; ovarian cyst.

Woman, æt. 38, married; ovarian enlargement.

Woman, æt. 52, change of life; affection of mind.

Man, æt. 65, weekly attacks for ten years; epilepsy.

⁴⁸ Relations. Antidoted by vegetable acids, oleaginous remedies, *Camphora*, *Nux vom.*, *Zincum*. It antidotes lead poisoning.

Compatible: after *Acon.* and *Spongia;* after *Eugenia jambos* in acne.

Compare: *Ambra*, *Amm. brom.*, *Bellad.* (but this drug is sthenic), *Camphora* (cholera collapse), *Gelsem.*, *Hyosc.*, *Natr. mur.* (mind), *Stramon.*, *Zincum*.

KALI CARBONICUM.

Potassium carbonate. K_2O, CO_2.

Provings by Hahnemann, Gersdorff, Goullon, Hartlaub, Nenning, Rummell and Robinson. See Allen's Encyclopedia, vol. 5, p. 281.

CLINICAL AUTHORITIES.—*Conjunctivitis and leucoma*, Terry, N. A. J. H., vol. 25, p. 308; *Blepharitis*, Schelling, Raue's Rec., 1872, p. 66; *Œdema of lids*, Norton's Opth. Therap., p. 103; *Toothache*, Schelling, Raue's Rec., 1872, p. 97; *Parotitis*, Hering, Rück. Kl. Erf., vol. 4, p. 53; *Affection of fauces*, Wesselhœft, Hom. Clin., vol. 4, p. 41; *Affection of throat*, Schelling, Hom. Clin., vol. 4, p. 89; *Cardialgia*, Schelling, Hom. Clin., vol. 4, p. 115; *Gastralgia*, Kunkel, Hom. Phys., vol. 6, p. 222; Allg. Hom. Ztg., vol. 112, p. 50; *Gastric disturbance*, Schelling, Hom. Clin., vol. 4, p. 94; Raue's Rec., 1875, p. 136; *Affection of stomach*, Curtis, N. A. J. H., vol. 8, p. 15; Schelling, Hom. Clin., vol. 4, p. 93; (2 cases) Schelling, B. J. H., vol. 32, p. 688; Pfander, Allg. Hom. Ztg., vol. 113, p. 203; Hofrichter, Rück. Kl. Erf., vol. 5, p. 312; *Hepatitis*, Houghton, Raue's Rec., 1872, p. 156; *Stitches in liver and lumbar region*, Houghton, Hom. Clin., vol. 4. p. 59; *Disease of liver*, Martin, Hom. Clin., vol. 1, p. 191; *Affection of liver*, Emmerich, Rück. Kl. Erf., vol. 1, p. 697; *Constipation*, Bernard and Strong, Stens, Raue's Rec., 1872, p. 150; *Hemorrhoids*, McNeil, Hom. Phys., vol. 2, p. 437; Smith, B. J. H., vol. 30, p. 394; Bönninghausen, Rück. Kl. Erf., vol. 5, p. 494; Gillet, Rück. Kl. Erf., vol. 1, p. 999; *Uterine affection*, Hartmann, Rück. Kl. Erf., vol. 2, p. 353; *Uterine hemorrhages*, Goullon, Hom. Clin., vol. 3, p. 129; *Menorrhagia*, Goullon, B. J. H., vol. 27, p. 683; *Menstrual affections*, Goullon, Hom. Clin., vol. 3, p. 130; *Menstrual disturbances*, Goullon, Rück. Kl. Erf., vol. 5, p. 591; *Scanty menses, Suppressed menses, Amenorrhœa, Dysmenorrhœa*, Hahnemann, Rückert, Rummel, Jahr, Rück. Kl. Erf., vol. 2, p. 235; *Nausea during pregnancy*, Wood, Raue's Rec., 1871, p. 161; *Abortion*, Goullon, Rück. Kl. Erf., vol. 2, p. 314; *Sickness during pregnancy*, Wood, Hom. Clin., vol. 3, p. 93; *Bronchitis*, Meyer, Rück. Kl. Erf., vol. 5, p. 684; *Asthma* (2 cases), Schelling, Raue's Rec., 1872, p. 112, Hom. Clin., vol. 4, p. 94; *Cough*, Berridge, Hom. Phys., vol. 6, p. 207; Martin, Trans. Hom. Med. Soc. Pa., 1880, p. 242, Hom. Clin., vol. 1, p. 192; Schelling, Hom. Clin., vol. 4, p. 90; Stens, Rück. Kl. Erf., vol. 5, pp. 685, 722; *Whooping cough*, Hering, Becker, Rück. Kl. Erf., vol. 3, p. 81; *Suffocative catarrh*, Schelling, Raue's Rec., 1874, p. 144; *Catarrh of chest*, Schelling, Raue's Rec., 1872, p. 111; *Chronic catarrh*, Skinner, Hom. Phys., vol. 5, p. 150; *Pleurisy*, Schelling, Raue's Rec., 1872, p. 122; Miller, Cin. Med. Adv., vol. 3, p. 380; *Pneumonia*, Goullon, Gross, Rück. Kl. Erf., vol. 3, p. 298; *Hydrothorax, Dropsy*, Heimann, Weber, B. J. H., vol. 34, p. 706; *Pneumonia*, Eidherr, Rück. Kl. Erf., vol. 5, p. 821; Lippe, Raue's Rec., 1875, p. 120; Sum, Raue's Rec., 1871, p. 100; *Phthisis*, Smith, Raue's P., p. 401; Stens, Raue's Rec., 1870, p. 193; *Consumption*, Lobethal, Kirschmann, Schelling, Rück. Kl. Erf., vol. 3, p. 372; *Lumbago* (2 cases), Farrington, Raue's Rec., 1874, p. 254; *Backache; Proctalgia during pregnancy*, Goullon, Rück. Kl. Erf., vol. 2, p. 383; *Affection of hips*, Müller, Rück. Kl. Erf., vol. 5, p. 915; *Morbus coxarius* (8 cases), McNeil, Cin. Med. Adv., vol. 6, p. 349, Organon, vol. 2, p. 238; *Spasmodic affections*, Emmerich,

Rück. Kl. Erf., vol. 4, p. 575; *Paresis*, Hartmann, Rück. Kl. Erf., vol. 4, p. 488; *Febrile attacks*, Schelling, Hom. Clin., vol. 4, p. 89; *Catarrhal fever*, Schelling, Raue's Rec., 1872, p. 234; *Ague*, Lippe, Hah. Mo., vol. 1, p. 122; Schelling, A. H. Z., 1869, p. 82; *Typhoid affection*, Goullon, Hom. Clin., vol. 3, p. 130, Raue's Rec., 1871, p. 199; *Puerperal fever*, Guernsey, Trans. Hom. Med. Soc. Pa., 1874, p. 399, and Obs., p. 633; *Dropsy*, Weber, Rück. Kl. Erf., vol. 4, 349; *Urticaria*, Rummel, Rück. Kl. Erf., vol. 4, 199; *Erysipelas*, Raue, Hom. Clin., vol. 3, p. 7–8.

¹ **Mind.** ▮Sudden attack of unconsciousness.

Ⅰ Ⅰ Cannot express herself; seems at a loss to know how to begin to say or do what she wishes. *θ*Puerperal mania.

▮Absentminded.

▮Dull, confused, stupid, as after intoxication.

Imagines seeing birds flying in room; he tries to catch them.

▮▮Great aversion to being alone.

▮Dread of labor.

▮Weeps much.

▮Alternating mood, at one time good and quiet, at another excited and angry at trifles; constantly in antagonism with herself; frequently hopeful, frequently despondent; frets about everything; peevish, impatient, contented with nothing. *θ*Melancholia.

Ⅰ Ⅰ Timid and apprehensive of future and about her disease.

▮Fear of being alone; fears she will die.

▮Anxiety with fear.

▮Despondency in open air; disappears on entering house.

▮Peevish, irritable; noise is disagreeable; easily startled, especially if touched; intolerance of human voice.

▮Irascible and passionate.

▮Very easily frightened; shrieks about imaginary appearances; starts when touched.

▮Is frightened and cries out whenever he is touched lightly on his feet.

▮Delirium in the night. *θ*Pleurisy.

² **Sensorium.** ▮Giddiness, nausea, pressure in stomach.

▮Vertigo: when rapidly turning head or body; evening and morning; on turning around; as if proceeding from stomach; loss of consciousness; frequent dulness of head as after intoxication, and as if ears were stopped up, with nausea almost unto vomiting; when walking; as if head was too light, must take hold on something; and vomiting; after eating, with heat in head, red face, darkness before eyes; sometimes one cheek hot the other cold; must lie down as soon as attack comes on, otherwise he is thrown down; before he falls he has stitching pain in forehead, root of nose and in eyes; attacks several times a day.

³**Inner Head.** ∎Pressure and drawing tearing in forehead, extending into eyes and root of nose.

∎Pressure in forehead, with photophobia.

❙❙Pressive headache in forehead, in afternoon, while walking, with peevishness.

πSensation in forehead as of a hot body having descended into it when stooping.

❙❙Drawing in forehead, in forenoon and at midnight.

❙❙Pressure and tension in forehead and eyes.

∎Pressing in front of head and temples, extending into eyes, with heat in face and head. θSick headache. θBlepharitis. θCatarrhal fever.

∎Stitches in forehead and temples, < stooping, moving head, eyes or jaw; > raising head and from heat.

∎Stitches into eyes and root of nose: with catarrh; before falling down with vertigo.

❙❙Pinching and tearing pain in l. temple at intervals.

❙One-sided headache, with nausea.

❙❙Tearing drawing in l. half of head.

❙❙Constant sensation of something loose in head, turning and twisting toward forehead.

∎Congestion to head, with throbbing and humming.

❙❙Congestion of blood to head, with intoxication arising from it.

∎Congestive and catarrhal headaches, with dry, hard cough.

∎Pressive headache.

∎Headache: from riding in a carriage; from coughing or sneezing; on awaking from sleep; from coryza; with nausea; with toothache; with backache; with intermittent; with great heaviness during menses.

∎Jerking in head from behind forward; dark before eyes, unconscious; > from drink of cold water; remains weak and nauseated.

∎Pressing pain in back of head.

∎Aching in occiput, toward nape of neck, > in open air.

∎Morning headache with vertigo, aching and stitches in occiput, felt only during motion; sharp, shooting pains from upper dorsal spine into occiput.

πViolent pressure over whole skull, down nape of neck, throbbing in head and whole body < by slightest contact, and increasing in paroxysms with violent nausea and vomiting of bile.

⁴**Outer Head.** ∎Liability of head to take cold from a draft, after being heated causing headache or toothache.

∎Painful tumors on scalp, like blood boils; < from pressure and motion, > from heat; itching as if in bones.

∎Wens on scalp.

∎Hair dry, brittle, falling off, mostly from temples, eye-

brows and beard; scalp itches and burns morning and
evening; oozes if scratched. *θ*Brain disease of children.
▮Great dryness of hair after nervous fevers.
▮Perspiration on forehead in morning.
⁵ **Sight and Eyes.** ▮Bright sparks, blue or green spots be-
fore eyes.
▮While reading or looking at a bright light: muscæ voli-
tantes; sharp stitches; fog before eyes.
▮Weakness of vision.
▮▮Eyes weak: after coition; after abortion; after measles.
▮▮Inclination to stare.
▮▮Painful sensitiveness of eyes to daylight; photophobia.
▮▮Lachrymation, shunning light; pain deep in eyes.
▮▮Small round ulcers on cornea with no photophobia.
▮▮Pannus, always < after a seminal emission.
▮▮Asthenopia with sticking and drawing together of lids
upon looking steadily at any object; burning, pressing
pain in eyes; borders of lids red and swollen; palpebral
fissure narrowed and palpebral conjunctiva hyperæmic;
constant photophobia, compelled to keep eyes closed
most of the time; < after using; slight rheumatism.
▮Milky, whitish spot near middle of r. cornea; vessels of
conjunctiva injected; sees with r. eye as if through fog
or smoke; when looking toward light lachrymation;
dizziness when stooping; cannot fix sight of any object
steadily without water running from eyes and feeling
of dizziness; artificial light appears to have rays all
around it; eye symptoms < morning; bloating after
meals; flatulency; obstinate constipation and stools too
large in size; cracking now and then in r. ear; expectoration of phlegm in morning with a salty taste. *θ*Conjunctivitis and leucoma.
▮▮Redness of white of eyes, with many vessels in it.
▮Smarting, burning, biting, stitching pain in eye.
▮▮Sharp tearing in r. orbit and eye at night.
▮▮Stitches in middle of eye.
▮▮Pressure in and above eyes.
▮Eyes painful on reading, as if pressed inward.
▮Corners of eyes ulcerate.
▮Soreness of external canthus, with burning pain.
▮Eyelids swollen; edges and canthi red; caruncula red
and swollen; lachrymation and pain from bright light;
pressing pain in front of head and temples into eyes,
with heat in face and head; loss of appetite; after eat-
ing pressure in stomach; belching; nausea and emptiness in stomach; gagging and vomiting up slime;
pressure and anxious feeling in chest; chilliness; cold
feet; evening fever, with thirst; weariness and heavi-

ness in limbs; face pale, dirty grey; restless sleep; great
deal of yawning through day. θBlepharitis.
∎Lids swollen and inflamed; agglutinated, especially
mornings.
∎Lids red, swollen; tarsi worse.
∎Eyelids swollen, also left cheek and upper lip.
∎Lids of r. eye inflamed, pain in eyes and inability to read.
∎∎Puffiness; swelling between eyebrows and lids, like a sac.
∎Enormous bag-like swellings under eyes. θErysipelas.
∎Œdema of lids, especially if accompanied by sticking
pains and heart indications.
∎Eyes sunken.
∎Sensation of coldness in lids.
⁶ **Hearing and Ears.** ∎∎Ringing, roaring, whizzing, singing,
cracking noises in ears.
∎Headache with noises in ear after a cold drink.
∎Hearing impaired, dull. θRheumatism.
∎∎Tearing in ears.
∎Stitches.from within outward; also with drawing behind
ears; otitis.
∎Face pale, sometimes flushed; head and r. ear hot; pain
stitch-like, drawing, especially behind ear; cheek swol-
len; little appetite; mouth dry; high fever with dizzi-
ness; chilliness, shuddering, some thirst but little desire
to drink; anxiety in chest; pulse accelerated, uneven;
weary in all the limbs.
∎∎Violent itching or tickling in ears.
∎∎Redness and heat of outer ear.
∎Right ear hot, left pale and cold. θGastritis.
∎Discharge of yellow liquid cerumen or pus.
∎Parotids, especially right, inflamed, swollen, hard.
⁷ **Smell and Nose.** ∎Dull sense of smell, especially from
catarrh.
∎Fluent coryza; excessive sneezing; pain in back, headache and lassitude.
∎∎Violent fluent coryza in evening, with frequent sneezing and headache, rough voice.
∎Dry coryza, with loss of voice or hoarseness; mucus in
throat, or sensation of a lump.
∎Dryness or stoppage of nose.
∎Obstruction of nose, making breathing through nostrils
impossible; > when walking in open air, returns in
room; itching in nose; fetid, yellow green discharge
from one nostril.
∎Coryza: thick yellowish discharge with great lassitude;
purulent, fetid discharge from one nostril; yellow, green
or bloody mucus; sore, crusty nostrils; complete closure
of nostrils.

▮Burning in nose; ulcerated nostrils; bloody, red nostrils every morning; external nose red, swollen; stinging pains.

▮Sore nose; mucous membrane swollen, covered with pimples and brown crusts; tip and wings red, swollen, with sore, stinging pain; headache; pain in stomach; nausea; belching; pulsation in abdomen; pain in limbs.

▮Nose thick and red.

▮▮Nose swollen, hard, red from tip to root.

▮▮Alae nasi red, swollen, suppurating, covered with yellow and grey crusts; burning pain. 'θStricture of œsophagus.

▮Frequent bleeding of nose.

▮Nosebleed: when washing face; every morning at 9.

▮▮Itching in nose.

⁸ Upper Face. ▮▮Paleness of face after a meal.

Face: red and hot; one cheek hot, the other cold; purple, bloated; dark red during cough, otherwise pale; pale, with weakness; sickly; with pale lips; sallow; grey; yellow; bloated, in morning.

▮▮Swelling of face, especially over eyes.

▮Stinging in cheeks; tearing stitches from a molar into forehead, eyes and temples.

▮Drawing pain in face.

▮▮Pimples on face and eyebrows, with redness and swelling.

▮Freckles; light brown spots; old warts; papulous eruptions.

⁹ Lower Face. ▮Upper lip swollen; bleeding rhagades.

▮▮Scurf upon upper lip.

▮▮Dry lips. θSick headache.

▮Lips: peel, chap, swell or ulcerate.

▮▮Itching on chin.

▮Hard swelling of submaxillary glands.

▮Swelling of lower jaw, with looseness of teeth and enlarged submaxillary glands.

¹⁰ Teeth and Gums. ▮Toothache, tearing, lancinating, with pains in facial bones.

▮Stitch pain and tearing from new molar into temple, front of head and eye; dizzy heaviness of head; bad alkaline smell from mouth; constant chilliness; dry skin, can't perspire; < from chewing. θToothache.

▮Stitches in teeth, with swelling of cheeks.

▮Pressive toothache in root of last hollow back tooth in evening.

▮Drawing toothache as soon as she gets into bed in evening, not during day.

▮Boring, pressive toothache, always after dinner, as if something got into tooth.

▮Toothache only when eating; throbbing; < when touched by anything cold or warm.

¡Teeth are loose.

¡Bad smell from teeth.

¹¹ **Taste and Tongue.** ¡Taste bitter; flat.

¡Tongue: white, with bad taste; after cold drinks; pale, greyish, in dyspepsia; coated grey, with sick headache.

¡Tongue swollen, covered with vesicles, tip burns as if raw, frænum sore.

¡Burning on tip of tongue, as if it was raw or covered with blisters.

¡Soreness of tip of tongue.

¡Painful pimple on tip of tongue.

¹² **Inner Mouth.** ¡Bad alkaline smell from mouth (toothache); smell like old cheese (scarlatina).

¡Foul taste in mouth; very slimy mouth.

¡¡Much saliva constantly in mouth.

¡Mouth dry: with increased saliva, in otitis; with stricture of œsophagus; in gastritis.

¡Dryness in mouth, without thirst, in evening.

¡Vesicles, painful, burning, all over inner mouth.

¡¡Sticking and biting in posterior portion of palate.

¡Chronic catarrhal inflammation of mouth and fauces.

¹³ **Throat.** ¡¡Sticking pain in pharynx, as if a fish bone was sticking in it, if he becomes cold.

¡Much mucus in fauces, which she is constantly obliged to remove by hawking; sharp stitches in eyes while reading and sewing.

¡Tenacious mucus in fauces and posterior of pharynx, mornings; difficult to hawk up; sensation as of a lump.

¡¡Scraping in throat, it feels dry, parched and rough.

¡¡Throat rough, with cough.

¡Crawling in throat, causing hemming and coughing, and a feeling of tightly adhering phlegm.

Throat feels as if squeezed, as if lungs came into throat.

¡Sensation as if a stick extended from throat to l. side of abdomen, as if stick had a ball on each end.

¡¡Difficult swallowing; food descends œsophagus slowly and small particles of food easily get into windpipe.

¡Stinging when swallowing; frequent desire to swallow saliva, but frequently cannot, causing a choking.

¡Pain in back when swallowing.

¡When swallowing, food remains half way, with gagging and vomiting. θStricture of œsophagus.

¡Pain in throat; dryness and sensation of something hard in swallowing; pain extended to stomach, burning, stitching, but only felt during deglutition; finally pain concentrated in centre of chest, where, in a small space, deglutition of food found an impediment, and remained fast, till it passed after a while with excruciating pain,

followed by rush of blood to head, vomituritio and nausea; when swallowing fluid, but especially solid food,
pressing, tensive pain at a point of chest, with sensation of a hard body preventing food from reaching stomach; simultaneously, burning, stitching pain
in back; three corresponding vertebræ always painful,
and patient shrieks when even slightly touched there;
cannot sleep on back during night; restless sleep, after
midnight; dry lips; dry mouth and throat; tongue
coated whitish grey; severe habitual headache; pressing
as of a stone, in forehead and vertex, every morning,
with vertigo.

▮Pointed, greyish yellow complexion; dull eyes, lids glued
together in morning; swelling of nose, hard, red, from
top to root, on tip, red, elevated; ulcerated nostrils, covered with yellowish brown crusts, with burning pains.

¹⁴ **Appetite, Thirst. Desires, Aversions.** ▮No appetite; disgust for food, or ravenous appetite.

▮Intense thirst.

▮Desire: for acids; for sugar and sweets.

▮Aversion to food, especially meat; it has a good taste
when he eats, yet he does not eat much.

▮Aversion to rye bread.

¹⁵ **Eating and Drinking.** ▮When eating: particles of food
easily get into windpipe; toothache.

▮Eating or drinking: < cough after measles.

▮During eating: sleepy.

After eating: burning from stomach to throat; colic renewed; abdomen distended; pressure and fulness in
stomach; stomach replete, especially after soup or coffee;
sour eructations; nausea, faintness, pressure in stomach
and gagging, with palpitation.

▮Wants to eat frequently on account of gone feeling in
stomach, but least food oppresses her. θSick headache.

▮When hungry, feels anxious, nauseated, nervous, tingling;
cough and palpitation > after breakfast.

Milk and warm food disagree.

¹⁶ **Hiccough, Belching, Nausea and Vomiting.** ▮Eructa-
tions sour; frequent in morning.

▮Uprisings of food and acids, following great uneasiness
starting from pit of stomach.

▮Uprising of water from stomach, much of which she expectorates.

▮Nausea: and loathing; from emotions; with anxiety
and faintness; after a meal; on every inward emotion;
during pregnancy.

▮Sick during a walk, no vomiting, feels as if she must lie
down and die; pregnancy.

‖Retching, vomiting of ingesta and slime; sour.
‖Vomiting of food and acids, with nausea.
¹⁷ **Scrobiculum and Stomach.** ‖‖Great sensitiveness of epi-
gastric region externally.
‖Throbbing in epigastric region, which is painful to touch.
‖Throbbing in pit of stomach, like a violent palpitation.
‖Emptiness and gone feeling in pit of stomach.
‖Stitches in pit of stomach; anxiety.
‖Pit of stomach swollen, tense, sensitive to touch.
‖Swollen feeling about whole epigastric region.
‖Painful sensation of emptiness in stomach, and after eat-
ing ever so little great feeling of fulness and pressure,
which soon gives way to sensation of goneness; burning
after eating, and rising from stomach to throat.
‖‖Stomach distended, sensitive; feels as if it would burst;
excessive flatulency; everything she eats or drinks
appears to be converted into gas.
‖Swelling of stomach and abdomen.
‖‖Constant feeling as if stomach was full of water.
‖Pressure in stomach like a heaviness, after eating.
‖Attacks of pressure in stomach, extending up into chest.
‖Burning acidity rising from stomach, with some spas-
modic constriction.
‖A feeling in stomach as if cut to pieces.
‖Violent throbbing and cutting in stomach.
‖‖Digging in stomach.
‖Pain in great cul de sac radiating to chest, to back and
extremities; pains in back and legs after eating.
‖Pressing, tensive pain, awakens at 2 A.M.
‖Stomach sore externally to pressure.
‖Severe cutting, lancinating pains in pit of stomach, <
night, and especially after midnight; must lean forward; mouth, throat and lips dry at night; rhagades on
lips; thirst off and on; pulse 100; constipation, discharges painful, or diarrhœa; sensitive spot in gastric
region on pressure. θGastralgia.
‖Pain in stomach, < stooping; pit of stomach bloated,
tense, hard and sensitive to touch; eats little, and even
this causes pressure in stomach; stool dry; urine red,
three times in night, the more the pressure the less it
flows; chilliness all the time; cold hands and feet, and
paleness of face. θGastricism.
‖Severe cardialgia, stomach not tolerating least amount of
food; vomiting and fainting; continual severe pressure,
bloatedness of stomach, in pit and around lower edge or
ribs, < from motion; pressure from tea and milk, which
is the only food she can take; eructations; vomiturition; pressure in the chest and back; pains in the

sacrum; horripilations; constant inclination to urinate; no sleep.

❚ Headache, pressing, tense, from occiput to forehead, beginning in morning after a restless sleep full of dreams; continuing more or less during day, with congestion to head; dim eyes and blue eyelids; at same time much nausea; pressure in stomach, < after eating; aversion to food; sensation of bloatedness and fulness of abdomen; beating in epigastrium; a few mouthfuls satisfy her, food causing fulness and bloatedness, with yawning; eructations; congestions; tongue coated white; urine pale, yellow, muddy; chilliness; malaise; cold feet; melancholia; buzzing in ears; stitches in chest and back; headache < during menses. *θ*Cardialgia and headache.

❚ After sleepless night headache with vertigo; pressure, tension in forehead and eyes; greyish coated tongue; thirst, dry lips, and total aversion to food; fulness in stomach and nausea; respiration difficult, anxious; features pale, pointed; eyes sunken; horripilations and chilliness; sometimes heat in head; no sleep; sensitive and irritable; hands and feet cold.

❚ Emptiness in stomach with desire to eat; after eating lightest kind of food, nausea, gagging and vomiting; throbbing in pit of stomach, almost taking her breath, with constant yawning; stool dry; stomach bloated, tense and painful to pressure; awakens early in morning with headache and dizziness, and feels nauseated at sight of food.

❚ Pit of stomach swollen, tense, sensitive to touch; deep in that region is felt a lump as large as a fist, quite sensitive to pressure; feet cold and œdematous; loss of appetite; cough with anxiousness; feels empty, gone in pit of stomach, but eating causes fulness, heaviness, tension in pit of stomach with difficult breathing; nausea with yawning, and throbbing in præcordial region; stool torpid, dry; palpitation of heart, ebullition with heat from abdomen to head; pulse weak and uneven, now quick, now slow; pain in back and small of back; weary in limbs; chilliness all day; restless sleep.

❚ Pressure and heaviness in stomach and chest, < in damp weather; desire to eat frequently, on account of sensation of goneness in stomach, but least food oppresses her, and the first morsel produces nausea, vomiturition and vomiting, followed again by sensation of emptiness and goneness in stomach; palpitations which nearly take her breath away; must yawn continually, so that tears run from eyes; stool dry; must get up several times during night to pass urine, which is pale, but muddy, as if mixed with dust; abdomen bloated, especially at pit, and painful to pressure, so that she hardly can bear pressure of clothing; takes a long while, in evening, to fall asleep, but then sleeps quietly; in morning, awakes with headache, vertigo, and even sight of food produces nausea.

▮Burning, pressure and aching in pit of stomach, extending over chest to pit of throat; after eating, cutting in l. side of stomach, and very painful grasping, extending over chest; in middle of chest feeling of a hard ball, with great pressure, extending to back; gulping up of phlegm relieves, but pain soon returns, with heavy beating in pit of stomach; frequent stitch pains and tearing in limbs; heat and ebullitions towards head; frequent chilliness and shuddering; cough < evening and morning, with greyish, greenish, lumpy expectoration; pulse small.

▮Everything she eats produces continual pressure; tension in stomach and pit of stomach; small portions of coffee or weak soup fill her up, with eructations; nausea and vomiturition; frequent headache and toothache; hot flashes, with abdominal pulsations; vertigo; continual chilliness; cold feet; internal chilliness, with constant inclination to micturate, but urine flows slowly and causes a burning sensation; stool dry, retarded; epigastrium bloated, tense, at pit hard and painful to least touch; respiration heavy, oppressed, especially when walking; when stooping, pain at pit of stomach <, respiration more oppressed; pain frequently moves to back; features pale, œdematous around eyes; sleep restless and dreamy; skin dry; is obliged to keep in bed.

▮Woman, æt. 35, after childbed, pressing, tensive pain in pit of stomach, wakening out of sleep about two or three o'clock A.M.; empty feeling in stomach; little eating or drinking causes fulness and pressure in stomach; lathoing, gagging, vomiting; pressure spreads to l. ribs, to liver and into back; is attended with belching, nausea, pressing pain in forepart of head into eyes, and chilliness and shuddering; face pale; eyelids swollen; tongue pale greyish; stomach bloated and hard, painful to pressure; pulse weak, uneven.

▮Boy, æt. 16, has gradually lost his appetite; all food he likes causes nausea; frequently, empty gone feeling in stomach; dryness of mouth; dry stool; turbid urine; face pale; eyes dim; pressure in front of head and eyes, with heat in head and flashes of heat; r. ear hot; l. ear pale and cold; after washing in cold water, red spots on

face; evening and morning dry cough with burning
in chest; feels week and constantly chilly, now.and then
stitch pains in limbs and about ribs; eruption of vesicles on back and thighs, which itch greatly in evening;
weakness of sight since measles; a fog before eyes when
reading.

❙A boy, æt. 11, vertigo, nausea, vomiting; after every
meal has vertigo, pain in forehead, heat of head, redness
of face, dimness of vision; cheeks, ears and forehead red,
eyes surrounded by rings and sunk in; one cheek often
hot, the other cold; if he does not at once lie down he
gets such severe vertigo that everything seems to be
whirling round, and even if he catches hold of something he falls to the ground, where he lies with staring
eyes, and objects seem distorted; before he falls has
shooting pain in forehead, root of nose and eyes; vertigo
chiefly when walking, stooping at work and on exertion,
also sometimes at night; had frequently to be carried
home from his work in fields; after attack, stupefaction,
loss of consciousness, sopor sometimes with delirium and
followed by exhaustion; pale, greyish yellow complexion, with dim, dull eyes, and grey, furred tongue; appetite not deficient, but nothing tastes good; after least
morsel feels too full, and can eat no more; pressive pains
in stomach and scrobiculus; rumbling in bowels, much
thirst, frequent yawning, urine scalds and is fetid; scrobiculus cordis distended, painful when pressed; at night
frequent desire to pass urine; diarrhœa; chilliness in
evening, often cough with much muco-purulent expectoration; difficult, anxious breathing, especially when
walking; sleep disturbed, full of dreams; in morning
exhausted, fetid smell from mouth, also noticed by day.

❙After drinking cold water while overheated, difficult respiration, formication, pressure in stomach, nausea and
vertigo; since then gastric derangement, vertigo, headache, noise in ears, rumbling in bowels, bellyache, eructations, empty feeling in stomach, debility; bad taste,
white tongue; feeling as if stomach was full of water,
wabbling when moving or stooping; staggering and
sensation of unsteadiness of heart when walking or driving, nausea, yawning, deep inspirations, fulness in scrobiculus cordis and beating there; frequent desire to
urinate, urine light yellow and turbid; sleep good, sleepy
by day; eyes red, constant chilliness, cannot get warm
even at his work; difficulty of perspiring; very weak.

❙Pyrosis after eating or drinking (especially cold water),
also at night; fluid regurgitated, tasted saltish, and often
like lime water; aching in epigastrium; pain in l. hypo-

chondrium, sharp aching or shooting, or with sense of dragging or weight, < at night; dragging or creeping in r. side, extending to shoulder; after eating, distension of stomach and abdomen; often throws up thick acid mucus; < from animal, and almost all vegetable food, except bread stuffs; frequent stinging burning aphthæ upon tongue, cheeks and inside of lips; sluggish bowels; hemorrhoids, often bleeding, with burning and tenesmus, and sore, swollen abdomen; head heavy and confused; rheumatic gnawing pains about shoulders and joints at night, < in damp and windy weather; has been in habit of taking enormous doses of magnesia.

▮Bloatedness of stomach, headache, chilliness, heat, nausea, thirst, bitter taste, gagging, vomiting; pressure in front of head and eyes; grey yellowish tongue; thirst; after eating, pressure and fulness of stomach, and loathing; breathing heavy; anxious; face pale; heat in head; no sleep.

▮Pressure in region of stomach, < in r. hypochondrium; pain < after meals, > after eating a very small quantity of food; pains generally < in morning, not extending very far and rarely going to back, mostly spreading over half of sternum when there occurs also oppression of breathing; marked relief of pain when assuming a straight position or when bending backward; sensitive to pressure in r. hypochondrium over region of stomach; every three to four days scanty, hard, lumpy stool; menses have not appeared for several months, leucorrhœal discharge every four weeks; emaciation. θPerforating ulcer.

▮▮Dyspepsia of aged persons rather inclined to obesity, or after great loss of vitality; repugnance to all food; constant chilliness, cold hands and feet; no sweat however great the heat.

[13] **Hypochondria.** ▮Feeling of heat, burning, pinching sticking in hepatic region.

▮Wrenching pain in liver on stooping.

▮Pains in liver through to back. θKeratitis.

▮▮Pressure extending towards liver, as if starting from r. breast, with throbbing in epigastric region, which is painful to touch.

▮Painful stitches in r. lumbar and region of liver, with tension across abdomen; stitches < on motion; must sit stooped forward, with elbows on knees, and face in palms of hands; when walking stooped forward with hands on knees. θHepatitis.

▮Stitch pain in r. side of chest through to shoulder; pressive, sprained pain in liver; can lie only on r. side; complete exhaustion; neither thirst nor appetite. θIcterus.

▮Pain in lower extremities; on lying down, cannot get her breath; stitching pain in r. side, commencing in back, and going through chest, < at night, whether lying down or rising; < in cold air; stitching pains in knee, which sometimes swell; stitching pain through r. shoulder and shoulder blade; appetite poor; stitching pains re-appear every year about time frost sets in; external warm applications cause the pains to move to other places. θDisease of liver with hydrothorax.

▮Painful stitches in r. lumbar region and region of liver, with tension across abdomen; stitches < on motion or deep inspiration, and particularly from any unguarded motion; > sitting stooped forward, elbows on knees and face resting on palms of hands; in moving about room stooped forward, steadying body by placing hands on knees to guard against any sudden motion. θAfter acute hepatitis.

▮Swelling of liver; abscess.

▮Icterus, biliary colic.

¹⁹ **Abdomen.** ▮Shooting and stitching pains in abdomen. θPhlegmasia dolens.

▮Epigastrium swollen, hard, sensitive; pulsations therein; pains in hepatic and umbilical region, also on both sides of inferior parts of stomach, down into bladder and testes.

▮Cutting, shooting, darting stitching all over abdomen.

▮▮Stitch pain in r. side of abdomen, < from motion.

▮Frequent, slight cutting about umbilicus.

▮▮Cutting pain in l. side of upper abdomen, extending from lower portion of l. chest, where there is a sticking at same time.

▮Cutting in abdomen, as if torn to pieces.

▮Cutting in intestines violent; must sit bent over, pressing with both hands, or lean far back for relief; cannot sit upright.

▮Cutting and drawing in abdomen, like false labor pains.

▮Frequent cutting in abdomen, as before diarrhœa.

▮Laborlike colic, with pain in back.

▮Colic, as if intestinal canal was full of water.

▮Throbbing in abdomen.

▮▮Heaviness and unrest in abdomen.

▮Feeling of coldness in abdomen, as if cold fluid passed through intestines, during menses.

▮▮Fulness, heat and great distension in abdomen, immediately after eating a little.

▮Tension across abdomen; heaviness, inactivity, coldness.

▮Hard distension of abdomen, with painfulness of umbilical region to touch.

ǀǀAbdomen distended with wind, after eating.
ǀIncarceration of flatus with colic.
ǀFeeling of tension of lower abdomen, and sensation of heaviness in it, while sitting and walking.
ǀǀPressure in lower part of abdomen on stooping.
ǀǀStitches in lower abdomen.
ǀAbdominal muscles painful to touch.
ǀStitches and painful bloatedness in groins.
ǀSwelling of inguinal glands. θNephritis.
ǀYellow scaly spots on abdomen and about nipples, becoming moist when scratched.
ǀAscites.

²⁰ **Stool and Rectum.** ǀǀDischarge of much flatus.
ǀDiarrhœa: painless, with rumbling in abdomen and burning at anus; only by day; chronic cases, with puffiness under eyebrows; chronic, of dyspeptics; alternating with constipation.
πSudden, vehement desire for stool as in diarrhœa, although stool is hard, with colic.
ǀInsufficient soft stool; after much pressure most of it remains.
ǀIneffectual urging to stool, with a feeling as if rectum was too weak to expel it.
ǀConstipation: in women whose abdominal organs are weak, in consequence of frequent miscarriages or multiple and difficult labors; cardiac palpitations; feeling of distension in breast; night sweats.
ǀStools: every eight to ten days, of large lumps; dry, too large in size; rectum inactive; feels distressed an hour or two before a passage; like sheep dung, passed with pain and exertion; light grey; frequent, soft, pale; yellowish or brownish, fecal; corrosive; soft, bloody; tough, dark, soft.
ǀBlood with stool.
ǀBefore stool: anxiety, distressed feeling; white mucous discharge; sudden and violent urging; colic; pinching deep in abdomen; rumbling; stitches in anus.
ǀDuring stool: paleness of face; cramps of stomach, nausea, eructation; pinching abdominal pain; colic; smarting at anus; nausea; rectum feels too weak to expel feces; painful straining extending into genitals; protrusion and distension of hemorrhoids, with pricking and burning.
ǀAfter stool: itching about anus; anus feels as if lacerated; burning at anus; pinching pains; stinging, burning, tearing, screwing, biting.
ǀAggravation: at night; at 3 or 4 A.M.; during day; in evening; day and night; after milk. θDiarrhœa.

▮Hemorrhoids; constipation due to inactivity of rectum; stool difficult, too large in size, accompanied by swelling and bleeding of hemorrhoids; discharge of blood from hemorrhoids during micturition.

▮Sensation as if anus was fissured; can scarcely convince patient to contrary : stinging, burning, tearing, screwing, itching, biting following even natural stool, setting patient almost crazy; walks floor back and forth for relief; cannot sleep at night on account of intolerable suffering; passage of feces difficult, owing to their great bulk. θHemorrhoids.

▮Feels as if red hot poker was being thrust up rectum; temporarily > by sitting in cold water, and by sitting on foot so as to press on anus; bowels loose; profuse discharge of blood. θHemorrhoids.

ⅠⅠBurning and griping in rectum.

▮Large painful hemorrhoids; > after riding.

▮Large discharge of blood from swollen hemorrhoids, with natural stool.

▮Protrusion of hemorrhoids during diarrhœalike stool, with needlelike stitches and burning for many hours.

▮Sore pain in hemorrhoids.

ⅠⅠInflammation, soreness, stitches and tingling, as from ascarides, in the varices.

▮Pain in hemorrhoids during cough.

▮Proctitis, with violent stitching pain.

In anus: lancinations; stitches; sticking; tearing; cutting; stitches; soreness; itching; crawling; burning.

▮Violent itching in anus and scrotum.

Ulcerated pimples at anus.

ⅠⅠAnal fistula.

ⅠⅠAscarides. θInfantile catarrh.

[21] **Urinary Organs.** ▮Stitches in region of the kidneys.

▮Tensive pain in l. kidney; swelling of inguinal glands; œdema of l. foot, extending gradually to r. and upwards over whole body; blackish urine, foams on shaking, on standing leaves a thick, reddish, slimy sediment; frequent soft, pale stools; after a blow on l. side, and remaining for hours in wet clothes. θNephritis.

▮Pressing; stitches, sometimes dull, at others acute; smarting in both renal regions; cutting tearing in neck and region of bladder; frequent urging to urinate, with slow discharge after long waiting and effort; frequent urination, urine at first increased, afterwards diminished; fiery, pale, greenish, dark yellow, muddy urine.

▮Violent cutting and tearing in bladder, neck of bladder and urethra.

▮Obliged to urinate frequently, but there is often pressure

on bladder a long while before urine comes; even at night is obliged to rise several times on account of it, though he drinks but little.

∎Frequent urination, especially at night, with much pressure and scanty emission.

∎Urine: hot, scanty, frequent, sediment red, slimy; blackish, foaming when shaken; turbid; greenish; fiery, diminished.

∎Burning in urethra during and after micturition.

∎Urine flows slowly, with soreness and burning.

∎Prostatic discharge after micturition.

₂₃ Male Sexual Organs. ∎Sexual desire excessive, with burning sensation, or deficient.

∣∣After coition, weak, especially the eyes.

∎Emissions, followed by great weakness.

∎Pollutions, with voluptuous dreams.

∎Copious, painful pollutions, with subsequent painful erections.

∎Swelling of testes and spermatic cords.

∎Scrotum feels as if bruised.

∎Dragging in l. testicle and penis.

∣∣Itching on scrotum.

₂₃ Female Sexual Organs. ∎Uterine tumor: with flatulency; stitching pains; spells of nausea; rising at night to urinate; dysuria; tendency to uterine hemorrhage

∎Pain in small of back as though it was pressed in from both sides, with laborlike colic and leucorrhœa; also during menses. θUterine displacement.

∎Uterine prolapsus and piles.

∎Stitching pains in and about uterus; laborlike colic, leucorrhœa; pain like a weight in small of back.

∎Stitching pains about tender uterus or all over abdomen at times. θHysteralgia.

∎Nausea, vomiting, stitches through abdomen; great weakness.

∣∣Chronic inflammatory states of womb, with nausea and vomiting.

∣∣Uterine spasms, especially with profuse menstruation and intermissions in wave of pulse.

∎Severe uterine spasms when menses should appear but do not; head heavy and dull; feels hot and restless; menses usually profuse.

∎Acrid, offensive smelling, vitiated menstrual discharge, with chilliness and cramping pains in abdomen.

∎Promotes expulsion of moles.

∎Feels very badly a week before catamenia; congestion to brain and chest, hot flashes, burning pain in region of hips, intermitting pulse, stitches in chest.

▮▮Menses too early, scanty, of a pungent odor, acrid, covering thighs with an itching eruption.

▮Menses too early, too profuse and long lasting.

▮Continual profuse menstrual hemorrhages.

▮Profuse and long continued menstration of bright red blood in females of sanguine temperament.

▮Menses suppressed, with anasarca or ascites.

▮After severe fright, three years previously, suppression of menses; frequent, severe pains in abdomen; tongue cherry red in color, sharp pains in l. hypochondrium, < walking, also prevents her sitting down; < in evening with difficult respiration; face now pale, again very red; frequent attacks of one-sided headache, particularly at times when menses should have appeared, with severe pains in l. side of forehead, which become throbbing in nature, particularly when working, and which cause tears to flow; headache in morning, > towards evening; pulse hard and full; frequent palpitation and epistaxis; lassitude and weakness in legs, < from slightest motion.

▮Amenorrhœic and menorrhagic symptoms due to organic affection of heart, deficiency of healthy blood; acrid discharges.

▮Menses entirely suppressed, or when menses do not appear at age of puberty; difficult first menses.

▮Before menses: swelling of cheeks and gums; sour eructations; shooting pains over abdomen; colicky pains; nettlerash; increased sexual desire, with sensation of thrill as during an embrace, especially on awaking in morning; sour eructations; shooting or crampy pains in abdomen; itching of vulva; nocturnal restlessness; chilliness.

▮▮Violent colicky pain in abdomen before menses appear, constipation during menses.

▮During menses: headache with heaviness; coryza; swelling of parotid glands; pains in back, loins and abdomen, head, ears and teeth; itching of skin, nettlerash; lassitude, sleepiness; restless, dreamful sleep; foul taste in mouth, eructation, nausea, vomiting, distension and rumbling in abdomen; excoriation between legs; heavy aching in small of back and down buttocks; cutting in abdomen; griping colic with pressure in abdomen and groins; painful weight in groins; severe backache when walking; pain in back as from a heavy weight; pudendum sore, burns and itches; pressure in small of back and forepart of lower abdomen, as if everything would push out at genitals.

▮Pain like a weight in small of back during menses.

■Great soreness about genitals, before, during and after menstruation.

■Sore pain in vagina during coition.

■Tearing in l. labium, extending through abdomen to chest; pinching pain in labia; stitches through vulva; soreness, gnawing, burning, itching in vulva. θVulvitis.

■Pimples on vulva.

■Mucous leucorrhœa.

²⁴ **Pregnancy. Parturition. Lactation.** ■During pregnancy, sickness coming on only during a walk, without vomiting, and accompanied by a feeling, as if she could lie down and die.

■Feels pulsation of all arteries, even down to tips of toes; feeling of emptiness in whole body, as if body was hollow; heavy and broken down feeling; it is only with greatest effort one can make any exertion.

■Vomiting, with a swoonlike failing of strength; much colicky, stitching pain in abdomen. θPregnancy.

■Back aches so badly while she is walking that she says "she feels as if she could lie down in the street" to obtain immediate rest and relief.

■Severe pains in small of back during pregnancy, particularly forcing and pressing in character, as if a heavy weight came into pelvis low down, occasionally becoming very annoying; also stitching, pressing proctalgia.

■■Abortion: impending, with pains from back into buttocks and thighs; discharge of coagula; habitual; during second or third month.

■After abortion, when there is great weakness of back and lower extremities, dry cough, long continued sweats, attacks of chilliness resembling ague, chronic inflammatory condition of uterus with nausea and vomiting.

■■Labor pains insufficient; violent backache, wants back pressed; bearing down from back into pelvis.

■Sharp, cutting pains across lumbar region, or passing off down buttocks, thus hindering labor; pulse weak.

■■The pains are stitching and shooting, or they are in the back, shooting down into glutei muscles or buttocks; or pass off down thighs.

■Easy confinement, but adherent placenta, which was removed eighteen hours after delivery of child; one week later a considerable metrorrhagia.

■Sixty hours after delivery, two chills, pricking, nettle-like pains over whole back where it touched bed; frequent shocks of a few seconds duration.

■Intense thirst, morning, noon and night continually; very rapid, small pulse; distressing cutting, shooting, darting and stitching pain all over abdomen, stitching

pains being in ascendency, come on during perfect rest,
and are not dependent upon motion of any kind; abdomen much distended; great exhaustion, with stupidity; does not seem to care for anything; urine scanty
and dark. θPuerperal fever.

❙Severe hemorrhage from uterus due to atony of blood
vessels, one week after labor.

❙After confinement : hemorrhage; hemorrhoids; peritonitis.

❙Tearing stitches in mammæ; on flow of milk.

❙Sequelæ following confinement and miscarriage, especially in weak, debilitated constitutions; weak back,
sweat, dry cough, prolonged metrorrhagia.

ⁿ **Voice and Larynx. Trachea and Bronchia.** ❙Aphonia,
with violent sneezing; complete hoarseness.

❙Scraping, dryness, parched feeling in larynx.

❙❙Roughness of throat.

❙Dry coryza; total loss of voice and hoarseness; collection
of mucus in throat and sensation of lump in throat;
convulsive and tickling cough at night; choking and
gagging unto vomiting, especially in morning.

❙Mucus seems to run from head to throat; hawks out easily
white, thick and tasteless mucus, < in early part of day;
breath offensive, < evening; catarrh alternates with
leucorrhœa, which is attended with backache, and is <
in morning. θChronic catarrh.

❙Chronic bronchitis when cold and damp have induced
vascular irritation ; severe, sometimes spasmodic, cough
day and night; effort to bring up a few lumps of greyish mucus often determines retching and vomiting;
breathing difficult and labored after frequent paroxysms
of coughing.

❙Dry cough as if membrane prevented breathing in
trachea, or as if some tough membrane was moved
about by cough, without being able to expectorate it.
θCough after measles.

ⁿ **Respiration.** ❙Weakness and weariness of chest, from
rapid walking.

❙❙Sensation as if there was no air in chest, and he could
not breathe.

❙Tension across chest, on expiration, while walking.

❙Stitches in chest, on inspiration.

❙❙Oppression of chest; shortness of breath in morning.

❙Spasmodic dyspnœa.

❙Suffocation from dryness of larynx.

❙❙Difficult, wheezing breathing.

❙Breathing labored ; after paroxysms of cough.

❙Dyspnœa, < from drinking, from motion, cannot walk
fast; arrest of breathing, awaking him at night.

❚Dyspnœa with violent and irregular beating of heart; pulsation all over body, especially in hysteric women.
❚❚Asthma; must lean forward with head on knees, < in morning.
❚Continual pressure after eating; tension in stomach and pit of stomach; small portions of coffee or weak soup fill her up; eructations; nausea and vomiturition; frequent headache and toothache; hot flashes with abdominal pulsations; vertigo; continual chilliness; cold feet; internal chilliness, with constant inclination to micturate, but urine flows slowly and causes burning sensation; stool dry, retarded; epigastrium bloated; tense, at pit hard, and painful to touch; respiration heavy, oppressed, especially when walking; when stooping, pain at pit of stomach <; respiration more oppressed; pain frequently moves over ribs to back; face pale, œdematous around eyes; sleep restless and full of dreams; skin dry. θAsthma.
❚Asthma, with habitual cough; paroxysm < during exertion or when walking; return every two or three hours, especially during evening and night; for several weeks paroxysms alternate with nightly diarrhœa, combined with loss of appetite, headache, nausea, dry cough, restless sleep, pressure in epigastrium, hands and arms covered with bluish red places, like ecchymosis; extremities very tired.
❚❚Terrible attacks of asthma; aggravation at 3 A.M.
ᵃ **Cough.** Cough: paroxysmal, from tickling in throat, larynx or bronchi, with dislodgement of tenacious mucus or pus, which must be swallowed; spasmodic, with gagging, or vomiting of ingesta and sour phlegm; tormenting, gets nothing up, sometimes feels as if a tough membrane was moved about, but would not loosen.
❚Cough affecting chest, caused by tickling in throat.
❚Convulsive and tickling cough at night. θCoryza.
During cough: sparks dart from eyes; rough pain in larynx; scratching and stinging in throat and chest; pain in abdomen and in hemorrhoidal tumors; stitches in rectum; nausea, retching, vomiting; stitches in r. side of chest (lower part); wheezing in chest; asthma.
❚❚Cough so violent as to cause vomiting.
❚Suffocative and choking cough at 5 A.M., as from dryness in larynx; cannot speak on account of cramp in chest, with redness of face and perspiration over whole body.
❚Evening and morning dry cough with burning in chest.
❚Great dryness of throat between 2 and 3 A.M.; awakes with a dry cough at 2 A.M.; coughs about an hour; scanty, yellow expectoration; cough causes gagging;

hard, caked swelling of l. submaxillary glands; pulse
86, weak.

❙❙Cough at 3 A.M., repeated every half hour.

❙Dry, hard cough, somewhat troublesome during night,
but much < at 4 A.M.; no expectoration; stitching pain
in l. side, which goes up back, when coughing or taking a long breath.

❙Dry cough at night, waking from sleep, with acute pain
in chest on coughing; little cough during day.

❙❙Dry cough with nightly diarrhœa.

❙Dry, hacking cough.   θMetrorrhagia.

❙Dry, short cough.   θPleurisy.

❙Fatiguing cough in evening.

❙Violent cough evenings, after lying some time in bed.

❙Awakened at night by cough.

❙Sensation of lump rolling over and over on coughing,
rising from r. abdomen to throat and back again.

❙Whooping cough: < at 3 A.M.; gagging and vomiting;
inflammation of lungs; baglike swelling between upper
lids and eyebrows.

❙Cough < by day and accompanied by pains in both sides
of abdomen like two knives going inward towards each
other, doubling her up, > by pressing with hands; constant raw pains in pit of stomach, < on coughing;
awakes between 5 and 6 A.M., with aggravation of cough
and pain in stomach and abdomen; sputa, smoke colored round lumps, a little streaked with blood, and come
flying out of mouth with force without effort; cough
causes sweat and exhaustion.

❙After measles, short, teasing cough, two or three paroxysms in rapid succession, dry, as if a membrane prevented breathing in trachea, or as if some tough mucus
was moved about by cough without being able to expectorate it; < eating or drinking; vomiting; pain in
lower part of chest where percussion is dull, with normal
sound in upper part; pressure in chest with fits of suffocation in morning; general malaise; heat; headache;
no appetite; dry stool; pale face; small and irregular
pulse; skin always dry.

❙After pneumonia: coughs up great masses of blood and
pus; night sweat; sleepless.

❙Short, teasing cough.

During evening cough, after lying down, he can raise better
if he turns from l. to r. side.

❙Dislodged mucus falls back into stomach.

❙Expectoration: tastes like old cheese; sourish; of small
round lumps; of blood streaked mucus; of pus.

᳁ **Inner Chest and Lungs.**   ❙Chest feels weak, faint from
walking fast.

❙Spasms of chest.

❙❙Cutting pain in chest: in evening, after lying down; does not know how she shall lie; < lying on r. side; in morning; in lower part of chest, especially in l. side; moving into epigastrium and leaving a stinging sensation in l. half of chest.

❙❙Stitches in sides of chest, on inspiration.

❙Stitching pain in lower portion of r. lung. θPleurisy.

❙Stitches beneath l. mamma, at times extending upward from low down in chest.

❙Stitches under l. mamma, and sometimes descending deep into chest; also in evening.

❘❘Dull, painful stitches in chest, from without inward, under l. clavicle, going off for a short while by pressing on parts in evening.

❙Dull stitches deep in l. chest under short ribs.

❙❙Sticking pressure in l. side of chest, on deep breathing.

❙Sticking pressure in r. side of chest.

❙Pressure in middle of chest, with gulping of watery phlegm; stricture of œsophagus.

❙Pressure in whole l. side of chest.

❙Pressure, heaviness, anxious feeling in chest.

❙Throbbing in l. side, near pit of stomach.

❙Chest becomes very sore, especially on talking.

❙Sore pain in upper part of chest, on breathing, touching, or lifting anything heavy.

❙Pain through lower third of r. chest to back.

❙Pain as if lower lobe of r. lung was adhering to ribs.

❙Dry cough day and night, with vomiting of ingesta and some phlegm; < after eating and drinking and in forenoon; during cough face gets dark red, otherwise it is pale; eyelids red and swollen; breathing short and anxious; heat, thirst without desire to drink; during day chilliness; cold extremities; crying all day; restless sleep, interrupted with crying and coughing; much yawning and sneezing; watery diarrhœa; discharge of worms. θCatarrh of chest.

❙Dyspnœa, < in spells, caused by cough, motion and drinking; breathing wheezing, labored, whistling during inspiration; face purple, bloated; region of stomach distended; arms twitch and hands move convulsively.

❙Difficult breathing, cannot walk fast; r. lung hepatized; pulse 106, small and hard; cannot lie on r. side, feels best lying on l. side. θPneumonia.

❙Pneumonia, with stitches through r. chest, hepatic inflammation; r. lung hepatized; < lying on r. side.

❙Pneumonia after measles; dry, hacking cough; fever; headache; stitches and pressing in chest; short breathing, wheezing, rattling; dry skin; great thirst; whitish grey tongue; loss of appetite; cough < towards morning, almost choking, < from eating or drinking, causing vomiting; pain in lower part of chest, with dull percussion sound; pulse small, and somewhat irregular; face pale; skin dry; stool dry.

∎Infantile pneumonia,´ much rattling during resolution.

∎During resolution; exudate considerable, and sometimes on both sides; great bubbling and rattling noise; great dyspnœa, preventing child from sleeping and drinking; puffiness, with cyanosis of hands and feet; tormenting cough, which, however, brings none of tough phlegm away; diarrhœa. θPneumonia.

∎Pleurisy: stitches in l. chest, with violent palpitation; dry cough, < 3 A.M.; stitches in lower r. lung; after *Acon.*, when severe stitching pains and difficult respiration continue or return; l. side particularly affected; palpitation of heart; dry, suppressed cough; exudation on r. side; during course of tuberculosis.

∎Predominant stitches; incipient pulmonary phthisis with exhausting, dry cough, short breathing; purulent expectoration, weakness and emaciation.

In beginning of phthisis, when there is occasional discharge of masses resembling pus; transient stitches through chest; dry, distressing cough; great debility and emaciation; during disorganizing stage of tubercles.

∎Profuse expectoration of whitish yellow pus with cough, 3–4 vessels being filled daily; < at night; pressure and heaviness in head; vertigo when moving; pinching and gripping in chest with pains about epigastrium and much cough; occasionally expectoration is difficult; whistling wheezing in chest; great dyspnœa; in afternoon much chilliness, in morning and at night fever with sweat; congestion; pains in limbs; tearing, stitching pains in eyes and ears, always on same side; obstinate constipation; prostration so great he must remain in bed; face earthy; pulse changeable; offensive smelling sweat; second stage. θPhthisis.

∎Stitching pain in temples, eyes, ears, teeth, chest and different parts of body; after dinner nausea, faintishness, sleep; about noon, chilliness; at night, heat; about 3 o'clock A.M., cough <; nursing mothers. θPhthisis.

∎After pneumonia, dry, spasmodic, distressing cough; great emaciation, eyes and cheeks sunken; great depression of mind and fear of death; painful oppression and scanty breath; cough, < after midnight, causing sleeplessness; cough short, hollow, painful, paroxysmal; expectoration of yellow pus, streaked with blood or containing small lumps of blood; great difficulty in expectorating loosened discharge; profuse night sweats; digestive disturbances; painful diarrhœa alternating with constipation; pressure in occiput.

▮Cough < from any exertion and < when lying down; green scabs are sometimes coughed up, and frequently hard, round, white masses fly from mouth when coughing or hawking; burning in top of head and soles of feet; sweaty palms; circumscribed red spot on one cheek; has attacks of gastric disorder which begin with belching of putrid gas, tasting like rotten eggs and ending with watery diarrhœa, < in morning; gets hungry and faint about 10 A.M.; contraction of heel cords; eruption of minute vesicles upon soles of feet; canker sores in mouth; gums bleed easily; trembling sensation through entire body, < through pelvic region; menses scanty and late; weeps very easily while stating her symptoms. θPhthisis.

▮Acts on lower part of r. lung.

▮Far advanced phthisis; expectoration of pus and blood; diarrhœa; night sweats; loss of appetite; falling away of intercostal spaces; prostration.

▮Pleuritis of tuberculous patients; affects especially clavicular region.

▮▮Persons suffering from ulceration of lungs can scarcely get well without this antipsoric. Hahnemann.

▮Far advanced hydrothorax; patient draws breath with difficulty and anxiety; hippocratic countenance.

Heart, Pulse and Circulation. ▮Stitches about heart and through to scapula.

▮Palpitation: in spells, taking his breath; frequent and violent; on least exertion; with ebullitions, on waking.

▮Pale greyish color of face; scanty menstruation; spell of palpitation of heart; pressure and heaviness in chest; evening chilliness; stitch pain and great anxiety in pit of stomach and through chest; throat as if squeezed together, as if lungs were in throat; good appetite, but after eating pressure in stomach and chest, and gagging; shudders frequently; has dizziness in walking; nausea; cold feet; pulse feeble, uneven.

▮Heart's action intermittent, irregular, tumultuous, weak.

▮Stitching pains in r. side, commencing in back and going through chest, < at night, when lying down or rising; dry, hard cough, especially < 3 A.M.; a blowing noise and a louder secondary tick of pulmonary artery; shortness of breath early in morning; dyspnœa during fast walking; great pain in chest, especially when talking; sharp aching behind sternum, when breathing; painful

throbbing in clavicle, shoulders, side of abdomen, etc.;
frequent intermission of beats of heart; crampy pain in
or about heart, as if it was hanging by bands firmly
drawn around; pain < taking strong inspiration, or
when coughing, not during exercise; burning in region
of heart; both arms go to sleep even after violent exercise; pulsative pains in upper arms, at intervals; cold
hands. θAngina pectoris.

▮After taking cold frequent desire to swallow saliva, but
often cannot do it, it then causes a choking in throat;
can swallow food and drink; heart beats quicker; he
feels weak; lying on r. side, heart feels suspended to l.
ribs and seems dragging them to r. side; pain as if
lower lobe of r. lung was adhering to ribs; difficulty
of breathing; has only been able to sleep sitting up,
otherwise saliva would run down throat; heart's action
irregular, tumultuous; systolic murmur loudest at apex.

▮Systolic murmur; stitch pains; second tick loud from
pulmonary stagnation; endocarditis.

▮In place of first tick, a blowing noise and a louder second
tick of pulmonary artery. θEndocarditis.

▮▮Insufficiency of mitral valves.

▮Pulse: rapid mornings, less so evenings; unequal, irregular; intermitting; slow and weak.

▮Ebullitions, with heat from abdomen to head; pulsations.

▮▮Tendency to fatty degeneration of heart.

³⁰ **Outer Chest.** ▮Falling away of intercostal spaces. θPul-
monary tuberculosis.

▮Small pimples on chest and back.

³¹ **Neck and Back.** Stiffness in nape of neck, morning in bed.

▮Back of neck stiff; shooting pains through chest; uvula
elongated.

▮Stiffness in l. nape and down l. inner scapula, < after
waking up and after laughing.

▮▮Stiffness between shoulder blades.

▮Neck feels large, clothing tight; congestion.

▮Swelling of cervical glands.

▮Tickling in glandular swelling of neck > on pressing
with cold hand.

▮▮Pimples on nape of neck.

▮Stitches in r. scapula on breathing.

▮Tearing in r. scapula, in morning.

Stinging pain as from blows and bruises, in r. scapula,
when in motion; may be felt as far as chest.

Violent stinging pain as from a sprain in l. scapula, extending into chest.

▮▮Stitch from apex of scapula to pit of stomach, during
fatiguing labor.

▮Burning tearing near r. side of spine, above small of back.
▮Drawing pain in small of back.
▮Pain in small of back < after standing or walking
▮Pain in small of back after a fall.
▮Feeling in morning as if small of back was pressed inward from both sides. *θ*Uterine displacement.
▮Hard pressure in small of back.
▮▮Sharp pains in small of back, with very acute laborlike pains running through to front at intervals of a few minutes, occasionally shooting down to glutei muscles.
▮▮Pressure or stitches in region of both kidneys.
▮▮Backache; while walking, she feels as if she must give up and lie down.
▮▮Bruised pain in back, during rest.
Occasional stitch from small of back, through l. side of abdomen, toward chest.
▮▮Sharp, stitching pains awaken him 3 A.M., he must get up and walk about; pains shoot from loins into nates; pulse weak, soft. *θ*Lumbago.
▮▮Stitching and shooting pains in back, shooting down into gluteal region or hips.
▮Back aches as if broken.
▮Tearing in lumbar muscles, impeding respiration.
▮Great weakness in small of back and lower limbs.
▮Stiffness and pain in small of back. *θ*Amenorrhœa.
▮Pain across sacrum like labor pains; feeling of tightening of skin of lower abdomen; feeling of weight in abdomen on walking, and especially on standing.
▮Gnawing in os coccygis.

⁵³ Upper Limbs. ▮▮Tearing in l. shoulder joint.
▮Pain, as from blows, under r. shoulder, when moving or touching it.
▮Cracking in shoulder joint, when moving or raising arm.
▮Axillary glands swollen, painful.
▮Sweat in axillæ.
▮▮Weakness and loss of power in arms.
▮Weakness in arms, mornings; arms feel numb, cold, go to sleep when lain on.
▮▮Pulsating pain in l. upper arm by pauses.
▮▮Drawing and tearing in elbows; stiffness.
▮Weakness, with cramps in hand and fingers; paresis.
▮▮Hands fall asleep.
▮Hands tremble when writing, mornings.
▮▮Laming pain in wrists.
▮Hands and arms covered with purplish spots.
▮▮Skin on hands rough and chapped.
▮Palms itch; vesicles form.
▮▮Dull, pressive tearing in hands, between thumb and index finger.

ı ıCramping of fingers while sewing.

ıBurning pain like glowing coals, two fingers of l. hand.

ı ıStitching tearing extending into finger joints.

ıFinger tips go to sleep early in morning.

ı ıSpreading vesicles on l. index finger; discharge watery.

[33] **Lower Limbs.** ıCrampy tearing in hip joint and knee; bruised pain when moving or sneezing. *θ*Coxalgia.

ıParalytic weakness in hip joint.

ıPains in r. leg, which is a fingers' breadth longer than l.; gluteo femoral fold almost obliterated; very weak, cannot stand alone, has not taken a step for eight months; spine curved; every change of position causes a pitiable cry. *θ*Morbus coxarius.

ıLeft lower extremity elongated about two fingers' breadth; gluteo femoral crease obliterated; knees slightly flexed as if anchylosed, permitting neither flexion nor extension of leg; violent lancinating pains in thigh and knee. *θ*Morbus coxarius.

ıFor last ten days would not walk ; considerable lengthening of r. lower extremity ; folds of nates almost obliterated; touch not painful. *θ*Morbus coxarius.

ıSharp drawing pains in r. knee and thigh ; affected leg about three fingers' breadth longer than sound one; nates flattened; movement of joint painful, although pressure caused no discomfort; pulse feverish; loss of appetite; tongue coated white; pains < at night; little sleep. *θ*Morbus coxarius.

ıPains and heaviness in l. thigh, < walking, and especially by forced marches; l. leg a finger's length longer than r., and head of femur partly forced out of acetabulum, threatening luxation. *θ*Morbus coxarius.

ı ıTwitching of thigh muscles. *θ*Coxalgia.

ıLower extremities frequently fall asleep.

ı ıFeeling of numbness and great inclination of whole r. leg to fall asleep.

ı ıParalytic drawing in whole thigh.

ı ıJerkings in muscles of thighs.

ıPains shoot down backs of thighs. *θ*Lumbago.

ı ıCramp in r. thigh and calf woke him twice at night.

ı ıSwelling, heat and redness of thighs. *θ*Pleurisy.

ıDifficulty in knees on going down stairs, and still more on going up.

ıDull pains in side of knee, walking or extending leg.

ı ıFrequent tearing in knees.

ıNightly rheumatic pains in legs.

ı ıRestlessness of legs in evening.

ı ıTearing in both tibiæ, with pain in periosteum when touched and a feeling of tension when walking.

। ।Drawing and tearing in bones of legs.

▮Drawing pain in tibia with aching in joints; ulcerative pain on pressure.

▮Burning and stinging in legs and feet.

▮Creepy chilly sensation on shins.

। ।Herpes on legs and thighs.

। ।Vesicles on tibia, with inflamed areola.

। ।Frequent tearing in ankles.

। ।Tearing on inside of foot and on sole.

▮Feet heavy, stiff; fall asleep after dinner.

▮Swelling of legs or of feet to ankles.

▮Feet cold in evening in bed.

▮Œdema of l. foot, extending to r. and upwards, becoming general. θNephritis.

▮Profuse fetid foot sweat; suppressed foot sweat.

। ।Tearing in toes; in first phalanx of great toe.

▮Stinging and burning in ball of great toe.

▮Violent itching on great toe, beneath nail, with pain when touched.

³⁴ Limbs in General. Pains mostly in upper arms and lower part of legs, < on going to sleep.

। ।Uneasiness in limbs, in evening; is obliged to move them about.

▮Heaviness in limbs; she is scarcely able to lift feet.

▮▮Jerking of legs on falling asleep.

▮Drawing, tearing, stitching pains in limbs.

। ।Limbs pain when resting them upon any object.

। ।Limbs fall asleep while lying.

। ।Pressive pain in joints.

। ।Sticking in joints and tendons.

▮Cracking in joints on motion.

▮Extremities very tired, with nightly diarrhœa and asthmatic cough.

▮Limbs tired and cold.

▮Puffiness; hands and feet cyanotic.

। ।Spasmodic contraction of fingers and toes.

³⁵ Rest. Position. Motion. Rest: bruised pain in back.

On lying down: cannot get her breath; cough <; stitching pains in r. side <; chill >.

After lying down: cutting pains in chest; does not know how she shall lie; during evening cough; can raise better if he turns from l. to r. side.

Cannot sleep on back in night.

Lying on r. side: pain in chest <; heart feels suspended to l. ribs.

Can lie only on r. side.

Cannot lie on r. side, feels best when lying on l. side.

When lying on arm: it feels numb, cold, goes to sleep.

Desire to lie down.

Must lie down: when vertigo comes on.

Could lie down in the street while walking, to obtain relief from backache.

If he does not at once lie down, he gets such a vertigo that everything seems to be whirling round, and even if he catches hold of something he falls to the ground, where he lies with staring eyes.

Cannot stand alone: r. leg longer than left.

Sitting: feeling of tension of lower abdomen; the only position in which patient could sleep; severe pain in l. hypochondrium.

Must sit stooped forward with elbows on knees, and face in palms of hands.

Must sit bent over pressing with both hands, or lean far back for relief, cannot sit upright, with backache.

Must lean forward: on account of severe pain in pit of stomach; asthma.

Stooping: stitches in forehead <; dizziness; pain at pit of stomach <; vertigo; wabbling in stomach; wrenching pain in liver; pressure in lower part of abdomen.

When assuming a straight position or when bending backward: marked relief of pain.

Raising head: stitches in forehead >.

Motion: headache with vertigo; < pain in tumors on scalp; severe pressure in stomach <; wabbling in stomach; stitches in lumbar region <; stitch pain in abdomen <; dyspnœa; stinging pain in r. scapula; of arm causes cracking in shoulder joint; causes bruised pain in legs; of joint of leg causes pain; cracking in joints; chilliness.

From slightest motion: lassitude and weakness in legs <.

Any exertion: asthma <; cough <; palpitation.

Rising: stitching pains in r. side <.

Moving head, eyes and jaw: stitches in forehead <.

Turning head or body: produces vertigo.

Raising arms: causes cracking of shoulder joints.

Scarcely able to lift foot: on account of heaviness of limbs.

Extending leg: causes dull pains in side of knee.

In moving about room: stooped forward steadying body by placing hands on knees to guard against any sudden motion.

Any unguarded motion: stitches <.

Walking: causes vertigo; obstruction in nose >; respiration oppressed; difficult, anxious breathing; sensation of unsteadiness of heart; feeling of tension of lower abdomen; pains in l. hypochondrium <; backache; brings on sickness during pregnancy; tension across chest, on expiration; respiration heavy, oppressed;

asthma <; dizziness; dyspnœa; pain in small of back
<: feels as though she must lie down; feels a tightness of
skin of abdomen; pain in thigh <; dull pain in knee;
feeling of tension in both tibiæ; irksome, limbs heavy;
walks floor back and forth for relief.

During a walk: sick, no vomiting.

Must get up and walk: on account of sharp, stitching
pains in back.

Going up and down stairs difficult: on account of knee
symptoms.

Rapid walking: weakness and weariness of chest.

During fatiguing labor: stitch from apex of scapula to
pit of stomach.

Violent exercise does not prevent arms from going asleep.

³⁶ **Nerves.** ∎Sudden shrieking; redness of face and eyes;
striking about with hands; grasping at head and chest,
and incoherent talk; sees figures, old repulsive persons
which fill her with fear; head hot, temperature of rest
of body being normal; spasmodic flexion of fingers; after
one to five minutes attack passes off, followed by headache, spasmodic constriction of chest and general sweat;
attacks come on several times during night or in daytime; several days before attack, headache, loss of appetite and nausea; during intermediate time perfectly
well. θHysteria.

∎∎Cannot bear to be touched; starts when touched ever so
lightly, especially on feet.

∎Twitching here and there in muscles.

∎Spasms, with full consciousness; puerperal spasms seem
to pass off with frequent eructations.

∎∎Frequent exhaustion, feels she must lie down or sit.

∎Whole body heavy or broken down; it is only with great
effort she can make any exertion.   θAfter labor.

∎Complete exhaustion. θIcterus. θTuberculosis.

∎∎Debility and desire to lie down.

∎Heaviness, especially of feet; walking becomes irksome.

∎Paresis; trembling.

∎Paralytic conditions which slowly and insidiously develop; attacks of vertigo in open air; finally paralysis
of lower limbs, upper limbs also becoming involved.

³⁷ **Sleep.** ∎Yawns continually. θSick headache. θBlepharitis.
θInfantile catarrh.

∎∎Great sleepiness: during day and early in evening;
while eating; after eating, with chilliness and yawning.

∎∎Unable to fall asleep before 11 or 12 o'clock.

∎∎Wakes about 1 or 2 A.M., cannot sleep again.

∎∎Awakening between 2 and 4 A.M., with nearly all ailments, but especially those of throat and chest.

∎Aroused by asthma.
∎No sleep; gastric ailments.
∎Restless sleep.
∎During sleep: starting; limbs twitch; gnashing teeth; crying; talking.
ⅠⅠFrequent awakening, with desire to urinate.
ⅠⅠAnxious dreams.
∎Dreams: of water; thieves; ghosts; diseases; dead people; misfortunes; erotic, imaginative, fantastic, sentimental.

ᴾᵉ Time. Morning: vertigo; headache with vertigo; scalp itches and burns; perspiration on forehead; eye symptoms <; expectoration of phlegm; eyelids agglutinated; face bloated; tenacious mucus in fauces; eructations; headache begins; cough <; dry cough, with burning; exhausted; pains in stomach generally <; headache on awaking; increased sexual desire, with sensation of thrill as during an embrace; intense thirst; choking and gagging unto vomiting; leucorrhœa <; shortness of breath; asthma <; dry cough with burning in chest; pressure in chest, with fits of suffocation; cough <; fever with sweat; gastric disorders; shortness of breath; pulse rapid; stiffness of neck; tearing in r. scapula; feeling as if small of back was pressed inward from both sides; weakness in arms; hands tremble when writing; finger tips go to sleep; chilliness; heat; sweat; headache rouses him.

2 A.M.: pressing tensive pain in stomach awakens; dry cough awakes him.

2 or 3 A.M.: awakened by tensive pain at pit of stomach; great dryness of throat; scarlet fever <.

Between 2 and 4 A.M. awakes with all ailments.

3 A.M.: terrible attacks of asthma; whooping cough <; dry cough <; stitching pain awakens him, must get up and walk; aggravation regularly.

At 3 or 4 A.M.: diarrhœa <.

5 A.M.: suffocating and choking cough.

Between 5 and 6 A.M. awakes with aggravation of cough.

9 A.M.: headache worst.

10 A.M.: gets hungry and faint.

Forenoon: dry cough <.

Noon: intense thirst; chilliness; headache >.

Early part of day: hawking of mucus.

During day: great deal·of yawning; toothache >; chilliness; sleepy; burning at anus; diarrhœa <; cough <; dry cough ; crying; sleepiness; frequent shudderings.

Day: severe cough.

Afternoon: drawing in forehead; much chilliness; nausea.

Evening: vertigo; scalp itches and burns; fever and thirst;

violent fluent coryza; pressive toothache; toothache in
bed; dryness in mouth; takes a long while to fall asleep;
cough <; dry cough with burning in chest; eruption
on back and thighs itches greatly; chilliness; diarrhœa
<; pains in l. hypochondrium <; headache >; offen-
sive breath <; asthma; dry cough with burning in
chest; fatiguing cough; violent cough after lying some
time in bed; stitches beneath l. mamma; dull stitches
in chest >; pulse less rapid; restlessness of legs; feet
cold; uneasiness of limbs; sleepiness; chills begin;
fever.

Night: delirium; sharp tearing in r. orbit and eye; cannot sleep on back; severe cutting, lancinating pain in
pit of stomach <; mouth, throat and lips dry; sleepless,
then headache; sometimes vertigo; frequent desire to
pass urine; sharp aching in hypochondrium <; rheumatic gnawing pains about shoulders and joints; stitching pain in r. side <; diarrhœa; cannot sleep on account
of intolerable suffering; obliged to urinate frequently;
restlessness; chilliness; intense thirst; convulsive and
tickling cough; severe cough; arrest of breathing awaking him; asthma; dry, hard cough somewhat troublesome, but much < at 4 A.M.; awakened by cough;
sweats; dry cough; expectoration <; fever with sweat;
heat; stitching pains in r. side <; pains in leg <; ulcers
bleeding.

Midnight: drawing in forehead.

After midnight: severe cutting pains in pit of stomach
<; cough <.

⁵⁰ Temperature and Weather. ‖Very much inclined to
take cold.

Heat: stitches in forehead and temples >; pain in tumors
on scalp >.

Warm applications: cause pain to move to other places.

Warm drinks: < sweat.

Warm room: chill >.

In room: obstruction of nose returns.

Open air: despondent; aching in occiput >; obstruction
in nose >; vertigo; chill <.

Change of air: sensitive to.

Anything cold or warm: < toothache.

Draft: easily gives cold, toothache and headache.

Windy weather: gnawing in shoulders and joints <.

Damp weather: pressure in stomach <; rheumatic gnawing about shoulders and joints <.

Washing face: causes nosebleed.

Washing in cold water: red spots on face.

Sitting in cold water: temporarily > feeling of red hot
poker thrust up rectum.

Cold water: drinking > jerking in head; while overheated, difficult respiration, pyrosis.
Cold air: stitching pain in r. side <.
When cold and damp have induced vascular irritation;
chronic bronchitis.

⁴⁰ **Fever.** ▮Frequent shuddering during day.
┃┃Great chilliness.
▮Chilly in morning, also about noon.
▮Chill: < outdoors; begins toward evening, > near
warm stove and after lying down.
▮Chilliness: after eating; on every motion, even in bed.
▮Chill after the pains. θLabor.
┃┃Cold hands and cold feet in bed.
┃Heat during morning hours, beginning in bed.
▮Heat with long yawning, stitching pain in head and chest,
pulsations in abdomen.
▮Internal heat, external chilliness.
┃┃Chill and heat, with dyspnœa.
▮Evening fever; chilly with thirst, then heat without
thirst; with violent, fluent coryza; later slight sweat,
with sound sleep.
▮Constant chilliness, violent thirst from internal heat; hot
hands; loathing of food.
▮Chill and fever, with oppression of breathing, constriction
of chest, pain in region of liver, thirst < during chill.
▮Entire want of perspiration.
▮Sweat: on every mental exertion, reading, writing; mostly
on upper parts; every night; all night without relief;
in morning; after eating; < by warm drinks; easily
excited by exercise; offensive or sour smelling; of axillæ
and perineum.
▮Night sweats, with cough. θAfter pneumonia. θPhthisis.
Type: quotidian; same time every day.
▮Intermittent fevers with whooping cough.
▮After taking cold in a draft of air, and becoming heated,
heaviness of limbs, tearing in whole body and head, roaring in ears, general coldness, during following night
sour smelling perspiration.
▮Chill severe, shaking him dreadfully for two hours; after
chill, nausea and vomiting of bile; during chill and
fever breathes very quick, from oppression of chest, cannot well talk on account of oppression; is not restless,
but suffers from anguish; lies quiet; much thirst; no
sleep, perspires all night; no appetite; pain in liver,
which seems to be smaller than usual. θAgue.
▮Fever, lasting from morning till noon, beginning with
chilliness, heat in head, headache, thirst, swelling and
redness of face, and lasting till noon, with loss of appe-

tite; afternoon free, with exception of debility and sensitiveness to change of air, ends at night with slight perspiration; during paroxysms, headache, stitches and
pressure in forehead and eyes; pains deep in eyes, with
photophobia and lachrymation; pain at first pressing,
then stitching, bringing tears to eyes; sparks before eyes,
and staring look; after half an hour, dimness and mist
before eyes; upper eyelids swollen; face red, hot; headache rouses him out of sleep in morning, < in intensity
up to 9 A.M.; thirst; roaring and swashing noises in ears;
towards noon >, but again < by taking solids or fluids
into stomach; for last two days it never ceased during
day and rendered nights sleepless; coughing or sneezing renders headache nearly unbearable.

▮Chill every morning till noon; slight perspiration at night;
headache; stitch pain and pressure in front of head
down into eyes; pain deep in eyes, with photophobia
and lachrymation; pain first pressing, then stitchlike,
causes to cry; flashes like lightning and sparks in eyes;
staring look; half an hour afterwards foggy and dark
before eyes; upper lids swollen; face red and hot; headache awakens him in morning out of sleep, < coughing
and sneezing; urine red yellow; stool dry.

▮Chilliness with headache; pressure and stitch pain in
front of head, in temples, extending into eyes; can
scarcely see; must shut eyes; vertigo; nausea; swelling of eyelids, of l. cheek and upper lip, with burning,
thirst and heat. θCatarrhal fever.

▮After catching cold, vomiting; headache; nervousness
and irritability; pale face; anorexia; pulse intermittent; disease finally becoming typhoid in character.

▮Intermitting pulse, vomiting, headache, nervousness,
easily frightened, pale, sickly complexion. θTyphoid.

⁴¹ **Attacks, Periodicity.** ▮Pains recur at 2 or 3 A.M., so that
he is unable to remain lying, and are < than during
day while moving about.

Two or three paroxysms of short, teasing cough in rapid
succession.

At intervals: pinching, tearing pain in l. temple; pulsative pains in upper arms; sharp pains runing from back
through to front of abdomen.

Every half hour after 3 A.M : cough.

Every two or three hours: asthma returns.

An hour or two before a passage: feels distressed.

Several times a day: vertigo.

Three times at night: urine passes.

Several times in one night or day: hysteria.

Twice in one night: awakened by cramps in r. thigh and
calf

Every morning: bloody, red nostrils; at 9 A.M., nosebleed;
   pressing in forehead and vertex, vertigo; chill till noon.
Nightly: diarrhœa; rheumatic pains in legs; sweats.
Every three or four days: scanty, hard, lumpy stool.
Every eight or ten days: stools of large lumps.
One week before catamenia: feels very badly.
Every four weeks: leucorrhœal discharge.
Every year when frost sets in: stitching pain reappears.
For two hours: violent chill.
From morning till noon: fever.
For two days: headache did not cease.
For last ten days: would not walk.
For several weeks: nightly diarrhœa.
For eight months: has not taken a step.

" **Locality and Direction.** Right: milky whitish spot near
   middle of cornea; sees as if through fog or smoke;
   cracking in ear; sharp tearing in orbit and eye; lids of
   eye inflamed; ear hot; parotid swollen, inflamed, hard;
   dragging or creeping on side; pressure < in hypochondrium; pressure as if starting from breast; painful
   stitches in lumbar region; stitch pain in side of chest
   through to shoulder; can lie only on side; stitching
   pain in r. side; stitching pain through shoulder and
   shoulder blade; stitch pain in side of abdomen; œdema
   of foot; as of lump rising from side of abdomen to
   throat; lying on side pain in chest <; stitching pain
   in lower portion of lung; sticking pressure in side of
   chest; pain through lower third of chest to back; pain
   as if lower lobe of lung was adhering to ribs; lung hepatized; cannot lie on side; stitches through chest; exudation in tuberculosis; stitching pains in side from back
   through to chest; lying on side heart feels suspended
   to l. ribs; stitches in scapula; tearing in scapula; stinging pain in scapula; burning tearing near side of spine;
   pains as from blows under shoulder; pains in leg; sharp
   drawing pains in knee and thigh; leg inclined to go to
   sleep; cramps in thigh and calf; œdema; swelling of
   parotid gland; swelling of face beginning at eye.
Left: pinching, tearing pain in temple; tearing drawing
   in half of head; cheek swollen; ear pale and cold;
   sensation as if a stick extended from throat to side of
   abdomen; cutting in side of stomach and pressure
   spreads to ribs; cutting pain in side of upper abdomen, extending from lower portion of chest; tensive
   pain in kidney; œdema of foot; dragging in testicle;
   severe pains in hypochondrium; severe pain in
   side of forehead; tearing in labium; hard caked
   swelling of submaxillary gland; stitching pain in

side; cutting pains in chest; stinging sensation in
half of chest; stitches beneath mamma; dull stitches
under clavicle; dull stitches deep in chest under short
ribs; sticking pressure in side of chest; pressure in
whole side of chest; throbbing in side, near pit of
stomach; feels best lying on l. side; stitches in chest;
when lying on r. side heart feels suspended to ribs and
seems dragging them to r. side; stiffness of nape and
down inner scapula; violent stinging pain in scapula;
stitch from small of back through side of abdomen;
tearing in shoulder joint; burning pain in two fingers;
spreading vesicles on index finger; leg little longer than
r.; pains and heaviness of thigh; œdema of foot;
erysipelatous inflammation on arm.

From r. to l. side: œdematous swelling under eyebrows.
From within outward: stitches in ear.
From without inward: stitches in chest.
From behind forward: jerking in head.
From upper to lower parts: rheumatism.

⁴³ **Sensations.** ▮Feeling of emptiness in whole body as if it
was hollow.

▮Stitches in stomach, abdomen and back.

▮▮Pains: stitching, darting, $<$ during rest and lying on
affected side.

☞ Sticking, stitching pains.

Pinching pain in internal parts.

▮Sensation of a lump rolling over and over on coughing,
rising from r. abdomen up to throat then back again.

Feeling as if bed was sinking from under her.

Vertigo, as if proceeding from stomach; dulness as after
intoxication and as if ears were stopped up; as if head
was too light; as of a hot body having descended into
it when stooping; as if something was loose in head;
itching as if in bones; sees as if through a fog; eyes as
if pressed inward; tip of tongue burns as if raw; as if a
fish bone was sticking in throat; as of a lump in pharynx; throat feels as if squeezed; as if lungs came into
throat; as if a stick with ball at each end extended from
throat to abdomen; pressing of a stone in forehead and
vertex; feels as if she must lie down; stomach feels as
if it would burst; as if stomach was full of water;
stomach feels as if it was cut to pieces; in middle of
chest feeling as of a hard ball; pressure as if starting
from r. breast; as if abdomen was torn to pieces; as if
intestinal canal was full of water; as if cold fluid
passed through intestines; as if rectum was too weak
to expel stool; anus feels as if lacerated; as if anus was
fissured; as if red hot poker was thrust up rectum;

scrotum feels as if bruised; small of back as though it
was pressed in from both sides; like a weight in small
of back; as if everything would push out at genitals; as
if she would lie down and die; as if body was hollow;
as if a heavy weight came down into pelvis low down;
dry cough as if a membrane prevented breathing, in
trachea, or as if some tough membrane was moved
about by cough; as if there was no air in chest; pain
like two knives going inward towards each other; as if
lower lobe of r. lung was adhering to ribs; throat as if
squeezed together; as if lungs were in throat; as if heart
was held by bands firmly drawn round; neck as if large;
tearing in r. scapula as from blows and bruises; stinging as from a sprain in l. scapula; back aches as if
broken; liver as if smaller than usual.

Pain: in forehead; in ears; deep in eyes; in teeth; in
back; from back into buttocks and thighs; in limbs;
in facial bones; in throat extending to stomach; in centre
of chest; in cul de sac radiating to chest; in stomach;
in sacrum; in small of back; in pit of stomach; in l.
hypochondrium; in liver; through to back; in lower
extremities; in hepatic and umbilical region; on both
sides of inferior parts of stomach down into bladder and
testes; in hemorrhoids during cough; in loins; in abdomen; in head; moves over ribs to back; on both sides
of abdomen; in lower part of chest where percussion is
dull; through lower third of r. chest to back; in small
of back; across sacrum; under r. shoulder; in r. leg; in
l. thigh; in region of liver.

Excruciating pain: in throat when swallowing.

Violent pain: in back.

Severe pain: in abdomen; in l. side of forehead; in small
of back.

Great pain: in chest.

Very acute laborlike pains: from back through to front.

Acute pain: in chest.

Sharp pains: in l. hypochondrium; in small of back.

Violent lancinating pain: in thigh and knee.

Lancinating: in teeth; in pit of stomach; in anus.

Sharp, cutting pain: across lumbar region or passing off
down buttocks.

Cutting: in stomach; in l. side of stomach; all over abdomen; l. side of abdomen from lower portion of l. chest;
in intestines; in anus; in neck and region of bladder;
in urethra; in chest.

Slight cutting: about umbilicus.

Tearing pain: in l. temple; in ears; in limbs; in anus;
neck and region of bladder; in urethra; in l. labium;

in r. scapula; in lumbar muscles; in l. shoulder joint; in elbows; in knees; in both tibiæ; in bones of legs; in ankle; in inside of foot and on soles; in toes; in first phalanx of great toe; in limbs; in whole body.

Tearing stitches: from a molar into forehead; in mammæ; in eyes; in ears; into finger joints.

Sharp tearing: in r. orbit.

Burning tearing: near r. side of spine.

Crampy tearing: in hip joint and knees.

Drawing tearing: in forehead; in eyes; in root of nose; in l. side of head; in bones of legs.

Dull, pressive tearing: in hands between thumb and index finger.

Shooting pain: in forehead; in root of nose and eyes; in epigastrium; in abdomen; over abdomen through chest; to glutei muscles; from loins into nates; down backs of thighs.

Sharp shooting pains: from upper dorsal spine into occiput.

Stitches: in forehead; in temples; in eyes; root of nose; in occiput; in eyes; in middle of eye; in ears; in teeth; in pit of stomach; in stomach; in back and chest; in r. lumbar and region of liver; in r. side; in lower abdomen; in groins; in the varices; in anus; in region of the kidneys; through abdomen; through vulva; in and about uterus; in rectum; in r. side of chest; beneath l. mamma, at times extending upwards from low down in chest; through r. chest; in l. chest; in lower lung; about heart through to scapula; in r. scapula; from apex of scapula to pit of stomach; in region of kidneys; from molar into temples; in r. side from back through to chest; in knees; in lower r. lung; in limbs; in abdomen.

Darting stitching: all over abdomen.

Transient stitches: through chest.

Occasional stitch: from small of back through l. side of abdomen, toward chest.

Dull stitches: in chest; deep in l. chest under short ribs.

Sticking: in posterior portion of palate; in pharynx; in hepatic region; in l. chest; in anus; in joints and tendons.

Sticking pressure: in l. side of chest; in r. side of chest.

Violent stinging pains: in l. scapula.

Stinging pains: in nose; in cheeks; when swallowing; in anus; in throat and chest; in r. scapula; in legs and feet; in ball of great toe; in joints and inner parts.

Stinging, burning aphthæ: upon tongue, cheeks and inside of lips.

Nettlelike pains: over whole back.

Pricking pains: over whole back.

Pricking: in hemorrhoids.

Beating: in epigastrium; in scrobiculus cordis.

Violent throbbing: in stomach.

Painful throbbing: in clavicle, shoulders, side of abdomen.

Throbbing: in head; whole body; in epigastric region; in pit of stomach; in præcordial region; in abdomen; in forehead; in l. side, near pit of stomach.

Pulsative pains: in upper arms.

Biting pain: in eyes; in posterior portion of palate; in anus.

Burning pain: in external canthus; in back; in region of hips; on two fingers of l. hand.

Pinching pain: in l. temple; in hepatic region; in abdomen; after stool; in labia; in chest.

Screwing: in anus.

Wrenching pain: in liver.

Griping: in abdomen.

Grasping: very painful, extending over chest.

Gripping: in chest.

Violent colicky pains: in abdomen.

Crampy pain: in or about heart; in abdomen.

Cramping: of hands while sewing.

Cramp: in r. thigh and calf.

Laborlike colic, with pain in back.

Gnawing: in vulva; in os coccygis.

Boring: in teeth.

Drawing: behind ears; in face; in teeth; in abdomen; in small of back; in elbows; in r. knee and thigh; in both legs; in tibiæ.

Dragging: in r. side, extending to shoulder; in l. testicle and penis.

Digging: in stomach.

Sore pain: in hemorrhoids; in vagina; upper chest.

Burning: in scalp; in eyes; in nose; on tip of tongue; all over inner mouth; from stomach to throat; in pit of stomach; in chest; of hemorrhoids; in hepatic region; at anus; in rectum; in urethra; in pudendum; in vulva; in top of head and soles of feet; in region of heart; in legs and feet; in ball of great toe; on skin; of herpes.

Soreness: in external canthus; of tip of tongue; in the varices; in anus; of pudendum; about genitals; in vulva; of chest.

Ulcerative pain: in legs.

Tensive pain: in pit of stomach; in l. kidney.

Bruised pain: in back; in hip joint and knee.

Pressing pain: in back of head; in eyes; in forepart of head into eyes; in chest.

Pressive pain: in forehèad; in root of tooth; in teeth; in chest; in stomach and scrobiculus; in liver; in limbs.
Sprained pain: in liver.
Rheumatic gnawing pains about shoulders and joints; in legs.
Sharp aching: behind sternum.
Constant raw pain: in pit of stomach.
Laming pain: in wrists.
Rough pain: in larynx.
Dull pains: in side of knee.
Heavy aching: in small of back and down buttocks.
Aching: in occiput; in pit of stomach; in epigastrium; in back; in joints of legs.
Severe pressure: in stomach; over whole skull; in small of back.
Pressure: in occiput; in stomach; in forehead, temples and eyes; in and above eyes; in chest; in pit of stomach; over chest to pit of throat; over chest, extending to back; spreads to l. ribs, to liver and back; in r. hypochondrium; in lower part of abdomen; in middle of chest; in side of chest; in region of kidneys; in scars.
Paralytic drawing: in whole thigh.
Heavy beating: in pit of stomach.
Jerking: in head; in muscles of thigh; of legs.
Smarting: in eyes; in both renal regions.
Tingling: in the varices.
Scraping: in larynx.
Scratching: in throat and chest.
Parched feeling: in larynx.
Tickling: in ears; in throat; in glandular swelling of neck.
Cracking: in ear.
Dryness: of nose; in mouth; in throat; in larynx.
Humming: in head.
Dulness: of head.
Sensation of lump rolling over and over, on coughing, rising from r. abdomen to throat and back again.
Sensation of lump in throat.
Sensation of unsteadiness of heart.
Uneasiness: of heart; of limbs.
Weakness: in arms; in hands and fingers.
Gone feeling: in pit of stomach.
Emptiness: in pit of stomach.
Painful weight: in groins.
Painful bloatedness: in groins.
Fulness: in stomach; of abdomen; in scrobiculus cordis.
Swollen feeling: about whole epigastric region.
Great distension in abdomen.
Tension: in stomach; in pit of stomach; in legs; in scars.

Constriction: of chest.

Heaviness: of head; of limbs; in stomach; in abdomen; of chest; of l. thigh; of feet.

Feeling of weight: in abdomen.

Feeling of tightening: of skin of lower abdomen.

Stiffness: in nape of neck; in l. nape and down l. inner scapula, between shoulder blades; small of back; feet.

Numbness of arms; of whole r. leg.

Crawling: in throat; in anus.

Trembling sensation: through entire body; < through pelvic region.

Violent itching: in anus and scrotum.

Itching: in tumors on scalp; of scalp; in ears; in nose; on chin; about anus; in anus; on scrotum; of vulva; of skin; in pudendum; of herpes; of warts.

Creeping: in r. side, extending to shoulder.

Creepy, chilly sensation on shins.

" **Tissues.**   ▮Paresis.

Twitching of muscles; muscles rigid; tremulous lassitude.

▮Atony of muscular tissue; disposition to easy overlifting.

▮▮Oppression of breathing accompanies most complaints.

▮▮Anæmia, with great debility, skin watery, milky white.

▮Easily takes cold.

▮Obesity.

▮Disposition to phlebitis.

▮Morbus coxarius.

▮Dropsical affections and paralysis of old persons.

▮Ascites in complication with liver and heart affections, especially of old people.

▮Body, legs and scrotum dropsically swollen.

▮Rheumatism, often attacking heart, generally going from upper to lower parts; painful swelling; •gout.

▮Stinging pains in joints and inner parts.

▮Swelling and induration of glands.

▮Bleeding, boring, burning, corroding ulcers; disposition to phlebitis; pus copious, bloody, ichorous, thin, watery.

▮Ulcers, bleeding at night.

▮Chronic catarrh, ozæna, with rheumatism or gout.

▮Emaciation.   θStricture of œsophagus.

" **Touch. Passive Motion. Injuries.** After a fall: first pain under l. shoulder, afterwards small of back, into thigh, bruised feeling between shoulder blades, sometimes in both arms.

Slightest contact: < violent pressure over whole skull.

Slightest touch, especially on feet: makes her start.

Cannot bear to be touched.

Touch: startles; causes pain which makes patient shriek; epigastric region painful; pit of stomach sensitive;

painfulness of umbilical region; abdominal muscles
painful; causes sore pain in upper part of chest; of
shoulder causes pain; causes tearing in both tibiæ; pain
in great toe; parotid gland tender.

Pressure: < pain in tumors on scalp; stomach sore externally; gastric region sensitive; stomach bloated and
painful; lump in pit of stomach sensitive; scrobiculus
cordis painful; r. hypochondrium sensitive; of hands
on abdomen > pain; dull stitches in chest >; tickling
in glandular swelling of neck >; causes no discomfort
in affected leg; ulcerative pain in tibia.

Can hardly bear pressure of clothing.

When resting limbs on any object, pains in them.

Driving: unsteadiness of heart.

Riding: < large painful hemorrhoids.

Riding in a carriage: causes headache.

After a blow on l. side: nephritis.

After a fall: pain in small of back.

" **Skin.** ı ıBurning in various places on skin, even under
axillæ, as from a mustard plaster.

ıDryness of skin; deficient perspiration.

ıSkin dry, itches; > from scratching.

ıHerpetic spots on face; old warts.

ıYellow, scaly spots over abdomen or around nipples.

ıBurning, itching herpes; moist after scratching.

Blotches after scratching; corrosive vesicles.

ıPersons inclined to pulmonary troubles; eruption dry at
first, but when scratched exuding a moisture. θEczema.

ıErysipelas.

ıFrom r. to l. side; œdematous swelling under eyebrows;
insensible and delirious; external cuticle peeling off,
but skin ıleft livid and purple; when touched ever so
slightly on feet, he jerks them up, much frightened;
talks of pigeons flying in room, which he tries to catch
with his hands; gets regularly < about 3 A.M. θErysipelas bullosum capitis, suppressed by salve.

ıSwelling of parotid gland, r. side; restlessness; groaning;
tossing about, < 2 or 3 A.M.   θScarlet fever.

ıScarlet fever with swelling of r. parotid, tender to touch,
mouth sore, lips and tongue black, painful, fetid, during desquamative stage.

ıSecondary erysipelas in an old lady, with chronic ulcers
on l. limb; swelling of face, beginning about r. eye, extending gradually downwards and also to l. eye and l.
side of face; enormous bags under both eyes; also erysipelatous inflammation on l. arm after being scratched
by a dog, whole lower arm and hand affected; headache; loss of appetite; fever.

∎Itching of warts.
∎∎Tension, pressure, rending in scars.

⁴⁷ Stages of Life, Constitution. ∎Suitable for the aged;
rather obese; lax fibre.
∎∎Dark hair, lax fibre, inclined to obesity.
∎Adapted to fleshy, aged people, and to complaints follow-
ing parturition; diseases characterized by stitching
pains.
∎∎Adapted to diseases of old people, dropsies and paralysis.
∎∎After loss of fluids, or of vitality, especially in anæmia.
Child, æt. 5 days; suffocative catarrh.
Girl, æt. 20 months, lymphatic blonde, very delicate; mor-
bus coxarius.
Child, æt. 2; catarrh on chest.
Child, æt. 3; morbus coxarius.
Girl, æt. 3½, suffering eight months; morbus coxarius.
Boy, æt. 5, lymphatic, badly nourished, limping for three
months; morbus coxarius.
Girl, æt. 6, after measles; cough.
Girl, æt. 6, good constitution, after measles; cough.
Girl, æt. 7, suffering six months; cough.
Girl, æt. 9, blonde, of rapid growth, affected last winter
with an offensive eruption on scalp which was allowed
to heal without treatment, mother asthmatic, every
week; spasmodic attacks.
Boy, æt. 11, four years ago had scarlet rash, which was
followed by general anasarca; affection of liver.
Boy, æt. 11, malaria nine months ago; typhoid symptoms.
Boy, æt. 11; affection of stomach.
Boy, æt. 11, lymphatic, pale, slight figure, suffering three
months; morbus coxarius.
Girl, æt. 12, good constitution, nervo-sanguine tempera-
ment; morbus coxarius.
Girl, æt. 13; pleurisy.
Boy, æt. 14, sanguine lymphatic, weakened by loss of
semen; morbus coxarius.
Boy, æt. 15, suffering four days; toothache.
Boy, æt. 15, sound constitution; febrile attacks.
Boy, æt. 16; dropsy.
Strong healthy girl, menses inclined to be late; urticaria.
Girl, æt. 19; amenorrhœa.
Girl, æt. 20, after severe fright, three years previously;
amenorrhœa.
Woman, æt. 20, delicate, suffering one year; asthma.
Servant girl, æt. 20, suffering one year; gastralgia.
Girl, æt. 20, blonde; affection of fauces.
Man, æt. 20, light hair, blue eyes, scrofulous; cough.
Man, æt. 20; erysipelas.

Girl, æt. 20, delicate constitution, one year ago had asthma
  and pain in joints, since then suffering; gastric disturbance.
Man, æt. 20, lymphatic, in bed six weeks; morbus coxarius.
Man, æt. 21, since tenth year suffering from cough with
  expectoration; phthisis.
Man, æt. 21; pneumonia.
Girl, æt. 21, blonde, weakly constitution; affection of throat.
Woman, æt. 23, blonde, mother of three children, tuberculous, one year ago had abdominal troubles, for which
  she took much quinine, since then ill; ulcer of stomach.
Woman, nervo-bilious temperament, seven years previously was in habit of taking enormous doses of magnesia to correct acidity of stomach during pregnancy,
  two years later confined again, and had prolapsus uteri
  and leucorrhœa; attacks of bilious colic for last three or
  four years; affection of stomach.
Woman, suffering six years; chronic catarrh.
Woman, after confinement, weakened by nursing, inclined
  to anæmia; metrorrhagia.
Woman, after great exertions from nursing sick children
  and taking cold; catarrhal fever.
Anæmic woman, after labor placenta retained by lower
  section of uterus, removed eighteen hours afterward by
  manipulation; uterine hemorrhage.
Woman, æt. 24, mother of three children, had inflamma-
  tion of eye and ulcer on cornea, during lactation; con-
  junctivitis and leucoma.
Seamstress, æt. 24, atrabilious constitution, menses scanty;
  cardialgia and headache.
Man, æt. 28, robust, after pneumonia; cough.
Woman, æt. 29; gastricism.
Woman, æt. 30, suffering one week; cough.
Woman, æt 32; palpitation of heart.
Woman, æt. 35, suffering eight days; affection of stomach.
Man, æt. 36, married; constipation.
Farmer, æt. 40; rheumatism.
Woman, æt. 42, weakly constitution; affection of stomach.
Woman, æt. 45, hard of hearing, rheumatic; gastric dis-
  order.
Mower, æt. 45, after drinking cold water while overheated;
  affection of stomach.
Woman, æt. 51, sallow, medium flesh, expression of intense
  suffering; hemorrhoids.
Man, æt, 60; ague.
Woman, æt. 60, seamstress, has frequently suffered with
  arthritic pains; blepharitis.
Woman, æt. 65; asthma.

Old woman; asthma.

Woman, æt. 67, for thirty years subject to arthritic attacks and severe paroxysms of pain in stomach, abdomen and limbs; cardialgia.

Woman, æt. 71, just recovering from acute hepatitis, complicated by passage of biliary calculi; stitches in liver and lumbar region.

[43] **Relations.** Antidoted by : *Camphora, Coffea, Spir. nitr. dulc.*

Compatible : following *Bryon., Lycop., Natr. mur., Nitr. ac. ;* preceding *Carbo veg., Phosphor., Fluor. ac.* (cocalgia), *Arsen., Lycop., Pulsat., Sepia, Sulphur.*

Complementary : *Carbo veg.*

Compare : *Natr. mur., Stannum.*

KALI CYANATUM.

Potassium Cyanide.   *K. C. N.*

Proved by Lembke in 1st and 2d triturations. Toxicological reports; see
Allen's Encyclopedia, vol. 5, p. 323.

CLINICAL AUTHORITIES.—*Neuralgic headache,* Cattell, B. J. H., vol. 11, p.
348; *Affection of chest,* Cattell, B. J. H., vol. 11, p. 39.

⁵Sight and Eyes. ! ! Double vision.
⁸Upper Face. ▮Agonizing attacks of neuralgic pains between temporal region and ciliary arch and maxilla,
with screaming and apparent loss of sensibility, as if
struck with apoplexy ; pulse 84; face flushed.
▮Severe neuralgic pains in temporal region and l. upper
jaw, daily at 4, increasing till 10, and ceasing at 4 P.M.,
in their interval anorexia, fever, headache.
▮Torturing neuralgic pains in orbital and supramaxillary
region, recurring daily at same hour, with much flushing of that side of face.
²³Inner Chest and Lungs. ▮Dulness on percussion ; respiration feeble, mixed with crepitus and bronchial
râles, on r. side below clavicle ; troublesome cough, preventing sleep at night.
³⁴Limbs in General. ▮Acute rheumatism in articulations.
³⁸Time. Night : cough prevents sleep.
⁴¹Attacks, Periodicity. Daily at 4 : severe neuralgic pains
in l. upper jaw, increasing till 10, ceasing at 4 P.M.
Daily at same hour : torturing neuralgic pains in orbital
and supramaxillary region.
⁴²Locality and Direction. Right : bronchial râle.
Left : severe neuralgic pains in upper jaw.
⁴³Sensations. As if struck with apoplexy.
Neuralgic pains : in orbital and supramaxillary region.
Agonizing attacks : of neuralgic pains between temporal
region and ciliary arch and maxilla.
Severe neuralgic pains : in temporal region and l. upper
jaw.
Acute rheumatism : in articulations.
⁴⁸Relations. Compare : *Cedron,* ▮*Stannum,* and *Platina* in
periodical neuralgia.

KALI FERROCYANATUM.

Potassium Ferrocyanide. $K_4FeCy_6.3H_2O = K_4FeC_6N_6.3H_2O.$

Proving by Bell. See Allen's Encyclopedia, vol. 5, p. 330.

CLINICAL AUTHORITIES.—*Menorrhagia; Debility;* Bell, Hahn. M., vol. 2, p. 44.

[1] **Mind.** Sad; inclination to weep.

[17] **Scrobiculum and Stomach.** [1] Acidity of stomach; sour eructations; much flatulence, sour or tasting of ingesta pressure at stomach after eating, accompanying symptoms of uterus.

[19] **Abdomen.** [1] Feeling of weakness and bearing down in bowels, particularly if bearing down extends to back.

[23] **Female Sexual Organs.** [1] Menses too frequent and too profuse, or late.
[1] Menorrhagia, three or four ounces a day, painless.
[11] Passive, painless flowing of blood of natural color, rather thin, and causing much debility.
[1] Leucorrhœa like pus, yellowish, creamlike, profuse, not irritating.
[11] Leucorrhœa only after menses, usually in daytime.
[1] Pain in small of back, accompanying leucorrhœa.

[24] **Pregnancy. Parturition. Lactation.** [1] Sensitiveness of lower part of abdomen to pressure, and womb very tender to touch of finger. *θ*Pregnancy.

[29] **Heart, Pulse and Circulation.** [11] Fatty heart, with weak, irregular pulse.
[11] Hypertrophy, with dilatation.
[1] Functional disorders of heart, with anæmia.

[31] **Neck and Back.** [1] Pain in small of back accompanying leucorrhœa.

[36] **Nerves.** Debility; paleness of lips, gums and whole skin; cold hands and feet; urine frequent, profuse, watery, and sometimes traces of coagulated blood; irregular, wandering, neuralgic pains; periodic neuralgia of head, following the sun.

[41] **Attacks, Periodicity.** Periodic neuralgia of head.

[48] **Sensations.** Pain: in small of back.
Irregular, wandering, neuralgic pains.
Periodic neuralgia: of head following the sun.
Pressure: at stomach after eating.

Weakness and bearing down: in bowels.
" Tissues. |Chlorosis, with cardiac debility.
" Touch. Passive Motion. Injuries. Touch: of finger,
    womb very sensitive.
Pressure: lower part of abdomen sensitive.
" Stages of Life, Constitution. Woman, æt. 35, delicate,
    brown hair, after confinement, suffering five months;
    menorrhagia.
" Relations. Compare: *Collin., Digit., Ferrum, Hydr. ac., Kali
    carb., Stannum* (sun headaches).

KALI IODATUM (HYDRIODICUM.)

Potassium Iodide.   *KI.*

Observations have been chiefly clinical, made on the sick with large doses of
the crude drug. See Allen's Encyclopedia, vol. 5, p. 331. It needs proving.

CLINICAL AUTHORITIES.—*Hydrocephalus*, Cattell, B. J. H., vol. 11, p. 345;
Syphilitic choroiditis; Disseminate choroiditis, Norton's Opth. Therap., p. 105; *Tumors
of orbit*, Wanstall, Norton's Opth. Therap., p. 104; *Paralysis of nervus abducens*,
Norton's Opth. Therap., p. 105; *Adhesions of middle ear*, Houghton, Raue's Rec.,
1875, p. 77; *Ozœna syphilitica*, Kafka, Raue's Rec., 1870, p. 124; *Eruption on face*,
Cattell, B. J. H., vol. 11, p. 346; *Diseased submaxillary gland*, McGeorge, Raue's
Rec., 1870, p. 140; *Diphtheria* (3 cases), Œhme; *Asthma*, Small, Raue's Rec.,
1873, p. 109; *Pleurisy*, Newton, Raue's Rec., 1873, p. 112; *Pleurisy with effusion*, Peters,
N. A. J. H., vol. 4, p. 536; *Pleurisy with exudation* (4 cases), Grubenmann, Allg.
Hom. Ztg., vol. 104, p. 3; *Dropsy of chest*, Peters, N. A. J. H., vol. 4, p. 563;
Pneumonia, Kafka, Raue's Rec., 1871, p. 100; Weber, Raue's Rec., 1874, p. 148;
Payne, Raue's Rec., 1870, p. 189; *Pleuro-pneumonia*, Gersdorff, N. E. M. G., vol.
1, p. 30; *Aneurism* (12 cases), Roberts, B. J. H., vol. 21, p. 494; *Sciatica*, Preston,
Raue's Rec., 1873, p. 202; *Gout*, Belcher, Hom. Rev., vol. 13, p. 152; Hirchel,
Raue's Rec., 1870, p. 280; *Epithelioma of tongue*, Petroz, Gilchrist, p. 161;
Syphilis, Grubenmann, Allg. Hom. Ztg., vol. 104, p. 4; McClelland, Raue's Path.,
p. 709.

[1] **Mind.** |Talkative, disposed to jest.
    | | Starts at every noise.
    | | Excited as if intoxicated.
    | Frantic excitation; catarrhal or mercurial headache.
    | | Inclined to be vexed, vehement, quarrelsome.
    | | Very great irritability and unwonted harshness of de-
      meanor; his children, to whom he is devotedly attached,

become burdensome to him; very passionate and spite-
ful temper; inclined to sadness and weeping, with con-
stant apprehension of impending evil. θMelancholia.
I I Torturing feeling of anguish preventing sleep.   ·
I I Whining; apprehensive as from threatened accident.
I Sadness and anxiety.   ·
I Intellectual weakness and paroxysms of dementia, accom-
panied by headache.

² **Sensorium.** Vertigo: with reeling, after meals.
On awaking, giddy, fluttering; must get up or smother.

³ **Inner Head.** I Hyperæmia in scrofula; also in weak or
tubercular patients; hammering in forehead; head
feels inflated; anxious, restless sleep.
I Congestion of brain from suppression of long standing
nasal discharge.
I I Heat in head, with burning and redness of face; beat-
ing in forehead and temples; > in open air.
I Terrible hammering pains in forepart of head, with sen-
sation as if brain was compressed from both sides, or
as though head was enlarged to three times its size.
I I Violent pain in frontal region.
I Feeling of heaviness in forehead.
I I Tearing or jerking stitches above l. eye, in frontal sinus.
I I Lancinating and darting over·l. eye and in l. temple.
I I Pains in sides of head, as if screwed in; > in open air.
I Irritating, offensive discharge, accompanied by boring,
tearing pains in temporal bone; during day a dull,
tense, numb feeling in affected side of head, during
night becomes intolerable; sudden shocks of pain.
I Pain in upper part of head, as if it would be forced asun-
der; that part of head hot to touch, though he is
generally chilly, and > by external warmth.
I Tensive, stinging, darting, lacerating pain in head.
I I Headache and heaviness in head, 5 A.M.; > after rising.
I Severe headache, with lachrymation.
I Catarrhal headaches with inflammation of mucous membranes of frontal sinuses; eyes, throat and chest.
I I Syphilitic or mercurial headaches.
I Headache, especially in occiput; coryza; pains in upper
maxilla and teeth.
I Acute hydrocephalus, with strabismus, labored respiration, convulsions; or with paralysis of r. side; dilated
immovable pupils; limbs of l. side in constant tremulous motion, hand being often drawn to head with an
undulatory, automatic movement; occasional convulsions and almost entire insensibility.
I Hydrocephalus; effusion; blindness; dilated pupils;
eyes staring, watery; crying out; vomiting.

'**Outer Head.** ∎Violent headache, hard lumps on cranium; after abuse of mercury; syphilis.
∎Periosteal syphilitic headache.
∎Scalp feels hot to touch.
∎Coldness of painful parts of head > by external warmth.
∎Scalp painful on scratching, as if ulcerated.
∎Great disposition for hair to change color and fall out.
'**Sight and Eyes.** ∎Vision dim and foggy; sees objects indistinctly.
∎Mistiness before eyes; after scrofulous ophthalmia or abuse of mercury.
∎Complete blindness, from effusion of water on brain, with dilated pupils, staring, watery eyes; frequent crying out and vomiting.
∎Sunken eyes, surrounded by blue rings.
∥Incipient glaucoma in syphilitic subjects; dull, discolored state of iris; burning in eyes, lachrymation, dilated pupils, amaurotic symptoms.
∎Irido-choroiditis, especially if syphilitic.
∎Choroiditis disseminata, especially if of syphilitic origin.
∎Fundus of r. eye shows extensive white patches (atrophy of choroid) and deposits of pigment; optic nerve hyperæmic, slight haziness of vitreous; commencing atrophic spots in choroid of l. eye and hyperæmia of nerve; R. v. $\frac{20}{70}$, improved to $\frac{20}{30}$.
∎Syphilitic choroiditis; excessive and variable amount of haziness of vitreous.
∎Syphilitic iritis, especially if inflammation is very severe and unyielding to influences of atropine; inflammatory process in iris so high, that pupil tends to contract, notwithstanding frequent instillation of strongest solutions of atropine; iris much swollen and aqueous more or less cloudy; ciliary injection very marked and of a bright angry appearance; pain may be severe, but is < at night; photophobia and lachrymation are variable.
∎∎Iritis syphilitica after abuse of mercury; aqueous cloudy; ciliary injection bright, angry looking; pains < at night.
∥Pupils dilated; eyes in constant motion.
∎Pustules on cornea; no photophobia, pain or redness.
∥Photophobia; constantly shields his eyes, and yet light does not seem to affect them much.
∎Conjunctiva of one or both eyes often affected; attack commences by more or less general or more or less rapid vascular injection, to which is speedily added a tumefaction of mucous membrane, and an infiltration, generally well marked, of submucous cellular tissue; considerable chemosis of eye and œdema of lids.

▮Chemosis; purulent secretion; eyes burn and are red
from lachrymation; scrofulous ophthalmia, especially
after mercury.

▮Œdema of lids with lachrymation; lower lids twitch.

▮Injection of conjunctivæ.

▮Injection and tumefaction of conjunctiva.

▮Great redness of mucous membrane of eyes, nose, throat
and palate, with profuse lachrymation. θAcute coryza.

▮Awoke in morning with dizziness, and afterwards had
three similar attacks; had had a severe cold; for two
days had noticed blurring of vision and diplopia which
had been steadily increasing and was only noticed
when looking to left; examination showed only slight
action of l. external rectus; syphilitic history. θParaly-
sis of l. nervus abducens.

▮Several tumors on entire upper border of l. orbit, firmly
adherent to bone and appearing to extend into orbit;
growths hard and encroached considerable upon upper
lid, especially at inner corner; painless, no inflammation and softening; syphilitic history.

▮Periostitis of orbit, especially if syphilitic; more or less
swelling extending even to temple, with œdema of lids;
pain may be intense or entirely absent.

▮▮Syphilitic affections of eye. .

⁶ **Hearing and Ears.** ▮▮Singing in ears.

▮Boring pain in ears; darting in ears (right).

▮▮Tearing in r. ear, which becomes sensitive; evening.

▮Otitis in rickety children with great tenderness of head.

▮After scarlet fever; r. and l. membranæ tympani depressed
and adhesions firm; throat tissues thick; tonsils hypertrophied with excessive catarrh, tympanum dilatable.

⁷ **Smell and Nose.** ▮▮Sensation of a leaflet at root of nose,
obstructing the smell.

▮▮Throbbing and burning pains in nasal and frontal
bones, with swelling.

▮▮Sensation of fulness in nose; beating pains in nasal bones.

▮Gnawing sensation in nasal bones, with lancinating and
boring pains, extending to forehead.

▮Acute coryza; great redness of mucous membrane of
eyes, nose, throat and palate, with profuse lachrymation,
violent sneezing, and running of water from nose; frequent irritation to cough and swelling of upper lids.

▮▮Repeated attacks of violent, acrid coryza from least
cold; violent sneezing, eyelids bloated, profuse lachrymation, stinging in ears, nose very tender; face red, ex-
pressing anguish and uneasiness; tongue white; nasal
voice; violent thirst; alternate heat and chill; urine
dark, hot; hammering in frontal region; sides of head
as if compressed, almost frantic; after much mercury.

¶Catarrhal inflammation of Schneiderian membrane in all
its continuations, frontal sinuses, Highmorian cavities
and fauces; red, swollen nose with continual secretion
of a watery, colorless, acrid fluid and violent painful
sneezing; swelling of eyelids; injected conjunctiva,
lachrymation; sticking pain in ears; red face, with
anxiety and restlessness; terrible, hammering pain in
forepart of head, with a sensation as though brain was
compressed from both sides, or as though head was
enlarged to three times its size; throwing about in bed;
frantic excitation; shaking for loathing; white coated
tongue; talking through nose; great thirst with fever,
which is marked by alternating hot and dry skin, and
then again body is drenched with sweat; heat prepon-
derates with intermitting shuddering and dark, hot
urine.
¶Ozæna syphilitica.
¶Discharge of watery, corroding mucus.
¶Nose red, swollen; discharge acrid, watery; tightening
root of nose. θSyphilis.
¶¶Accumulation of very tenacious mucus in nostrils.
¶Purulent nasal secretion.
¶¶Discharge from nose of greenish black, or yellow
matter, of foul and sickening smell; decomposed green-
ish red blood
¶Chronic catarrh: chilliness and nightly rheumatic pains
in limbs; of frontal sinuses; scrofulous or syphilitic.
¶Ulceration of septum. θOzæna.
¶Ulceration of internal nose, involving frontal sinuses
and antrum Highmori.
¶Syphilitic ozæna after abuse of mercury with pain in shin
bones, especially at night. θOzæna.
¶¶Violent epistaxis, after mercury.
⁸ Upper Face. ¶¶Anxious expression with restlessness.
¶Paleness of face; face colorless during spasmodic attacks.
¶Face red, burning. θCongestion to head. θPneumonia.
¶Stinging darting in left cheek with coryza; after abuse
of mercury; antrum of Highmore affected.
¶Swelling of face and tongue, especially after mercury.
¶Eruption on face; subcutaneous cellular tissue swollen,
forming small tumors like tubercles; violent pain in
both orbital processes, and across forehead; l. nostril
ulcerated within and excoriated without, with occasional troublesome yellow discharge which concretes
upon it; pallid, leaden hue of face; slightly curved
concavity down centre of nose, from ulceration of
septum.
⁹ Lower Face. ¶¶Upper lip, nose, mouth and fauces hyper-
sensitive.

ǀ ǀ Dry, chapped lips.

ǀ ǀ Lips covered with viscid mucus in morning.

ǀ ǀ Blotches: on cheeks, surrounded by swelling and redness; at corners of mouth.

ǀ ǀ Gnawing in both sides of lower jaw.

ǀ ǀ Small pustule on chin, discharging water.

ǀ Chin drawn to r. side, a running sore under ramus of
jaw, bleeding easily and profusely if scab is removed;
dizziness, head feels full at times and then nose bleeds;
eyes weak; stinging pain in r. ear and r. submaxillary
gland; sharp pain in chest when moving about, > by
sitting down; cramp pains in stomach; constipation;
menses scanty, pale, regular; breath fetid; sweats much;
restless at night; has been salivated. θDiseased submaxillary gland.

ǀ ǀ Enlargement and suppuration of submaxillary gland.

¹⁰ **Teeth and Gums.** ǀ Grumbling in teeth and face; copious
saliva; thirst; violent darting in ears; abscess of antrum.

ǀ Teeth feel elongated; painful in evening.

ǀ Teeth decayed; gnawing pains; gums swollen; > from
warmth; < from cold; evening, and 4 to 5 A.M.

ǀ Gums ulcerated as after mercury; bloody saliva, smells
like onions, with sensation as if a worm was crawling
at root of tooth.

ǀ Ulcerative pain and swelling of gums; decayed teeth;
gumboils; gums recede from loose teeth.

¹¹ **Taste and Tongue.** ǀ ǀ Food has no taste or tastes like straw.

ǀ Rancid taste in mouth, after eating or drinking.

ǀ ǀ Bitter sweet taste; morning after waking.

ǀ Bitterness in mouth and throat, going off after breakfast.

ǀ Tongue white.

ǀ Impression of teeth on swollen tongue; after mercury.

ǀ Burning on tip of tongue; vesicles.

ǀ Ulceration of tongue and mouth.

ǀ Epithelioma of tongue.

¹² **Inner Mouth.** ǀ ǀ Numbness of mouth; morning on waking.

ǀ Dryness of mouth.

ǀ Dryness and bitterness in pharynx and mouth.

ǀ Heat in whole mouth, with swelling.

ǀ Very offensive odor from mouth.

ǀ Copious salivation.

ǀ Violent ptyalism, with irregular, superficial ulceration of
mucous lining of mouth; surface looks white, as if covered with milk.

ǀ Viscid, saltish saliva during pregnancy.

ǀ Bloody saliva, with sweetish taste in mouth.

ǀ ǀ Ulceration of mucous membrane of mouth.

ǀ ǀ Irregular ulcers, looking as if coated with milk; burning vesicles; on tongue, after mercury; stomacace.

[13] **Throat.** ❙Ulceration of velum palati; in scrofulous subjects.
❙❙Uvula swollen and elongated; mucous membrane as if œdematous.
❙Feeling of dryness and itching in throat with burning at epigastrium, copious salivation; running from nose; intense injection of conjunctivæ, and lachrymation.
❙❙Roughness and dryness of throat; cough.
❙❙Pain and dryness in throat and stomach.
❙Dryness of throat, enlarged tonsils and papulæ on face; copious salivation, especially if from mercury.
❙❙Stinging and a sort of painful pressure when swallowing or talking.
❙❙Increased mucus; choking sensation as if something had lodged in throat; going off after hawking up piece of thick mucus.
❙❙Terrible pain at root of tongue, night before going to sleep; pain extends to both sides of throat, with fear of death; sensation as if spasm would close pharynx.
❙Follicular inflammation; laryngeal irritation, dry cough; burning tickling in throat, secondary syphilis or tertiary, with deposits in throat.
❙Chronic pharyngitis.
❙Chills; fever; pain in throat; pulse, 135; skin hot; exudate on both tonsils. θDiphtheria.
❙On second day, headache; general indisposition; languor and fever; fauces very red; uvula swollen and elongated; tonsils covered with exudate. θDiphtheria.
❙Hard lump from right angle of lower jaw to larynx and trachea, intermittent beating of carotid; face pale, anxious; dyspnœa; mucous râles; submaxillary gland enlarged with purulent infiltration around.
❙Goitre (sensitive to contact).
❙Submaxillary glands swollen, suppurating.

[14] **Appetite, Thirst. Desires, Aversions.** ❙Food has no taste; tastes like straw.
❙Loss of appetite; emaciation.
❙Anorexia.
❙Thirst; excessive day and night; with nausea, vomiting and bloated abdomen.

[15] **Eating and Drinking.** After eating: bitter taste > (after breakfast); emptiness and qualmish feeling not going off.
After food or drink: rancid taste.
❙Cold milk makes all symptoms worse.

[16] **Hiccough, Belching, Nausea and Vomiting.** ❙Hiccough; evening.
❙Gulping up of large quantities of air.
❙❙Eructations momentarily > burning and pressure in stomach.

∎Heartburn with flatulence.

∎Nausea.

∎Violent vomiting, with accumulation of saliva.

¹⁷ **Scrobiculum and Stomach.** ∎Burning in pit of stomach.

ιιEmpty, cold feeling, not > by eating.

∎Throbbing, painful burning in stomach; cutting and burning around navel like a coal of fire; rumbling and shrill noises in stomach; belching. θGastritis.

∎Degeneration of mucous membrane of stomach, with vomiting, heartburn, emaciation and diarrhœa.

∎Phlegmasia of stomach and intestines.

¹⁸ **Hypochondria.** ιιDarting in r. hypochondrium, and a similar dart in side of abdomen, when talking.

∎Syphilitic affections of liver.

∎Swollen spleen after intermittent fever.

¹⁹ **Abdomen.** ∎Sudden, painful bloating of abdomen or about navel, followed by diarrhœa.

∎Cutting and burning around umbilicus.

ιιAbdominal sufferings extend into groins and thighs.

∎Inguinal glands swollen; gonorrhœa or chancre.

∎After mercurial treatment; ulcerating bubo, with fistulous openings, and discharge of dark, thin, offensive, corroding ichor.

²⁰ **Stool and Rectum.** ∎Light green, yellow, watery stools.

∎Diarrhœa and tenesmus, with pain in small of back, as if in a vice; after mercury.

∎Chronic diarrhœa in syphilitic or mercurial subjects.

∎Obstinate constipation; stools hard and scanty.

∎Serous mucus from rectum.

∎Syphilitic affection, like cancer, of rectum.

²¹ **Urinary Organs.** ∎Morbus Brightii, with gout or mercurio-syphilis; granulated kidney.

∎Urine dark, scanty; painful; sediment dirty yellow; heat in head; malaise; chilliness from small of back up over body; flushes; small of back feels bruised; darting pains in renal region. θNephritis.

∎Burning pain in kidneys, and bladder feels swollen.

∎Urine suppressed. θPneumonia.

ιιRetention of urine; prostate enlarged.

∎Painful urging to urinate; disappears when menses come.

Urine: increased, unquenchable thirst; copious, frequent, pale and watery; red as blood; streaked with blood.

∎Enuresis at night, in scrofulous and syphilitic children.

²² **Male Sexual Organs.** ∎Sexual desire diminished; testes atrophied.

∎Penis swollen, inflamed; constant semi-erections and sexual desire.

∎Muco-purulent discharge from urethra, with burning in urethra, and sometimes discharge of blood.

❙Thick, green gonorrhœal discharge ; no pain.

❙Chronic urethritis, with secretion.

❙Gangrenous chancre.

❙Extensive swelling of glans penis with paraphimosis.

❙Obstinate vegetation on glans penis.

❙Spermatic cords thickened; secondary syphilis.

❙Orchitis and syphilitic ulcers on scrotum.

❙❙Syphilis; especially with indolent, swollen glands; deep chancres, hard edges; buboes ulcerating with fistulous openings; thin, offensive, corrosive, ichorous discharge or suppuration slow, difficult, curdy, after abuse of mercury.

²²**Female Sexual Organs.** ❙Severe burning, tearing and twitching pains in ovarian region, especially r. side; sensation of swelling and congestion of ovaries, with pain as from a corrosive tumor there.

❙Fibroid tumors, subinvolution, hypertrophy and enlargement of uterus, predisposing to hemorrhage; dysmenorrhœa, constant leucorrhœa; emaciation; prostration.

❙❙Before menses: frequent urging to urinate.

❙During menses: thighs feel as if squeezed; pains go into thighs; chilly, " goose flesh " all over with heat in head; bruised pains in groins and small of back, < sitting.

❙Dysmenorrhœa with great urging to urinate, disappearing with onset of flow; < from cold milk; pressing in groins obliging her to bend double.

❙Menses: too early; late and more profuse than usual; too scanty, in fleshy women; suppressed.

❙Ulcerated mucous tubercles, or thick, scabby eruption on labia; chancre.

❙Itching and burning of vulva and thighs.

❙Discharge of mucus from vagina.

❙Leucorrhœa: watery, acrid, corrosive, with biting in pudendum; milky white; like washings of meat; green or yellow; putrid.

❙Tumor of breast.

❙Atrophy of mammæ.

²⁴**Pregnancy. Parturition. Lactation.** ❙Galactorrhœa.

²⁵**Voice and Larynx. Trachea and Bronchia.** ❙Voice nasal. *θ*Catarrh *θ*Bronchitis.

❙Loss of voice.

❙Hoarseness, pain in chest, oppressed breathing, pain in eyes with cough; coryza; pains in limbs; influenza after abuse of mercury.

❙Mucous membrane of rima glottidis and upper part of larynx, œdematous.

❙❙Raw pain in larynx, as if from granulations.

∎Arytænoids of purplish color, tumefied and granular; follicular ulceration; voice hoarse; sounds above middle key impossible; dry cough; sensation of dryness, burning and tickling in larynx.

∎Awakened, especially 5 A.M., with dry throat, oppression, loss of voice; glands swollen. θSpasmodic croup of scrofulous children.

∎∎Awakens with choking, can scarcely breathe; choking spells, œdema of larynx.

∎Rough feeling in trachea, compelling hawking.

∎Laryngophthisis.

²⁴Respiration. ∎No air enters lungs; epigastrium sunken; face livid; laryngeal obstruction.

Had to get up, thinking he would be smothered.

∎Oppression of breathing, awaking patient in morning hours, especially in œdema of lungs.

∎Asthma in young people that have not gotten their growth, with many rheumatic symptoms about chest, and sleeplessness.

²⁷Cough. ∎Cough from constant irritation in throat; suffocative; larynx swollen; short, dry, occasioned by roughness; dry, with feeling of soreness in larynx, evening or several successive mornings; with expectoration of mucus; syphilitic cases.

∎Cough dry, hacking; later copious, green sputum.

∎Deep, hollow cough, with whitish and greenish expectoration, and tearing out pain, starting from ensiform cartilage.

∎Hoarse cough, with pain through breast.

∎∎Expectoration greenish, copious; looks like soapsuds. θPneumonia. θŒdema pulmonum.

²⁸Inner Chest and Lungs. ∎Fine transient stitches deep in middle of chest.

∎Violent stitches in middle of sternum, extending to shoulders.

∎Stitches through sternum to back, or deep in chest, while walking.

∎Pleuritic stitches; effusion. θPneumonia. θBright's disease.

∎Pain as from soreness, with sticking deep in chest, in region of r. lower rib, in evening.

∎Sharp pain through r. lung from nipple.

∎Pains through lungs; tired and weak; fluttering at heart; nervous. θUlcer on leg.

∎Pains in chest as if cut to pieces.

∎After a cold; great difficulty of breathing, inability to lie down in comfort, and not at all on r. side; heart displaced, beats violently; l. side filled with fluid; complete dulness and great resistance on percussion; l.

chest enlarged and bulging; absence of respiratory sounds. θDropsy of chest.

∎Pleuritic effusion in l. chest, in front extending up to third rib, behind as far as spine of scapula; absolute dulness on percussion and entire absence of respiratory sounds; heart pressed to r. side; catarrhal inflammation in upper portion of r. chest; despite the great compression of l. lung dyspnœa is not very great when lying quietly; great weakness, cannot sit up without assistance, and must be held during examination; night sweats; loss of appetite; thirst; fever; pulse 108; great mental depression, anæmia and emaciation.

∎Subacute pleurisy and effusion into chest; l. side of chest nearly two-thirds filled with fluid.

∎Pneumonia, first stage; also later for congestion of brain; face bloated, bluish; lower jaw dropped; pulse irregular, intermittent; limbs as if paralyzed; urine suppressed; complete hepatization; awoke suddenly with great oppression; apoplectic congestion to head.

∎∎Hepatization of r. lung; bronchial respiration, bronchophony, dulness on percussion; abundant expectoration of white froth, resembling soapsuds. θPneumonia.

∎Upper part of l. lung infiltrated, spreading to r. lung; face collapsed; constant delirium. θPneumonia.

∎After great bodily exertion, shaking chill; deep sleep, out of which he could not be roused; lies upon back, snoring loudly, eyes closed, injected conjunctiva, hot head, dry tongue, bluish lips, sunken lower jaw; bluish finger nails; irregular, intermitting pulse; extremities, when raised, fell back as if paralyzed; dull percussion sound in both clavicular region, on r. down to third, on l. down to second rib; bronchial breathing, crepitation; no cough, but on putting ear to chest, loud snoring appeared to come out of these parts as if through a tube; urine suppressed. θBilateral croupous pneumonia.

∎Lobular pneumonia; fever, localized pain, painful breathing.

∎Ptyalism, ulcerated lips and tongue, sordes excessive; great prostration; short breathing; must lie on back; serous effusion in r. pleura; hepatization of lower two-thirds of r. lung. θPleuro-pneumonia.

∎∎Phthisis pituitosa, with purulent or green sputum; exhausting night sweats and loose stools.

∎∎Œdema pulmonum: with pneumonia; secondary to morbus Brightii: sputum like soapsuds, green.

²⁹ **Heart, Pulse and Circulation.** ∎Fluttering on awaking, giddy; must get up, fearing otherwise he will smother. Fluttering of heart and nervousness; feels very weak.

❙Palpitation, < while walking.

❙Darting pains in heart, when walking; after abuse of mercury; after repeated endocarditis.

❙Valvular defects after repeated endocarditis, especially affecting r. ventricle, which gradually becomes dilated; stupor, and loss of breath; greatly annoying palpitations; pulse quick, but varying every moment; tumultuous, violent, intermitting and irregular action of heart and pulse, with tensive pain across chest.

❙Pulse accelerated; frequent.

: Aneurism : of arch of aorta; of carotid; at point of origin of carotid and subclavian; of innominate artery.

³¹ **Neck and Back.** ❙Glandular swellings on neck; rachitis.

❙Swelling of whole thyroid gland, increasing very rapidly, sensitive to touch and pressure.

: Bronchocele; when enlargement of thyroid is due to hypertrophy, not to cystic formation or other causes.

❙Submaxillary glands swollen, suppurating.

❙Small of back feels as if in a vice, very painful, not allowing to lie still at night or in daytime; has to sit in bent position.

❙Darts in small of back; meningitis; abuse of mercury.

❙❙Stitches in small of back when sitting.

❙❙Moving produces intense pain in small of back; chronic rheumatism of chest and back.

❙Bruised pain in lumbar region, < sitting bent; stitches.

❙❙Chills from sacrum up over back.

❙Pain in os coccygis, as from a fall.

❙Meningeal inflammation after abuse of mercury, or secondary syphilis.

³² **Upper Limbs.** ❙Left shoulder feels bruised.

❙❙Pain in shoulder as if lame, only during motion.

❙❙Tendons of r. shoulder feel stretched, swollen, < during motion or from touch.

❙❙Tearing in shoulder and then in ear.

❙❙Tearing pain in elbows, shoulders, and r. wrist.

❙❙Tearing and contraction in inner surface of ring finger; it remains some time bent; also in thumb and index finger. θRheumatism. θGout.

❙Tip of thumb ulcerates and turns yellow.

³³ **Lower Limbs.** ❙Gnawing in hip bones; darting in l. hip at every step, forcing him to limp.

❙Gnawing, aching, tearing pains in r. thigh and leg; a darting from point where sciatic nerve leaves pelvis, to within ten inches of popliteal space, then interrupted to appear about middle and outer side of calf, continuing to external malleolus and heel; motion at first painful, is after a moment more bearable; she walked, leaning toward affected side, as much as though femur had been dislocated above acetabulum, when standing an inch and a half from floor; < at night, not able to remain in bed; pain in thigh, leg and knee joint, excruciating when lying down, eliciting screams; gave up bed for several weeks, occupying a chair, in a semi-reclining position; emaciated and prostrated from want of rest and pain; pains bearable during day, < in evening, > in open air; violent jerking of limb and muscles of thigh; pain < in knee, tearing and lacerating.

∎Pain > by walking and flexing leg; < from standing, sitting or lying in bed. θSciatica.

∎Tearing and pain in left femur.

❘❘Tearing darting in thighs, joints, big toe; < at night and lying on r. or suffering side, or on back.

∎Tearing in r. thigh and knee, awakens him at night, < lying on affected side or back. θSciatica.

∎Tearing in l. knee, as if in periosteum; knee feels swollen during night.

∎Knee doughy, spongy, no fluctuation; skin red in spots and hot; gnawing, boring or tearing, < at night, must often change position; white swelling.

❘❘Violent gnawing pain in l. leg, as if in periosteum.

∎Cramps in calves; after mercury.

∎Acute gout in both feet.

∎Pain as if bruised in left instep.

∎Ulcerative pain in heels and toes.

⁵⁴ Limbs in General. ∎Tearing, darting pains; periosteum attacked; from mercurialization or syphilis; rheumatism; gout.

∎Violent rheumatic pains in limbs every evening and night, with preceding chilliness.

∎Rheumatism < at night, and lying on suffering side or on back; jerking of tendons; contractions; restless sleep; loss of appetite; emaciation; tearing, darting pains.

∎Lies upon back with bent knees; arms drawn to thorax; immovable and stiff in all joints; joints of knees, feet, shoulders and elbows filled with solid exudate; tendons as hard as bone and stiff; fingers drawn tightly to palms of hands and joints all swollen; involuntary jerking of limbs, < night; completely helpless, must be fed like a child; emaciated to skin and bone; loss of appetite; could not sleep without opiates; pain in back and gouty pains in joints. θGout.

⁵⁵ Rest. Position. Motion. Lying down: difficult breathing; excruciating pains in lower limbs.

Lies upon back, snoring loudly.

Must lie on back: short breathing.

Lies on back with bent knees; arms drawn to thorax; immovable in all joints.

Lying on r. side or on back: pains <.

Cannot lie still: on account of pain in small of back; pain in lower limbs.

Must get up or smother.

Sitting: pain in chest >; pain in back; stitching in small of back; pain in leg <.

Sits up in chair in semi-reclining position, on account of pains in lower limbs.

Cannot sit up without assistance; great weakness.

Siting bent: < bruised pain in lumbar region.

Obliged to bend double: on account of pain in groins.

Has to sit double: on account of pain in back.

Standing: pains in leg <.

Must change position: on account of tearing in knee.

After rising: heaviness and pain in head >.

Motion: at first painful in lower limbs after a moment is more bearable.

Moving: sharp pain in chest; intense pain in small of back; pain in shoulders; tendons of shoulders feel stretched.

Throwing about: in bed.

Restless: moving about.

Walking: stitches in back, sternum and chest; palpitation <; darting pains in heart; pain in leg >.

Great bodily exertion: shaking chill.

Nerves. ❙Subsultus tendinum, or contractions of muscles and tendons.

❙Restless moving about.

❙Great general debility; exhaustion.

❙❙Chorea of rheumatic origin.

❙Paralysis of any of muscles dependent upon syphilitic periostitis.

❙Hemiplegia; paralysis; spinal meningitis.

Sleep. ❙❙Frequent yawning without drowsiness.

❙Sleepy and drowsy.

❙Sleepless from anguish; restless; horrid dreams.

❙❙Loud weeping in sleep, but unconscious of it.

❙Awaking: suddenly, pneumonia, croup; as if smothering; heart fluttering; bitter taste.

Time. Morning: awoke with dizziness; lips covered with viscid mucus; bitter taste; numbness of mouth; awakening with dry throat, oppression, loss of voice; awakes with choking; soreness of larynx.

5 A.M.: heaviness of head.

Afternoon: chill, sweat.

During day: dull, tense, numb.feeling in affected part of
head; thirst; pains bearable.

4 to 7 P.M.: chilly with thirst.

6 to 8 P.M.: drowsy.

Evening: tearing in r. ear; teeth painful; hiccough; soreness of larynx; sticking in region of lower rib; pains
in limbs <.

Night: pain becomes intolerable; pain in eye <; syphilitic ozæna with pain; restless; terrible pain at root of
tongue; thirst; enuresis; sweats; pain in lower limbs <;
pains <; knee feels swollen; tearing in knee; rheumatism; jerking of limbs; chilly; pains make him frantic.

³⁹ Temperature and Weather. ❙Irresistible desire for the
open air; walking in open air does not fatigue.

Warmth: external, >; general chilliness; teeth >;
lumps on cranium >; coldness of scalp >.

Can get warm in bed, but not from heat of stove.

Open air: heat in head >; pains in head >; pains in
limbs >; coryza <.

Cold: teeth <.

⁴⁰ Fever. ❙Chilly, with thirst (4–7 P.M.), or all night, with
shaking and frequent waking; can get warm in bed,
but not from heat of stove.

❙From lower part of back upward and through whole
body; 6–8 P.M.; drowsy.

❙Shaking chill at night, sleepy, with frequent waking; so
chilly at night that she could not get warm.

❙Chilliness predominates, fever marked by hot flushes,
but little perspiration, very much aggravated at night.

❙At times chilly, with dry skin; at others profuse sweat.

❙Flushes of heat, with dulness of head.

Heat then sweat; afternoon.

Sweat in afternoon; skin at times dry; at others profuse
sweat; night sweats.

❙Intermittent fever; thirst with chill; chill not > by
warmth; mouth dry; anasarca; scrofula.

❙Catarrhal fevers.

⁴¹ Attacks, Periodicity. Every evening: violent rheumatic
pains in limbs.

Every night: rheumatic pains in limbs.

⁴² Locality and Direction. Right: paralysis of side; fundus
of eye; tearing in ear; membrana tympani depressed;
chin drawn to side; stinging pain in ear and submaxillary gland; darting in hypochondrium; pain in ovarian region; sharp pain through lung; cannot lie on
side on account of difficulty of breathing; heart pressed
to side; catarrhal inflammation in upper part of chest;
lung infiltrated; serous effusion of pleura; hepatization

of lower two-thirds of lung; valvular defects; tendons of shoulder feel stretched; tearing in wrist; pain in thigh and leg; lying on side pains <; tearing in thigh and knee.

Left: stitches above eye; darting over eye; in temple; limbs of this side in constant tremulous motion; atrophic spots in choroid of eye; diplopia only noticed when looking to slight action of external rectus; paralysis of nervous abducens; several tumors on upper border of orbit; membrana tympani depressed; nostril ulcerated within, excoriated without; side of chest filled with fluid; chest enlarged; pleuritic effusion of chest; lung compressed; lung infiltrated; shoulder feels bruised; darting in hip; pain in femur; tearing in knee; knee feels swollen; violent pain in leg; pain in instep.

[43] **Sensations.** Excited as if intoxicated; as if brain was compressed from both sides; as though head was enlarged to three times its size; head as if screwed in; as if head would be forced asunder; scalp as if ulcerated; as if a leaflet was at root of nose; as if a worm was crawling at root of tooth; surface of mouth as if covered with milk; as if something had lodged in throat; as if spasm would close pharynx; back as if in a vice; pain in ovaries as from a tumor; thighs feel as if squeezed; pain in larynx as if from granulations; pain as from soreness in chest; chest as if cut to pieces; limbs as if paralyzed; loud snoring appeared to come out of chest as if through a tube; shoulder as if lame; pain in os coccygis as from a fall; tearing in knee as if in periosteum; as if bruised in l. instep.

Pains: in sides of head; in upper part of head; in upper maxilla and teeth; in throat; in stomach; in small of back; in ovarian region; into thighs; in chest; in eyes; through breast; in region of lower ribs; through lungs; in shoulder; in os coccygis; in thigh, leg and knee joint; in l. femur; in back.

Terrible pain: at root of tongue.

Intense pain: in small of back.

Excruciating pain: in thigh, leg and knee joint.

Intolerable nocturnal bone pains.

Violent pain: in frontal region; in both orbital processes; across forehead.

Severe: headache with lachrymation; pain in eyes.

Sharp pain: in chest; through r. lung from nipple.

Tearing: above l. eye; in r. ear; in shoulder; in elbow; in r. wrist; in inner surface of ring finger; in thumb; in index finger; in r. thigh and leg; in knee; in l. femur; in thighs, joints, big toe; in l. knee.

Severe burning, tearing, twitching pain: in ovarian region.

Tearing out pain: starting from ensiform cartilage.

Boring, tearing pains: in temporal bone; in knee.

Boring pain: in ears; in nasal bones.

Ulcerative pain: in gums; in heels and toes.

Beating: in forehead; in temples; in nasal bones; of carotids.

Throbbing pain: in nasal and frontal bones; in stomach.

Hammering: in forehead.

Darting: above l. eye and in l. temple; in ears; in l. cheek; in r. hypochondrium; in side of abdomen; in renal region; in heart; in small of back; from where sciatic nerve leaves pelvis to within ten inches of popliteal space, then interrupted to appear about middle and outer calf, and to external malleolus and heel.

Lancinating: over l. eye and in l. temple; in nasal bones to forehead; in throat.

Lacerating pain: in knee.

Cutting: around navel.

Violent stitches: in middle of sternum.

Stitches: through sternum to back; deep in chest; in small of back.

Jerking stitches: above l. eye; in frontal sinus.

Fine transient stitches: deep in middle of chest.

Sticking pains: in ears; in larynx.

Jerking: violent, of limb and muscles of thigh.

Acute gout: in both feet.

Violent rheumatic pains: in limbs.

Sudden shocks of pain: in head.

Gnawing: in nasal bones; in both sides of lower jaw; in teeth; in r. thigh and leg; in knee; in l. leg.

Cramp pains: in stomach.

Cramps: in calves.

Rheumatic pains: in limbs; in chest and back.

Gouty pains: in joints.

Bruised pains: in groins and small of back; in lumbar region; in shoulder.

Tensive, stinging, darting, lacerating pain: in head.

Tensive pain: across chest.

Aching: in r. thigh and leg.

Grumbling: in teeth and face.

Stinging: in ears; in l. cheek; in r. submaxillary gland; in throat.

Painful burning: in stomach.

Burning tickling: in throat.

Burning: of face; in eyes; in nasal and frontal bones; on tip of tongue; at epigastrium; in stomach; in pit of

stomach; around navel; in kidneys; in urethra; in
larynx.
Biting: in pudendum. .
Soreness: of larynx.
Heat: in whole mouth; in head.
Painful bloating: around navel.
Pressing: in groins; in stomach.
Tightening: at root of nose.
Stretched feeling: in tendons of r. shoulder.
Painful: urging to urinate; syphilitic nodes; breathing.
Numbness of mouth.
Dull, tense, numb feeling: in affected part of head.
Rough feeling: in trachea.
Dryness: of mouth; of pharynx; of throat; in stomach;
in larynx.
Fulness: of nose.
Heaviness: in forehead.
Itching of throat; of herpes on face.
" Tissues. ❙Emaciation and loss of appetite.
❙Purpura hemorrhagica.
❙Hemorrhage from nose, lungs, rectum.
❙Discharges from mucous surfaces thin, ichorous, corro-
sive, or green.
❙❙Chronic periosteal rheumatism of syphilitic or mercu-
rial origin; intolerable nocturnal bone pains, driving
patient to despair.
❙Chronic arthritis, with considerable spurious anchylosis.
❙❙Swelling of bones and periosteum, with nocturnal pains.
❙Diseases of periosteum and capsular ligaments of joints.
❙❙Bony tumors; interstitial distension of bones; pains <
at night.
❙❙Caries and necrosis after syphilis and abuse of mercury.
❙Gout and rheumatism; synovitis.
❙Painful syphilitic nodes.
❙❙Glands: swollen; goitre; bronchial, submaxillary,
ulcerating; atrophied; interstitial infiltration.
❙❙Glands suppurate; discharge thin, corrosive, or curdy;
indolent, with hard edges.
❙❙Glands atrophy; especially testes and mammæ.
❙Dropsy from pressure from swollen glands.
❙Distends all tissues by interstitial infiltration; œdema;
enlarged glands; tophi; exostoses; swelling of bones.
❙Ulcers: vegetations bleed easily and are unhealthy;
canceroid; deep; involving bone structure.
❙Scrofula.
❙❙Rupia syphilitica.
❙Condylomata of long standing in cachectic subjects.
❙Condyloma accuminatum after chancre.

❙Bubo very hard with curdy, offensive discharge, if suppurating; thickening of spermatic cord; ulceration of
nose, mouth and throat, with corroding, burning discharge; lancinating pains in throat; system depressed;
effusion of serum into cellular tissue; induration of
liver. θSyphilis.

❙After abuse of mercury: tuberculous pustules in face;
roseola on chest and extremities; discolored, large
ulcers on skin; bone swelling; nightly bone pain;
bloody stools, with tenesmus; falling out of hair.
θSyphilis.

❙Secondary syphilis, especially after abuse of mercury or
combined with scrofula; buboes, chancres, with hard
edges, thin, corrosive or curdy pus; deep eating ulcers.

❙Especially useful in tertiary syphilis.

Skin. ❙Itching herpes on face.

❙Purpura hemorrhagica.

❙❙Roseola spots. θSyphilis.

A kind of *erythema nodosum*, in three cases, consisting of
red, urticaria-like elevations, appearing on face, neck,
arms and legs, and preceded by itching, leaving, after
disappearing, infiltrated spots; they were observed only
during the winter.

❙❙Papulous eruption; with dryness of throat.

❙Papulæ worse on face, shoulders and back; dry throat.

❙Tubercles on face.

❙Tubercular syphilitic skin eruption.

❙Itchlike pimples and vesicles.

❙Herpes, size of dime, on cheek.

❙❙Eczema cruris; pityriasis capitis.

❙❙Small boils on neck, face, scalp, back, chest, suppurating; often leaving scars.

❙Pustulous eruption often umbilicated and leaving scars.

❙Syphilitic eruptions, chiefly in cachectic persons, pustular
or squamose.

❙Furuncular eruption, epidemic, of various sizes, from a
small pustule to a large boil; often this latter becomes
carbuncular and is generally surrounded by little
pustules.

A kind of hard tumors, especially on legs, dark color,
yellow pustules interwoven; basis hard and painful to
pressure, only their navel-like centre is not painful;
surrounded by a red halo; after discharging they
gradually sank in space of a month or even a whole
year, when they finally covered themselves with thick
crusts which remained for a long time.

❙Rupia; impetiginous eruption; herpetic eruption; eruption simulating acne.

▮Ecthymatous eruption.

⁴⁷ **Stages of Life. Constitution.** ▮▮Scrofulous patients; especially if syphilis or mercurialization is superadded.

Girl, æt. 5; dropsy of chest.

Girl, æt. 10; diphtheria.

Boy, after scarlet fever; adhesions of middle ear.

Girl, æt. 15, rapid growth, small chested; pleuritic exudation.

Girl, æt. 18; disease of submaxillary gland.

Girl, æt. 20; sciatica.

Young lady, no history of syphilis; disseminate choroiditis.

Man, æt. 23; pleuritic exudation.

Woman, æt. 25, in good circumstances, in fifth month of pregnancy; pleurisy with exudation.

Man, æt. 32; pneumonia.

Man, æt. 36, thin and delicate; pleurisy.

Man, æt. 38; diphtheria.

Colored women, syphilitic history; tumors of orbit.

Man, æt. 40, had syphilis; paralysis of nervus abducens.

Woman, æt. 46, weak constitution; pleuritic exudation.

Man, æt. 50, suffering one week; pleuro-pneumonia.

Man, æt. 85; bilateral croupous pneumonia.

⁴⁸ **Relations.** Antidoted by: *Hepar.*

It antidotes: *Mercur.*, lead poisoning.

Compare: *Arsen., Bellad., Conium* (knee), ▮▮*Hepar,* ▮▮*Iodum,* ▮*Laches.,* ▮▮*Mercur., Mezer., Pulsat., Silica, Sulphur.*

KALI MURIATICUM.

Potassium Chloride.   *KCl.*

The clinical symptoms of Kali chloricum (potassium chlorate) of which we have provings by Martin and Tully (see Allen's Encyclopedia, vol. 5, p. 316), are deemed sufficiently similar to those of Schuessler's Tissue Remedies to be included herein.

CLINICAL AUTHORITIES.—*Insanity,* Kurtz, Rück. Kl. Erf., vol. 5, p. 272; *Loss of vision of r. eye,* Schuessler, p. 96; *Chorio-retinitis,* Woodyatt, Norton's Oph. Therap., p. 107; *Parenchymatous keratitis,* Norton's Oph. Therap., p. 106; *Faceache,* Herber, Frank, Meyer, Rück. Kl. Erf., vol. 1, p. 424; *Faceache,* Martin (2 cases), Rück. Kl. Erf., vol. 1, p. 424; *Paralysis of r. facial nerve,* Cramoisy, Org., vol. 3, p. 112; *Caries of teeth,* Neumann, A. H. O., vol. 10, p. 310; *Affection of mouth,* Liedbeck, Rück. Kl. Erf., vol. 1, p. 507; *Stomatitis, ulcers in mouth,* Henoch, Hirsch, Lauri, Rück. Kl. Erf., vol. 5, p. 219; *Stomatitis ulcerosa,* Windelband, B. J. H., vol. 36, p. 366; *Angina,* Goullon, Raue's Rec., 1870, p. 142; *Diphtheria,* Goullon, Œhme's Therap.; *Dysentery,* Bigler, Raue's Rec., 1875, p. 8; *Nephritis,* Windelband, B. J. H., vol. 36, p. 366; *Albuminuria,* Sanders, Trans. Am. Inst. Hom., 1883, p. 669; *Catarrh of bladder,* Edlefsen, N. A. J. H., vol. 26, p. 134; *Gonorrhœa,* Windelband, B. J. H., vol. 36, p. 366; *Suppurating buboes,* Windelband, B. J. H., vol. 36, p. 366; *Leucorrhœa,* Schuessler; Windelband, B. J. H., vol. 36, p. 366; *Croup,* Schuessler; *Whooping cough,* Ameke, B. J. H., vol. 36, p. 366; *Catarrhal pneumonia,* Breuer, Allg. Hom. Ztg., vol. 105, p. 171; *Catarrhal phthisis,* Morgan, Trans. Hom. Med. Soc. Pa., 1880, p. 231; *Facial paralysis,* Drysdale, Hughes; *Open carcinoma* (locally), Burow, A. H. O., vol. 10, p. 310; *Infantile syphilis,* Hughes; *Variola,* Burow, A. H. O., vol. 10, p. 810; *Read,* N. A. J. H., vol. 10, p. 176.

[1] **Mind.** Sad, apathetic, with chilliness in evening.

   ❙Alternate states of sadness and cheerfulness, associated with congestion, > from nosebleed.

   ❙Habitual loss of appetite; patient absolutely refuses to take food, or imagines he must starve. θInsanity.

[2] **Sensorium.** A glass of wine or beer intoxicates easily.

   Confusion of head, also in occiput, with a peculiar sensation in cervical muscles.

   Vertigo: after violent exercise, with congestion to head; with headache.

[3] **Inner Head.** Tightness in occiput, sneezing and coryza.

   Aching in l. side of temple.

   ❙❙Headache: extending into jaws; in evening; in occiput; with vomiting, hawking up of milk white mucus.

   ❙❙Sick headache; white coated tongue, or vomiting of white phlegm.

⁴ **Outer Head.** Pains in head and face, with hawking up of white mucus.

Catarrh of frontal cavities; tumors.

πMarked increase of dandruff, falling in small white flakes over coat collar, accompanied by itching.

▮Crusta lactea, sore or scaldhead of children.

⁵ **Sight and Eyes.** ı ıLuminous appearance before eyes when coughing or sneezing.

ı ıCongestion to eyes, they feel irritated; redness in evening with some pain.

▮Irritable retina.

▮While walking through fields covered with snow, sudden severe pain in r. eye, followed at once by blindness, saw nothing with r. eye, all seemed smoke and mist; l. eye became gradually weaker from month to month; but little of retina can be seen, there being a kind of mist over it, which seemed to spread from vitreous humor over background of eye; retina dim and misty, veins forming a dark network; in some places indistinctly defined spots, some larger than others, appearing like residue of extravasated blood; arteries scarcely visible, and seemed pale and contracted.

▮Dimness of r. eye, he could not read a newspaper; cornea, iris and pupil normal; no external redness; vitreous rather hazy, with some black shreds suspended in it, having very limited motion on rotating eye; optic nerve and bloodvessels normal; inside the disk, a large, irregular, atrophic spot, involving choroid and retina, surrounded by several small ones; edges irregular and pigmented; sclerotic seen white through their centres; choroid adjacent, congested and thickened; some vessels lost in infiltrated part to appear on other side; a dull pain, occasionally, in eye and over brow, with an ill defined feeling of contraction around eye; vision $\frac{30}{200}$; Snellen 11 slowly deciphered. At the end of a month vision rose to $\frac{20}{70}$ and Snellen 3 was read at five inches; a year afterwards the man could read Snellen 2½, distant vision $\frac{20}{70}$, but under Kali mur. for a week it was again $\frac{20}{70}$. The patient's business engagements prevented longer treatment. (Improved.) θChorio-retinitis.

▮Parenchymatous keratitis; for three months there had been an infiltration into r. cornea, which commenced at outer side and extended over whole cornea; could only count fingers; occasional pain, moderate photophobia and redness; pupil dilated slowly and incompletely, though regularly, and contracted quickly.

▮Retinal exudation.

ı ıConjunctivitis and keratitis, with formation of small

superficial blisters; small ulcers on cornea following a blister; feeling of sand in eye; white mucous secretion or yellowish green pus from eyes.

||Opaque spots on eye; leucoma.

❙On lower edge of l. cornea, a little blister from which a bundle of small veins run; feeling of sand in eye; edges of eyelids scabby.

❙❙Conjunctivitis and keratitis (scrofulous) with a formation of phlyctenulæ, but only superficial.

||Suppurating points on edges of eyelids; edges scabby; yellow crusts of pus on edges of lids.

Secretion: yellowish green, purulent; white, mucous.

⁶ Hearing and Ears. Deafness: from swelling of internal ear; from swelling of Eustachian tubes and tympanic cavity; with swelling of glands, or cracking noise on blowing nose, or white coated tongue.

||Earache; with gray or white furred tongue; with swelling of glands; with swelling of throat, or cracking noise in ear when swallowing.

⁷ Smell and Nose. Bleeding of nose: at night; from r. nostril. Tension and tensive drawing in cheeks inducing desire to sneeze, with cramp in malar muscles.

||Stopped or dry coryza.

❙Violent coryza, sneezing and profuse secretion of mucus; twitching of masseter muscles; catarrh after mercury.

White mucous discharge in coryza, catarrh of frontal sinuses.

Cold: stuffy, in head, with whitish grey tongue; with white, non-transparent, or yellowish discharge.

❙Hawking of mucus from posterior nares.

⁸ Upper Face. ❙Suffering expression of face. θStomacace.

||Bloated face; sickly expression.

||Flushes of heat.

❙Increased sensitiveness of whole face, with irritation in root of nose, twitchings in corners of eyes; after mercury.

❙Lightning-like attacks of pain in face, gradually growing more frequent; l. side of face fiery red, with twitching and trembling in muscles of face, lachrymation, throbbing of temporal artery; < speaking, chewing, eating fruit or anything sour; excited by least touch.

||Cramplike drawing in cheeks, extending to articulation of jaws; tearing in upper jaw; after abuse of mercury.

||Faceache, with swelling of gums or cheek.

❙Paralysis of r. facial nerve; difficulty of speaking, eating and whistling; could not puff out cheeks, because lips could not be held firm on r. side of face; mouth oblique in laughing or speaking; neither wrinkles nor contractions of muscles on paralyzed side.

❙Facial paralysis, beginning with faceache; tenderness on touch or pressure of affected side.

Pimple on forehead, face, and between lips and chin.

Spots in face.

⁹ **Lower Face.** ❘❘Tension and tensive drawing in cheeks, inducing a desire to sneeze; cramp in malar muscles.

❘❘Cramplike drawing in cheeks, extending to articulation of jaw, with stinging in jaw and teeth.

❘❘Mumps, without fever.

Twitching in muscles of lower jaw.

❘❘Swelling of lips; after mercury.

❘❘Pimples on lips; chapped lips from cold.

❘❘Barber's itch.

¹⁰ **Teeth and Gums.** ❘❘Dulness of teeth; toothache in upper jaw.

❘❘Toothache with swelling of gums and flow of saliva.

❘❘Painful caries of teeth.

❙Gums: inflamed, bright red; very sensitive; bleed easily.

❙❙Scorbutis, especially after mercury; offensive smell.

❘❘Ulceration of edges of gums.

❙Gumboil, before suppuration.

¹¹ **Taste and Tongue.** ❙Taste: disagreeable; saltish; sour; bitter sour; stinging burning, sourish; brassy after mercury.

❘❘Bitter taste with feeling of coldness on tongue, removed after breakfast and dinner.

❙Tongue coated: thin, white, not mucous; dirty yellow in stomacace; white, or only in middle; after diarrhœa.

❙White fur on tongue of syphilitic origin.

❘❘Coldness on tongue and in pharynx.

❘❘Burning, stinging blisters on tongue and in buccal cavity.

Inflammation of tongue.

❙Cannot talk; epithelioma.

¹² **Inner Mouth.** ❙Heat and dryness; peeling off of lips.

❙Breath excessively fetid, in ulceration and diphtheria.

❘❘Accumulation of mucus.

❘❘Saliva flows freely; profuse and acid; tasting brassy.

❘❘Stinging burning with sour taste in mouth. ·

❘❘Pain, with swelling of gums and cheeks.

❙❙Aphthæ and stomatitis, simple or ulcerative.

❙Sore mouth, with spongy, bleeding gums, patches in fauces and on pharynx, like diphtheria or follicular disease; fetor unbearable.

❙❙Most acute ulcerative and follicular stomatitis; whole mucous surface red and tumid, and in cheeks, lips, etc., were numerous grey based ulcers.

❙Follicular ulcers on inside of lips and dorsum of tongue; mouth full of saliva; glands enlarged and tender, in cachectic people.

▌Severe pain throughout whole body; dimness of vision, letters appear smaller when reading; sensitive, lachrymose; their gums become sensitive and foul smelling, bleeding easily and discharging pus; heat and dryness in mouth with salivation; earthy color of face; face bloated; lips hot, swollen, epithelium being thrown off in scabs; general lassitude; feels more tired in morning than evening; attacks periodical, lasting eight to nine days.

▌Stomatitis ulcerosa; mercurial or scrofulous; gums swollen, easily bleeding, and usually projecting from a set of bad teeth; fetor oris; salivation; aphthous ulcers on tongue and cheeks, particularly in children.

▌Aphthæ, thrush of little children or nursing mothers, without great flow of saliva.

▌Ulceration in mouth which had perforated cheeks.

▌Whitish exudation on mucous membrane of mouth.

❘❘Epithelial degeneration of mucous membrane of mouth; a forerunner of cancer.

▌Epithelioma; ulceration had reached face.

▌Tongue swollen filling cavity of mouth; bears impression of several parts of mouth; ulcerated places deep enough to admit end of little finger; discharge ichorous, terribly offensive; small, superficial ulcers, painful on sides; hard, somewhat elastic places on tongue; color deep violet. θEpithelioma and hypertrophy.

[13] **Throat.** ❘❘Roughness; dryness of fauces.

▌Dryness of throat and chest, with violent cough, as from vapor of sulphur.

❘❘Cynanche tonsillaris.

▌Tonsillitis, with much swelling.

▌A syphilitic fur in cavity of mouth and fauces.

▌Tonsils swollen, cover white or whitish grey.

▌Catarrh of mucous membrane of fauces, tonsils and pharynx, with white exudation.

Pharynx feels cold.

▌▌Hawks up cheesy lumps about size of a split pea, having a disgusting odor and taste. θFollicular pharyngitis.

▌Angina, beginning with white points on opening of ducts of glands, threatening diphtheritis.

▌Pain on swallowing; < on one side; considerable redness of fauces; frequently white, diphtheritic patches on tonsils; dirty coated tongue; fever; chilliness; suffering expression of face; fetor oris. θAngina.

▌▌Croupous, diphtheritic exudations.

❘❘Diphtheritis, if fauces are not swollen.

▌Diphtheria: with offensive effluvia; invading larynx.

❘❘Numerous grey ulcers in mouth and throat; excessive

secretion of tough, stringy saliva; epistaxis; ravenous
hunger followed by total anorexia; dryness and pain in
throat, with difficult swallowing (beginning paralysis of
glosso-pharyngeal nerve); excessive micturition; hæmaturia; albuminuria; hoarse voice; incessant cough and
difficult respiration; chest pressed together and watery
froth exuding from mouth. θDiphtheria.

❚On fourth day, pulse 120, bad sleep, little appetite; entire
fauces filled with exudate; violent pain in throat; strong
fetor oris; in morning a fainting fit. θDiphtheritis.

❚Secondary syphilis affecting fauces.

¹⁴ **Appetite, Thirst. Desires, Aversions.** ❙❙Violent hunger
between regular periods of eating.

❙❙Canine hunger in attacks, > after drinking water.

❙❙Want of appetite; increased thirst.

¹⁵ **Eating and Drinking.** ❙❙Beer and wine intoxicate easily.

❙❙After eating breakfast and dinner, bitter taste renewed.

¹⁶ **Hiccough, Belching, Nausea and Vomiting.** Eructations: empty; sourish; alternating with pains in chest
and abdomen.

❙❙Gagging and gulping up white mucus.

❙❙Loathing with shivering; nausea with eructations.

❙❙Vomiting: of white slime; of blood.

¹⁷ **Scrobiculum and Stomach.** ❙❙Cutting in stomach.

❙❙Pressure, with empty feeling in stomach; chilliness;
listlessness.

❙❙White or greyish coated tongue, pain or heavy feeling
on r. side over liver; fatty food disagrees; eyes look
large and projecting. θDyspepsia.

❙❙Gastritis: from taking too hot drinks; second stage,
white coated tongue.

❙❙Hemorrhage from stomach.

¹⁸ **Hypochondria.** ❙❙Tensive pressure in region of liver, disappearing after emission of flatus.

❙❙Painful pressure in region of spleen.

❚Portal congestion and enlarged liver; emptiness in stomach; pain in r. side, light yellow color of evacuations,
white or greyish furred tongue, constipation; hemorrhoidal complaints.

❙❙Liver disease with dropsy.

¹⁹ **Abdomen.** ❙❙Colic in pelvic region; diarrhœa; shifting of
flatulence.

❙❙Chill, resulting in catarrh of duodenum, white coated
tongue; stools light colored. θJaundice.

❚Peritonitis.

❚Suppurating buboes.

²⁰ **Stool and Rectum.** ❚Diarrhœa: after fatty food, pastry,
etc.; evacuations light colored, white or slimy; white

coated tongue; painful, passing nothing but mucus; in typhoid fever, stools like pale yellow ochre; bloody, or bloody mucus.

ı ıHard, dry stool, latter part mixed with mucus.

ıStool so dry it almost crumbles.

ıConstipation through want of bile from sluggish liver; light colored stools.

ı ıConstant pains in rectum.

ı ıDysentery; much blood passing with the slime.

ıPains in abdomen, cutting as if from knives; calls to stool every fifteen or twenty minutes, with tenesmus extorting cries; evacuations consist of only a tea or tablespoonful of blood. θDysentery. .

ıHemorrhoidal bleeding; dark, thick blood.

ı ıSyphilitic complaints about the anus.

ı ıChafing or rawness of skin in children.

ı ıAscarides, threadworms.

²¹ **Urinary Organs.** ı ıInflammation of kidneys, catarrhal or croupy.

ıNephritis parenchymatosa; much albumen in urine.

ı ıKidney disease with dropsy.

ı ıInflammation of bladder with violent fever.

ıAcute and chronic catarrh of bladder.

ıCystitis, second stage, when swelling has set in; discharge of thick white mucus.

ı ıChronic catarrh of bladder.

ıTurbid urine; dirty yellow sediment. θNephritis.

ı ıItching in urethra.

ıDiabetes, excessive and sugary urine; stomach and liver deranged, grey or white coating on tongue; dry and light colored stools from want of bile; pain in kidneys.

²² **Male Sexual Organs.** ıVoluptuous dreams with violent emissions.

ıViolent erections with emissions and itching of scrotum.

ıSexual desire diminished, with chilliness and apathy.

ı ıItching in urethra.

ıOrchitis from suppressed gonorrhœa.

ıPost-gonorrhœal induration of left testicle, from abuse of injections of *Cuprum sulph.*

ı ıHydrocele in little children.

ı ıGonorrhœa of glans or urethra; second stage, with chordee.

ıGleet combined with eczema (latent or visible), or a disposition to glandular swellings. θGonorrhœa.

ıSoft chancre.

ıAfter chancre, pointy condylomata on corona glandis.

ıChronic syphilis.

ı ıSuppurative bubo.

²³ Female Sexual Organs. Menses: delayed too long or suppressed; too early or lasting too long; excessive, dark clotted, or tough, black, like tar; too frequent.

▮Hemorrhages from womb.

▮Leucorrhœa: mild and white; not transparent; obstinate and acrid.

²⁴ Pregnancy. Parturition. Lactation. ▮Morning sickness, with vomiting of white phlegm.

▮Albuminuria in gestation.

▮▮Threatened abortion.

▮First stage of puerperal fever.

▮Mastitis, weed, gathering breast, before formation of pus.

²⁵ Voice and Larynx. Trachea and Bronchia. ▮Hoarseness.

▮▮Fever, loud barking cough, restlessness at night with much rough and hard coughing; dry heat and great oppression. θSpurious croup.

▮Croup, membranous exudation.

▮Bronchitis, second stage, when thick phlegm forms.

²⁶ Respiration. ▮▮Constriction of chest as from vapors of sulphur.

▮▮Oppressed breathing.

▮Bronchial asthma when secretion is white.

▮Asthma; mucus, white and hard to cough up, tongue whitish or furred greyish.

²⁷ Cough. ▮▮Violent cough with coryza.

▮▮Dryness of throat and chest with violent cough as from vapor of sulphur.

▮Acute, short, spasmodic cough.

▮Cough, stomachy, noisy, with protruded appearance of eyes, or itching at anus.

▮Croupy cough; hard, white coated tongue.

▮Whooping cough, much opaque, white mucus.

Cough: in consumption, with thick white sputa, white coated tongue; white or yellowish white phlegm.

▮▮Sputa white as milk.

▮Yellowish green mucous discharge from lungs.

²⁸ Inner Chest and Lungs. ▮▮Oppression of chest, with violent beating of heart, sometimes preceded by rush of blood to chest or attended by a sensation as if lungs were tied with a thread.

▮Constriction of chest with palpitation of heart.

▮Constriction in chest, as from vapor of sulphur.

▮Pleurisy, second stage; plastic exudation.

▮Cold in chest, with thick white or yellowish sputa.

▮Lung disease, expectoration whitish, thick, or yellowish white and slimy; tongue frequently coated with white fur at back.

▮Inflammation of lungs, second stage; tongue white coated.

▮▮Catarrhal pneumonia, r. side.

Croupy inflammation of lungs.

Catarrhal phthisis, affecting small space in upper r. lung, with crackling respiration (audible at night to herself), dulness on percussion; paleness; emaciation; fever slight; cough with greenish expectoration.

Hemorrhage from lungs.

30 Heart, Pulse and Circulation. Palpitation of heart, with constriction of chest.

Perceptible but not accelerated beating of heart, with coldness in cardiac region.

Violent but uniform beating of heart; oppression of chest, cold feet.

Palpitation of heart, with sensation of coldness in region of heart.

Palpitation from excessive flow of blood to heart; in hypertrophic conditions.

Pericarditis, second stage.

Heart disease causing dropsy.

Pulse accelerated, or soft and sluggish, not synchronous with beats of heart.

Right pulse full, soft, sluggish (68), intermitting every twenty-five or thirty beats, not synchronous with beats of heart (80), l. pulse being at same time small, soft, easily compressible.

Embolus; for that condition of blood which favors the formation of clots (fibrinous), which causes plugs.

31 Neck and Back. Glands of neck swollen.

32 Upper Limbs. Coldness in arm; internal coldness in r. arm.

Drawing, tearing in wrist joints or tearing ir r. wrist joint along ulna.

After dancing and cooling drafts from r. side, a stiff neck and pain in shoulder when moving r. arm; next night so bad that she had to cry out; three months later, cannot move arm, it causes pain in shoulder and shoulder blade; elbow and hand somewhat movable; fingers numb and powerless; pains are a continuous pressing; dry heat or letting sun shine on it, does good; cannot bear tight clothes or to lie on affected side.

Tenalgia crepitans.

Phlyctænoidal pimples on backs of hands.

Warts on hands.

Itching pimples with small vesicles on dorsa of hands.

33 Lower Limbs. Inflammation of hip joint.

Hip joint disease, second stage, when swelling commences or is present.

Drawing in thigh.

Violent darting in r. knee.

ı ıSwelling of leg below knee; cold and very hard, and looked as if ready to burst; almost twice its usual size.

ıChronic persistent swelling of feet and lower limbs, swelling soft at first, afterwards hard to touch, without pain or redness; itchy; at one stage snowy white and shining; swelling less perceptible in morning than in evening; great tension, with a feeling as if it would burst.

ı ıCramp in leg.

ıUlcers on legs with callous edges.

ıCold feet, with palpitation of heart.

ıFresh chilblains; bunion.

ıIngrown toenails.

³⁴ **Limbs in General.** Lameness: rheumatic; with shiny, red swellings; chronic, caused by rheumatism of joints.

ıRheumatic pains.

ıAcute articular rheumatism.

ıAll joints swollen, could not stay in bed a single night.

ıChilblains on hands or feet or any part.

³⁵ **Rest. Position. Motion.** When moving r. arm: pain in shoulder.

Violent exercise: vertigo with congestion to head.

³⁶ **Nerves.** ıGreat weakness; with diarrhœa.

ıTwitchings of muscles, especially about face and head; < after abuse of mercury.

ı ıConvulsions followed by delirium.

ıEpilepsy, if occurring with, or after suppression of eczema.

ıAsthma; white mucus and hard to cough up.

ıRheumatic paralysis.

³⁷ **Sleep.** ı ıSomnolence.

ı ıSnoring and oppression of breathing; restless sleep with anxious dreams, towards morning.

³⁸ **Time.** Toward morning: restless sleep with anxious dreams.

Morning: feels more tired than evening; fainting fit; sickness; swelling in limbs >.

Evening: chilliness; headache; redness of eyes, with pain; swelling in limbs <.

Night: bleeding of nose; restlessness, with much rough and hard coughing; crackling respiration audible to herself; could not stay in bed a single night on account of swollen joints; delirium; itching.

³⁹ **Temperature and Weather.** In bed: itching of whole body.

Dry heat and letting sun shine on arm does good.

Cooling drafts, after dancing: stiff neck and pain in shoulder.

Cold: chaps hands and lips.

⁴⁰ **Fever.** ı ıShivering all over; or over back and neck, with warm feet.

ı ıContinual chilliness with rigidity of hands.

∎Chill with vomiting of white (not transparent) mucus.
❘❘Chilly in open air; in afternoon.
❘❘Febrile condition, violent beating of pulse and heart.
❘❘Intolerable heat in head.
∎Intermittent fever; fur at back of tongue greyish or white; vomiting of white (not transparent) mucus.
∎Inflammation of peritoneum, pleura, and serous membranes of brain and pericardium.
∎Childbed fever.
∎Grey or white deposit on tongue; diarrhœa, with light yellow ochre colored evacuations; abdominal tenderness and swelling. ⊘Typhoid fever.

⁴¹ **Attacks, Periodicity.** Every fifteen or twenty minutes: calls to stool.
Periodical attacks lasting eight to nine days: severe pain throughout whole body.
Twenty-four hours: rash disappears.
For three months: infiltration into r. cornea.
Three months after taking cold: cannot move arm; it causes pain in shoulder and shoulder blade.

⁴² **Locality and Direction.** Right: dimness of eye; bleeding from nostril; paralysis of facial nerve; lips could not be held firm on side of face; heavy feeling on side over liver; pain in side; catarrhal pneumonia; catarrhal phthisis affecting small space in upper lung; pulse full, soft, sluggish; internal coldness in arm; tearing in wrist joint; stiff neck and pain in shoulder when moving arm; violent darting in knee; pimples in corner of mouth.
Left: aching in side of temple; eye became gradually weaker from month to month; blister on lower edge of cornea; side of face fiery red; pulse small, soft, easily compressible.

⁴³ **Sensations.** As if sand was in eye; as if leg would burst; as if lungs were tied with a thread.
Pains: in head and face; on swallowing < on one side; in throat; in rectum; in abdomen; in kidneys; in shoulder when moving arm; in shoulder blade; of gums and cheeks; in chest; in abdomen; on r. side over liver; in r. side.
Violent pain: in throat.
Severe pain: throughout whole body.
Sudden severe pain: in r. eye.
Violent darting: in r. knee.
Lightning-like attacks of pain: in face.
Tearing: in upper jaw.
Cutting: in stomach; in abdomen.
Drawing tearing: in wrist joints; along ulna.

Cramplike drawing: in cheeks.
Throbbing: of temporal artery.
Colic: in pelvic region.
Tensive drawing: in cheeks.
Drawing: in thigh.
Rheumatism: of joints.
Aching: in l. side of temple; extending from head into jaws; in face; in teeth.
Stinging burning: taste; blisters on tongue.
Stinging: in jaw and teeth.
Twitching: in corners of eyes.
Irritation: in root of nose.
Dull pain: in eye and over brow.
Painful pressure: in region of spleen.
Tensive pressure: in region of liver.
Pressure, with empty feeling in stomach.
Constriction: of chest.
Heavy feeling: on r. side over liver.
Oppression: of chest.
Tightness: in occiput.
Peculiar sensation: in cervical muscles.
Dryness: in mouth; of fauces; of throat and chest.
Confusion: of head; in occiput.
Emptiness: in stomach.
Itching: in urethra; of scrotum; on tongue; at anus; of whole body.
Internal coldness: in r. arm.
Coldness: in cardiac region; in arms.

" **Tissues.** ⅠⅠDisturbed action of vasomotor nerves, congestions, with tension, or coldness.

   ▮Congestions; in second stage, interstitial exudation;
   causes swelling or enlargement of parts, white coated
   tongue or white sputa.

   ▮Hemorrhage, blood clotted, black, thick, viscid.

   ⅠⅠInflammation of lymphatic vessels; acute glandular infiltration; hard swellings.

   ▮Inflammation of serous membranes in second stage of
   peritonitis, pleuritis and pericarditis; acute articular
   rheumatism and inflammation of lungs.

   ▮Discharges of thick, white or yellowish, slimy mucus,
   from nose, ear, eyes, or any passage lined with mucous
   membrane.

   ▮Mucus white, like milk-glass.

   ▮Fibrous exudation on mucous membranes.

   ▮Exudations, fibrinous, in interstitial connective tissues,
   causing swelling and enlargement of these parts.

   ▮Exudations, after inflammation, with effusion of lymph.

   ▮Sticky exudations.

।।Fibrinous exudations, glandular infiltration, and inflammatory infiltration of skin, causing swelling of part, arising from a disturbed balance of organic (albuminoid) basis in cells and of molecules of potassium chloride, or muscle salt, which stands in biological relation to albuminoid substances—*i. e.*, fibrine.

।Hard, scorbutic infiltration of subcutaneous tissue.

।Croupous and diphtheritic exudations.

।।Diseases which arise from want of this salt are marked either by exudations (swellings), torpor of liver, or by casting off of effete albuminoid substance, as seen in white coating of tongue, or whitish secretions and expectorations.

Dysentery, diphtheria, laryngeal croup, croupous pneumonia, fibrous exudation in interstitial connective tissue (*e. g.*, mastitis), acute infiltrations of lymphatic glands, infiltrated inflammations of skin with or without vesiculation (erysipelas, etc.).

।Adhesions, recent, consequent on inflammations; fibrinous exudations arising from excessive blood pressure on walls of bloodvessels.

।If swelling remains on bruised parts.

।Cuts, with swelling.

।Proud flesh.

।।Causes diminution and shrinking of granulations, resorption of adjacent infiltrations, diminution of secretion and of sensitiveness, and revival of drooping spirits. *θ*Open carcinoma (locally).

।Carbuncles, for swelling.

।Abscess, second stage, or when swelling (interstitial exudation) takes place.

।Acute or chronic articular rheumatism.

।Rheumatic, gouty pains.

।Dropsy: from obstruction of bile ducts and enlargement of liver; from weakness of heart; with palpitation.

Liquid drawn off whitish; white mucus in sediment of urine.

।Ascites; anasarca; sequela of fever.

।Many disorders, especially cutaneous eruptions, resulting from use of bad lymph in vaccination (*Silica*).

।Condylomata; warty excrescences.

।।Scorbutic mouth; especially after mercury; chronic scorbutus; scurvy.

।Infantile or chronic syphilis.

" Touch. Passive Motion. Injuries. Touch: excites lightning-like attacks of pain in face.

Cannot bear tight clothes or lie on affected side.

Injuries, from falls, blows, etc., with swelling of parts; chilblains; burns; proud flesh after mechanical injuries.

⁴⁶ Skin. ׀׀Itching of whole body, in bed.
  ׀Jaundice caused by gastro-duodenal catarrh.
  ׀Erythema; swelling present; white coated tongue.
  ׀Excoriation, chafing of skin, especially if inclined to
     scab, tongue whitish.
  ׀Intertrigo of infants.
  ׀Chapped hands or lips from cold.
  ׀׀Papulæ, small, red; pimples on thigh and in r. corner
     of mouth; small vesicles on extremities filled with pus,
     red areolæ, not itching much.
  ׀׀Rash, with single pimples.
  ׀Pimples on face, neck, etc., caused by disturbed action of
     follicular glands.
  ׀Eruption with white scales.
  ׀Eruption of blisters. θIntermittent.
  ׀Eruptions: pustules, pimples; discharging a whitish
     mattery substance; on skin (rash), if connected with
     stomach derangement; white coated tongue, accom-
     panied by deranged menstrual period.
  ׀Blisters arising from burns.
  ׀Little blisters on skin, filled with lymph. θIntermittent.
  ׀Vesicles, with seroso-fibrinous contents.
  ׀Herpes Zoster.
  ׀Eczema: arising after vaccination with bad vaccine
     lymph; from suppressed or deranged uterine functions;
     oozing from inflamed skin; of white secretions from skin.
  ׀Mealy scurf.
  ׀Greenish, brownish, yellow crusts.
  ׀Milk crust.
  ׀Inflammation of skin, with subcutaneous swelling.
  ׀Festers, gatherings in any part; boils.
  ׀׀Proud flesh in ulcers.
  ׀Miliary and venereal symptoms.
  ׀Barber's itch.
  ׀׀Chilblains; recently contracted.
  Inflamed flaws in nails.
  Lupus.
  ׀׀Erysipelas bullosa.
  ׀Vesicular erysipelas and shingles.
  ׀׀Chicken pox.
  ׀Measles; hoarse cough, glandular swellings, furred tongue,
     white or grey deposit; after effects: diarrhœa, whitish,
     or light colored loose stools, white tongue, deafness from
     swellings, etc.
  ׀Variola.
  ׀Attack of slight scarlatina, rash disappearing after
     scarcely twenty-four hours; throat symptoms which
     threatened to be severe disappeared in three or four days;

on seventh day almost complete retention of urine set in, although child drank a good deal; urine albuminous; feet swollen; abdomen greatly distended; high fever; delirium at night.

⁴⁷ Stages of Life, Constitution. ▪Mercurialized patients when a scorbutic state has been created.

Boy, æt. 1½; catarrhal pneumonia.

Girl, æt. 7; blisters on cornea, scabby eyelids.

Boy, æt. 7; croup.

Man, æt. 23, increased dandruff.

Woman, æt. 24, blonde, suffering five years; affection of mouth.

Woman, æt. 29, melancholic, suffering from mental disturbance, and chronic affection of liver; faceache.

Woman, æt. 33, married; catarrhal phthisis.

Man, æt. 35; parenchymatous keratitis.

Woman, æt. 36, suffering from chronic affection of liver, after mental disturbance; faceache.

Man, æt. 36, suffering for two years; chorio-retinitis.

Man, suffering three days; dysentery.

Woman, æt, 44, gouty; faceache.

Woman, æt. 56, always wore blue spectacles, three years ago, while walking through fields covered with snow, on which sun was shining brightly; sudden loss of vision of r. eye.

⁴⁸ Relations. Antidoted by: *Bellad., Calc. sulph., Hydrast., Pulsat.*

It antidotes: *Mercur.*, especially when scorbutic state of blood exists.

Compatible: after *Ferr. phos.* in glossitis, bloody vomiting, cystitis, croup, tussis and pertussis, heart diseases, pleuritis, pneumonia, typhus, skin inflammations, rheumatism, and mechanical. injuries; follows *Kali phos.* in ear diseases and suppresséd menses; is followed by *Kali sulph.* in syphilis, cramp and inflammations; is followed by *Silica* in mastitis and syphilis.

Compare: *Apis, Arsen., Bellad., Bryon., Cadmium.* (constricted chest), *Calc. phos.* (lupus), *Iodium, Iris, Mercur., Merc. dulc.* (eustachian tube troubles), *Mur. ac., Natr. mur., Nitr. ac., Pulsat., Rhus tox., Spongia, Sulphur, Thuja.*

KALI NITRICUM.

Nitre.   *KNO₃.*

Proved by Hahnemann and his provers, also by Engler, Hecker, Heister-
bergkh, Kneschke, Kummer, Richter, Siebenhaar, Jörg, Assman, Alexander, Rummell, Schroeder, Lier, Frinzelberger, Nicol, Traub, Frank,Muhlenbein, and others.
See Allen's Encyclopedia, vol. 5, p. 855.

CLINICAL AUTHORITIES.—*Polypus of nose,* Kippal, Org., vol. 3, p. 96; *Use in
dysentery,* Gauwerky, Rück. Kl. Erf., vol. 5, p. 446; *Pains in chest,* Gregg, p. 20;
Affections of chest, Arnold, Rück. Kl. Erf., vol. 5, p. 823; *Pneumonia,* Hocking,
Raue's Rec., 1874, p. 149; *Anthrodynia,* Cattell, B. J. H., vol. 11, p. 349; *Rheumatism,* Cattell, B. J. H., vol. 11, p. 349.

¹ **Mind.** Depression; anxiety; peevishness; delirium.
² **Sensorium.** I I Fainting fits, with vertigo in morning when
          standing, > when sitting down; afterwards obscuration
          of sight, with great weakness and drowsiness; pain in
          small of back and constriction in abdomen; staggering
          gait, with vertigo. θVertigo.
³ **Inner Head.** I I Headache in vertex on rising.
⁷ **Smell and Nose.** I I Sore pain and swollen feeling in r.
          nostril, painful on pressure.
          ▮Mucous polyp of r. side, very large, and distending nose.
          ▮Polypus of r. nostril, growing more rapidly after each
          attack of headache, which was > by camphor.
⁸ **Upper Face.** Small pustules on face.
¹¹ **Taste and Tongue.** Sour taste.
          Tongue coated white.
¹² **Inner Mouth.** Fetid odor from mouth.
¹⁴ **Appetite, Thirst. Desires, Aversions.** Little appetite,
          with much thirst.
          ▮Thirst, drinks a sip at a time for want of breath.
¹⁷ **Scrobiculum and Stomach.** I I Faintlike weakness about
          pit of stomach.
¹⁹ **Abdomen.** Violent colic, more in r. side of abdomen, > by
          emission of flatus.
          I I Stitching and sticking pain; abdomen swollen and very
          tender to touch; coldness of lower extremities; numb
          and stiff feeling of affected parts, as if they were made
          of wood. θPeritonitis.
²⁰ **Stool and Rectum.** ▮Diarrhœa after eating veal.
          Stools: watery; thin, fecal; bloody; soft or diarrhœa-like;
          sluggish; hard, like sheep dung.

Before stool: violent colic; urging.

During stool: cutting colic in whole intestinal canal; tenesmus.

After stool; cutting colic: tenesmus; burning and stinging in anus.

Frequent pressing in rectum.

In dysentery, after *Acon.*, when latter fails to remove cutting pain, great thirst and icy coldness of feet; followed well by *Nux*.

²¹ **Urinary Organs.** ▮Frequent urging to urinate, at first only a few drops, then usual stream.

▮Burning in urethra while urinating, and greatly diminished urine.

▮Profuse emission of urine, as clear as water. θDiabetes insipidus.

²² **Female Sexual Organs.** ▮▮Suppression of menses.

▮Menstrual blood black as ink, with much suffering.

▮Thin, white, mucous leucorrhœa, with pain in small of back, as if bruised.

²³ **Inner Chest and Lungs.** Violent stitch in upper part of sternum, from without inward, on l. side.

Stitches in middle of chest, extending to both sides and toward axilla, when walking (during menses).

Stitches in l. side of chest, toward back, and below l. mamma.

Sticking below short ribs of r. side, toward back, apparently behind liver.

▮Stitching pains in chest greatly impeding respiration.

▮Congestion to lungs in tuberculosis.

▮Severe stitches in l. side of chest in evening, causing shortness of breath; severe cough, with expectoration of blood; synochal fever; full, hard and quick pulse; heaviness and dulness of head; delayed, hard stool; red or turbid urine; great and constant thirst. θLung affections.

▮Pneumonia, with excessive heat and thirst, > by copious perspiration and profuse hemorrhage.

▮Relapse induced by exposure; distressing dyspnœa; cannot lie with head low; wants to be fanned to keep from suffocating; thirst, drinks only sip at time for want of breath; pulse rapid; cough, with purulent expectoration. θPneumonia.

▮Severe, acute pains in chest, cutting like a knife, and shooting from centre of sternum to armpit and sides of chest below; cough and expectoration. θSuppressed syphilis.

▮Oppression of chest in phthisical subjects, when constant irritation to cough and expectoration, often bloody in character, causes an evening fever with hot hands and cheeks.

❙Useful in all stages of phthisis, but particularly for acute exacerbations with much cough, dull headache and severe pain in chest; cough caused by tickling in middle of chest, very severe, taking away breath, with audible palpitation of heart, expectoration often mixed with coagulated blood.

⁰ Heart, Pulse and Circulation. ❙Acute rheumatism, with endocarditis.

³² Upper Limbs. Pimples on r. forearm, discharge water when scratched.

Boil at lower part of thumb.

³¹ Limbs in General. ❙Anthrodynia in several joints.

Formication in hands and feet.

³⁵ Rest. Position. Motion. Cannot lie with head low, on account of dyspnœa.

Standing: vertigo.

Sitting down: vertigo >; debility <.

Rising: headache on vertex.

Walking: stitches in middle of chest.

Gentle motion: debility >.

³⁶ Nerves. Debility felt more when sitting than during gentle motion.

³⁷ Sleep. Sleep restless, with nightmare.

Insomnia after midnight; light morning sleep.

❙❙On awaking, pain in small of back.

³⁸ Time. Aggravation: 3 A.M.

Morning: vertigo; light sleep.

Evening: severe stitches in l. chest; fever with hot hands and cheeks.

After midnight: insomnia.

⁴² Locality and Direction. Right: sore pain and swollen feeling in nostril; mucous polyp in side of nostril; violent colic more in side of abdomen; sticking below short ribs; pimples on forearm.

Left: violent stitches on side of sternum; or stitch in side of chest.

From without inward: violent stitch in sternum.

⁴³ Sensations. As if parts of whole body were made of wood.

Pain: in small of back; in vertex.

Severe pain: in chest.

Cutting: pains in chest; colic, in intestinal canal.

Shooting pains: from centre of sternum to armpit and sides of chest below.

Violent stitch: in upper part of sternum.

Stitches: in middle of chest; in l. side of chest and below mamma.

Stitching and sticking pains in abdomen.
Sticking: below short ribs of r. side.
Violent colic: in r. side of abdomen.
Burning and stinging: in anus.
Burning: in urethra.
Sore pain: in r. nostril.
Pressing: in rectum.
Constriction: in abdomen.
Swollen feeling: in r. nostril.
Heaviness and dulness: of head.
Faintlike weakness: about pit of stomach.
Numb and stiff feeling: of affected parts.
Tickling: in middle of chest.
Formication: in hands and feet.
Coldness: of lower extremities.

" **Tissues.** ▪Acute rheumatism, with endocarditis.

" **Touch. Passive Motion. Injuries.** Touch: abdomen very tender.
Pressure: nostril painful.

" **Skin.** Vesicles full of thin yellow fluid.

" **Stages of Life, Constitution.** Asthmatic constitutions.
Girl; polypus.
Man, æt. 35, syphilitic subject; pains in chest.
Woman, æt. 72; pneumonia.

" **Relations.** Compare: *Lycop.* in lung affections; *Canthar.* and *Camphora* in renal diseases

KALI PERMANGANICUM.

Permanganate of Potash.   2 $KMnO_4$.

Proved by H. C. Allen. See Allen's Encyclopedia, vol. 5, p. 351.

CLINICAL AUTHORITIES.—*Ulcerated throat,* Woodgate, Hom. Rev., vol. 12, pp. 151, 152; *Diphtheria* (2 cases), Sprague, A. H. O., vol. 4, p. 360; Allen, A. H. O., vol. 3, p. 352; Nichol, Œhme's Therap., p. 45; B. J. H., vol. 34, p. 336.

[13] **Throat.** ∎Sanious discharge from nares.
∎Tonsils and soft palate swollen and inflamed; patches of whitish ulceration on tonsils; pain in swallowing; glands of neck tender. θUlcerated throat.
∎Tonsils swollen, and on each patches of ulceration of yellowish color; much pain internally and externally.
∎Diphtheria, with ulceration, and gangrenous suppuration with fetid odor.
∎Violent headache; throat swollen and painful, profuse salivation; cervical glands swollen and painful; fauces covered with peculiar wash leather, greyish membrane; breath offensive from beginning, and thin, watery, sanious fluid escaping from nares excoriating upper lip; dark colored offensive diarrhœa; vomiting; fluids taken by mouth return through nose; general prostration. θDiphtheria.
∎Comatose state; prostration extreme; nares completely plugged, fetor intolerable; pulse intermitting. θDiphtheria.
∎Pharynx swollen very much and covered with a yellowish membrane; high fever; unable to speak or swallow; pulse 135; furred tongue; fetid breath. θDiphtheria.
∎Pharynx covered with yellowish pseudo-membrane, not very firmly attached; extreme fetor of breath; inability to swallow; pulse 140 and feeble; great prostration. θDiphtheria.
∎Underneath a fetid, scablike membrane considerable erosion of mucous membrane. θDiphtheria.
∎Odor of breath unbearable; fluids taken by mouth returned by nose; general and excessive prostration; great dyspnœa; foul diphtheritic exudations all over fauces.
[27] **Cough.** ∎∎Expectoration very fetid.
[47] **Stages of Life, Constitution.** Girl, æt 3; diphtheria. Girl, æt. 6, suffering one week; diphtheria.

Girl, æt. 7; diphtheria.
Girl, æt. 9, stout build; diphtheria.
Girl, æt. 16; ulcerated throat.
Woman, æt. 25, cook; ulcerated throat.

KALI PHOSPHORICUM.

Phosphate of Potash. K_2HPO_4.

One of the constituents of the human body, obtainable from calcined bones.
Also obtained by adding carbonate of potassium to dilute phosphoric acid.
One of the Twelve Tissue Remedies, introduced by Schuessler.
This valuable medicine needs proving on the healthy; so far we have but the
suggestions of Schuessler, and results of limited clinical experience.

CLINICAL AUTHORITIES.—*Mental alienation*, Amberg, Schuessler's Tissue Rem-
edies, p. 70; *Melancholia religiosa*, Amberg, Schuessler; *Headache*, Wesselhœft,
Schuessler, p. 29; *Neuralgia of face*, Wesselhœft, Schuessler, p. 29; *Stomatitis*, Rapp,
Schuessler, p. 43; *Cholerine*, Schuessler, p. 84; *Enuresis*, Crowell, Schuessler, p. 64;
Amberg, Allg. Hom. Ztg., vol. 103, p. 84; *Asthma*, Rapp, Schuessler, p. 63.

¹ **Mind.** ❚Loss of memory, or weak memory.
  ❙❙Quiet delirium. θDysentery. θPneumonia.
  ❙❙Delirium tremens; horrors of drunkards; fear, sleeplessness, restlessness and suspicion; rambling talk; endeavors to grasp or avoid visionary images.
  ❚Says she is eternally and irretrievably damned; continually weeping and crying, wringing her hands, pulling
   to pieces and tearing her clothing, as well as bed covering; does not recognize her surroundings; no sleep;
   staring eyes; often must be held by two persons; food
   and medicine must be forcibly administered. θMelancholia religiosa.
  ❙❙Anxiety, nervous dread without special cause, gloomy
   moods, fancies, taking dark views of things, dark forebodings.
  ❚Melancholia and other similar ailments, which arise from
   deranged mental function, caused by overstrain of mind,
   or from exhausting drainings affecting nerve centres of
   spinal cord.
  ❙❙Sighing or moaning, also when occurring during sleep.
  ❙❙Whining and fretful disposition in children and adults.
  ❚Crying or screaming in children, from undue sensitiveness.
  ❙❙Hysterical fits of laughter and crying; yawning.

I I Shyness, excessive blushing, from undue sensitiveness.
I I Vexation, restlessness and irritability.
I Easily frightened, and inclined to fear.
I Depression of spirits and lassitude.
I Profound hypochondria and melancholia, weariness of
    life and fear of death, suspiciousness, weeping mood.
I I Dread of noise, oversensitiveness to noise and light.
I I Homesickness, morbid activity of memory, haunted by
    visions of past, and longing after them.

² Sensorium. I Concussion of brain.
    I I Nervous vertigo; cerebral anæmia.

³ Inner Head. I Excruciating nervous headache, with great
    sensitiveness to noise, during menses.
    I I Pains and weight at back of head, with feeling of weari-
    ness and exhaustion.
    I Headache of students; brain fag from overwork.
    I I Headache > by motion.
    I I Softening of brain; early stage; hydrocephalus.
    I I Brain affections with diarrhœa smelling like carrion.

⁵ Sight and Eyes. I I Weak sight; from exhausted condition
    of optic nerve; strabismus; after diphtheria.
    Excited, staring appearance of eyes.
    Drooping of eyelids.

⁶ Hearing and Ears. I I Deafness, from want of nervous per-
    ception, weakness, or exhaustion of auditory nerve.
    I Noises in ears from nervous exhaustion; nervous roaring.
    I I Ulceration of membrana tympani and middle ear sup-
    purations, with foul discharge.
    I I Atrophic conditions of nerve.

⁷ Smell and Nose. I I Epistaxis; from predisposition or
    weakness; ozæna.
    I I Hay fever with nervous irritability.

⁶ Upper Face. I I Face livid and sunken, with hollow eyes.
    I Neuralgia in r. side of face, proceeding from hollow teeth,
    > by cold applications.
    I I Facial neuralgia; great weakness after attack.
    I I Loss of power in muscles of face, causing contortions, or
    an involuntary twist of mouth. θParalysis.

¹⁰ Teeth and Gums. I I Chattering of teeth, nervous.
    I I Toothache of highly nervous, delicate, pale, irritable,
    sensitive persons.
    I I Bright red border, easily bleeding gums; scorbutic.

¹¹ Taste and Tongue. I I Tongue: coated, like stale, brownish,
    liquid mustard; offensive breath; excessively dry in
    morning, feeling as if it would cleave to roof of mouth.

¹² Inner Mouth. I I Breath offensive, fetid; stomatitis.
    I I Gums spongy and receding.
    I Noma.

[13] **Throat.** I I Diphtheria, with marked, putrid, gangrenous condition, and fearful stench from mouth; malignant.

[14] **Appetite, Thirst. Desires, Aversions.** I I Excessive hungry feeling, soon after eating, caused by nervous depression or weakness.

[16] **Hiccough, Belching, Nausea and Vomiting.** I Inordinate appetite; wants to eat almost every hour; very tired and enervated.

[17] **Scrobiculum and Stomach.** I I Sweat during meals, with feeling of weakness at pit of stomach; "gone sensation."
I I Indigestion with great nervous depression; faint feeling.
I I Inflammation of stomach; failing strength, dryness of tongue.

[18] **Hypochondria.** I I Affection of spleen; leucæmia lienalis.

[19] **Abdomen.** I I Flatulence with distress about heart.
I I Inflammatory colic of horses with incipient gangrene.
I I Abdominal herniæ and prolapsus; in weak persons.

[20] **Stool and Rectum.** I I Diarrhœa: painless, watery; with heavy odor; occasioned by fright and other causes depressing and exhausting nerves; putrid, carrionlike stools; great prostration.
I I Delirium, dryness of tongue, tympanites; carrionlike odor of discharges; dysentery; pure blood is discharged.
I Stools: like rice water; offensive, ichorous; pure blood.
I Vomiting and diarrhœa; painful cramps in calves; rice water stools. θCholera.
I I Cholera (second stage) caused by affection of nerves of intestinal canal.
I Putrid and typhoid dysentery.

[21] **Urinary Organs.** I I Bright's disease; depressed condition of nerves; sleeplessness, irritability, weary feeling.
I I Diabetes; nervous weakness; breath peculiar, with haylike odor, thirst, emaciation, often voracious hunger, all consequent on liver derangement.
I I Inflammation of bladder; asthenic condition.
I I Catarrh of bladder; vomiting, paleness of face, loss of strength and dryness of tongue.
I I Paralysis of sphincter, inability to retain urine, generally of old people.
I Incontinence of urine, from paralysis of sphincter.
I Obstinate enuresis; general weakness.

[22] **Male Sexual Organs.** I I Phagedenic chancre; balanitis.

[23] **Female Sexual Organs.** I I Catamenia: premature and profuse in nervous subjects; too scanty; too profuse, with heavy odor, dark red, or blackish red, thin and not coagulating.
I I Amenorrhœa, retention or delay of monthly flow, with depression of spirits, lassitude, and general nervous debility.

²¹ **Pregnancy. Partutition. Lactation.** Labor pains: feeble and ineffectual; spurious.

ııMastitis, pus brownish, dirty looking, with heavy odor; adynamic condition; gangrenous, bad colored, bad smelling pus.

ııChildbed fever with absurd notions or mania.

ııSecond stage of puerperal fever.

²³ **Voice and Larynx. Trachea and Bronchia.** ııSpeech slow, becoming inarticulate; creeping paralysis.

ııRecent paralysis of vocal cords.

ııHoarseness from overexertion of voice.

ııCroup, last stage; extreme weakness, pale or livid countenance.

²¹ **Respiration.** ııNervous asthma with depression; asthma after most moderate use of food; asthma with sallow features, sunken eyes, emaciation.

ıShortness of breath; asthmatic when going up stairs.

²⁷ **Cough.** ıWhooping cough in highly nervous patients, or great exhaustion.

²⁸ **Inner Chest and Lungs.** ıPain in lower part of l. thorax, < on coughing; slight catarrhal cough; tongue dry; pulse frequent, small and intermittent; no appetite; great weakness.

ııŒdema pulmonum; dyspnœa, spasmodic cough, with expectoration of frothy, serous masses; lassitude and prostration; livid countenance.

²⁹ **Heart, Pulse and Circulation.** ııPalpitation: from nervous causes; on ascending, with shortness of breath; with nervousness, anxiety; with sleeplessness.

ıIntermittent action of heart: with morbid, nervous sensitiveness; from violent emotions, grief, care.

ııFainting, from weak action of heart.

ııPulse intermittent, irregular.

ııSluggish circulation, in sensitive, nervous subjects; to strengthen heart's action.

³¹ **Neck and Back.** ıSpinal anæmia from exhausting diseases.

ıSoftening of spinal cord, loss of power, stumbles and trips.

ıParalytic or rheumatic lameness, stiffness after rest, > by gentle motion.

³³ **Lower Limbs.** ııRheumatic or neuralgic affections of sciatic nerve, > from motion.

ıFor two days drawing, laming pain in sole of foot; affected place size of silver dollar, bluish.

ııChilblains, if recent.

³⁴ **Limbs in General.** ııParalyzing pain in limbs, > by motion and external warmth.

³⁵ **Rest. Position. Motion.** During rest: tearing, paralytic pains <.

After rest: stiffness; severe rheumatism.

Rising: neuralgic pains <; paralytic pains <.

Beginning to move: paralytic pains <.

Motion: headache >; rheumatic affection >; paralytic pains >.

Gentle exercise: neuralgic pains >; stiffness >; rheumatism >.

Going up stairs: shortness of breath.

" Nerves. I IStarting on being touched, or at sudden noises.

I IUndue irritability, after exhausting diarrhœa or long continued use of purgatives.

I IDisposition to feel bodily pains too acutely.

I Nervous attacks, from sudden or intense emotion, or from smothering passion; in highly nervous and excitable persons; also feeling as of a ball rising in throat.

I IFits, from fright, with pallid or livid countenance.

I ISpasmodic attacks; face pale and sunken, body and limbs cold, violent palpitation θEpilepsy.

I INervous affections, when occurring without reasonable causes, such as impatience, irritability, dwelling upon grievances, merriment becoming oppressive, shedding tears about trifles, making mountains out of mole hills.

I Neuralgia, much reduced constitutions, paralyzing pains.

I INeuralgic pains, > with gentle exercise, < on rising.

I Sciatica.

I Paroxysms of pain followed by great weakness.

I IFeeling of faintness; lassitude and palpitation.

I General debility, with nervousness and irritability.

I IAdynamic typhoid condition.

I ICollapse, with livid countenance and low pulse.

' ITearing, paralytic pains in nerves, most during rest, > from motion without exertion, especially felt after rising from sitting, or on beginning to move.

I ILameness: recent, paralytic, from exhaustion of nerves, with stiffness after rest, yielding to gentle exercise; rheumatic; rigidity of muscles.

I Creeping paralysis; course of disease slow; tendency to wasting, with loss of sense of touch.

I IShock of paralysis, with morbid sensibility, or a bruised and painful feeling in part affected, or rigidity of paralyzed limbs.

I Paralysis dependent on exhaustion of nerve power in recent cases, as after diphtheria.

I IParalytic states, nasal voice, strabismus, etc., after diphtheria.

I IAtrophic paralysis.

I IInfantile paralysis recent, and if connected with teething.

I ISoftening of spinal cord, idiopathic, with gradual deadening of nerves.

" Sleep. I IYawning: excessive, unnatural; hysterical.

ı ıSleeplessness: after worry or excitement; from nervous
causes; simple wakefulness.

ı ıNight terrors, in children awakening with fright and
screaming; somnambulism.

ı ıNoises in head on falling asleep, feeling as if a rocket had
passed through head.

³⁸ Time. Morning: tongue dry; rheumatism.

³⁹ Temperature and Weather. External warmth: > paralytic pain in limbs.

Cold applications: neuralgia >.

⁴⁰ Fever. ı ıTyphus or typhoid fevers; haggard face, pulse
whizzing or very small.

ı Ileo-typhus.

ı ıIntermittent fever; sweat profuse and exhausting, fetid.

ı ıIn yellow fever; if *Carbo veg.* is not sufficient.

ıExcessive, exhausting, strong smelling sweats.

⁴¹ Attacks, Periodicity. Almost every hour: wants to eat.

For two days: drawing, laming pain in sole of foot.

⁴² Locality and Direction. Right: neuralgia of face.

Left: pain in lower part of thorax.

⁴³ Sensations. As if tongue would cleave to roof of mouth;
as of a ball rising in throat; as if a rocket had passed
through head.

Pains: at back of head; in lower part of l. thorax.

Lancinating nervous headache.

Tearing, paralytic pains: in nerves.

Paralyzing pain: in limbs.

Painful cramps: in calves.

Drawing, laming pains: in sole of foot.

Rheumatic or neuralgic affections: of sciatic nerve.

Neuralgia: in r. side of face.

Bruised and painful feeling: in part affected.

Dryness: of tongue.

Weight: at back of head.

⁴⁴ Tissues. ı ıFunction of brain cells depressed. θAfter concussion.

All ailments which arise from or denote a want of nerve
power; hence nervous prostration, exhaustion, nervous
rigors; also all affections in which brain, and conse-
quently mind, shows want of vigor.

ı ıInsanity, mania or other mental derangement; from
exhausted or depressed condition of brain or nerve cells,
showing itself in perverted function.

ı ıAnæmia or leucæmia, caused by long lasting mental
depression, poverty of blood from continuous influences
depressing mind or nerves.

ıToo rapid decay of blood corpuscles.

ıHemorrhages; blood not coagulating, thin, blackish or
light red.

⦁Septic hemorrhages; stench from mouth and stomach; discharges smelling like carrion; putrid gangrene; prostration.

⦁Scorbutus, gangrene, noma or stomatitis, gangrenous angina, phagedenic chancre, offensive, carrionlike diarrhœa, adynamic or typhoid conditions.

⦁Fatty metamorphosis in muscular fibres.

ı ıAtrophy, wasting disease, putrid smelling stools.

ı ıRheumatism, acute and chronic, with pains disappearing on moving about, severe in morning after rest, and on first rising from sitting position.

⦁Rachitis with atrophy; profuse, discolored, foul smelling diarrhœa; violent thirst; sometimes discolored vomiting; brown covering of teeth, etc.

ı ıSuppurations, dirty, foul, ichorous fetid matter.

ı ıCancer, encephaloid, medullary, soft (brainlike convolutions), chiefly occurring in young.

⦁Noma.

ı ıChancre, phagedenic.

ı ıPurpura hemorrhagica.

⁴⁵ Touch. Passive Motion. Injuries. Touch: causes him to start.

Mechanical injuries: ichorous discharge, gangrene.

⁴⁶ Skin. ı ıUrticaria.

ı ıVesicles; with bloody ichorous contents.

ı ıGreasy, offensive smelling crusts or scales.

ı ıSkin diseases with bad smelling discharge.

⦁Scarlet fever: putrid condition of throat; typhoidal.

ı ıSmallpox; adynamia and decomposition of blood.

⦁Offensive ulcers; bad colored, ichorous, bad smelling.

ı ıPemphigus malignus.

⁴⁷ Stages of Life, Constitution. Pale, sensitive, irritable persons.

Atrophic conditions in old people.

Girl, æt. 7; enuresis.

Woman, æt. 33, pale and thin; neuralgia of face.

Woman, æt. 44, formerly neither inclined to piety nor fanaticism; melancholia religiosa.

Man, æt. 60; enuresis.

Man, æt. 80; mental alienation.

⁴⁸ Relations. Compare: *Arsen., Baptis., Carbo veg., China, Ignat., Kreos., Laches., Mur. ac., Phosphor., Phytol., Pulsat., Rhus tox.*

Compatible: *Cyclam.,* disordered mental conditions; *Kali mur.,* in puerperal fever; *Magnes. phos.,* bladder troubles; *Zinc. phos.,* incipient paralysis of brain, with nephritic irritation; *Natr. mur., Nitr. ac.,* hemorrhages.

After weakening diseases, mushrooms, by virtue of containing *Kali phos.,* rapidly restore muscle and nerve tissue.

KALI SULPHURICUM.

Sulphate of Potash. $K_2 SO_4$.

One of the Twelve Tissue Remedies introduced by Schuessler. Needs proving.

CLINICAL AUTHORITIES.— *Vertigo*, Schlegelmann, Schuessler's Biochem., p. 75; *Falling off of hair*, Wesselhœft, Schuessler's Tissue Remedies, p. 27; *Ear affection*, Wesselhœft, Schüssler's Tissue Remedies, p. 25; *Disease of antrum Highmori*, Wesselhœft, Schuessler's Tissue Remedies, p. 26; *Ozœna*, Wesselhœft, Schuessler's Tissue Remedies, p. 27; *Whooping cough*, Wesselhœft, Schuessler's Tissue Remedies, p. 25; *Whooping cough*, Knerr, Schuessler's Tissue Remedies, p. 26; *Chorea* (13 cases), Cattell, B. J. H., vol. 11, p. 343; *Articular rheumatism*, Schlegelmann, Schuessler's Biochem., p. 75; *Epithelioma* (2 cases), Orth, Schuessler's Biochem., p. 68; *Itch eruption in children*, Cattell, B. J. H., vol. 11, p. 352; *Ivy poisoning* (Rhus tox.), Wesselhœft, Schuessler's Tissue Remedies, p. 26.

² Sensorium. ❙Dreadful vertigo, especially on rising from lying, on standing from sitting, and when looking upwards; every moment in fear of falling and dare not leave her room.

³ Inner Head. ❘❘Rheumatic headache, < in warm room and in evening, > in open air.

⁴ Outer Head. ❘❘Great pain on moving head from side to side or backwards; can move it forward without pain.
❙Yellow scales (dandruff) on scalp.
❙Bald spot as large as a silver dollar on l. side of head; hair falls out easily when combing, all over head, also hair of beard. θAfter gonorrhœa.
❙Copious scaling of scalp, moist and sticky.
❙Yellow dandruff.

⁵ Sight and Eyes. ❘❘Purulent or yellow mucus in eye diseases.
❙Catarrh of conjunctiva, with yellow secretion.
❘❘Ophthalmia neonatorum.
❙Eyelids, with thin, yellow crusts.
❙Discharge from eyes yellow, slimy, or sticky watery.
❘❘Cataract.

⁶ Hearing and Ears. ❙Deafness caused by catarrh and swelling of Eustachian tube and middle ear.
❙Watery, mattery discharge from ear; yellow slimy tongue.
❙Secretion of thin, yellow, sticky fluid after inflammation.
❙Brown offensive secretion from r. ear; polypoid excrescence closes meatus near opening; entirely deaf in r. ear for eight weeks.

∎Stinking otorrhœa of four years' standing.

Smell and Nose. ∎Taste and smell lost. *θ*Ozæna.

∎Coryza, yellow mucous discharge.

∎Thick, yellow, offensive discharge, alternating with watery discharge for eighteen months; l. nostril <; catamenia every three weeks; takes cold easily. *θ*Ozæna.

∎About once a week a thick, dark brown, semi-fluid accumulation of pus formed in upper l. nostril, on being blown out emitted a terrible stench; about a month previous a piece of carious bone was taken from antrum Highmori, through an upper l. alveolus, from which a tooth had been drawn four years previous.

∎Old catarrh with yellowish viscous secretion.

⁸ **Upper Face.** ∎Faceache, < in warm room and in evening; > in cool or open air.

∣∣Epithelioma on r. cheek, extending from lower eyelid to ala nasi; size of a silver dollar; ulcerating stage; indurated base and wall-like, hard, elevated edges (greatly improved).

∎Epithelioma, size of half dollar, situated on r. side of nose just under canthus of eye; eye sympathetically affected, either through extension of disease process, or through irritating discharge, entrance of which was facilitated by a slight destruction of edge of lower lid at canthus; conjunctivitis palpebrarum et bulbi, with haziness of cornea.

⁹ **Lower Face.** ∣∣Blistered lips and mouth. *θ*Whooping cough.

∣∣Lower lip swollen. *θ*Epithelioma.

¹⁰ **Teeth and Gums.** ∎Toothache < in warm room and toward evening, > in cool open air.

¹¹ **Taste and Tongue.** ∣∣Loss of taste. *θ*Ozæna.

∣∣Insipid, pappy taste.

∎Tongue: coated with yellow mucus; yellow, slimy, sometimes with whitish edge.

¹⁷ **Scrobiculum and Stomach.** ∎Sensation of faintness at stomach, and befogged feeling in head, fearing to lose her reason.

∣∣Pressure and feeling of fulness in stomach with a yellow mucous coating on tongue.

∣∣Indigestion, with sensation of pressure as of a load, and fulness at pit of stomach. *θ*Dyspepsia.

∣∣Chronic catarrh of stomach; yellow, slimy coated tongue.

∎Catarrh of stomach and duodenum, with a yellow coated tongue; jaundice from it.

¹⁹ **Abdomen.** ∎Gastro-duodenal catarrh; jaundice.

∎Hard and tympanitic abdomen. *θ*Whooping cough.

²⁰ **Stool and Rectum.** ∣∣Diarrhœa: yellow, slimy or watery mattery stools.

❙Black, thin, offensive stools. θWhooping cough.

❙Habitual constipation with coated tongue.

❙Hemorrhoids with catarrh of stomach and yellow, mucus coated tongue.

²² **Male Sexual Organs.** ❙Gonorrhœa of glans or urethra; discharge purulent, yellow mucous, or greenish.

❙Orchitis after suppression of gonorrhœa.

❙Gleet.

²³ **Female Sexual Organs.** ❙Menstruation, too late and too scanty, with a feeling of weight and fulness in abdomen.

❙❙Catamenia every three weeks. θOzæna.

❙❙Headache during catamenia.

❙❙Metrorrhagia.

❙Leucorrhœa yellowish, or watery mattery.

²⁵ **Voice and Larynx. Trachea and Bronchia.** ❙❙Hoarseness after taking cold.

❙Bronchitis, if mucus is distinctly yellow and slimy, thin, or watery mattery and profuse.

❙Yellow mucus coughed up without great exertion. θBronchitic asthma.

²⁷ **Cough.** ❙Whooping cough, with retching, without vomiting; inflammatory catarrhal stage; decidedly yellow, slimy expectoration.

❙Last stage of whooping cough; blistered lips and mouth; black, thin, offensive stools five times a day, hard, tympanitic abdomen; wasted to a shadow, given up to die.

❙Coarse râles; cannot cough up large amount of mucus. θPneumonia.

❙Yellow mucous expectoration.

²⁸ **Inner Chest and Lungs.** ❙Inflammation of lungs, with wheezing; if yellow, loose rattling phlegm be coughed up with difficulty, or sputa consist of watery matter.

❙❙Pneumonia with coarse râles, cannot cough up mucus.

³¹ **Neck and Back.** ❙❙Pains in back, nape of neck, or in limbs; periodical < in evening, or in warm room; > in cool or open air.

❙Backache and pains in limbs; < in warm room and towards evening, > in cool open air.

❙❙Stiff neck, head inclined towards l.; shoulder raised.

³² **Upper Limbs.** ❙❙Eruption in l. axilla, about neck and on back of both hands (Rhus poisoning).

❙Scaly eruption mostly on arms, > from hot water.

³³ **Lower Limbs.** ❙Varicose ulcer on r. leg just above instep, after kick of a horse three years ago; eight inches in circumference, concave, dark blue, emitting a stinking odor.

³⁴ **Limbs in General.** Pain in limbs.

Acute and wandering rheumatism of joints.

∎After being chilled while overheated, frightful pains in r. shoulder and violent fever; pains leave shoulder and attack l. knee, then go from joint to joint, and again several joints affected at a time; maddening pains, unceasing, day and night. θArticular rheumatism.

∎Pains passing from joint to joint; serous exudations.

³⁵ Rest. Position. Motion. Rising from lying: dreadful vertigo.

Sitting: dreadful vertigo.

Standing: dreadful vertigo.

Moving head from side to side or backwards: great pain.

³⁶ Nerves. ∎Chorea.

³⁷ Sleep. ∣∣Very vivid dreams.

³⁸ Time. Evening: rheumatic headache <; faceache <; toothache <; pains in back and limbs <.

³⁹ Temperature and Weather. Pains grow < in warm room and in evening; > in open, cool air.

Hot water: scaly eruption on arms >.

Warm room: rheumatic headache <; faceache <; toothache <; pains in back, neck and limbs <.

After being chilled while overheated: frightful pains in r. shoulder.

Open air: rheumatic headache >; faceache >; toothache >; pains in back, neck and limbs >.

Cold water: eruption >.

⁴⁰ Fever. ∣∣Intermittent fever with yellow, slimy coated tongue.

∎Rheumatic fever; pains shifting, wandering.

⁴¹ Attacks, Periodicity. Five times a day: black, thin, offensive stools.

Periodical pains: in back, neck and limbs < in evening.

About once a week: a thick, dark brown semi-fluid accumulation of pus formed in upper l. nostril.

Every three weeks: catamenia.

For eight weeks: entirely deaf in r. ear.

For eight months: effects of ivy poisoning.

For eighteen months: thick, yellow, offensive discharge from nose.

Four years' standing: stinking otorrhœa.

⁴² Locality and Direction. Right: brown offensive secretion from ear; entirely deaf for eight weeks; epithelioma on cheek; epithelioma on side of nose; varicose ulcer on leg just above instep; frightful pains in shoulder.

Left: bald spot on side of head; a thick dark brown semi-fluid accumulation of pus formed in upper nostril; a piece of carious bone was taken from antrum Highmori through an upper alveolus; head inclined to shoulder; eruption in axilla; pains leave shoulder and attack knee.

⁴³ Sensations. Pressure as of a load: at pit of stomach.

Pains: in back; nape of neck; in limbs.

Maddening pains: in joints.

Frightful pains: in r. shoulder; in l. knee; from joint to
joint.

Great pain: in head.

Acute and wandering rheumatism of joints.

Rheumatic headache.

Pressure: in stomach.

Feeling of fulness: in stomach; at pit of stomach; in
abdomen.

Befogged feeling: in head.

Faintness: at stomach.

Burning, itching papular eruption.

Itching pimples arising singly on skin.

" **Tissues.** ।।Its sphere of action is in lymphatic vessels;
when there is a lack of this substance, a yellow mucous
catarrh arises or a yellow sticky discharge from isolated
places on membranes.

Secretions from mucous membranes yellowish; green.

Catarrhs, colds, with yellow, slimy secretions or expectoration of watery matter.

Inflammations, with yellow, slimy or serous secretions.

In third stage of inflammation, resolution, when a yellow
mucous discharge occurs.

Effusions, watery mattery; favors resorption.

Fungoid inflammation of joints; white swelling.

।Migratory rheumatism of joints.

।।Wasted to a shadow.   θWhooping cough.

Epithelioma; soft polypi.

Ailments accompanied by desquamation, peeling off
skin, or with itching pimples arising singly on skin.

" **Touch.   Passive Motion.   Injuries.** After kick of a
horse three years ago: varicose ulcer on r. leg.

" **Skin.** ।।Jaundice caused by gastro-duodenal catarrh.

।Suppressed rash of measles or other eruptive diseases,
with harsh and dry skin.

।।Abundant scaling of epidermis.

।।Promotes desquamation after erysipelas; accelerates removal of scabs in smallpox.

।।Scarlet fever; stage of desquamation.

।Burning, itching, papular eruption exuding puslike
moisture.

।Recurring eruption of fine red pimples running together,
presenting a red, swollen appearance; a thoroughly
alkaline fluid oozes out copiously; after subsiding cuticle comes off in fine scales; itches and stings intensely
>; formerly by cold water, lately by hot.

।Scurfs, scaling, chapping.

Sores on skin, with yellow, sticky secretions on limited portions, or discharges of thin, watery matter, sometimes with peeling of surrounding skin.

I I Epithelial cancer, discharge thin, yellow, serous.

I Eczema, or skin affections; discharge decidedly yellow, slimy, sometimes sticky or watery mattery; when suddenly suppressed.

I Effects of ivy poisoning (Rhus tox.) for eight months; , repeatedly broke out with small, hard, herpetic vesicles, forming a thin scab, with itching and some moisture; eruption appears in l. axilla, about neck and on back of both hands; she has a sensation of faintness at stomach and befogged feeling in head, fearing to lose her reason; very vivid dreams.

I I Nettlerash, with or without yellow, slimy tongue, generally caused by indigestion.

I Itch eruption in children.

I Chafing of children.

I Diseased condition of nails, shown in interrupted growth.

⁴⁷ **Stages of Life, Constitution.** Child, æt. 18 months; whooping cough.

Boy, æt. 10, small, dark, lean; whooping cough.

Girl, æt. 19, light complexion, scrofulous; ear affection.

Woman, æt. 25, single, dark complexion, suffering eight months; ivy poisoning (Rhus tox.).

Woman, æt. 25, married, dark complexion; ozæna.

Man, æt. 26, healthy, powerful; articular rheumatism.

Man, æt. 27, dark; falling off of hair, after gonorrhœa.

Man, æt. 30, light complexion; disease of antrum Highmori.

Man, æt. 33, light complexion; ozæna.

Woman, æt. 54; vertigo.

Man, æt. 55, factory operative, ulcer on side of nose for four years, at first there was a somewhat reddened spot which was moderately elevated, and which became afterward covered with a horny crust, which later, dropping off, left an ulcer which steadily increased in depth and breadth; epithelioma.

Widow, æt 70, suffering for years; epithelioma.

⁴⁸ **Relations.** Compare: *Kali mur.*, in deafness, hoarseness, pertussis; *Natr. mur.*, in deafness, pains in stomach, coarse râles, profuse exudations.

Compatible: *Acet. ac.*, in itching and redness of skin; *Arsen., Calc. ostr., Hepar, Pulsat., Rhus tox., Sepia, Silica, Sulphur.*

KAOLIN.

Porcelain or China Clay.   *Alumina Silicata.*

CLINICAL AUTHORITIES.—*Croup*, Searle, Elliott, A. II. O., vol. 8, p. 128;
Lilienthal, Raue's Rec., 1871, p. 80; Searle, Elliott, Parker, Raue's Rec., 1872, p.
106; Landesmann, Raue's Rec., 1870, p. 171; Boyce, Times Retros., vol. 3, p. 29.

[7] **Smell and Nose.** ❚Nostrils feel sore; scabs form in nose;
scanty and blood streaked secretion.

[13] **Throat.** ❚Membrane covering both sides of throat. θDiphtheria.

❚ Fever, headache in forehead, with flushed face and sore
throat; r. tonsil and arch of velum covered with heavy,
yellowish white membrane; breath fetid; great prostration. θDiphtheria. (In alternation with Bellad.)

[25] **Voice and Larynx. Trachea and Bronchia.** ❚Husky
voice, metallic, rasping breathing and suffocative cough.

❚Croupous inflammation in lower part of larynx or in
upper part of trachea.

❚Awoke from sleep with croupy cough; voice husky, later
sunk to whisper; sawing sound during both expiration
and inspiration; high fever. θCroup.

❚Voice a little husky; during night very feverish; next
day skin felt dry; wanted to be carried about; appetite
diminished; very little cough; on auscultation, metallic,
rasping sound increasing toward evening; suffocating
spells. θCroup.

❚Croup, with labored, sawing respiration, after failure of
Acon., Hepar, Spongia, Bromium, Phosphor. and Iodum.

❚Croup, after failure of Spongia.

[38] **Time.** Towards evening: metallic, rasping sound increased.
Night: very feverish.

[42] **Locality and Direction.** Right: tonsil and arch of velum
covered with heavy, yellowish white membrane.

[45] **Sensations.** Pain: in forehead.

Soreness: of nostrils; of throat.

Dryness: of skin.

[47] **Stages of Life, Constitution.** Boy, æt. 16 months, strong
and healthy parentage; croup.

Child, æt. 4; diphtheria.

Boy, æt. 4; croup.

Girl, æt. 5; croup.

Boy, æt. 5; croup.

Young woman, subject to repeated attacks; diphtheria.

KALMIA LATIFOLIA.

Mountain Laurel. *Ericaceæ.*

An evergreen shrub, found on rocky hills, flowering in May and June.
The tincture is prepared from the fresh leaves.

Introduced by Hering and proved by himself, Kummer, Behler, Bute, Clark, Haeseler, Williamson, Freitag, Reichelm and others. See Allen's Encyclopedia, vol. 5, p. 388.

CLINICAL AUTHORITIES.—*Sun headache*, Thayer, N. E. M. G., vol. 9, p. 149; *Retinitis albuminurica*, Allen, Norton's Oph. Therap., p. 107; *Sclero-choroiditis anterior*, Allen, Norton's Oph. Therap., p. 107; *Sclerotitis*, Boyle, Allg. Hom. Ztg., vol. 112, p. 77; *Neuralgia oculorum*, Johnson, A. H. O., vol. 1, p. 168; *Chronic sore throat*, Clifton, Times Retros., vol. 3, p. 29; *Pressure in epigastrium*, Hansen, Allg. Hom. Ztg., vol, 113, p. 62; *Gastralgia*, Clifton, Times Retros., vol. 3, p. 29; *Abdominal neuralgia* (5 cases), Cushing, Times Retros., vol. 2, p. 14; Ring, Raue's Rec., 1874, p. 260; *Bright's disease*, Macy, A. H. Rev., vol. 3, p. 364; *Angina pectoris*, Clifton, Times Retros., vol. 3, p. 29; *Endocarditis*, Dunham, Dunham's Lectures, p. 194; *Heart disease*, Hering, MSS.; Dunham, MSS.; Siegrist, Raue's Rec., 1875, p. 127; *False pleurisy*, Pretsch, A. H. Rev., vol. 1, p. 326; *Neuralgia*, Clifton, Times Retros., vol. 3, p. 29; Ball, N. A. J. H., vol. 3, p. 92; *Neuralgia of spine*, Sonnenschmidt, MSS.; *Acute articular rheumatism*, Clifton, Times Retros., vol. 3, p. 29; *Rheumatism*, Pretsch, A. H. Rev., vol. 1, pp. 325–6; Boyce, Org., vol. 1, p. 323.

[1] **Mind.** ❚In a recumbent posture, mental faculties and memory perfect, but on attempting to move, vertigo.
❚Anxiety with palpitation.
Toward evening and next forenoon very cross.

[2] **Sensorium.** ❚Vertigo: with headache, blindness, pains in limbs and weariness; while stooping and looking down.
❚Vertigo: with aching in face. θNeuralgia.
❚Giddiness, with headache and nausea.

[3] **Inner Head.** ❚Pulsating headache in forehead.
Pain in forehead in morning when waking, < after rising.
❚Aching in forehead, followed by rending in bones of r. or l. side of face; shooting downward into eye teeth; moving backward down neck and outwardly on both sides; succeeded by pain in l. shoulder; rending in bones of legs to feet.
❙❙Pain over r. eye; giddiness; eyes weak and watery.
❙❙Pressing pain on a small spot on r. side of head.
❚Headache internally, with sensation, when turning, of something loose in head, diagonally across top.

∎A cracking in head frightens him, it ends in a sound in ears like blowing a horn.

∎A shuddering without coldness commences with cracking as if surcharged with electricity.

∎Severe pressing headache, < and > with sun.

∎Sensation of heat in head in morning.

∎Dulness in head; headache; backache.

∎Neuralgic paroxysmal pains.

∎Headache < in evening and in open air.

⁴ Outer Head. ∎Pain from back of neck up over scalp to top of head and temples, also affecting face r. side; tender to touch; pain shooting twitching; sometimes in spots; > from cold, < from heat; every afternoon, last with great severity, through night. θNeuralgia.

∎Rheumatic pain in scalp.

⁵ Sight and Eyes. ∎Glimmering before eyes.

∎Everything black before eye when he looks downward; nausea and eructations of wind (in morning).

∎Dull, weak eyes.

∎Retinitis albuminurica, occurring during pregnancy; pains in back.

∎Nephritic retinitis accompanied by much pain in back, as if it would break.

∎Sclera inflamed, vitreous perfectly filled with exudation, and glimmering before eye, especially on reading with the other. θSclero-choroiditis anterior.

∎Sclerotitis, particularly in rheumatic subjects; eyeball painful on motion.

∎Parenchymatous keratitis.

∎Severe pain in r. eye, extending to forehead; commences at sunrise, < until noon; then > and leaves at sunset. θNeuralgia oculorum. (After *Acon.* and *Bellad.* failed.)

∎Pressure in r. eye (evening); also above r. eye.

∎Stitches in eyes, ears, fingers and feet.

∎Itching in eyes; when rubbing them they sting.

∎∎Pain in eyes, which makes it painful to turn them.

∎∎Sensation of stiffness in muscles around eyes, and of eyelids.

∎∎Asthenopia; stiff, drawing sensation in muscles upon moving eyes.

∎Eye symptoms < evening and in open air.

⁶ Hearing and Ears. ∎Stitches in and behind r. ear; in neck and thighs, at night.

∎Sound like blowing a horn, after cracking in head.

∎∎Meniére's disease.

⁷ Smell and Nose. ∎Coryza: with increased sense of smell; with sneezing, dulness, headache and hoarseness.

∎Tearing in root of nose and nasal bones, with nausea.

⁸ **Upper Face.** Face: red, with throbbing headache; pale. ■Anxious expression of countenance. *θ*Rheumatism of heart.

■Flushing of face, with vertigo. *θ*Neuralgia.

❘❘Pressing pains in r. side of face, especially between eye and nose.

■Prosopalgia, right sided; pains rending; agonizing; stupefying or threatening delirium.

■Fothergill's faceache.

■Severe neuralgia in r. cheek, with alkaline taste in mouth.

■Facial neuralgia, involving teeth of upper jaw, but not from caries.

■After exposure to cold, pains in r. side of head, ear and face, and even going down to arm, sometimes attended with numbness, or succeeded by numbness in parts affected; pains sticking, teasing, pressing, or shooting in a downward direction; pains occur at irregular times, continue for no definite period, coming suddenly or gradually, and leaving as uncertainly; < by worry or mental exertion; > by food. *θ*Neuralgia.

■Facial neuralgia after zoster.

❘❘Face itches at night.

❘❘Roughness of cheeks (during every Summer).

⁹ **Lower Face.** ■Lips swollen, dry and stiff.

❘❘Cracked lips with dry skin.

❘❘Stinging in jawbones.

❘❘Tired feeling in chewing muscles.

■Stitches and tearing in lower jaw.

¹⁰ **Teeth and Gums.** ■Teeth tender, with neuralgia of face. ■Pressing pain in molars, late in evening.

¹¹ **Taste and Tongue.** ❘❘Bitter taste with nausea, > after eating.

■Tongue: white, dry; sore l. side; hurts when talking.

■Stitches in tongue.

¹² **Inner Mouth.** ■Tingling in salivary glands, immediately after eating, with sense of fermentation in œsophagus and copious salivation.

■Sublingual salivary gland inflamed.

¹³ **Throat.** ■Throat feels swollen; sensation as if a ball was rising.

■Sensation of dryness in throat, difficult deglutition, thirst.

■Pressure in throat; stitches in eyes and nausea.

■Great dryness of throat, with aching pains, the dryness causing frequent cough. *θ*Chronic syphilitic sore throat.

¹⁵ **Eating and Drinking.** ■Pains > by food. *θ*Neuralgia.

¹⁶ **Hiccough, Belching, Nausea and Vomiting.** ■Eructations of wind. *θ*Angina pectoris. *θ*Gastralgia.

■Nausea, everything becomes black before eyes, pressure

in throat, incarcerated flatus, oppression of breathing,
rheumatic pains in limbs.

| | Wine relieves vomiting.

¹⁷ **Scrobiculum and Stomach.** ∎Pressure in pit of stomach,
like a marble; < sitting in a stooping position, > sitting erect; sensation as if something would be pressed
off below pit of stomach.

∎Pit of stomach sore to touch.

∎Pains < sitting bent, yet a feeling as if to do so was
necessary, > by sitting or standing upright; crampy
pain, with eructations of wind, palpitation of heart.
*θ*Gastralgia.

¹⁸ **Hypochondria.** ∎Pains in region of liver.

¹⁹ **Abdomen.** ∎Incarcerated flatus, with nausea.

∎Sensation of weakness in abdomen, extending to throat;
> by eructation.

∎Sudden pains in paroxysms, across abdomen above umbilicus, from lower border of liver, downward toward
left, then ceasing in r. side; < from motion and from
lying on either side, obliged to lie on back; > when
sitting up. *θ*Abdominal neuralgia.

∎Neuralgia of bowels in married women.

²⁰ **Stool and Rectum.** ∎Stool like mush, easily discharged,
as if glazed, followed by pressure on rectum.

∎Diarrhœa, with dulness, dizziness, weariness, nausea and
bellyache.

²¹ **Urinary Organs.** ∎Frequent micturition of large quanti-
ties of yellow urine.

∎Profuse micturition > headache.

∎Albuminuria; also with pains in lower limbs.

∎Abdomen greatly distended; extremities, especially lower
ones, swollen; much difficulty in standing and walking;
urine scanty, high colored, 5 per cent. albumen, fibrinous casts, large epithelial scales, one prismatic crystal
of triple phosphate; vertigo; occasional pain in head;
much pain in lower extremities; complexion sallow and
skin unnaturally dry. *θ*Bright's disease.

²² **Female Sexual Organs.** ∎Menses too soon; regular, but
painful.

∎During menses, pain in limbs, loins, back and interior
of thighs.

∎Suppressed menses, with severe neuralgic pains throughout whole body.

∎Leucorrhœa yellowish; one week after menses; symptoms < then.

²³ **Voice and Larynx. Trachea and Bronchia.** ∎Pressure
as if some one squeezed throat with thumb and finger.

∎Noise as from spasm in glottis when breathing.

| | Hoarseness, with coryza.

¶Tickling in trachea.

²⁶ **Respiration.** ¶Difficult and oppressed breathing; throat feels swollen, nausea. θRheumatism.

¶Oppressed and short breathed, which obliges him to breathe quickly, involuntarily.

¶Oppressed breathing, with palpitation of heart, anxiety.

¶Dyspnœa and pain. θAngina pectoris.

²⁷ **Cough.**. ¶Frequent cough, caused by dryness or scraping in throat.

¶Expectoration easy, smooth, grey; tasting putrid; saltish.

²⁸ **Inner Chest and Lungs.** ¶Feverish heat, with great pain in chest; < when breathing and from slightest motion.

¶Pain in chest as from a sprain.

¶Shooting through chest above heart into shoulder blade; pain in l. arm.

¶Stitches in lower part of chest.

²⁹ **Heart, Pulse and Circulation.** ¶Fluttering of heart.

¶Palpitation of heart, with anxiety and oppressed breathing; with faint feeling.

¶Palpitation up into throat, after going to bed; trembling all over; < lying on l. side; > lying on back; anxiety.

¶Palpitation, dyspnœa, pain in limbs, stitch in lower part of chest; right sided prosopalgia.

¶Heart's action very tumultuous, rapid and visible.

¶Attacks of angina pectoris. θFatty degeneration of heart.

¶Angina pectoris; slow, feeble pulse; eructations of wind, dyspnœa and pain.

¶Severe pain in cardiac region, with slow, small pulse. θHypertrophy with dilation and aortic obstruction.

¶¶Paroxysms of anguish about heart, dyspnœa, febrile excitement; rheumatic endocarditis, with consequent hypertrophy and valvular disease.

¶Pressure like a marble from epigastrium toward heart, with a strong, quick heart beat; every beat has a strumming as if it would burst, along sternum to throat; third or fourth beat harder, followed by an intermission.

¶Pressure behind middle of sternum, < morning and evening, and when stooping; palpitation of heart with anxiety; pulse regular; first sound of heart somewhat harsh; pressure behind sternum and in epigastrium, > sitting erect; as if something was being pressed away from under sternum.

¶Severe palpitation of heart, with constriction of throat, < from motion, deep inspiration, or holding breath; pressure and stitching in region of heart; severe one sided, tearing headache, < over eye and in bulbus oculi; during attack anxiety and shortness of breath; between

attacks, dry cough; first sound of heart strongly accentu-
ated and often intermitting; (ictus cordis) impulse of
heart plainly visible, lifting stethoscope; pulse intermittent; pressure in epigastrium, < in bent position,
> sitting erect; pressing down sensation in epigastrium.

❙❙Wandering rheumatic pains in region of heart, extending down l. arm.

❙Shooting, stabbing pain from heart through to l. scapula,
causing violent beating of heart. θRheumatism.

❙Pains suddenly leave extremities and go to heart; shooting, stabbing pain, through to l. scapula, causing
violent beating of heart, with anxious expression of
countenance, quick but weak pulse and difficult breathing. θRheumatism.

❙Articular rheumatism has been treated externally, and
cardiac symptoms ensue.

❙❙Heart disease, after frequent attacks of rheumatism, or
alternating with it.

❙❙Hypertrophy and valvular insufficiency, or thickening,
after rheumatism, paroxysms of anguish about heart,
with dyspnœa and febrile excitement.

❙Propped up in bed, with anxious expression of face, livid
hue of countenance; visible, tumultuous and very rapid
action of heart; after acute rheumatism. θEndocarditis.

❙Quickened but weak pulse. θRheumatism of heart.

❙Pulse: slow, weak; arms feel weak; scarcely perceptible,
limbs cold; irregular.

❙Remarkable slowness of pulse, 48 in minute. θNeuralgia.

❙Slow, small pulse. θHypertrophy of heart.

❙Pulse slow and feeble. θAngina pectoris.

❙Pulse very slow. θDysmenorrhœa.

❙Very feeble pulse, 40 beats per minute.

²⁰ **Outer Chest.** ❙❙Pleuritis falsa in winter season.

❙High fever; breathing oppressed, must lie quietly on
back, every motion attended with violent pains in
thorax, back and axillary joints. θRheumatism of
muscles of thorax and back.

²¹ **Neck and Back.** ❙Muscles of neck sore to touch and on
moving them.

❙Pains from neck down arm to little and fourth finger;
neck tender to touch; pains paroxysmal, < in early
part of night, and attended by stiffness; marked slowness of pulse, 48 beats per minute. θNeuralgia.

❙Violent pain in upper three dorsal vertebræ, extending
through shoulder blades.

❙Sensation of lameness in back, evening in bed.

❙Constant pain in spine, sometimes < in lumbar region,
with great heat and burning.

∎Feeling of paralysis in sacrum.
∎Aching across joints.
³² Upper Limbs. ∎Pain in shoulders.
∎Deltoid rheumatism, especially on r. side.
∎Stitches in lower part of l. shoulder blade.
∎Paroxysmal pains in r. arm. θNeuralgia.
∎Pains in l. arm.
∎Rheumatic pains in arms.
∎Cracking in elbow joint.
∎Stitches in hands; hands feel as if they had been sprained.
∎Pain in l. wrist, causing hand to feel paralyzed.
∣∣Erysipelatous eruption on hands extending further.
∎Weakness in arms; pulse slow.
³³ Lower Limbs. ∎Tearing pain from hip down leg to feet.
∎Rheumatic pains in leg from hip down.
∎Pains in lower extremities.
∎Rheumatic pains in r. leg, extending as far as toes, in
morning.
∎Stitches: externally on knee; in feet, soles, toes, big toe.
∎Sensation of weakness in calves.
∎Feet feel sprained.
∎Unable to walk; ankles swollen; pains, though mostly
confined to ankles, shift about from joint to joint.
θChronic rheumatism.
³⁴ Limbs in General. ∎Rheumatism often attacks heart, and
generally goes from upper to lower parts; pains shift
suddenly.
∎Rheumatic pains, mostly in upper arms and lower parts
of legs; < when going to sleep.
∎Joints hot, red, swollen. θAcute rheumatism.
∎Acute articular rheumatism; pains shift about from point
to point, especially when beginning in upper extremities and subsequently felt in lower; joints hot, red and
swollen; pains < on least motion and during evening,
or soon after going to bed; rheumatoid pains from sudden chill or exposure to cold wind.
∎Arms feel weak, limbs cold.
³⁵ Rest. Position. Motion. ∎Pains <: sitting bent, yet a
feeling as if to do so was necessary, but > by sitting or
standing upright. θGastralgia.
∎Pains < on least motion. θAcute rheumatism.
In a recumbent posture: mental faculties and memory
perfect, but on attempting to move vertigo.
Lying on l. side, palpitation <.
Lying on back: palpitation >.
Must lie on back: on account of oppressed breathing; ab-
dominal neuralgia.
Sitting in a stooping position: pressure in pit of stomach
<; palpitation <.

Sitting erect: pressure in pit of stomach, pains across abdomen >; pressure behind sternum >; palpitation >.

Stooping: vertigo; pressure behind sternum <.

After rising: pain in forehead <.

Standing: difficult on account of swelling of lower extremities.

Stands up and walks in his sleep.

Motion: of eyeballs causes pain; pains across abdomen <; slightest, pain in chest <; palpitation <; attended with violent pains in thorax, back and axillary joints; of muscles of neck painful; pains <.

Turning head: sensation as of something loose in it.

Walking: difficult on account of swelling of lower extremities.

Shuns all exertion; weariness in all muscles.

Unable to walk: ankles swollen; can hardly go up stairs.

³⁶ Nerves. ∎Weariness in all muscles; shuns all exertion, can hardly go up stairs.

∎Weary and giddy, with diarrhœa.

∎∎Weakness the only general symptom with neuralgia.

∎Trembling, thrilling, strumming, with palpitation.

∎Weakness and paralytic condition of limbs.

³⁷ Sleep. ∎∎Restless sleep, turns often.

∎Periosteal pains prevent sleep.

While sleeping stands up and walks about; talks in sleep.

Dreams: racking his brains; fantastic; of murder.

³⁸ Time. ∎Pains < during early part of night, or soon after going to sleep. θNeuralgia. θAcute rheumatism.

Morning: pain in forehead; heat in head; nausea and eructations of wind; pressure behind sternum <; rheumatic pains in r. leg.

Towards evening and next forenoon: very cross.

Evening: headache <; pressure in r. eye; eye symptoms <; pressing pain in molars; pressure behind sternum; lameness of back; pains <.

Night: headache; stitches in neck and thighs; face itches; early part, pains from neck down arms.

³⁹ Temperature and Weather. Pains are felt from a sudden chill, or exposure to a sudden wind. θAcute rheumatism. θNeuralgia.

Heat: pain in head <.

With sun: headache < and >; pain in r. eye < and >.

Open air: headache <; eyes <.

Cold: pain in head >.

After exposure to cold: pain in r. side of head, ear and face; rheumatoid pains.

⁴⁰ Fever. ∎∎Chilliness, with coldness; shaking chill in cold air; chills run over back.

∎Febrile excitement. θEndocarditis.

∣∣General heat; with burning and pain in back and loins.

∣∣Cold sweat.

⁴¹ **Attacks, Periodicity.** ∎Pain occurring at irregular times, continuing for no definite period, coming suddenly or gradually, and leaving as uncertainly. θNeuralgia.

Paroxysmal pains: in head; across abdomen above umbilicus; from neck down arms; in arms.

Every afternoon: headache, lasts through night.

Every Summer: roughness of cheeks.

One week after menses: leucorrhœa.

⁴² **Locality and Direction.** Right: rending in bones of side of face; pain over eye; pressing pain on a small spot on side of head, severe pain in eye; pressure in eye, above eye; stitches in and behind ear; pressing pains in side of face; prosopalgia; severe neuralgia; pains in side of head, face and ear; deltoid rheumatism <; pains in arm; rheumatic pain in leg.

Left: rending in bones of side of face; pain in shoulder; tongue sore on side; pain in arm; lying on side palpitation <; wandering rheumatic pains down arm; shooting pains from heart through to scapula; stitches in lower part of shoulder blade; pains in arm; pain in wrist.

Downward: pain shooting into eye teeth; pain across abdomen from lower border of liver down to left, then ceasing in r. side.

Moving backward: pain down neck and outwardly on both sides.

∎Pains change places. θRheumatism.

Pains move downward: head; bones of face; from ear to arm; down spine; down leg; arm to fingers.

Pains move upward: neck over head; ball in throat; lower limbs, then upper.

⁴³ **Sensations.** Sensation as if body was surcharged with electricity.

As of something loose in head diagonally across top; a shuddering without coldness commences with cracking, as if surcharged with electricity; as if back would break; as if a ball was rising in throat; as if something would be pressed off below pit of stomach; stool as if glazed; as if some one squeezed throat with thumb and finger; pain in chest as from a sprain; pressure like a marble from epigastrium towards heart; a cracking in head frightens him, it ends in a sound in ears like blowing a horn; every heart beat has a strumming as if it would burst, along sternum to throat; as if something was being pressed away from under sternum;

hands as if they had been sprained; feet as if sprained; as if furuncles would form here and there.

Pains: in limbs; in forehead; in l. shoulder; over r. eye; in head; in back; from back of neck up over scalp to top of head and temples; in eyeball; in eyes; in r. side of head, ear and face; in region of liver; in lower limbs; in loins; in interior of thighs; in chest; in l. arm; suddenly leave extremities and go to heart; from neck down arm to little and fourth finger; in spine; in l. wrist, causing hand to feel paralyzed.

Sudden pains in paroxysms: across abdomen, above umbilicus, from lower border of liver, downward toward left; in r. arm.

Anguish: about heart.

Violent pain: in upper three dorsal vertebræ.

Severe pain: in r. eye to forehead; in cardiac region.

Great pain: in chest.

Much pain: in lower extremities.

Tearing: in root of nose and nasal bones; in lower jaw; in one side of head from hip down leg to feet.

Rending: in bones of r. or l. side of face; in bones of legs to feet.

Shooting, stabbing pain: from heart through to l. scapula.

Shooting, twitching pain: over head.

Shooting: downward into eye teeth; through chest above heart into shoulder.

Stitches: in eyes, ears, fingers and feet; in and behind r. ear; in neck and thighs; in lower jaw; in tongue; in lower part of chest; in lower part of shoulder blade; in hands; externally on knee; in feet, soles, toes, big toe.

Stitching: in region of heart.

Stitching, tearing, pressing or shooting pains: in a downward direction in face.

Stinging: in jawbones.

Pricking sensation: in skin.

Rheumatic pain: in scalp; in heart; in limbs; in region of heart, extending down l. arm; in arms; in leg from hip down; in r. leg; shift from joint to joint; mostly in upper arms and lower parts of legs: all over body.

Severe neuralgia: in r. cheek; throughout whole body.

Neuralgic paroxysmal pains: in head.

Neuralgia: in bowels.

Throbbing headache.

Pulsating headache: in forehead.

Aching: in face; in forehead; in throat; across loins.

Severe pressing headache.

Pressing pain: on a small spot on r. side of head; in r. side of face; in molars.

Pressure: in r. eye; above r. eye; in throat; in pit of stomach; from epigastrium to heart; behind sternum; in region of heart.

Burning: in spine.

Great heat: in spine.

Heat: in head.

Soreness: of l. side of tongue.

Dryness: in throat.

Dulness: in head.

Swollen feeling: in throat.

Constriction: of throat.

Stiff, drawing sensation: in muscles on moving eyes.

Rigidity of skin.

Numbness: in affected parts after pain.

Feeling of paralysis: in sacrum.

Stiffness: of muscles around eyes and of eyelids.

Lameness: in back.

Weakness: in abdomen extending to throat; in calves.

Tired feeling: in chewing muscles.

Cracking: in elbow joints.

Tingling: in salivary glands.

Tickling: in trachea.

Itching: in eyes; in face.

" Tissues. ▮Acute rheumatism, going from joint to joint; violent fever; pains intense; ankles most painful and swollen; < from least movement.

▮Rheumatic pains all over body.

▮Pains shifting, pains suddenly changing position; tendency to metastasis to heart. θRheumatism.

▮Every joint and every muscle of body affected; high fever; every attempt to move attended with excruciating pains; afterwards paralysis of arms and legs. θRheumatism.

▮Dropsy from cold with rheumatic complaints.

" Touch. Passive Motion. Injuries. Touch: face tender; pit of stomach sore; muscles of neck sore.

Rubbing: eyes causes stinging.

" Skin. ▮▮Sensation of rigidity of skin.

▮▮Pricking sensation in skin, with moderate sweat.

▮▮Dry skin.

▮Erysipelatous, inflamed eruption on hand (similar to eruption caused by *Rhus tox.*), with oppressed breathing.

▮▮Eruption like itch.

▮▮Red, inflamed places here and there, exceedingly painful, as if furuncles would form.

" Stages of Life, Constitution. Girl, æt. 10, scrofulous diathesis, suffering three months; Bright's disease.

Girl, æt. 10, suffering ten days; endocarditis.

Boy, æt. 12; rheumatism.

Young German; chronic rheumatism.

Servant girl, suffering three months; sun headache.

Woman, suffering one week; neuralgia.

Man, æt. 27, fourth attack within ten years, each attack lasting from two to four months; neuralgia oculorum.

Man, æt. 33, formerly treated for ulcer of stomach; pressure in epigastrium.

Man, æt. 47, rheumatic; pressure in epigastrium.

Relations. Antidoted by : *Acon.*, *Bellad.*

Compare: *Bellad.* (throbbing head, erysipelas); *Benz. ac.* (gout, valvular disease); *Calc. ostr.* (cardiac hypertrophy); *Diosc.* (gastralgia); *Kali bich.* (catarrhs, rheumatism); *Lith. carb.* (valvular disease); *Lycop.* (rheumatic gout, urinary symptoms); *Natr. mur.* (hemiopia); *Pulsat.*, rheumatism, shifting pains; *Rhus tox.* (rheumatism); *Spigel.* (rheumatic endocarditis).

KOBALTUM.

Cobalt.   *Co.*

A metal known to Hohenheim in the fourteenth century. Derives its name from the German word *Kobold*, signifying mischievous spirit, so named by the miners who considered it a profitless ore. It is found in conjunction with nickel from which it has to be separated, a process first taught in 1807 by a chemist named Lougier, improved by Liebig in 1848, and perfected by Genth, a Philadelphia chemist, who produced absolutely pure Kobalt in 1850.

From this chemically pure Kobalt Hering made his proving in July, 1850.

Further provings were made by Koller, Lippe, Jones and Sparhawk. See Allen's Encyclopedia, vol. 5, p. 361.

CLINICAL AUTHORITIES.—Hering, Lippe, Pehrson, MSS.

[1] **Mind.** Great exhilaration of spirits, vivacity and rapid flow of thoughts.

Desire for study.

Indisposed to mental and physical labor; low spirited; thinks too little of himself.

All mental excitement increases sufferings.

[2] **Sensorium.** Dizziness; dulness; feeling as if head grew large (during stool).

[3] **Inner Head.** Pain in forehead, with uneasiness in stomach.

Frontal or occipital pain, < from stooping.

Dull, pressive pain in temples.

At every jar, feels as if top of head would come off.

Frontal headache, with pain back of eyes.

Headache in morning, with beating and sore aching.

Headache when getting up from sitting.

4 Outer Head. Great itching on hairy scalp, in beard and under chin, burning when scratching.

Sore pimples along edge of hair back of head.

5 Sight and Eyes. Dim vision; darting pains in eyes when writing, feeling when opening lids, as if little strings were holding them together and snapping.

Flickering before eyes when reading; letters look blurred.

Darting, shooting pains in eyes, from bright light.

Eyes ache at night.

Lachrymation and pain from cold air; sensation as of sand under lids.

Smarting in lids when using eyes.

6 Hearing and Ears. Aching, humming in l. ear.

Stinging through l. ear from roof of mouth.

7 Smell and Nose. Putrid, sickish smell before nose.

Watery discharge, with sneezing.

Nose feels obstructed.

Left nostril feels dry; filled with scales; itching.

8 Upper Face. ▮Red hard lumps on r. cheek.

9 Lower Face. Peeling of lips, with soreness and bleeding.

·Disposition to keep jaws tightly closed.

Large boils, very painful, on chin and l. lower jaw.

▮A large furuncle in region of l. lower jaw.

10 Teeth and Gums. ▮▮Pain in hollow teeth, they feel too long; gums swollen, tender, as if ulcerated; < from cold air.

11 Taste and Tongue. Flat taste; bad taste, with belching in morning.

Tongue coated white; cracks across middle.

12 Inner Mouth. Pricking, stinging in roof of mouth, extending to l. ear.

Constant watery secretion, with frequent swallowing.

13 Throat. Soreness, with rawness when hawking.

Dryness and soreness, mornings.

Hawking up thick, white mucus, which fills throat, in morning.

Feeling of fulness, from stomach to throat.

14 Appetite, Thirst. Desires, Aversions. Diminished appetite, especially for supper.

15 Hiccough, Belching, Nausea and Vomiting. Hiccough after eating, with soreness in pit of stomach.

Belching of wind, mornings and after stool.

Rising of sour or bitter water, with pain in stomach; afterward, dryness in throat.

ı ıQualmishness, with fulness of stomach.

Nausea, with pain in forehead.

¹⁷ **Scrobiculum and Stomach.** Pain in stomach and abdomen after eating, uneasiness; must move about.

Stomach feels as if it contained undigested food.

ı ıFulness in stomach, extending to throat; qualmishness.

Soreness when inspiring deeply, or from hiccough.

¹⁸ **Hypochondria.** Shooting, stitching from region of liver down into thigh.

ıShooting pains in hepatic region and sharp pain in region of spleen, < on taking a deep inspiration; fulness in abdomen after a slight meal; constant dropping of blood with stool. θHepatic derangement.

Sharp pain in splenic region, < when inspiring deeply.

¹⁹ **Abdomen.** Abdomen feels empty about umbilicus.

Cutting before stool.

Rumbling in abdomen.

Fulness in abdomen after a light meal.

Colic at 5 A.M., followed by large stool and tenesmus.

²⁰ **Stool and Rectum.** Urgent desire for stool while walking, < when standing; stool profuse, watery, spouting.

Stool large, soft, with tenesmus and aching in sphincter ani; severe colicky pain in lower part of abdomen; tenesmus after stool; during stool, dizziness.

ıCostiveness alternating with diarrhœa.

ı ıFeces like hazelnuts, with dulness in head.

Pressure in rectum.

ı ıConstant dropping of blood from anus (stools not bloody).

²¹ **Urinary Organs.** ı ıScanty urine.

Albuminuria.

Frequent discharge of small quantities of urine.

Increased secretion of pale urine, frequent urination in morning, after drinking coffee.

Scanty urine, with greasy pellicle; yellow flocculent, or red sediment, and strong, pungent smell.

Smarting in end of urethra during micturition.

Burning in urethra.

²² **Male Sexual Organs.** ıFrequent nocturnal emissions, with lewd dreams; only partial or no erections; impotence.

ıSeminal emissions at night, with headache and backache.

ıImpotence and emissions without erections.

Severe pain in r. testicle, > after urinating.

ı ıSecondary gonorrhœa, with a greenish discharge.

Yellow brown spots on genitals (and abdomen).

²⁵ **Voice and Larynx.   Trachea and Bronchia.** Stitches in anterior part of larynx.

²⁶ **Respiration.** Frequent sighing.

On taking a deep inspiration, stitches in chest, soreness in stomach and pain in spleen.

²⁷ **Cough.** Cough, with soreness in throat and rawness when hawking.

Short, hacking cough, with expectoration of bright red blood, which seemingly comes from larynx.

Expectoration of thick, tough mucus, mixed with blood, with fulness and pressive pain in larynx; scratching, rawness and burning in throat, and a disposition to keep jaws tightly closed; < from pressure, empty deglutition and cold water.

Copious expectoration of sweetish, frothy, white mucus, with lumps in it.

²⁸ **Inner Chest and Lungs.** Deep stitches in lower part of chest, mostly l. side, from deep inspiration.

ı ıThrough chest fulness of stomach to throat.

²¹ **Neck and Back.** Pain, between shoulders, in lumbar region and small of back.

ı ıAching pain in small of back, or spine; < sitting, > rising, walking or lying down.

ıı Backache, with seminal emissions.

πPain along spine, and from sacrum down through legs into feet, < while sitting.

²² **Upper Limbs.** Aching in wrist joints, with occasional stitches.

²³ **Lower Limbs.** πPain in upper part of r. hip bone, < sitting.

Shooting into thigh from liver.

Excessive weakness of knees.

Foot sweat between toes, smelling sour or like soleleather.

Flushes of heat along legs.

Stitches in legs.

Jerks in limbs when falling asleep.

Trembling of limbs, especially legs, aching when sitting.

Pricking, as of needles, in feet.

²¹ **Limbs in General.** Bruised pain in all limbs.

Stitches in arms and legs.

²⁵ **Rest. Position. Motion.** Lying down: backache >.

Sitting: aching in back <; pain along spine; pain in hip bone <.

Standing: desire for stool <.

Rising from sitting: headache, backache >.

Stooping: frontal and occipital pain <.

Walking: urgent desire for stool; backache >.

Must move about: pain in stomach with uneasiness.

²⁷ **Sleep.** ı Distressing drowsiness, in evening, sleeps ten to eleven hours and still hardly able to get up in morning.

ı ıDisturbed, unrefreshing sleep.

Wakeful; can do with less sleep.

On rising, pain in head and small of back.

ıLewd dreams, emissions; only partial or no erections.

³⁸ Time. Morning: headache with beating and sore aching;
belching and bad taste; dryness and soreness of throat;
hawking up thick white mucus; frequent urinating.
5 A.M.: colic.
Evening: distressing drowsiness.
Night: eyes ache; seminal emissions.

³⁹ Temperature and Weather. Getting warm in bed: itching all over.
Cold air: lachrymation and pain in eyes; pain in teeth <.

⁴⁰ Fever. Chilly from 11 to 12 A.M.; headache, with nausea
and languor from noon to 2 P.M., then fever and sweat.
Chilliness, with yawning, from 4 to 5 P.M.; feels dull and
weak, with aversion to mental exertion.
Flushes of heat: with sweat; along legs.

⁴¹ Attacks, Periodicity. 11 to 12 A.M.: chilly.
From noon to 2 P.M.: nausea and languor.
From 4 to 5 P.M.: chilliness with yawning.

⁴² Locality and Direction. Right: red, hard lumps on cheek;
severe pain in testicle; pain in upper part of hip bone.
Left: aching, humming in ear; stinging through ear to
roof of mouth; larger boils on lower jaw; large furuncle
in region of lower jaw; stitches in side of chest.

⁴³ Sensations. As if head grew large; as if top of head
would come off; as if little strings were holding eyelids
together; as of sand under lids; teeth feel too long;
gums as if ulcerated; stomach as if it contained undigested food: pricking as of needles in feet.
Pain: in forehead; in head; in occiput; back of eyes;
in stomach; in forehead; in abdomen; in back;
in spleen; between shoulders; in lumbar region; in
small of back; along spine; from sacrum down through
legs into feet; in upper part of r. hip bone.
Severe pain: in r. testicle.
Sharp pain: in region of spleen.
Shooting: in eyes; from region of liver down into thigh;
in hepatic region; into thigh from liver.
Cutting: in abdomen.
Darting: in eyes.
Severe colicky pain: in lower part of abdomen.
Stitches: in anterior part of larynx; in chest; in wrist
joints; in legs; in arms.
Stitching: from region of liver down into thigh.
Stinging: through l. ear from roof of mouth.
Burning: on hairy parts of head when scratched; in ure-
thra; in throat.
Sore aching: in head.
Soreness: of lips; of throat; in pit of stomach; in stomach.
Smarting: in lids; in end of urethra.

Pressive pain: in larynx.

Bruised pain: in all limbs.

Aching: in eyes at night; in l. ear; in small of back; in wrist joints; in legs; in sphincter ani.

Beating: in head.

Pricking: in roof of mouth.

Dryness: of throat.

Pressure: in rectum.

Dull, pressive pain: in temples.

Fulness: from stomach to throat; in abdomen; in larynx.

Itching: on hairy scalp; in beard and under chin; in l. nostril; all over.

" Touch. Passive Motion. Injuries. Pressure: disposition to keep jaws tightly closed <.

At every jar: feels as if top of head would come off.

" Skin. Much itching all over, when getting warm in bed.

Pimples on shoulders, pit of stomach and buttocks; bleed easily when scratched.

" Relations. Compare *Agnus cast.*, impotency; *Zincum*, pain in back < while sitting.

KREOSOTUM.

A product of distillation of wood tar.

Provings by Syrbius, Hartung, Sen. and Jun., Immisch, Lange, Koch, Heinemann, Lunderstadt, Wahle, Eichhorn, Thomas. See Allen's Encyclopedia, vol. 5, p. 408.

Additional verified symptoms from provings by Hering and Kummer, MSS.

CLINICAL AUTHORITIES.—*Difficulty of hearing during menstruation*, McClatchey, Trans. Hom. Med. Soc. Pa., 1881, p. 157; *Syphilitic deafness*, Teste, B. J. H., vol. 29, p. 780; *Cancerous tumor on lower lip*, Thompson, Raue's Rec., 1872, p. 97; *Curious teeth*, Liedbeck, Rück. Kl. Erf., vol. 1, p. 463; *Hemorrhage after extraction of tooth*, Kleinert, Rück. Kl. Erf., vol. 5, p. 859; *Vomiting*, Wahle, Rück. Kl. Erf., vol. 1, p. 557; *Gastromalacia*, Kreuss, Rummel, Goullon, Krummacher, Arnold, Rück. Kl. Erf., vol. 1, p. 605; *Painful, hard spot in stomach*, Wahle, Rück. Kl. Erf., vol. 1, p. 637; *Diarrhœa*, Kurz, Rück. Kl. Erf., vol. 1, p. 836; *Enuresis*, Perrussell, Raue's Rec., 1871, p. 187; Bœnninghausen, Sommer, Rampal, Rück. Kl. Erf., vol. 2, p. 43; *Chronic ovarian affection*, Pröll, B. J. H., vol. 34, p. 737; *Uterine affection*, Wahle, Rück. Kl. Erf., vol. 2, p. 354; Reisig, Rück. Kl. Erf., vol. 2, p. 354; *Uterine affections in middle-aged women*, Kurtz, Rück. Kl. Erf., vol. 2, p. 354; *Ulcers on neck of uterus*, Wahle, Rück. Kl. Erf., vol. 2, p. 353; *Cauliflower excrescences around os uteri*, Neidhard, Org., vol. 2, p. 105; *Menorrhagia*, Gülzon, Allg. Hom. Ztg., vol. 103, p. 51; *Wesselhœft*, Hom. Clin., vol. 4, p. 87; Raue's Rec., 1872, p. 178; *Leucorrhœa*, Landrey, B. J. H., vol. 29, p. 166; Molin, Rück. Kl. Erf., vol. 2, p. 363; *Puerperal metritis*, Bentsch, Rück. Kl. Erf., vol. 2, p. 448; *Perichondritic laryngismus*, Unsin, Rück. Kl. Erf., vol. 5, p. 740; *Whooping cough*, A. R., Rück. Kl. Erf., vol. 5, p. 723; *Hemorrhage from lungs*, Wahle, Rück. Kl. Erf., vol. 3, p. 217; *Consumption*, Frank, Kurtz, Lobethal, Schron, Rück. Kl. Erf., vol. 3, pp. 377-379; *Phthisis* (2 cases), Wahle, Rück. Kl. Erf., vol. 3 p. 218; *Gangrene of lungs*, Willard, Trans. Hom. Med. Soc. Pa., 1876, p. 297; *Hemorrhages*, Trinks, B. J. H., vol. 29, p. 318.

[1] **Mind.** Stupid feeling in head; vacant gaze; neither seeing nor hearing.

Frequent vanishing or failure of thought.

I I Weakness of memory; forgetfulness. θAfter nosebleed.

I I Thinks herself well. θMetritis.

❚Sorrowful mood, inclined to weep, or longing for death; music and similar emotional causes impel him to weep.

Anxious, apprehensive mood.

Ill humor; moroseness; peevishness; ill temper, obstinacy.

❚Fretful, irritable, agitated, screams nights. θBronchitis during dentition.

Excited condition; ailments from emotions.

Confounding ideas; also in puerperal fever with putridity. Seeks for unpleasant things and broods over them.

² Sensorium. Stupefaction, dizziness and vacancy in head, with complete loss of thought, sight and hearing.

Painful dulness of head, as after a carouse.

Vertigo: mornings, in open air, with staggering like from drunkenness, must hold on to something; passes off in room; danger of falling on turning round quickly.

Roaring in head.

³ Inner Head. Throbbing and beating in forehead from l. side of head.

Dull feeling in head as from a board across forehead.

Pulsation in forehead and vertex, when awaking in morning, with heat in face.

Chronic periodic headache in forehead, piercing pain; wheals or swellings on scalp.

Heaviness or pressure in various parts of head, with sensation as if brain would force through forehead.

Occipital headache; much pain and soreness.

Headache: after a carouse; with sleepiness; tearing, drawing and jerking pains; jerking, tearing, sticking, burning pains in anterior part of head; semilateral and extending to cheeks, jaws, teeth and neck; induced by talking, moving, sitting up or lying on side not affected, with great excitability and nervous irritability.

⁴ Outer Head. Eruptions on forehead, as with drunkards.

Falling off of hair.

Sensibility of scalp to touch, and when hair is combed.

Scales in large, indurated masses fall off freely.

Scald head.

⁵ Sight and Eyes. Dimsighted: as if looking through gauze; as if something was floating before eyes, obliging to wipe them constantly.

Staring, dull, lifeless and stupid look.

Itching and smarting sensation in eyes, on edges of lids; < rubbing.

Suggilation on conjunctiva of r. eye.

Burning and redness of conjunctiva.

Acute aggravations of chronic keratitis; hot, smarting lachrymation.

Blenorrhœa of conjunctiva, with moderately profuse discharge and much smarting in eyes.

Heat in eyes, with ulceration.

Burning heat in eyes, with tears, < by bright light.

Hot, acrid, smarting tears, like salt water; < in a bright light, on rubbing eyes and early morning.

Slight inflammation of Meibomian glands.

Eyes sunken, with blue rings around, or protruding.

❚❚Chronic swelling of eyelids and their margins; agglutination of lids.
❙❙Uncontrollable twitching of lids.

ᵎHearing and Ears. ❙Hardness of hearing with buzzing.
❙Roaring in head; also humming and difficulty of hear-
ing before and during menses.
❙Girl, æt. 9, syphilitic deafness; teeth wedge shaped; old
looking; had snuffles when a baby; attacks of vomiting.
❙Stitches in ears; otitis.
❙Heat, burning, swelling and redness of l. outer ear, pro-
ceeding from a pimple in concha, stiffness and pain in ·
l. side of neck, shoulder and arm.
❙❙Itching in ears.
❙Humid tetter on ears, with swelling of cervical glands
and livid grey complexion.
❙❙Affections of external ear.

ᵗSmell and Nose. ❙❙Subjective putrid smell with loss of
appetite; in morning, on awaking.
❙Nosebleed: with heaviness and throbbing in forehead,
sleepiness; thin, bright red blood.
❙Frequent sneezing: especially in morning; with stoppage
of nose; rough and scraping sensation in throat; with
dry, nasal catarrh.
Nasal secretion thick.
❙❙Catarrh fluent or dry, with much sneezing.
❙Chronic catarrh with old people.
❙Epithelial cancer on right ala nasi.
❙❙Lupus on nose; l. side.

ᵃUpper Face. ❙Sick, suffering expression; old looking
children.
❙Complexion: wretched; earthy; livid; pale, green, with
swelling of cervical glands; pale, bloated; coppery ap-
pearance.
❙Burning pains; < from talking or exertion, > lying on
affected side; nervous, excitable.
❙Face cold, of pale, bluish tinge, especially on temples and
around nose and mouth.
❙Flushes of heat, with circumscribed redness of cheeks.
❙Face hot, cheeks red, feet cold.
❙Great heat and brown redness of face (during siesta), with
throbbing in cheeks and forehead, and frequent mictu-
rition.
❙❙Scaly herpes on eyelids, cheeks and around mouth.
❙Acne in face.

ᵎLower Face. ❙Dry lips, peeling off, easily cracked.
❙Wants to moisten lips frequently, without being thirsty.
❙❙Tumor, size of a pea, on lower lip, with acrid, watery
ichor, making surrounding parts sore.

| | Eruption on under lip.

| | Pustulous pimples, with yellow scabs on chin and cheek.

10 Teeth and Gums. | | Bad odor from decayed teeth.

|| Toothache: extending to temples and to l. side of face; drawing, extending to inner ear and temples; caused by caries.

| | Teeth wedge shaped. θSyphilitic deafness.

| | Great restlessness, wants to be in motion all the time, and screams whole night. θDentition.

|| Teeth show dark specks and begin to decay as soon as they appear.

|| Gums: bluish red, soft, spongy, easily bleeding, inflamed, ulcerated, scorbutic.

| Protruding gums infiltrated with dark watery fluid.

| After extraction of tooth, persistent oozing of dark, slightly coagulated blood, finally checked by application of alum; hemorrhage reappeared at shorter or longer intervals, at first only from teeth, later entirely from nose, continuing one year, and causing great debility.

| Absorption of gums and alveolar process.

11 Taste and Tongue. | | Bitter or flat taste.

| Bitter taste, especially in throat

| | Everything eaten tastes bitter; bitter taste of food, not perceived until just as it is being swallowed.

| Tongue dry; with mucous coating; coated white.

12 Inner Mouth. || Putrid odor from mouth.

13 Throat. | | Pressure on r. side of throat when swallowing.

| Scraping in throat, with roughness and dryness.

| | Small, round, bluish red spots (petechiæ) on throat.

| Diphtheria; malignant form, when confined to fauces, with terrible fetor oris.

| Fever, vomiting, loss of appetite, restless sleep, general languor, swelling of glands; three days later, suddenly, very much exudate in fauces; fetor oris. θDiphtheria.

| Scrofulous and lymphatic patients, with black softening and decomposition of mucous membrane, with atony and extension of softening, especially towards œsophagus. θDiphtheria.

11 Appetite, Thirst. Desires, Aversions. | Greedy drinking followed by vomiting; great thirst.

| Keen appetite, especially for meat; craves smoked meats.

| | Loss of appetite, aversion to meat, vomits after it.

| Desire for spirituous drinks, weakening leucorrhœa.

| | Stomach aches, from acid food.

15 Eating and Drinking. || Water, after it is swallowed, tastes bitter.

Worse from eating cold food; > from warm diet.

Dares not remain fasting.

[16] **Hiccough, Belching, Nausea and Vomiting.** ▮Belching and hiccough, especially when sitting up or being carried.

▮Belching: sour; empty; after dinner, with throwing off of frothy saliva, and with scraping roughness in throat.

▮Deep and lasting disgust for food in convalescents.

▮Nausea: during pregnancy; constant inclination to vomit without doing so; with chilliness morning and evening.

▮▮Vomiting: of sweetish water; of undigested food; in evening of all food eaten during day; of undigested food two or three hours after eating; with dimness of vision; of everything eaten; of large quantities of sour, acrid fluid, or of white, foamy mucus.

▮▮Continuous vomiting and straining to vomit.

▮Sympathetic vomiting, as of phthisis, of cancer of liver or uterus, of pregnancy, and of chronic kidney disease.

▮Seasickness.

[17] **Scrobiculum and Stomach.** ▮Cold feeling at epigastrium internally, as if cold water or ice was there.

▮Feeling of fulness, as after having eaten too much.

▮Tension over stomach and scrobiculum; tight clothing is intolerable.

▮▮Painful hard spot, at or to left of stomach.

▮Malignant induration, fungus and ulcers of stomach; painless gastromalacia; pressing, gnawing, ulcerative pain in stomach, with hæmatemesis.

▮Gastromalacia, preceded by great restlessness and sleeplessness, and accompanied by vomiting and diarrhœa.

▮Sudden vomiting of all food, soon followed by lienteric stools; slimy coating on tongue; rapid and extreme emaciation; constant whining; sleeplessness. θGastromalacia.

▮For several weeks diarrhœa, finally smelling cadaverous; vomiting; extreme blueness of face, as from nervous congestion. θGastromalacia.

▮Rapid emaciation in children, vomiting, intense thirst, bloating in region of stomach, greyish white or chopped offensive stools. θGastromalacia.

▮Very frequent and sudden vomiting of food; frequent hiccough, belching, especially when raised up; remarkably rapid emaciation of whole body, but particularly of neck and face; bluish pale appearance of face, especially about temples, nose and mouth; dull, staring, vacant look, eyes sunken, surrounded by blue rings; coldness of face and hands; drowsiness, with half open eyes; feeble whining; quick, scarcely perceptible pulse; red, slightly elevated eruption on l. forearm. θGastromalacia.

[18] **Hypochondria.** ▮Stitches in region of liver. θPregnancy.

∎Bruised pain in region of liver, with sensation of fulness.

ǀǀConstriction of hypochondria, cannot tolerate tight clothing.

ǀǀPressure in region of spleen; spleen painful to pressure.

¹⁹ Abdomen. ǀǀUlcerative pain in abdomen.

ǀǀPain in region of umbilicus.

ǀǀSensation of contraction in abdomen, as if a hard twisted ball was lying in umbilical region.

∎Distension of abdomen, as after a copious meal.

∎Abdomen distended and tense, like a drum.

∎Burning in bowels.

∎Laborlike pains in abdomen, with drawing in upper abdomen, extending to small of back and pressing toward lumbar vertebræ, with flushes of heat in face, palpitation of heart, frequent pulse and ineffectual urging to urinate, finally small quantities of hot urine are passed; after paroxysm chill, and discharge of milky leucorrhœa.

ǀǀSore pain in abdomen during deep inhalation.

ǀǀShattering sensation in abdomen.

∎Painful sensation of coldness in abdomen; icy coldness in epigastrium. θDyspepsia.

∎Violent abdominal spasms, < in groins.

∎Colic, resembling pains of labor.

∎Tabes mesenterica, with hypertrophied glands in fleshy, flabby subjects.

²⁰ Stool and Rectum. Stools: watery; papescent; dark brown; watery, putrid, containing undigested food; greyish or white, chopped, very fetid; frequent, greenish, watery; cadaverous smelling.

ǀǀIneffectual painful urging to stool.

ǀǀConstipation, stool hard, expelled after much pressing.

∎Cramplike pain in rectum during stool.

∎Children struggle and scream during act of defecation, and seem as if they would go into fits.

∎Diarrhœa in nursing infants during dentition.

∎Diarrhœa, with vomiting; continued vomiting, straining to vomit predominates; child resists tightening of anything around abdomen, which increases restlessness and pain; much thirst; gums hot; coldness of hands and feet.

∎Cholera infantum, second and third stages, with bloody, shreddy, mucous evacuations, with or without oppressiveness, gagging, dull, leaden countenance, somnolence; incipient hydrocephaloid.

∎Constant vomiting and greedy drinking; belching or hiccoughing when carried. θCholera infantum.

∎Much blood, often in clots, in diarrhœic, thin, fetid stools, which are always followed by great prostration. θTyphus.

∎Stitches in rectum, extending towards l. groin.

∎Constriction of rectum in case of uterine cancer.

²¹ **Urinary Organs.** ∎∎Frequent urgency to urinate, with copious, pale discharge; at night cannot get out of bed quick enough.

∎Diminished secretion, though drinking much.

∎Urine: chestnut brown; clouded; reddish, with red sediment; depositing white sediment; colorless; fetid; alkaline.

∎Wets bed at night, wakes with urging, but cannot retain urine, or dreams he is urinating in a decent manner.

∎Urine flows during deep, first sleep, from which child is roused with difficulty. θEnuresis nocturna.

∎Chronic enuresis; patient thin, emaciated.

∎∎Smarting and burning in pudenda during and after micturition.

∎Diabetes mellitus.

²² **Male Sexual Organs.** ∎∎Sexual desire too weak.

∎Burning in genitals, during coition, with swelling of penis next day.

∎Prepuce bluish black with hemorrhage and gangrene. θSyphilis.

²³ **Female Sexual Organs.** ∎After chill menses suppressed for six months; unable to lie on either side; dull pain in region of ovaries, could not bear strong pressure; morning urine colorless; brownish yellow, acrid leucorrhœa; constipation. θChronic ovarian affection.

∎During coition, burning in parts, followed next day by discharge of dark blood.

∎Hard lump on neck of uterus; ulcerative pain during coition.

∎Ulcerative pain in cervix uteri.

∎Severe pain in small of back and uterine region, extending to thighs; deep in pelvis burning as of red hot coals; whimpering and whining; discharge of offensive blood in large clots; vagina swollen and burning hot, mucous membrane greatly puffed; uterus high up, neck hard and swollen; at orifice of uterus small, warty growths; parts extremely irritable and painful to touch; externally, fundus of uterus swollen, painful like a blood boil on slightest touch; pulse small and hard; great debility; sleeplessness.

∎Painful pressure towards genitals; stitches, from small of back through pelvis to external genitals; constant burning pain in small of back; bland leucorrhœa finally acrid, watery, occasionally ichorous, bloody, with pungent, offensive smell; severe pain during coition, with fear and trembling at thought of it; general aggrava-

tion during menstruation; sick, suffering appearance;
prostration from least exertion; > during rest; dwindling and falling away of mammæ, with small, hard,
painful lumps in them; cervix scirrhous, hard and very
painful to touch; os open, almost everted, inner surface
like cauliflower; pulse small, weak, 100; anxious, fearful.
∎Putrid state of womb after childbirth.
∎∎Inveterate ulcers on neck of uterus.
∎Uterine affections of middle aged women; long lasting
leucorrhœa, or frequently recurring uterine hemorrhages, both accompanied by pressing sensations; finally
discharges become offensive, bloody and watery,
acrid, ichorous or clotted; burning, occasionally
stitching in back and lower abdomen; on standing sensation as if a load was resting in pelvis; coition painful; general aggravation during menstruation; examination painful; vagina hot, mucous membrane puffed
and follicles often hypertrophied; at mouth of uterus
warty or cauliflower excrescences.
∎Cancer of uterus (much improved).
∎Menses: too early, too profuse and too protracted; succeeded by an acrid smelling, bloody ichor, with itching
and biting in parts; more or less pain during flow, but
much < after it; flow intermits, at times almost ceasing,
then recommencing; in third month of pregnancy.
∎Menses very profuse; blood clotted; sometimes with uterine pain, and always a week too late, with severe headache before and during menses.
∎Menorrhagia, < lying, > getting up and walking about.
∎Before menses: hardness of hearing; foamy eructation or
vomiting of mucus; bloatedness; griping about navel;
burning in back; leucorrhœa; excitement and restlessness; looks swollen as if pregnant.
∎Buzzing in head, before, during and after menses.
∎∎Severe headache before and during menses.
∎Catamenia with uterine pain.
∎During menses: hardness of hearing; rushing sound in
ears; humming and pressing outwards in head; stitches
in side; cutting pain in abdomen; borborygmi; diar-
rhœa; chills; sweat on chest and back.
∎Painful urging toward genitals.
∎Bearing down and weight in pelvis; as if something
was coming out of vagina; < by motion.
∎She thinks she is almost well when the discharge reap-
pears. θMenses. θMetrorrhagia.
∎∎Her hemorrhage seems to pass into a corrosive, ichorous
discharge, and then to freshen up again and go on.
After menses: laborlike abdominal cramps; uterus ten-

der; constricting pain in vagina, followed by fluor
albus; prolapsus.

❚Metrorrhagia: blood dark and offensive; in large clots;
fainting; pulseless.

❚Metrorrhagia continuing four weeks; fainting and pulseless; discharge dark and offensive.

❚Constant flow of thin, watery and offensive blood, <
lying; emaciation; debility. θMenorrhagia.

❚❚Leucorrhœa: putrid, acrid, corrosive; stains clothing
yellow, stiffens like starch; mild or acrid, causing much
itching; milky, after coccyodynia; < between menses;
or for a few days before menses; with great weakness;
< standing or walking, not sitting; flowing like menses.

❚❚Discharge from vagina frequently looks quite white, and
then had odor of green corn.

❚Bland, yellow leucorrhœa, preceding each urination, with
frequent desire to micturate.

❚Drawing pains along coccyx down to rectum and vagina,
where a spasmodic, contractive pain is felt; > when
rising from sitting; subsequent milky leucorrhœa.

❚Sterile from leucorrhœa.

❚Electric-like stitches in vagina, seem to come from abdomen, always make her start.

❚Voluptuous itching deep in vagina.

❚❚Violent itching of vagina, so that she is obliged to rub
it; posteriorly there is smarting; external genitals
swollen, hot and hard; on urinating, vagina pains as if
sore; in evening.

❚❚Corrosive itching in vulva; sore and burning after
scratching.

❚❚Scirrhus of vagina, painful to slight touch.

❚Burning and swelling of labia.

❚Violent itching between labia and thighs.

❚Aphthous or inflammatory state of external parts, symp-
tomatic of ovarian or uterine disease.

²¹ **Pregnancy. Parturition. Lactation.** ❚❚During pregnancy: nausea and vomiting; ptyalism; vomiting of
sweetish water before breakfast; vomiting after supper;
metrorrhagia threatening abortion (third month); leucorrhœa; tightness across pit of stomach.

❚❚Lochia: blackish, lumpy, very offensive; excoriating;
almost ceasing, freshen up again; persistent, brown and
offensive.

❚Chill, then general heat, finally sweat; pulse soft and
quick; trembling, anxiety, confusion of mind, weakness
of memory, thinks herself well; lochia dark, lumpy and
very offensive; vagina moist, not very hot; abdomen
soft and sensitive; constipation. θPuerperal fever.

∎Mammæ: stitches; dwindling away; small, hard, painful lumps in them; hard, bluish red and covered with little scurfy protuberances, from which blood oozes whenever scurf is removed.

²⁵ **Voice and Larynx. Trachea and Bronchia.** ∎Scraping and roughness in throat; hoarseness, ceasing in morning, after sneezing.

∎Perichondritis of larynx, septic form, with softening and degeneration affecting mucous membrane of larynx, and particularly that of œsophagus.

∎Heavy pressure on sternum. θBronchitis.

∎Bronchial irritation accompanying dentition; child extremely fretful, irritable, much agitated, and screaming in night.

∎Chronic bronchial and laryngeal catarrh, with hoarseness; hawking mucus from trachea and bronchi, sometimes bloody, especially that from trachea; heavy pressure on sternum when turning over in bed in morning; < on approach of warm weather; no cough.

²⁶ **Respiration.** ∎Shortness of breath, heaviness, anxiety, frequent desire to take a deep breath; chest feels bruised, as if beaten; as if sternum was being crushed in. θNervous asthma.

²⁷ **Cough.** Cough: whistling; dry; tormenting; evening, in bed; caused by crawling below larynx, or, as if in upper bronchi; with dyspnœa; convulsive, with desire to vomit; dry, spasmodic, in morning, causing retching; concussion of abdomen and escape of urine; with easily detached white expectoration; scraping, with profuse, thick, yellow, or white mucous expectoration; dry, wheezing, hollow; during dentition; with pain in chest and sternum, compelling to press hand on it; stitches and soreness in chest.

∎Aggravation of cough: morning and evening; while exhaling; from motion; from music; when awaking, when lying on side or turning in bed.

∎During cough: scratching in throat; stitches and bruised pain in chest; asthma; jarring of abdomen; retching; discharge of urine; chills and heat; sleepiness.

∎After coughing spell, copious, purulent expectoration.

∎Periodical blood spitting, greenish yellow, puslike sputa.

∎Expectoration: white; thick yellow; black coagulated blood.

∎Frequent blood spitting, severe pains in chest, afternoon fever, and morning sweat.

∎Fatiguing cough with old people, copious sputa.

∎Violent winter cough of old people, with spasmodic turns at night, and very copious light colored mucous sputa; pain or pressure referable to sternum.

▮Whooping cough.

▮Cough for several weeks; vomiting of tough, white
phlegm with the cough, sometimes of a yellowish color;
cough < in evening and morning; after lying down
and from exercise; crawling below larynx, which excites cough; perspires after coughing and feels weak;
stomach swells in evening, has to unfasten clothes;
sometimes sneezes when he coughs.

²⁸ **Inner Chest and Lungs.** ▮Dreadful burning in chest;
constriction.

▮Stitches: in l. chest, just over heart; across chest, during morning till noon; first in l. then in r. chest; in r.
chest, interrupting breathing; under scapula.

▮Acute stitches in middle of chest, < during inspiration,
attended with feeling of lameness and extending to
elbow joint across r. shoulder, where pains are most violent on lifting arms; chronic leucorrhœa.

▮Pains in chest, > from pressure.

▮Anxious feeling of heaviness and oppression in chest.

▮Breath quick and labored, puffing of cheeks and violent
working of nostrils. θPneumonia.

▮Periodic attacks of blood spitting, with fever, and expectoration of greenish yellow pus; pains in chest; can lie
only on one side. θPhthisis.

▮Suddenly seized with cough and expectoration of blood;
lies in bed, greatly emaciated; is afraid to open mouth;
heaviness and oppression of chest; constipation; during
night coughed up much black blood; appetite lost; pulse
weak, suppressed, intermittent; face greyish yellow.

▮Coughing spells every Autumn and Spring, with expectoration of yellowish green pus and blood, fever and inability to lie on one side. θPhthisis.

▮After whooping cough, accompanied by inflammatory
affection of lungs and larynx, phthisis purulenta; with
every paroxysm of cough, expectoration of a large mass
of pus, followed by such great prostration that he can
hardly speak; severe evening exacerbations; loss of
appetite; emaciation; must stay in bed. θConsumption.

▮After neglected pulmonary catarrh, severe, persistent,
spasmodic cough, often attended by vomiting; expectoration, profuse, slimy and purulent; must sit up nearly
all night; constant stitches in l. chest; bitter taste in
mouth; fetor oris; frequent greenish, watery diarrhœa;
hectic fever. θConsumption.

▮Must stay in bed; face and body greatly emaciated;
cough with profuse and frequent expectoration; frequent
blood spitting; severe pains in chest; fever in afternoon; sweats in morning; consumption.

❙Emaciation; intense hectic fever; night sweats; shortness of breath; dry, teasing cough; great debility.
❚❙Gangrene of lungs.

²⁹ **Heart, Pulse and Circulation.** ❙Anxiety at heart; op-
pression of breathing.
❙❙Stitches: over heart; in heart.
❙Pulsation in all arteries, when at rest.
Pulse: small, weak and quick; soft, quick and trembling;
small and hard; slow; rapid, scarcely perceptible; falls
from eighty to sixty, even to forty-seven.
❙❙Pulse small and weak, with orgasm of blood.

³¹ **Neck and Back.** ❙Glands of neck swollen.
❙❙Pain in back: at night; < when lying.
❙Pain as if small of back would break; < during rest, >
from motion.
❙Pain in small of back and sacral region, like labor pains;
urging to urinate and ineffectual desire for stool.
❙Spasmodic drawing from behind forward, into genitals,
or down into thighs; stitches. θCancer uteri.
❙Drawing pain along coccyx to rectum and vagina, where
a spasmodic, contractive pain is felt.
❙❙Continuous burning in small of back.

³² **Upper Limbs.** ❙❙Pain in shoulders as if they had been
uncovered all night.
❙Scapulæ as if bruised.
❙Stitches in arm, from shoulder joint through to fingers,
which feel as if asleep, without power or feeling.
❙❙Pain as if bruised when touched inner side of upper arm.
❙❙Pain in elbow joint, as if tendons were too short.
Slightly elevated red blotches on l. forearm.
❙❙Pain in ulnar muscles, extending to little finger; cramp-
like in l. arm; drawing, with lameness in right.
❙❙Fingers become white and insensible, especially in
morning after rising.
❙❙Left thumb pains as if sprained and stiff.
❙❙Cracking of skin of hands.

³³ **Lower Limbs.** ❙❙Bruised pain on crest of ilium, as if from
a heavy burden, or after running; stitches from same
through abdomen; pain in same and in lumbar vertebræ, in morning, as if tired.
❙Pain in l. hip joint, as if luxated; as if leg was too long
when standing.
❙Boring pain in r. hip, alternating with numbness and
loss of sensation of whole thigh. θRheumatic gout.
❙❙Tingling or buzzing sensation in lower limbs.
❙Pain in whole leg, as from an ulcer.
❙❙Sensation as if knee joint would suddenly give way.
❙❙Alternate swelling of knee joints and wrists, with sensa-
tion of numbness and rigidity of limbs.

ı ıSwelling and stiffness of feet; white, cold swelling.
ı ıStitches in r. ankle and l. heel.
ı ıUlcerative pain in soles; burning itching in soles.
³⁴ **Limbs in General.** ıAlternate swelling of knees and joints
of hands, with disagreeable sensation of numbness and
stiffness in limbs. θRheumatic gout.
ıPain in all limbs, as if beaten, or as after a long walk;
lassitude or heaviness with drowsiness.
ıStitches in joints.
ı ıRed, scaly skin on bends of knees, like herpes.
ı ıSkin on extremities dry and rough.
³⁵ **Rest.   Position.   Motion.**   Rest: symptoms of female or-
gans >; pulsation in all arteries; pain in back <;
restlessness <; chill <; seems to increase pains.
During repose: a sensation as if all parts of body were in
motion.
Lying down: cough <; pain in back <.
Lying on side: cough <.
Lying on side not affected: causes pains in anterior part
of head; burning pains in upper face.
Can lie only on one side: phthisis.
Unable to lie on either side.
Sitting: leucorrhœa >.
Must sit up nearly all night: cough.
Sitting up: causes pains in anterior part of head; belching
and hiccough.
Standing: sensation as if a load was resting on pelvis;
leucorrhœa <.
Rising from sitting up: contractive pain in vagina >.
Least exertion: causes great prostration; faintness.
Motion: causes pains in anterior part of head; bearing
down and weight in pelvis <; cough <; pains in back
>; restlessness >.
Wants to be in motion all the time.
She cannot keep quiet after getting up from sleep.
Turning over in bed: heavy pressure on sternum; cough <.
Turning around quickly: danger of falling.
Lifting arms: pains most violent.
Walking: leucorrhœa <.
Staggering, must hold on to something: vertigo.
³⁶ **Nerves.** ıGeneral weakness and prostration; great debility.
ıFaintness in morning, when rising earlier than usual.
ıFatigue from least exertion.
ıWeariness, as if from too long a foot journey.
ı ıProstration, with sleeplessness.
ı ıGreat restlessness and excitation of whole body, < in
repose than during motion.
Spasms during dentition; swelling over a tooth not quite
through.

‖Child moans constantly, or dozes with half open eyes, or is cross and sleepless; during dentition.

‖Very severe, old, neuralgic affections, with tearing pain.'

‖Perfect depression of trophic nervous system.

³⁷ Sleep. ‖Great drowsiness, with frequent yawning.

Sleeplessness, < before midnight.

‖‖Will only sleep when caressed and fondled.

‖Tosses about all night, without any apparent cause.

‖Starting, when scarcely fallen asleep.

‖‖Laughs aloud during sleep.

‖Dreams: of crying; of falling from a height; of being out in a snow storm; of being poisoned; of bright fire; of very dirty (clothes) wash; that he is urinating, and awakes to find the dream a reality.

‖Very difficult to waken child out of sleep. θEnuresis.

‖Generally better after sleep.

³⁸ Time. Morning: vertigo; pulsation of forehead and vertex; hot, acrid tears; loss of appetite; frequent sneezing; chilliness after sneezing; hoarseness >; turning over in bed pressure on sternum; dry, spasmodic cough; cough <; sweat; stitches across chest; fingers white and insensible; pain in lumbar vertebræ; faintness; sweat.

Afternoon: fever.

Evening: chilliness; vomiting; vagina as if sore; cough <; stomach swells; exacerbations; itching drives him almost wild; herpes on palms of hands, in ears, elbows, knuckles and malleoli <.

Before midnight: sleeplessness <.

Night: screaming; cannot get out of bed quick enough to urinate; wets bed; spasmodic cough; coughed up much black blood; sweats; pain in back; tosses about.

³⁹ Temperature and Weather. Warmth: herpes >.

On approach of warm weather: heavy pressure on sternum.

Open air: vertigo; herpes <.

⁴⁰ Fever. ‖‖Transient chill without thirst.

‖‖Chill, predominating when at rest.

‖‖Shaking chill, with severe flushes of heat in face, red face and icy cold feet; after the chill, thirst.

‖‖Chill: great bodily restlessness; alternating with heat.

‖Coldness of face and hands.

‖Heat mostly in face.

‖Flushes of heat, with circumscribed redness of face.

‖‖Sweat scant and only during morning, with heat and redness of cheeks.

‖Putrid fever.

⁴¹ Attacks, Periodicity. Periodic: headache; blood spitting.

Two or three hours after eating: vomiting of food.

For several weeks: diarrhœa.
Before and during menses: humming and difficulty of
hearing; headache; buzzing in head.
For six months: suppression of menses.
Every Autumn and Spring: coughing spell.
Winter: cough.
For one year: hemorrhage from teeth and nose.
Day after coition: swelling of penis; discharge of blood.

⁴² Locality and Direction. Right: suggilation on conjunctiva of eye; pressure on side of throat; stitches in chest;
lameness in elbow joint and shoulder; drawing and
lameness in arm; boring pain in hip; stitches in ankle.
Left: throbbing and beating in side of head; heat,
burning, swelling and redness of outer ear; stiffness of
neck; lupus on nose; toothache extending to side of
face; slightly elevated eruption on forearm; stitches in
groin; stitches in chest; red blotches on forearm;
cramplike pain in arm; pain in hip joint; stitches in
heel.
First l. then r.: stitches in chest; pain in wrists.
From behind forwards: drawing into genitals.
Stitching downward; pressing inward.

⁴³ Sensations. As if a board was across forehead; as if brain
would force through forehead; as if looking through
gauze; as if something was floating before eyes; as if
cold water or ice was in epigastrium; as if a hard
twisted ball was lying in umbilical region; as if children would go into fits during defecation; burning as of
red hot coals deep in pelvis; as if a load was resting on
pelvis; as if something was coming out of vagina; vagina as if sore; chest as if beaten; as if sternum was
being crushed in; as if small of back would break; as
if shoulders had been uncovered all night; scapulæ as
if bruised; fingers as if asleep; inner side of upper arm
as if bruised; as if tendons of elbow joint were too short;
l. thumb as if sprained; as of a heavy burden on crest
of ilium; lumbar vertebræ as if tired; hip joint as if
luxated; as if leg was too long when standing; pain
in leg as if from an ulcer; as if knee joint would suddenly give way; limbs as if beaten, or as if after a long
walk; weariness as if from too long a foot journey; sensation in skin as from ulceration.
Pain: in occiput; in l. side of neck, shoulder and arm; in
teeth extending to temples and l. side of face; in region
of umbilicus; in uterus; in vagina; in chest and
sternum; in small of back and sacral region; in shoulders; in arm; in elbow joint; in ulnar muscles; in l.
thumb; in abdomen and lumbar vertebræ; in l. hip
joint; in whole leg; in all limbs.

Violent pain: elbow joint across r. shoulder.
Severe pain: in head; in small of back and uterine re-
    gion, extending to thighs; during coition; in chest.
Violent spasms: in groins.
Cutting: in abdomen.
Tearing, drawing, jerking pains: in head.
Piercing: in head.
Stitches: in ear; in region of liver; in rectum; from
    small of back through pelvis to external genitals; in
    side; in chest; just over heart; across chest; in r.
    chest; under scapula; in middle of chest; in heart;
    from back into genitals; in arm from shoulder joint
    through to fingers; from crest of ilium through abdo-
    men; in r. ankle and l. heel; in joints.
Electric-like stitches: in vagina.
Stitching: in back and lower abdomen; in chin and cheeks.
Ulcerative pain: in abdomen; during coition, in cervix
    uteri; in soles.
Pressing, gnawing, ulcerative pain: in stomach.
Drawing: in teeth, extending to temples and inner ear;
    in upper abdomen; along coccyx down to rectum and
    vagina; from behind forward into genitals or down into
    thighs; in r. arm.
Griping: about navel.
Cramplike pain: in rectum; in l. arm.
Laborlike pains: in abdomen.
Contractive pain: in vagina.
Colic: in abdomen.
Throbbing and beating: in forehead; in cheeks.
Burning pain: in r. hip.
Bruised pain: in region of liver; on crest of ilium.
Shattering sensation: in abdomen.
Rheumatic pains: in joints.
Pulsation: in forehead and vertex.
Burning pains: in face; in small of back.
Sore pain: in abdomen.
Burning: of conjunctiva; of outer ear; in bowels; in
    pudenda; in genitals; in female sexual organs; in back
    and lower abdomen; of vagina; of labia; in chest; in
    small of back.
Soreness: in head; in chest.
Smarting: in eyes; in pudenda; in vagina.
Biting: of female organs.
Heat: in face; in eyes.
Constriction: hypochondria; rectum; vagina; chest.
Painful dulness: of head.
Dull pain: in region of ovaries.
Painful pressure: towards genitals.

Painful hard spot: at l. of stomach; in mammæ.
Scratching: in throat.
Rough and scraping sensation: in throat.
Dull feeling: in head.
Fulness: in stomach; in region of liver.
Tightness: across pit of stomach.
Contraction: in abdomen.
Bearing down and weight: in pelvis.
Pressure: on sternum; in region of spleen.
Anxious heaviness and oppression: in chest; at heart.
Heaviness or pressure: in various parts of head; of fore-
head; on r. side of throat.
Stiffness: of l. side of neck, shoulder and arm; in limbs.
Stupid feeling: in head.
Numbness: of thigh.
Roaring: in head.
Buzzing: in head.
Tingling and buzzing: in lower limbs.
Crawling: below larynx.
Burning itching: in soles.
Voluptuous itching: deep in vagina.
Itching: in eyes; in ears; of female organs; from leucor-
rhœa; in vagina; between labia and thighs.
Painful sensation of coldness: in abdomen.
" **Tissues.** ❙Hemorrhages; small wounds bleed much.
❙Profuse, passive hemorrhages, epistaxis, hæmoptysis and
hæmaturia.
❙Typhoid hemorrhages, with fetid stools, followed by great
prostration.
❙Fetid evacuations and excoriation of mucous surfaces
generally; skin wrinkled; restless and sleepless nights.
❙Profuse and offensive secretions of mucous membranes
and ulcerations of same, with greatly depressed vitality.
❙Rheumatic pains in joints, also stitches, most of hip and
knee; numbness of whole limb as if asleep.
❙Rapid emaciation.
❙Scrofulous and psoric affections.
❙Spongy, burning ulcers; pus acrid, ichorous, fetid, yellow.
❙Gangrenous, cancerous and putrefying ulcers.
❙Epithelioma; carcinoma ventriculi or uteri.
❙Carbuncle.
❙Tendency to decomposition; great irritability, < at rest.
θAnthrax.
" **Touch. Passive Motion. Injuries.** Touch: scalp sen-
sitive; orifice of uterus painful; fundus of uterus pain-
ful like a blood boil; cervix scirrhus very painful; on
inner side of upper arm, pain.
Pressure: region of spleen sensitive, in region of ovaries
unbearable; of hand > pain in chest and sternum.

Rubbing: smarting in eyes <; hot, acrid tears.

Tight clothing is intolerable: constriction of hypochondria.

" Skin. **Itching**; toward evening so violent as to drive one almost wild.

Wheals like urticaria.

Sensation in skin as from ulceration, especially on face and chin.

Eruption of nodosities and blisters like bug bites.

Eruption dry as well as moist, in almost all parts of body, especially on backs of hands and feet, in palms, in ears, in popliteal region, and on knuckles of hands, with much itching.

Large, greasy looking, pockshaped pustules, over whole body; skin tense, shining, deep red; greasy moisture.

Painless, pustular eruption all over body, especially on chin and cheeks; sticking pain.

Watery or sero-purulent herpes, on back of hands and fingers and joints, itching violently towards evening.

Herpes in palms of hands, in ears, elbows, knuckles and malleoli, < evenings and in open air, > from warmth.

Old ulcers, painful, putrid.

Skin remarkably pale.

" Stages of Life, Constitution. Dark complexion, slight, lean.

Complexion livid, disposition sad, irritable.

Often indicated for old women.

Torpid, leuco-phlegmatic temperament.

Old looking children, hard to awaken.

Child, æt. 6 weeks, bottle-fed; gastromalacia.

Girl, æt. 3 months; gastromalacia.

Boy, æt. 6 months, bottle-fed; gastromalacia.

Boy, æt. 2½, weak, delicate, irritable and wilful; suffering nine months; diarrhœa.

Girl, æt. 5, blonde, delicate; enuresis.

Child; daily attacks of vomiting.

Girl, æt. 8, two sisters sick with violent diphtheritis; diphtheria.

Girl, æt. 9, had snuffles when a baby, teeth wedge shaped, very old looking, syphilitic dyscrasia; deafness.

Boy, æt. 10, strong; hemorrhage after extraction of tooth.

Girl, æt. 13, tall for her age, fair, blonde, delicate; menstrual ailment.

Boy, æt. 18, dark complexioned, slight and lean, stature ill developed, suffering since childhood; enuresis.

Girl, æt. 18, suffering 3 months; consumption.

Man, æt. 18, weak, poor circumstances, suffering since childhood; incontinence of urine.

Girl, æt. 20; consumption.

Woman, æt. 25, brunette, with bright red complexion and not very mild disposition; chronic ovarian affection.

Woman, æt. 26, full blooded, after two abortions, a birth, then two more abortions; affection of uterus.

Young woman, after difficult labor, two years ago; attacks of vomiting.

Young woman, scrofulous; frequent attacks of pneumonia.

Woman, phlegmatic, mother of four children; puerperal metritis.

Man, æt. 30, tall, good constitution, cheerful disposition; hemorrhage from lungs.

Woman, æt. 32, married, suffering ten years; leucorrhœa.

Woman, æt. 33, small build, childless; uterine affection.

Woman, æt. 40, mother of three children; menorrhagia.

Woman, æt. 41; rheumatism.

Tailor, æt. 46, weak, drunkard; consumption.

Woman, æt. 50; painful, hard spot in stomach.

Relations. Antidoted by: *Acon.* (vascular erethism); *Nux vom.* (violent pulsations in every part of body).

Compatible: before *Sulphur;* before *Arsen.*, in cancer; frequently followed well by *Bellad.*, *Calc. ostr.*, *Kali carb.*, *Lycop.*, *Nitr. ac.*, *Rhus tox.*, *Sepia.*

Incompatible: *Carbo veg.*

Compare: *Ant. tart.*, *Carbo an.*, *Graphit.*, *Hepar*, *Iodum*, *Ipec.*, *Laches.*, *Mercur.*, *Petrol.*, *Phosphor.*

LAC CANINUM.

Dogs' Milk.

The use of dogs' milk in medicine is of ancient date. "Dioscorides, Rhasis, Pliny and Sextus recommend it for the removal of the dead fœtus. Sammonicus and Sextus praise it in photophobia and otitis. Pliny claims that it cures ulceration of the internal os. It was considered an antidote to deadly poisons."

The remedy was revived by Reisig, of New York, who used it successfully in the treatment of diphtheria. After Reisig the remedy was used by Bayard and by Swan, to whose indefatigable exertions we owe the present status of this valuable medicine. Swan's potencies were prepared from Reisig's 17th.

Provings (with potencies from the 30th upwards) by Laura Morgan, Hazlitt, Miss W., Mr. J. L. H., H. K., Mrs. Wheelwright, White, Grant, Swan, Taylor and family, and numerous others. See Swan's Materia Medica of Nosodes and Morbific Products, 1888, arranged by Berridge.

CLINICAL AUTHORITIES.— *Sensation of film before eyes,* Swan, Raue's Rec., 1875, p. 61 ; *Sore throat,* Fowler, Org., vol. 3, p. 102 ; Biegler, Hom. Phys., vol. 6, p. 410 ; Hills, Hah. Mon , vol. 10, p. 279 ; Gale, Hom. Phys., vol. 2, p. 69 ; *Diphtheritic sore throat,* Carr, Org., vol. 2, p. 204 ; Baillie, Raue's Rec., 1874, p. 112 ; *Diphtheria* (4 cases), Hiller, Org., vol. 3, p. 339 ; Swan, Times Retros., vol. 3, p. 29 ; Hills, Payne, Cin. Med. Adv., vol. 5, pp. 83, 84 ; Lippe, Org., vol. 1, p. 364 ; Finch, Wildes, Wesselhœft, Nichols, Cin. Med. Adv., vol. 5, pp. 178–182 ; *Croupal diphtheria,* Wesselhœft, Org., vol. 3, p. 362 ; *Affection of stomach,* Hiller, Org., vol. 2, p. 288 ; *Syphilitic ulceration of penis,* Lippe, Org., vol. 2, p. 342 ; *Injurious effects of weaning,* Gramm, T. H. M. S. Pa., 1884 p. 47 ; *Parenchymatous metritis,* Biegler, MSS. ; *Sciatica and sore throat,* Swan, Hom. Phys., vol. 6, p. 411 ; *Rickets* (4 cases), Bernard, Times Retros., vol. 3, p. 29 ; *Sciatica and rheumatism,* Hiller, Org., vol. 3, p. 338 ; *Acute rheumatism,* Lippe, Org., vol. 2, p. 484 ; *Rheumatism,* Butler, Hom. Phys. ; *Nervous affection,* Berridge, Hom. Phys., vol. 3, p. 217 ; *Acute neuralgia,* Hiller, Org., vol. 3, p. 338.

[1] **Mind.** ❚Very forgetful ; in writing, uses too many words or not the right ones ; very nervous.

❚Omits final letter or letters of a word, when writing ; in speaking substitutes name of object seen, instead of object thought of.

❚Very absentminded ; makes purchases and walks off without them ; goes to post a letter, brings it home in her hand.

❚Cannot collect her thoughts ; confused feeling.

❚Very restless ; cannot concentrate her thoughts or mind to read ; wants to leave everything as soon as it is commenced.

❚Is impressed with idea that all she says is a lie.

Every time a symptom appears she feels very confident that it is not attributable to medicine, but that it is some settled disease.

❚Sensation as if she was going deranged, when sitting still and thinking; sometimes she has most horrible sights presented to her mental vision (not always snakes), feels horribly afraid that they will take objective form and show themselves to her natural eye.

ⅠⅠThinks she is looked down upon by everyone, that she is of no importance in life.

ⅠⅠImagines he wears some one else's nose. θDiphtheria.

❚Imagines to be dirty.

❚Imagines she sees spiders. θDiphtheria.

Woke at daylight feeling that she is a loathsome, horrible mass of disease (while the breasts were affected); could not bear to look at any portion of her body, not even hands, as it intensified feeling of disgust and horror; could not bear to have any one part of her body touch another, had to keep even fingers apart; felt that if she could not in some way get out of her body, she should soon become crazy.

ⅠⅠAfter inhaling gas for extraction of teeth, very strange sensation in head (such as he felt when going off under gas); sometimes imagines heart or breathing are going to stop, or otherwise frightens himself, and this makes heart beat violently; occasionally very depressed, and fancies he is going out of his mind.

Sensation or delusion as if surrounded by myriads of snakes, some running like lightning up and down inside of skin; some that are inside feel long and thin; fears to put her feet on floor, lest she should tread on them and make them squirm and wind around her legs; is afraid to look behind her, for fear that she will see snakes there, does not dream of them and is seldom troubled with them after dark; on going to bed she was afraid to shut her eyes for fear that a large snake, the size of her arm, would hit her in the face.

Worries herself lest pimples which appear during menses will prove to be little snakes, and twine and twist around each other.

On lying down either by day or night begins to think how horrible it would be if a very sharp pain, like a knife, should go through her, and thought of it causes great mental distress.

ⅠⅠAttacks of rage, cursing and swearing at slightest provocation.

ⅠⅠCannot bear to be left alone for an instant. θDiphtheria.

ⅠⅠNo desire to live.

Sits and looks under chairs, table, sofa and everything in room, expecting yet dreading to see some terrible monster creep forth and feeling all the time, that, if it does, it will drive her raving mad; she is not afraid in dark, it is only in light where she can imagine that she can see them.

ⅠⅠFits of weeping two or three times a day.   θParenchymatous metritis.

ⅠⅠChild cries and screams all the time, especially at night, and will not be pacified in any way.

ⅠⅠWhen paroxysms of intense nervousness come on, feels like tearing off her clothes; takes off her rings; cannot bear anything to touch her, especially over l. ovarian region, from which she frequently lifts bed clothes.

ⅠHad to keep her fingers apart from each other.

ⅠDepression of spirits, doubts her ability and success, thinks she will have heart disease and die of it.

ⅠChronic "blue" condition; everything seems so dark that it can grow no darker.

ⅠⅠGloomy feelings, < as headache gets worse. θParenchymatous metritis.

ⅠⅠFears she will become unable to perform her duties.

ⅠⅠFear of death, with anxious expression of countenance.

ⅠⅠVery nervous; constant dread; a feeling as if she was going to become unconscious. θDiphtheria.

ⅠⅠWakes distressed, and obliged to rise and occupy herself in some manner; fears she will be crazy. θParenchymatous metritis.

Has great fear of falling down stairs at times.

ⅠVery cross and irritable only while headache lasts.

ⅠⅠWhen awake, very irritable and cries constantly.

ⅠⅠFeels insulted because she thinks she is looked down upon by everyone.

ⅠIntense ugliness and hatefulness; writes to her best friends all sorts of mean and contemptible things.

ⅠⅠEasily excited. θParenchymatous metritis.

ⅠⅠToo excited to allow examination of throat.

ⅠⅠFeels weak, and nerves so thoroughly out of order, that she cannot bear one finger to touch another. θNervous throat affection.

ⅠⅠExceedingly nervous and irritable.   θParenchymatous metritis.

ⅠⅠVery easily startled. θParenchymatous metritis.

² **Sensorium.** ⅠDizzy sensation with slight nausea.

ⅠⅠAfter inhaling diphtheritic breath, light headed, with tingling on vertex and slight sore throat.

ⅠⅠConstant noise in head, very confusing; < at night and at menses. θParenchymatous metritis.

ıı Wakes at night with sensation as if bed was in motion;
noise in head bad beyond description; first thought on
waking that headboard was swaying, and so occasion-
ing distress, but found it arose from internal causes.
θParenchymatous metritis.

³ **Inner Head.** ∎Frontal headache.

∎On going into cold wind, terrible pain in forehead as if
it would split open, > on going into warm room.

ıı After midnight, very severe frontal headache, and a
piercing pain on vertex. θTyphoid pneumonia.

ıı Headache both frontal and occipital, < by turning eyeballs upwards.

ıı Headache over eyes, < when sewing. θPharyngitis.

∎Headache: in afternoon, principally over l. eye; over l.
eye on first awaking.

ıı Pains and throbbing in temples. θDyspepsia.

ıı Headaches, mostly through temples, darting, stabbing;
sometimes begin on r. side, and sometimes on l.; always
going from one side to other.

∎Pains in head during day, first on one side, then on
other; seem perfectly unbearable; > on first going
into air.

ıı Headache from below eyes over whole head and top of
shoulder. θParenchymatous metritis.

ıı Severe pressure on brain. θParenchymatous metritis.

∎Arose in morning with heavy, dull, frontal headache, and
at 9 A.M., severe sharp pain on top of head, coming from
nape of neck, then stretching across head forward; pain
so severe that he presses top of head with hands; neck
stiffened; bending head forward, or lying down, causes
congestion, increasing pain; again, pains subside for
short time, and begin anew, either in front part of head,
or in nape of neck, or all over head at once; when pain
is frontal it causes lachrymation. θAcute neuralgia.

ıı Frequently wakes with sick headache, which seems to
commence at nape. θNervous throat affection.

ıı Sick headaches, beginning in nape; pain settling gradually in r. or l. forehead.

ıı Darting pains from occiput to forehead; beating. θParenchymatous metritis.

ıı Headaches seem unbearable, and are attended by pain
in lumbar region; all pains cease as soon as throat gets
worse. θDiphtheria.

∎Headache < by noise or talking, > by keeping quiet;
confused feeling in head.

⁴ **Outer Head.** Head very sore and itches almost all the time.

Sore pimples on scalp which discharge and form a scab;
extremely painful when touched or on combing hair.

⁵ **Sight and Eyes.** ❘❘Eyes sensitive to light. θRheumatism.
❘❘❘Must have light, yet is intolerant of sunlight. θDiphtheria.
▮Tendency in retina to retain impression of objects, especially of colors; or somewhat of object last looked at is
projected into next.
While looking at an object, appears to see just beyond or
out of axis of vision, an object passing across field of
sight; but on adjusting eye to see it, is gone; it always
appears as a small object, ❘❘like a rat or bird, sometimes
on floor, at others in air.
❘❘Sees faces before her eyes, < in dark; the face that
haunts her most is one that she has really seen.
❘❘Sees big eyes and creeping things. θDiphtheria.
❘❘Difficulty in distinguishing objects; in reading, letters
run together. θAfter diphtheria.
▮When reading, page does not look clear, but seems covered with various pale spots of red, yellow, green and
other colors.
❘❘When looking in a mirror by gaslight, after exerting
eyes, sees a green spot or a green band before her l. eye,
the band slanting downward from l. eye to r. cheek.
θGlaucoma.
❘❘Square or round green spots or brown spots before l.
eye, when sun is bright; sometimes bright spots before
l. eye. θCataract.
❘❘Frequent sensation of a film before eyes, with vertigo,
and while thus suffering would see a small dark object,
like a mouse or bird, coming up to her left.
❘❘Film over eyes from reading or looking closely.
❘❘Eyes blurred. θParenchymatous metritis.
❘❘Heavy pain in eyeballs, with outward pressure.
❘❘Burning in l. eye. θRheumatism.
❘❘Eyes watery and discharging. θDiphtheria.
❘❘Eyes dull and lustreless. θDiphtheria.
❘❘Dark brown areolae under eyes. θRetarded menses.
❘❘Non-œdematous swelling of upper and lower lids; pink
color of lower lids, most noticeable on r. θDiphtheria.
❘❘Heaviness of l. upper eyelid, with pain above l. eye.
▮Upper eyelids very heavy, could scarcely keep eyes open.
❘❘Agglutination of l. eyelids. θRheumatism.

⁶ **Hearing and Ears.** ❘❘Sounds seem very far off.
Pain in both ears; noises; as if ears were full.
❘❘Deafness from hereditary syphilis.
❘❘Green odorless discharge.

⁷ **Smell and Nose.** ❘❘Nose cold. θDiphtheria.
▮Fluids escape through nose while drinking. θDiphtheria.
❘❘Epistaxis: when speaking or swallowing; at 4 P.M., re-
turning at intervals. θDiphtheria.

▮Considerable sneezing.

▮Head so stuffed she can hardly breathe.

▮Stuffed feeling in head, as of a severe cold in head.

▮▮One side of nose stuffed up, the other free and discharging thin mucus at times and thin blood; these conditions alternate, first one nostril stopped up and the other fluent, and vice versa. θDiphtheria.

▮Nasal discharge, excoriating nostrils and upper lip.

▮▮Coryza, with discharge of thick white mucus.

▮Fluent catarrh from both nostrils, with sensation of fulness of upper part of nose.

▮Coryza; constant watery discharge from nose, excoriating nostrils and upper lips.

▮▮Profuse nocturnal nasal discharge, like gonorrhœa, staining pillow greenish yellow.

▮▮Nose became so bad that there was fear of destruction of bones; bloody pus discharged several times daily; nasal bones sore on pressure.

▮Sore on r. side of septum of nose; next day nose sore, constant inclination to pick at it and get scab off.

▮▮Two very angry gatherings, one under l. side of nose, and one on upper l. nostril; both came to a head, and discharged matter and blood, and afterwards scabbed over; before discharge shooting pain. θSick headache.

8 **Upper Face.** ▮▮Face indicates great anxiety. θDiphtheria.

▮▮Countenance pale and careworn. θDiphtheria.

▮▮Face very red, and then suddenly pale.

▮Face flushed; cheeks red. θDiphtheria.

▮▮Face flushed, swollen and hot; burns, feels dry.

▮Dark brown areolæ under eyes. θRetarded menses.

▮▮In morning, l. superior maxillary feels sore; most of time there is dull pain, < by exertion; sometimes throbbing pain, burning, throbbing, aching heat, sensation of fulness; cannot wear her false teeth from soreness and swelling of maxillary; an exacerbation of pain leaves face very sore; pains > by warm applications, but only cold applications > soreness.

9 **Lower Face.** ▮▮Red circular spot below r. malar bone, burning to touch. θDyspepsia.

▮▮Flushes on l. cheek. θDyspepsia.

▮Lips dry and peeling off; dry and parched, but mouth constantly full of frothy saliva.

▮▮Seems to affect lower lip most, and blisters and fever sores on lips are amenable to its influence.

▮▮Jaw cracks while eating. θDyspepsia.

▮▮Submaxillary glands swollen. θDiphtheria.

▮▮Swelling of l. parotid, with sore throat and loss of appetite.

▮▮Parotid gland first attacked, and disease extends to other glands of neck; throat and sides of neck not tender to external touch. *θ*Diphtheria.

 ||Swelling of parotid passes from r. to l., but more often from l. to r.

¹⁰ Teeth and Gums. ||Paroxysmal gnawing pain in l. upper canine, temporarily yields to any cold application. *θ*Sick headache.

 ||Gums swollen, ulcerated, retracted, bleeding, teeth loose; caused by defective nutrition and exposure.

¹¹ Taste and Tongue. ||Nothing tastes natural, except salt food. *θ*Epulis.

 ❚Putrid taste in mouth. *θ*Diphtheria.

 ||Tongue generally red and moist. *θ*Diphtheria.

 ❚Tongue coated whitish, except edges, which are red.

 ❚Tongue coated, dirty looking, centre to root.

 ❚Tongue furred whitish at edges, centre and root darker.

 ||Tongue: heavily coated, and dry to the tip; dirty coated, yellowish white and slimy; dry; thickly coated, greyish white. *θ*Diphtheria.

 ❚Tongue coated whitish grey, having an underlying bluish look.

 ||Slight yellow coating on tongue. *θ*Diphtheria.

 ❚Tongue coated brown.

 ||Difficulty in articulating, owing to a semi-paretic state of tongue, causing stuttering if she talks fast; has to speak very slowly.

¹² Inner Mouth. ||Peculiar rattle in mouth, right along tongue; on attempting to hawk her mouth clear, mucous rattled along tongue quickly and continually; utterance was so indistinct as to be unintelligible, and every word she tried to speak was accompanied by this quick and continuous rattle along tongue. *θ*Diphtheria.

 ||Breath offensive, putrid. *θ*Diphtheria.

 ||Mouth dry and parched; drinks little and often.

 ❚Mouth very dry without thirst.

 ❚Mucus in mouth, < after eating, and in open air.

 ❚Mouth full of frothy mucus; inclination to swallow.

 ❚Increase in quantity of saliva which is slightly viscid.

 ❚Mouth constantly full of frothy saliva, lips dry, parched.

 ||Constant spitting and drooling, very profuse, making chin and breast sore. *θ*Diphtheria.

 ❚During sleep, saliva runs from mouth, so as to wet pillow.

 ||Stomatitis; stomacace; cancrum oris; nursing sore mouth.

¹³ Throat. ||Throat very sensitive to touch externally.

 ||Sensation as if throat was closing and she would choke, sensation is between throat and nose; feels as if something in throat was either enlarged or relaxed; desires to keep mouth open lest she should choke; sometimes

cannot swallow, because there seems to be a kind of muscular contraction in throat.

I I Paralytic symptoms strongly marked; as soon as he went to sleep, would stop breathing, and was only kept alive by keeping him awake; apparently respiration was kept up by voluntary effort. θDiphtheria.

I I Talking is very difficult, and there is a disposition to talk through nose. θNervous throat affection.

I I Swallowing very difficult, painful, almost impossible.

I I Uvula elongated and very much swollen, diphtheritic coating on it; tonsils swollen and coated; back of throat patched, extending up to hard palate; odor offensive and diphtheritic.

I Constant inclination to swallow, causes pain extending to both ears.

I Pricking sensation in throat, as if full of sticks.

I I Pricking and cutting pains through tonsils on swallowing, shooting up to ears. θDiphtheria.

I Pain in throat pushes toward l. ear.

I I On swallowing, acute pain at one time on r. side of throat, and again on l. side. θDiphtheria.

I I Throat > after drinking cold or warm; < by empty swallowing. θDiphtheria.

I I Throat feels stiff as a board. θDiphtheria.

I I Throat sensitive. θParenchymatous metritis.

I Tickling and sense of constriction in upper part of throat, causing constant dry, hacking cough.

I Feeling of lump in throat, which goes down when swallowing, but returns; throat < on r. side.

I I Sensation of ball or round body in l. side of throat, and feeling that it could be removed with a knife.

I I Marked sensation of lump in throat on l. side, when swallowing; pain extends to ear. θDiphtheria.

I I Sensation of lump in r. side of throat, with a feeling that she could take hold of it with her fingers and pull it out; accompanied by a very annoying pricking, stitching feeling; constant inclination to swallow saliva, which causes soreness of throat.

I I Lump on l. side of pharynx below tonsil, causing an enlargement that filled each arch of palate, nearly to r. side.

I I Most pain when swallowing solids, no aversion to cold drink; when swallowing solid food, it seems to pass over a lump, with sore and aching pains extending to and into l. ear. θDiphtheria.

I Soreness of throat commences with a tickling.

I Throat feels raw.

I I Sensation of rawness, commencing usually on l. side of throat. θDiphtheria.

▮Throat feels dry, husky, as if scalded by hot fluid.

ııThroat has a burnt and drawn feeling as from caustic.

▮Pain in r. side of throat in region of tonsil. θAcute
rheumatism.

ııWakes with throat and mouth painfully dry. θParenchymatous metritis.

ııThroat very dry and sore, much inflamed, < r. side;
palate red, uvula elongated; very painful deglutition.

ııThroat sore, œdematous, puffed, tonsils badly swollen.

▮Especially shining, glazed and red appearance of throat.
θSyphilis.

ııSore throat, pains in whole body and limbs, severe headache. θDiphtheria.

▮Throat very sore on l. side; painful to external pressure
both sides.

ııSore throat on r. side, low down, and extending up to
ear; pain when swallowing; sensitive to external pressure; slight coryza.

ııThroat sore, swollen, red and glistening. θDiphtheria.

ııSore spot in l. side of throat, only at night, removed by
1 A.M.; next night same on r. side of throat; after 1 A.M.
returned no more.

▮Crusts on skin, with greyish yellow matter under them;
mucous follicles of throat raised and swollen, and covered with whitish, cream colored mucus; bloody pus discharged from nose several times a day; nasal bones sore
to pressure. θSore throat.

▮Partial suppression of urine; throat sore and of an œdematous, puffy appearance; next morning, pulse 130; temperature 102; tonsils badly swollen; great indisposition
to take food or drink. θSore throat.

▮▮Soreness of throat commences with a tickling sensation,
which causes constant cough; then a sensation of a lump
on one side, causing constant deglutition; this condition
entirely ceases, only to commence on the opposite side,
and often alternates, again returning to its first condition; these sore throats are very apt to begin and end
with menses.

ııSore throat just before menses for several years ever
since diphtheria; small yellowish white patches of exudation on tonsil of affected side, with great difficulty of
swallowing, and sharp pains moving up into ear; these
patches are also present on back of throat and uvula;
some are quite yellow and some are white; scraping
them off makes them bleed.

▮Throat very sore, pain extending to chest; dry and sore;
deep red color on either side of throat opposite tonsils.

▮Shortly before going to bed, throat began to feel raw and

sore; did not sleep well; next morning, throat felt full
and sore, somewhat < on r. side; this condition continued two days, when it seemed to continue downward
to chest.

▮On waking in morning, throat felt as if there were lumps
in it like two eggs, and sore all the time, especially when
swallowing; cold water seemed to > momentarily; in
evening, examination revealed both tonsils much swollen and very red, l. most, and distinct patches on l. tonsil.

▮Right tonsil red and swollen; pain in tonsil of gnawing
character; < at night; dreams of snake in bed.

▮▮Tonsils inflamed and very sore, red and shining, almost
closing throat; dryness of fauces and throat; swelling
of submaxillary glands.   θTonsillitis.

▮Quinsy, just ready to discharge, disappeared without discharging, in an unusually short time; the trouble had
been changing from one side to other and back again;
has not returned.

▮Sore throat, rapidly growing <; fever; difficult swallowing; r. side <; r. tonsil intensely inflamed, bright red
and greatly enlarged, and a yellowish grey spot on inner
surface; whole pharynx, uvula and velum much inflamed; spot became larger, and others formed in pharynx; l. tonsil became nearly as large as r.; fetid breath;
subsequently a bright scarlet eruption on face, neck,
hands and chest, like scarlatina; almost total inability
to swallow, especially fluids; aversion to liquids, particularly water.

▯▯Quinsy; suppuration ran from l. tonsil to r., then from
r. to l., then back again to r., then both tonsils equally;
and again one tonsil would > and the other grow
<; whole posterior portion of throat was an œdema-
tous swelling, rising up like an insurmountable barrier;
thick tough pieces of diphtheritic membrane were coming away, and new membranes constantly reforming;
swelling in throat so large and tense that mouth could
not be closed.

▯▯Mucous follicles raised or swollen, and covered with a
whitish, cream colored mucus.

▯▯Whole membrane of throat swollen, dark red, with grey
patches and small, irregular shaped ulcers; membrane
peeled off occasionally; articulation and deglutition
intensely painful; < after sleep.

▯▯White ulcers on tonsils.

▮Sore throat, beginning at l. tonsil, swollen and ulcerated;
throat feels swollen and raw, pricking and cutting pains
shoot through tonsils when swallowing; submaxillary
glands swollen, sore and aching pain in l. ear; most

pain when swallowing solids; food seems to pass over a lump, no aversion to cold drink; while drinking, fluid escaped through nose.

ı ıSore throat commencing on l. tonsil, which was swollen and ulcerated, and presented a depression covered by a white patch; the disease later extended to palate and r. tonsil, the parts red and shining.

ı ıThroat highly inflamed, swollen, almost closed, grey diphtheric spots on l. side of throat.

ı ıSore throat, ulcer on inner side of each tonsil, tonsils red and slightly enlarged, rest of throat dry. θDiphtheria.

ı ıUlcers increase in size and number, but neighboring membrane looks clearer. θDiphtheria.

ı ıSmall, round or irregular, grey white ulcers on tonsils and fauces, both sides. θDiphtheria.

ı ıTonsils swollen as almost to close throat. θQuinsy.

ı ıRight tonsil covered with ash grey membrane extending along free palatine border to uvula, which it had already involved; room loaded with diphtheritic odor; next day membrane had passed centre, involving whole arch of palate, and reaching far down on l. tonsil.

ı ıRight tonsil raw, swollen; grey white membrane there and on fauces. θDiphtheria.

ı ıWhole of r. tonsil covered with diphtheritic patch.

ı ıBoth tonsils swollen and covered with spots of exudation, like the mould on preserves.

ı ıTongue, fauces, tonsils, all swollen and covered with a dirty coating. θDiphtheria.

ı ıOn each tonsil a very thick exudation, covering nearly entire surface; while examining a large piece of membrane was accidentally detached from one tonsil, followed by considerable hemorrhage.

ı ıThroat very sore, tonsils enlarged, especially l., very large white patches; tonsils and pharynx deep purple red; putrid odor from throat; after patches were expectorated, they left throat very sore, raw and bloody.

ı ıThroat very sore, < l. side; large greenish ulcers on both tonsils, surrounded by grey white exudation, parts not covered are a deep purple red; swelling externally on both sides; after exudation on tonsils disappeared, a raw, bloody surface was left. θDiphtheria.

ı ıWhite patches, like eggs of flies, on both tonsils, extending thence to back of throat; tonsils enlarged and deep red; felt she would suffocate at night from full feeling in throat, which prevented sleep; swallowing toast gave some pain, but seemed to clear throat; drinking caused more pain in throat, and she had to gulp it down.

ı ıGargling with warm water brought up a stringy mucus.

॥Whole membrane of throat highly inflamed, swollen,
and glands enlarged on both sides. θDiphtheria.

॥False membrane in throat, thick, grey, or slightly yellow, or dark and almost black, or white and glistening,
almost like mother of pearl, or fish scales.

॥Dark red, angry streaks of capillaries in fauces, giving
place to shining, glistening deposit, or tough membrane;
half arches filled with sticky, fetid saliva.

■■Diphtheritic membrane white like china; mucous membrane of throat glistening as if varnished; membranes
leave one side and go to other repeatedly; desire for
warm drinks, which may return through nose; post-
diphtheritic paralysis.

■Glossy, shining appearance; disposition on part of membrane to change its position in fauces. θCroupous diphtheria.

॥Ulcers on throat shine like silver gloss, symptoms went
from side to side; croupy symptoms not well marked;
after exudation was cleared off, a deep excavation was
left. θDiphtheria.

॥Diphtheritic deposits look as if varnished; exudations
migratory, now here, now there. θDiphtheritic croup.

॥Thick membranous mass lying on soft palate, l. side;
diphtheritic masses covering uvula and posterior wall
of throat; next day, membrane on soft palate thicker,
dirty brown on uvula and posterior walls and pillars of
throat, much more extensive and offensive; very difficult deglutition; a large membranous mass, which
threatened suffocation, having been removed by forceps;
on following morning a second membrane had taken
place of first, and walls of throat were covered with a
dirty grey exudation; uvula almost black, and coarse
shreds of membrane hanging from it.

■In morning throat very sore; r. tonsil covered with
ulcers and patches, which extended over palate and
covered l. tonsil; next day membrane extended across
posterior wall of pharynx; uvula elongated, accompanied by chilliness, high fever, pains in head, back
and limbs, great restlessness and extreme prostration.

॥Throat sore, but little swelling, tonsils very slightly
enlarged; soreness of throat, first chiefly r., then l.; well
marked diphtheritic membrane on both sides of throat
situated on an inflamed red base, $\frac{3}{4}$ inch long, $\frac{1}{2}$ inch
wide, $\frac{1}{8}$ inch thick, and the same length and width as
at the base; anterior edge a dirty yellow; centre more
organized, pearly, glistening, white like cartilage; membrane on r. side seems more firm and dense, and disappeared later.

■Severe chills, headache, pain in back and limbs, restlessness and sore throat; three days later r. tonsil covered
with ashy grey membrane, extending along free palatine
border to uvula, which it had already involved; peculiar
diphtheritic odor in room; pulse small; skin clammy;
rapid vital exhaustion; next day membrane involved
whole arch of palate and passed down to l. tonsil. θDiphtheria (after failure of *Phytol.* and *Lycop.*).

■Roof of mouth and back wall of pharynx coated with
a greyish yellow deposit, greater part of which soon
disappeared, lasting only about an hour; throat very
much > by noon, deposit had nearly disappeared, but <
again by night.

||Throat covered with diphtheritic membrane; uvula
elongated, swollen and covered with black and white or
grey diphtheritic deposit; back of throat, extending to
hard palate, all covered; breath very offensive; l. side
of neck swollen and almost even with jaw; great difficulty in swallowing; after throat began to improve, disease seemed to work through whole alimentary canal,
for uvula and parts were very much swollen, and every
little while there would be involuntary discharges of
diphtheritic matter from uvula and rectum.

■Patch of diphtheritic membrane appeared first on r. tonsil, then on l., and frequently alternated sides; swelling
of neck (submaxillary and lymphatic glands) also alternated in like manner; < during and after a cold storm
from northeast; tickling in throat when drinking; one
side of nose stuffed up, the other free and discharging
thin mucus at times and thin blood; this condition of
nose also alternated; non-œdematous swelling of eyelids, pink color of under lid, particularly of r. eye;
breathing hoarse and croupy, at times entire stoppage
of breath; often snoring, and only possible through
mouth; obstinate constipation, frequent desire, with
darting pains in rectum, no power to expel; stool
large in size, whitish, rough, scaly, hard; could not bear
to be left alone an instant; saw big eyes and creeping
things; must have light, yet is intolerant to light of
sun; urine scanty, infrequent, no desire, coffee colored;
80 per cent. of albumen and much mucus; quantity
less than a gill in twenty-four hours. θDiphtheria.

■Fever; bathed in warm perspiration, especially about face,
neck and hands; anxious expression; eyes watery and
discharging; wants to sit up in mother's arms; cries
and desists at every attempt to nurse; reaches for water,
yet refuses to take it; respiration hoarse; crying whispered and broken, often no sound at all; pulse 170;

tongue, fauces and tonsils swollen and covered with
dirty coating; drooling from mouth; throat tender to
touch externally; thick, dirty grey diphtheritic membrane, covering free border of epiglottis, and extending
off to each side; child refuses to swallow and sputters
out the medicine, some returning through nose. *θ*Diphtheria.

∎Soreness of throat, accompanied by intense heat; pulse
scarcely to be counted; prostration so complete that
patient refused even to make an effort to take medicine;
temperature 102.6°; great sensitiveness of throat externally; symptoms < after sleep; very thick exudate,
covering nearly entire surface of each tonsil, which, if
forcibly removed, is followed by considerable hemorrhage. *θ*Diphtheria (after failure of *Laches.*).

∎Throat highly inflamed, swollen, almost closed; grey,
diphtheritic patches on l. side of throat; difficult breathing, at times suffocative spells; pulse 140; face flushed,
swollen and hot; tongue dry and thickly coated, greyish white. *θ*Diphtheria.

∎On third day r. tonsil swollen and on it a small diphtheritic patch, rest of throat inflamed; on fourth day both
tonsils swollen and covered with diphtheritic patches,
with difficult deglutition; high fever, restlessness, cried
out and talked in sleep; complained of pains in head,
back and limbs; bright scarlet redness on chest and
around neck, which, on fifth day, extended all over
body and legs; disease now at highest point; skin, in
large patches, assumed a dark red color bordering on
purple; whole body swollen; membrane, swelling and
soreness < on r. side; deglutition impossible; refusing
to drink while complaining of intense thirst; characteristic fetor in room; soreness on r. side decreased and
commenced on l.; l. tonsil and posterior wall of pharynx covered with membrane; posterior nares invaded;
marked sensation of lump in throat on l. side, when
swallowing, with pain extending to l. ear; tongue coated
dirty, yellow white and slimy; absence of prostration;
improvement commenced on seventh day and remedy
was discontinued. *θ*Diphtheria.

∎Pains in limbs, small of back and head disappear, and
throat becomes more painful, but looks better; often
ulcers increase in size and number, but neighboring
membrane looks clearer; < by empty deglutition;
throat feels stiff; > after drinking, warm or cold, no
thirst, but dry mouth; pain pushes toward l. ear; r.
tonsil raw, swollen, grey white membrane there and on
fauces; epistaxis when speaking or swallowing, in one

case; sweat all over; great exhaustion with poisoned
feeling; frequent micturition, urine dark; restless, legs
and whole body; face burns dry; constant spitting,
drooling; ulcers small, round or irregular, grey white;
voice hoarse, interrupted by weakness and hoarseness.
θDiphtheria.
ı ıThroat filled with substance that looked like "smear
kase;" throat, tongue, roof of mouth, gums and cheeks
completely lined with this substance; mouth and throat
filled with loose particles; horrible odor. θPost-scarla-
tinal diphtheria.
ıHeaviness, and stomach bloated and tender; enlargement of tonsils, l. tonsil <; feels weak; cannot eat or
drink anything without pain in pit of stomach; shortness of breath and general languor. θAfter diphtheria.
ı ıMembrane would leave throat, and a very severe interstitial hemorrhage of bright red blood would ensue;
hemorrhage would slowly improve, and membrane appear again in throat; these had continued to alternate
for several days. θDiphtheria.
ı ıFalse membrane, thick grey, yellow or dark, surrounding mucous membrane dark or bright, may be < on
either side, or inflammation shift from side to side, generally < on l.
ı ıFalse membrane, thick, yellowish grey, often greenish.
ı ıPharyngeal inflammation, with wholesale destruction
of epithelium, viscidity of saliva, heat of palms; absolute
necessity for constant change of position.
ı ıThick, dirty grey diphtheritic membrane covering free
border of epiglottis, and extending off to each side.
ı ıUvula pretty free from membrane, but intensely sore
and bleeds   θDiphtheria.
ıUvula coated (in seven cases).
.ı ıAfter membrane exfoliates, mucous membrane appears
raw and bloody, with increased deglutition.
ı ıIn most cases of diphtheria, the throat symptoms begin
on r. side.
ı ıInflammation, ulcers and swelling shift from side to side,
generally < on l. θDiphtheria.
ı ıDiphtheritic and diphtheritic croup; membranous croup.
¹⁴ **Appetite, Thirst. Desires, Aversions.** ıNo appetite.
θDyspepsia. θAcute rheumatism. θDiphtheria.
ı ıAppetite and strength failing; dislike to food, especially
fat or greasy. θParenchymatous metritis.
No appetite or thirst. θDiphtheria.
ı ıThirst for little at a time, but often, as throat is so dry
and hot. θDiphtheria.
ı ıThirst. θAcute rheumatism.

। ।Great thirst for large quantities, often.

❙Desire for highly seasoned dishes, which is very unusual; has used pepper, mustard and salt freely.

। ।Desire for warmish water with a pinch of salt in.

। ।Craves milk and drinks much of it. *θ*Diphtheria.

। ।Aversion to liquids, especially water. *θ*Diphtheria.

¹⁶ **Hiccough, Belching, Nausea and Vomiting.** ❙❙Great faintness of stomach and nausea. *θ*Metritis.

❙Nausea, with headache, on waking; all morning.

। ।Nausea at beginning of diphtheria.

। ।The almost constant diphtheritic discharges from mouth and nose nearly ceased, and she almost immediately had spells of sickness of stomach, and would occasionally vomit pieces of membrane. *θ*Diphtheria.

। ।Frequent attacks of severe vomiting, and when not so, always feeling of nausea, and fear to eat. *θ*Sick headache.

¹⁷ **Scrobiculum and Stomach.** ❙Weak, sinking feeling in stomach pit, on waking in morning.

। ।Gnawing, hungry feeling, not > by eating; everything she eats, except fish, makes her worse; the thought of milk makes her sick. *θ*Sick headache.

❙Dyspeptic pain, as from a stone, or undigested food, in stomach pit at 9.45 P.M.; followed by a stabbing pain in r. lung, just below nipple.

❙Burning in epigastric region ; feeling of weight and pressure of stone in stomach ; very thirsty ; abdomen swollen and burning, with bearing down pains therein ; mucous, yellow, liquid stools; pulse 100; pains and throbbing in temples; flushes on l. cheek ; red, circular spot below r. malar bone, burning to touch ; no appetite, cannot bear food ; jaw cracks while eating. *θ*Affection of stomach.

। ।Stomach tender and bloated ; cannot eat or drink anything without pain in stomach pit. *θ*After diphtheria.

। ।Beating in stomach and bowels.

। ।Severe throbbing in region of solar plexus ; when it becomes very severe, which it did daily for hours at a time, it would seem to extend or continue upwards to head, when dizziness and lightness of head would supervene, requiring her to lie down at once, otherwise she would fall violently to the floor.

। ।Gastralgia or cardialgia, < at menses, so she would drop to the floor, comes and goes suddenly.

¹⁸ **Hypochondria.** । ।Severe burning pain in r. hypochondriac and iliac region and corresponding part of back, extending across back to l. side of abdomen ; < when on feet or when fatigued, > when lying down.

¹⁹ **Abdomen.** ❙Abdomen very hard and swollen, in evening.

ı ıAbdomen swollen and burning, with bearing down pains therein.

ı ıExtreme heat in abdomen.

ıSevere shooting pain in abdomen, passing in all directions.

∎Pressure from within outwards, as if contents of abdomen would be forced outwards, just above pelvis.

ı ıIntense sharp pain in l. side of abdomen, with nausea while leaning forward.

ı ıPain and burning in l. side of abdomen and pelvis, with weight and dragging on that side; clothes feel heavy.

∎Pain in pelvis, principally in r. ovarian region.

∎Headache over l. eye on first waking, and great pain in pelvis, most marked at r. ovary.

∎Pains in abdomen intermittent.

ı ıPain in abdomen, < leaning forward; > leaning back.

ı ıSmarting in r. groin; pains seem to be in pelvic bones, uterus and limbs. θParenchymatous metritis.

∎Very acute pain in l. groin, extending up l. side to crest of ilium, > by stool; sometimes pain is in track of colon.

ı ıFeeling of tension in l. groin, do not want to walk or stand as it increases sensation, > by flexing leg on abdomen.

²⁰ Stool and Rectum. ı ıMucous yellow liquid stools.

∎Constipation. θAcute rheumatism.

ı ıObstinate constipation; frequent desire with darting pains in rectum, no power to expel; stool large, whitish, rough, scaly, hard. θDiphtheria.

²¹ Urinary Organs. ∎Constant desire to urinate, urine scanty.

∎Constant desire to urinate, passing large quantities frequently; at night she dreams of urinating, and wakes to find an immediate necessity.

ı ıConstant desire to urinate, with intense pain. θUrethral chancre.

∎Constant inclination to urinate, which was restrained as urination caused intense pain when coming in contact with vulva.

∎Urine unusually frequent and dark.

' ıUrine frequent: especially at night; scanty, high colored; red sediment.

ı ıUrine very scanty and dark. θAcute rheumatism.

∎Urine dark, heavily loaded with thick reddish sediment that adhered in different colored circles to bottom and sides of vessel.

ı ıGreat difficulty in urinating. θDiphtheria.

ı ıUrinating only once in twenty-four hours, and then copiously, but with some difficulty and slight irritation. θDiphtheria.

ı ıUrine scanty, infrequent, coffee colored, no desire to

urinate, quantity less than a gill in twenty-four hours-
eighty per cent. albumen, with much mucus.

ı ıNo urine for forty-seven and three-quarter hours, blad,
der pretty full, parts fearfully swollen, and irritation on
urination very great. θDiphtheria.

ı ı Urine partially suppressed. θTonsillitis.

Male Sexual Organs. ı ı Large chancre on dorsum of penis,
with a fungoid bacteric mass covering whole of corona
glandis, which was first of a glossy, shining, white appearance, and later covered with a fungus, looking like
fully developed aphthæ; edges of swollen prepuce covered with nodosities and itching.

ı Penis enormously swollen, and a chancre on glans like
a cauliflower excrescence, over half an inch in diameter;
it was red, smooth and glistening; no pain; in a week
there appeared two more small chancres, deep, sharp
edges, clean, and with same shining appearance.
θSyphilis.

ı ı Small sore at entrance of urethra; kept getting <; prepuce involved for about half inch, and parts of glans
around urethra an open ulcer, exhaling most fetid smell,
and with most excruciating pain; hemorrhage at 10 P.M.
every evening, and during day when removing dress-
ings; constant desire to urinate, with intense pain; no
sleep for a fortnight, red, glistening appearance.

ı Prepuce involved for about an eighth of an inch, and
parts of glans penis around urethra an open ulcer exhaling most fetid smell; pain excruciating; hemorrhages
at ten every evening and during day when removing
dressing; desire to urinate constant, and accompanied
by intense pain; had not slept for a fortnight; red, glistening appearance of ulcer. θSyphilitic ulceration of
penis.

ı Chancre on prepuce l. side of frænum, granulating rapidly
from centre to circumference.

ı ı Buboes and chancres.

ı ı When gonorrhœa is >, catarrh sets in

ı ı Gonorrhœal pains, intermittent, in front, middle or posterior part of urethra.

Female Sexual Organs. Heat in ovarian and uterine
region (with menses); inflammatory and congestive condition of ovaries before menses, especially of r. ovary,
with extreme soreness and sensitiveness, which makes
every motion and position, even breath, painful.

ı ı Pain in abdomen principally in r. ovarian region.

ı ı Sharp pain in r. ovary.

ı In afternoon, sharp pains in r. ovarian region, not constant but intermittent.

▮Severe pain in r. ovarian region, > by flow of bright red blood.

▮Pain in l. ovarian region; across lower part of abdomen.

⼁⼁Constant burning pain in l. ovarian region, extending from l. leg even to foot. θOvaralgia.

⼁⼁Sharp pains beginning in l. ovary, and darting like lightning either towards r. ovarian region, or else up l. side and down arm, or sometimes down both thighs; but most generally down l. leg to foot, which is numb; pains act something like labor pains, and are accompanied by great restlessness of legs and arms, and great aching in lumbar region; on fifth day after premature labor.

▮Inflammatory and congested condition of uterus, with extreme soreness and tenderness, that made every motion, position, and even breath, painful.

⼁⼁Parenchymatous metritis (two cases), in one, uterus three times as large as natural, round as a ball, and body very hard, cervix obliterated by altered form of body; uterus sensitive.

⼁⼁Much pain before and after menses, severe headache and entire prostration for first day or so. θMetritis.

⼁⼁Sharp, lancinating pains like knives cutting upwards from os uteri, and as these were being relieved, sensation as of needles darting upwards in uterus.

⼁⼁Pain in uterine region, passing down inside of thighs, half way to knees, and r. leg feels numb.

▮Pains in uterine region, all day, no particular direction except down inner side of thigh half way to knees.

⼁⼁Severe pain in entire uterine region, with profuse discharge of yellow, brown and bloody leucorrhœa, two weeks after menses; intense pain and enlargement of l. ovary, which could be seen protruding.

▮Blood bright red and stringy, hot as fire, coming in gushes and clotting easily; constant bearing down pain, as if everything would come out of vulva. θUterine hemorrhage.

⼁⼁Uterine hemorrhage for six weeks; ovarian pains alternated sides, as did the chronic headache.

⼁⼁Retroverted uterus.

⼁⼁Menses: fourteen days too soon, profuse; seven days too soon; flow came in gushes, scanty, intermittent, bright red and stringy, preceded by much flatulence from bowels; very stringy and sticky, cannot get rid of them.

⼁⼁Great engorgment of breasts, with sensitiveness to touch, precede menses.

⼁⼁Menses nearly ceased; at menses much pain in r. thigh and uterus, constant desire for stool, very low spirited. θParenchymatous metritis.

∎Dysmenorrhœa, abdomen sensitive even to weight of clothing; flatus from vagina.

∎Membranous dysmenorrhœa.

∎∎Sore throats are very apt to begin and end with menstruation.

∎Leucorrhœa, very profuse during day, none at night; discharge whitish and watery; pain in small of back; very irritable; < standing or walking.

∣∣Bearing down as though everything would fall out through vagina, with very frequent desire to urinate, and smarting in urethra.

∎Escape of flatus from vagina.

∣∣Great swelling of l. labia and terrible pain while urinating; from gonorrhœa.

∎Itching in l. side of labia, with rough eruptive condition on l. side of vagina, with acrid leucorrhœa; excoriating.

∎Raw and bad smelling sores between labia and thighs, in folds of skin; < when walking, would rather keep still all the time; sores are covered with disgusting white exudation.

∣∣Foul smell from genitals. θHerpes.

∣∣Pressure on labia causes a slight flow of blood; menstruation commenced entirely normal.

∎Intense painful soreness of vulva, extending to anus, coming on very suddenly about noon, and lasting for about two hours; came again during evening; could not walk, stand or sit; > by lying on back and separating knees as far as possible.

∣∣Great irritation about vulva and rectum. θDiphtheria.

∎Urination causes intense pain in vulva, when even least drop of urine comes in contact with it.

∎Itching of vulva.

∣∣Breasts very sore and painful, with sharp, darting pain in r. ovarian region extending downwards to knee, very painful and must keep leg flexed. θAfter miscarriage at sixth month.

∎Breasts very sore, sensitive to least pressure; dull, constant, aching pain in them all evening.   ·

∎Breasts very painful, but no lumps; pains are caused by least jar; has to hold breasts firmly when going up or down stairs; breasts < towards evening, pressure of her arm, in natural position, caused considerable pain.

∎Breasts very painful and sore; feel as if full of hard lumps, very painful when going up or down stairs.

∣∣Soreness and enlargement of breasts.

∎Breasts seem very full.

∎Constant pain in nipples.

₂₄ Pregnancy. Parturition. Lactation. ∣∣Afterpains very severe, and shooting down into thighs.

I I Knots and cakes in breast, after miscarriage.

I I Galactorrhœa.

I I Loss of milk while nursing, without known cause.

I I Serviceable in almost all cases where it is required to dry
up milk.

I I Given for an ulcerated throat to a nursing woman, it
cured throat and nearly dried up milk.

ᵛ Voice and Larynx. Trachea and Bronchia.   I I Loss of
voice.   *θ*Pharyngitis.

I I Throat troubles her much if she reads aloud or talks
more than usual; it seems almost as though it was
stopping up, and she feels very hoarse, but has no soreness; there is a feeling of fulness and choking.

I I Unable to speak loud; distressed feeling while speaking.

I I Respiration hoarse, crying was whispered and broken,
often no sound at all.   *θ*Diphtheria.

I Slight hoarseness, with now and then a change of voice,
after walking, but soon passing away.

I I Excessive hoarseness, and tickling, choking sensation,
> moving about.

I I Voice hoarse and husky; interrupted by weakness and
hoarseness.

I I Larynx sensitive to pressure.   *θ*Diphtheria.

I I Constriction in lower part of larynx, like a finger across
throat; feeling as of a bar across back of throat.

ᵛ Respiration.   I I Difficult breathing; during evening had
several suffocating spells.   *θ*Diphtheria.

I I Terrible dyspnœa immediately after sleep, first on l. side
of chest; dyspnœa compelled her to be lifted upright
with violent exertion to get breath; sharp pain in region
of heart with each attack.   *θ*Acute rheumatism.

I I Breathing hoarse and croupy, and at times an entire
stoppage of breath, when it would resume with a violent effort.   *θ*Diphtheria.

I I Breathing often snoring and only possible through
mouth.   *θ*Diphtheria.

I I Short breath.   *θ*After diphtheria.

I I Great difficulty in breathing, could not lie down flat.

I I Breathing very labored.

I I Loud snoring during sleep.

I I Sensation as if breath would leave her when lying
down and trying to sleep; has to jump up and stir
around for an hour or so every night.

ᵛ Cough.   I Tickling sensation in throat causing cough; in
afternoon quite hoarse.

I Cough from tickling in upper anterior part of larynx, <
talking and lying down.

I I Cough caused by irritation in upper part of throat, <

lying down at night, also after eating and drinking and
after talking; with soreness of l. side of throat and constant desire to urinate.

ı ıCough on taking a long breath, not when swallowing.

ı ıHard, metallic cough.

ı ıCroupy cough, a dry, hoarse bark, penetrating through
closed doors all over house. *θ*Diphtheria.

ı ıCough and dyspnœa.

ı ıConstant cough, accompanying soreness. *θ*Diphtheria.

ı ıExpectoration of profuse, sticky, tough, white mucus in
masses, with coryza.

²⁸ **Inner Chest and Lungs.** ı ıSharp, incisive pain between
scapulæ, passing through to sternum, with a sense of
pressure or constriction of chest in afternoon.

ı ıTrembling, jerking and fluttering through lungs, with
numb, prickling sensation all over body, legs and arms.

ı ıPulse so rapid it could scarcely be counted. *θ*Diphtheria.

ı ıPulse 130. *θ*Tonsillitis.

ı Pulse quick, full and strong, with pain in chest and throat.

ı ıPulse of little volume. *θ*Diphtheria.

ı ıPulse 130, wiry, weak.

ı ıPulse: quick and feeble; 100; 120; 140; 170; 130–140;
almost gone.

ı ıPulse 117. *θ*Diphtheria.

ı ıPulse rapid, quick. *θ*Acute rheumatism.

ı ıHeart beats rapidly from slight causes. *θ*Parenchymatous metritis.

³¹ **Neck and Back.** ı ıNeck stiff. *θ*Rheumatism. *θ*Neuralgic headache. *θ*Diphtheria.

ı ıPain in back of neck. *θ*Diphtheria.

ı ıWandering pains in nape with stiffness. *θ*Rheumatism.

ı ıNeck aches, making her want to bend head forwards;
entire spine sensitive. *θ*Parenchymatous metritis.

ı ıSpine aches from base of brain to coccyx. *θ*Pharyngitis.

ı ıHeat, pain and beating in small of back. *θ*Metritis.

ı ıPain in back. *θ*Diphtheria.

Wakes with severe pain in lower part of back, it is often
five minutes before she can straighten; pain leaves her
when she has been about work a short time, not returning till morning. *θ*Nervous throat affection.

ı ıIntense, unbearable pain across supersacral region, extending to r. natis and down r. sciatic nerve; pain so
severe as to prevent sleep or rest; at same time diphtheritic sore throat on r. side, with sensation of a lump,
could not swallow solid food.

³² **Upper Limbs.** ı Fetid perspiration in axillæ, staining
linen brown.

ı After exposure to draft in evening: sudden violent pains

in r. shoulder so severe that she was unable to raise the
arm, as if disabled by dislocation. θAcute rheumatism.
ı ı Pain in l. shoulder extending across to r.; could scarcely
move arm. θPharyngitis.
ı ı Neuralgic pains in shoulders, l. then r.; then vice versa.
ı ı Pain in one or other shoulder. θRheumatism.
ı ı Shoulders and arms ache. θParenchymatous metritis.
ı ı Partial paralysis of l. arm, unable to raise hand to head ;
on attempting to do so was seized with sharp pains in
arm below shoulder.
ı ı Left hand bloats and is numb, with trembling, jerking
and fluttering through lungs; numb, pricking sensation
all over body, arms and legs.
ıSharp pain in l. hand, l. arm as if asleep.
ı ı Trembling of l. hand, as in paralysis agitans.
ı ı Fingers extremely cold but not rest of hands.
ı ı Two warts on little finger.
³³ **Lower Limbs.** ı ı Almost constant pain in r. hip. θMetritis.
ı ı Pain in r. hip and leg while walking, with a trembling
of leg, and slight feeling of uncertainty, particularly on
going down stairs. θParenchymatous metritis.
ı ı Articular rheumatism in r. hip and knee joints, especially former; she was seated in an arm chair, unable
to move, complaining of bruised, smarting, lancinating
pains in both joints and in lumbar region, with swelling of affected joints; pains < by slightest motion at
night, by touch and by pressure of bed clothes;
next day pains and swelling had gone to l. hip and
knee joints, leaving r. almost free; the ensuing day they
had almost entirely disappeared from l. hip and knee
joints and had again attacked r. hip and knee; complaining, moaning and sighing on account of her sufferings and probable termination of her illness.
ıRheumatic pains in l. hip and along sciatic nerve; wandering pains in nape of neck, with stiffness; pains in
one or other shoulder; pain above l. eye and heaviness
of eyelid; burning in eye; agglutination of eyelids; sensitiveness to light. θSciatica and rheumatism.
ıIntense, unbearable pain across supersacral region, extending to r. natis and down r. sciatic nerve; pain so
severe as to prevent sleep or rest. θSciatica.
ı ı Partial paralysis of r. leg from miscarriage; has to use
a cane; r. ovary sore by spells and pain darts down leg,
sometimes to foot; leg feels numb and stiff, but cannot
keep it still any length of time; feels better by flexing
it on abdomen.
ı ı Can only walk with assistance of a cane. θHip disease.
ı ı Cannot walk any distance; trembling through r. thigh,

and feeling as though entire lower portion of body was
giving way; felt as though something was strained
across lower part of bowels. θParenchymatous metritis.
ιιSciatica.

ιιLimbs cold to knees. θDiphtheria.

ιBruised pain in soles of feet, stiffness of ankle, knee and
hip joints, and occasionally intense pains which move
upwards; pain in ankle joints as of a dull plug pushing;
joints stiff and sore, tender to touch, < from heat and
least motion; later knees and then hips became involved; at first the l. ankle was attacked, and then, after
some hours suffering, the r., with relief to l., and so on
with knees and hips; chest affected, terrible dyspnœa
coming on immediately after sleep, first on l. side; compelled her to be lifted upright with violent exertion to
get breath, sharp pain in cardiac region; urine scanty
and dark; pain in r. side of throat; generally < at 5
P.M. θAcute rheumatism.

ιιAfter exposure to cold night air when drunk, sharp,
darting pains, < by any motion, with swelling in r. knee
and r. ankle; next day joints of l. knee, l. ankle, l. hand,
extremely painful, moderately swollen, slightly red;
ensuing day, l. ankle and knee better, but r. shoulder
and elbow similarly affected.

ιNumb pains chiefly in ankles, < while quiet, with
swelling; veins of ankles distended; > while extreme
heat is applied. θRheumatism.

ιιEcthyma: a sore breaks out on r. leg, excessive itching,
inflammation, then swelling, blisters form and suppuration sets in; afterwards clear lymph, then discharge of
matter; then scabs and scales, turning eventually into a
branlike desquamation; scars have left discolored skin.

ιιRestlessness in legs.

ιιCramps in feet.

" Limbs in General.   ιιAching pains in limbs and back.
ιPains in limbs as if beaten. θPharyngitis.

. ιιBruised pains in soles making it difficult to walk; in
twelve days pains suddenly left soles, and appeared in
r. knee joint, being smarting, lancinating, with light
swelling of joint; could not move affected limb, as least
motion < pains, as did touch and pressure of bedclothes; on following day l. knee joint affected in same
way, r. >; on ensuing day r. again affected, with relief
to l.; afterwards hip joints attacked alternately with
same symptoms, alternating like these in pains and
swelling, l. joints one day with > of r., and vice versa;
also lancinating pains in l. side of chest; after four days
wrist joints affected, first r., with same symptoms as

those of lower extremities, symptoms of one side of
body alternating with those of other; not able to move
himself in bed, lancinating pains made him cry out;
constipation, sleeplessness, no fever; pains and swelling
< every evening, night, by movement, touch and press-
ure of bedclothes; numb pains chiefly in ankles <.
| | Burning of hands and feet at night. θOvaralgia.

⁵ Rest. Position. Motion. Rest: headache >.

Lying on back: with hands over face, falls asleep; separating knees as far as possible > soreness of vulva.

Lying down: thinks how horrible it would be if a very
sharp pain, like a knife, should go through her; causes
congestion; cough <; does not seem to touch bed.

Could not lie flat: great difficulty in breathing.

Sitting: as if she was going deranged.

Bending head forward: causes congestion.

Leaning forward: nausea; pain in abdomen <.

Leaning back: pain in abdomen >.

Standing: leucorrhœa <.

Cannot find comfortable position in bed, there is no way
she can put her hands that they do not bother her.

Motion: painful on account of soreness of ovarian region;
> hoarseness; pains in hip and knee joints <; sore-
ness of joints <; sharp, darting pains in knee and
ankle <; pain in knee <.

Flexing leg on abdomen: tension in groin >.

Cannot straighten herself: pain in back.

Could not raise arm: pain in shoulder.

Exertion: dull pain in l. superior maxillary.

Must jump up and stir about to > feeling as if breath
would leave her.

Walking: leucorrhœa <; sores between labia and thighs
<; pain in r. leg; felt as if walking on air.

Does not want to walk or stand: sensation in groin <.

Going up or down stairs: causes pain in breasts.

Going down stairs: trembling of leg.

⁵ Nerves. ▮Restlessness. θDiphtheria.

▮No inclination for least exertion, would like to do nothing
but sleep; much lassitude.

| | Heaviness, weakness, general languor. θAfter diphtheria.

| | Profound depression of vitality. θDiphtheria.

▮General weakness and prostration very marked.

| | Great exhaustion, with "poisoned" feeling. θDiphtheria.

| | Profound prostration, to extent of refusing to make effort
to take a dose of medicine. θDiphtheria.

| | In morning so much prostrated that she could not turn
in bed; so tired. θDiphtheria.

| | Very weak. θDiphtheria.

ı ıSinking spells every morning, attended with great nervousness. θParenchymatous metritis.

ı ıOften feels as if she would lose use of limbs. θNervous
throat affection.

ı ıChild partially paralyzed after diphtheria; could not
walk; pain all over, cough, aphonia, loss of appetite,
emaciation.

ı ıWhen walking seems to be walking on air; when lying
does not seem to touch bed.

ıSuffering from very unpleasant nervous symptoms; not
in low spirits, but weak, and nerves so thoroughly out
of order that she cannot bear one finger to touch the
other, and often feels as though she should lose use of
her limbs; sensation as if throat was closing, sensation
is between throat and nose; feels as if something in
throat was either enlarged or relaxed, and has a desire
to keep mouth open; talking difficult; disposition to
talk through nose; sometimes cannot swallow, because
there seems to be a kind of muscular contraction in
throat; sleep restless, frequently wakes with sick headache, which seems to commence at nape; wakes with
severe pain at lower part of back; pain leaves when
about work a short time, does not return until next
morning; nerves very much' overwrought, afraid of
being unable to perform duties. θNervous affection.

³⁷ **Sleep.** ı ıGreat desire to sleep. θDiphtheria.

ı ıCried out and talked in sleep. θDiphtheria.

ı ıSleeplessness from emotional strain, with entire nervous
debility.

ıCannot find any comfortable position in bed ; there is no
way she can put her hands that they do not bother her;
falls asleep at last on her face.

ıVery restless at night; very difficult to get into a comfortable position ; generally goes to sleep lying on back
with hands over head.

ıSleep disturbed, very wakeful; limbs cold all night.

ı ıSleep prevented by being very cold for one hour after
retiring, with great nervousness.

ıVery restless all night; could not keep clothes over her.

ı ıSleepless and crying continually.

ı ıRestless sleep at night, bad dreams. θMetritis.

ı ıDreamed a large snake was in bed. θTonsillitis.

ıGot to sleep late; profuse sweat during sleep; felt feverish all night; in morning > in every way.

ı ıAt night lies with l. leg flexed on thigh, and thigh on
pelvis; restless; < after sleep. θOvaralgia.

ıDreams frequently that she is urinating, and wakes to
find herself on point of doing so, requiring immediate
relief.

ı ı Dreams of going on a journey, and was separated from party, and had to walk a long distance, and arrived at station just in time to see train start off.

ı ı Aggravation of symptoms after sleep. θDiphtheria.

³⁸ Time. Morning: dull, frontal headache; l. superior maxillary feels sore; nausea, weak, sinking feeling in stomach pit; much prostration.

4 A.M.: copious epistaxis.

9 A.M: sharp pain on top of head.

Noon: throat >; soreness of vulva comes suddenly.

Day: pains in head.

Afternoon: headache; hoarseness; constriction of chest.

Evening: abdomen hard and swollen; intense soreness of vulva; aching in breasts.

9.45 P.M.: dyspeptic pain in stomach pit.

Night: constant noise in head <; sensation as if bed was in motion; sore spot in l. side of throat removed by 1 A.M.; next night same on r. side; pain in tonsil; gnawing <; felt she would suffocate; throat <; dreams of urinating; urine frequent; rheumatic pains <; burning of hands and feet; very restless; limbs cold.

After midnight: very severe frontal headache.

³⁹ Temperature and Weather. Heat: soreness of joints <; pains in ankles > while heat is applied.

Warm room: pain in forehead >.

Warm applications: pains in superior maxillary >.

Open air: headache >; mucus in mouth <.

Exposure to draft: severe pain in r. shoulder.

Cold night air: sharp, darting pains in knee and ankle.

During and after a cold northeast storm: throat <.

Cold winds: terrible pain in forehead.

Washing: causes pain in herpetic eruption.

Cold applications: soreness of superior maxillary >; pain in upper canines >.

Cold water: sore throat momentarily >.

⁴⁰ Fever. ı ı Severe chills. θDiphtheria.

ı ı Fever and chills for a few days, and up and down every few hours.

∎ Feels feverish.

∎ Intense fever on waking in morning, with perspiration.

ı ı Fever, and bathed in warm perspiration, especially about face, neck and hands. θDiphtheria.

ı ı Intense heat. θDiphtheria.

ı ı Moderate fever. θDiphtheria.

ı ı Fever. θDiphtheria θAcute rheumatism.

ı ı High fever. θDiphtheria.

ı ı Dry, hot skin. θDiphtheria.

ı ı Fever returning every afternoon. θDiphtheria.

ı ı Temperature 102.   θTonsillitis.
ı ı Temperature 102⅜.   θDiphtheria.
ı ı Temperature 103¼.   θDiphtheria.
ı ı Temperature 103.   θAcute rheumatism.
ı ı Sweat all over.   θDiphtheria.
ı ı Skin clammy.   θDiphtheria.
ı Exhausting sweats; after sleep.
ı ı Wakes in night in cold perspiration, with fearful fore-
    boding.   θParenchymatous metritis.
ı ı Perspired considerably through night, sweat having a
    rank smell.   θAcute rheumatism.
⁴¹ Attacks, Periodicity.   ı ı Aggravation morning of one day,
    evening of next.   θDiphtheria.
  Paroxysmal pain: in l. upper canine.
  Intermittent pains: in r. ovarian region.
  At times: fear of falling down stairs; stoppage of breath
  At intervals: copious epistaxis.
  Several times daily: bloody pus from nose.
  Lasting two hours: soreness of vulva.
  Two or three times a day: fits of weeping.
  Once in twenty-four hours: urinating.
  Daily for hours: severe throbbing in region of solar plexus.
  Every morning: sinking spells.
  Every evening, 10 P.M.: hemorrhage from urethra.
  Every night: sensation as if breath would leave her pains
    in wrists and knees <.
  Forty-seven and three-quarter hours: no urine.
  For two days: sore throat.
  For several days: alternately membrane appears in throat,
    then a severe interstitial hemorrhage.
  Third day: tonsil swollen and on it a small patch.
  Fourth day: both tonsils swollen.
  Fifth day: rash extended all over arms and legs.
  For six weeks: uterine hemorrhage.
  For several years, ever since diphtheria: sore throat just
    before menses.
⁴² Locality and Direction.   Right: pain in head beginning
    on side; pink color of lower lid; sore on side of septum;
    red circular spot below malar bone; acute pain on side
    of throat; throat < on side; sensation of lump in side
    of throat; pain in region of tonsil; throat much in-
    flamed on side; throat sore; sore spot on side of throat;
    tonsil red and swollen; side of throat <; tonsil intensely
    inflamed; tonsil covered with ash grey membrane; ton-
    sil raw, swollen; diphtheritic symptoms begin on side;
    stabbing pain in lung; burning pain in hypochondriac
    and iliac region; pain in ovarian region; smarting in
    groin; sharp pain in ovary; numbness of leg; much

pain in thigh; pain down sciatic nerve; pains in shoulder; pain in hip; pain in leg; rheumatism in hip; partial paralysis of leg; trembling through thigh; swelling in knee and ankle; sore on leg; swelling of knee joint.

Left: pain over eye; sees green band before eye, slanting downward to r. cheek; spots before eye; burning in eye; heaviness of upper lids; pain over eye; agglutination of lids; gathering under side of nose; superior maxillary feels sore; flushes on cheek; swelling of parotid; pain in upper canine; pain on side of throat; sensation of ball or round body in side of throat; feeling of lump in side of throat; lump in side of pharynx; pain from throat to ear; rawness on side of throat; throat very sore; sore spot in side of throat; patches on tonsil; diphtheritic spots in throat; large patches on tonsil; thick, membranous mass lying on side of soft palate; neck swollen; pain crossing from r. iliac region to l. side of abdomen; intense pain in side of abdomen; burning in side of abdomen; acute pain in groin extending up to side of crest of ilium; tension in groin; chancre on prepuce side of frænum; pain in ovarian region; sharp pain down leg from ovary, enlargement of ovary; swelling of labia; itching in side of labia; eruptive condition on side of vagina; terrible dyspnœa; pain in shoulder; partial paralysis of arm; hand bloats and is numb; sharp pain in hand; arm as if asleep; trembling of hand; pain in ankle, knee and hand.

From l. to r.: neuralgic pains in shoulders.

From r. to l.: swelling of parotid.

From within outwards: pressure in abdomen.

Alternating sides: throat symptoms; articular rheumatism in lower limbs; bruised pain in ankles; pains in ankles, knees and elbows; swelling and ulcers.

❚❚Erratic disposition of symptoms; pains constantly flying from one part to another.

" Sensations. As if she was going deranged; as if surrounded by myriads of snakes; as if bed was in motion; as if forehead would split open; as if ears were full; as if throat was closing; as if something in throat was either enlarged or relaxed; throat as if full of sticks; as if a lump was in throat; as of a ball or round body in l. side of throat; as of a lump in r. side of throat, with a feeling that she could take hold of it with her fingers and pull it out; throat as if scalded by hot fluid; throat as if burnt by caustic; throat felt as if there were lumps in it like two eggs; diphtheritic deposit looks as if varnished; pain as from a stone in stomach pit; as if contents of abdomen would be forced outwards; as of needles darting upwards in uterus; as if everything would come out at vulva; breasts as if full of hard lumps; as if throat was stopped up; as if a finger was across throat; as of a bar across back of throat; as if breath would leave her when lying down; l. arm as if asleep; as of a dull plug pushing in ankle joint; pain in limbs as if they had been beaten; feels as if she would lose use of limbs; when walking, as if walking on air; when lying in bed, as if she did not touch it; as if throat was closing; as if an insect was crawling on shoulders, neck and hands.

Pain: over eyes; in temples; above l. eye; in both ears; in r. side of throat; in whole body and limbs; in chest; in tonsils; in head, back and limbs; in pit of stomach; in l. side of abdomen and pelvis; in ovaries; in abdomen; in track of colon; in uterine region and down thighs; in r. thigh and uterus; in small of back; in nipples; in chest and throat; in back of neck; from l. shoulder to r.; in r. hip and leg; in labia.

Excruciating pain: in prepuce.

Unbearable pain: in head; across supraorbital region.

Violent pain: in r. shoulder.

Terrible pain: in vertex; in l. labia while urinating.

Very severe pain: in forehead; in head; in r. ovarian region; in entire uterine region; in lower part of back.

Intense pain: in urethra; in l. ovary; in vulva.

Intense sharp pain: in l. side of abdomen.

Acute pain: on r. side of throat then in l.; in l. groin, extending to l. side to crest of ilium.

Sharp, incisive pain: between scapulæ, passing through to sternum.

Sharp pain: on top of head coming from nape of neck; in arm below shoulder; in l. hand; in cardiac region; in r. ovarian region; beginning in l. ovary and darting like lightning either towards r. ovarian region, or else up l. side and down arm, or sometimes down both thighs, generally down l. leg to foot; in region of heart.

Sharp pains like knives: cutting upwards from os uteri.

Lancinating: in chest.

Cutting: through tonsils.

Stabbing: in r. lung.

Darting stabbing: from one side of head to other.

Darting: from occiput to forehead; in rectum; in r. ovarian region; in knees and ankles.

Shooting: to ears; in abdomen; down into thighs.

Piercing: on vertex.

Beating: from occiput to forehead; in stomach and bowels; in small of back.

Throbbing: in temples; in region of solar plexus.

Bruised, smarting, lancinating pains: in both joints and in lumbar region; in l. hip.

Bruised pain: in soles of feet.

Pricking stitching: in throat.

Bearing down pains: in abdomen.

Neuralgic pains: in shoulders.

Burning: in r. hypochondriac region and corresponding part in back; in l. ovarian region.

Aching: in throat; in l. ear; in lumbar region; in breasts; in neck; in whole spine; in arms and shoulders; in limbs and back.

Rheumatic pain: in r. hip; knee joints; l. hip; along sciatic nerve.

Wandering pains: in nape with stiffness.

Gnawing pain: in l. upper canine; in tonsil.

Heavy dull pain: in forehead.

Heavy pain: in eyeballs.

Severe pressure: on brain.

Sick headache: beginning in nape gradually settling in r. or l. forehead.

Intense painful soreness: of vulva extending to anus.

Smarting: in r. groin; in urethra.

Intense heat: of throat; of palms; of abdomen.

Burning: in l. eye: in epigastric region; in abdomen; in hands and feet.

Soreness: of head; of pimples on scalp; on r. side of septum of nose; of l. superior maxillary; of throat; of uvula; of r. ovary; of uterus; of breasts.

Heat: in small of back.

Rawness: in throat.

Sensitiveness: of entire spine.

Trembling, jerking, fluttering: through lungs, with numb, prickling sensation all over body, legs and arms.

Burnt and drawn feeling: in throat.

Distressed feeling in throat: when speaking.

Poisoned feeling.

Pressure: from within outwards in abdomen.

Stuffed feeling: in head.

Feeling of fulness and choking: in throat.

Weight and dragging: in l. side of abdomen.

Constriction: in upper part of throat; of chest.

Tension: in groin.

Stiff feeling: in throat.

Stiffness: of ankle, knee and hip joints.

Numbness: of leg.

Pricking: in throat; through tonsils; all over body, arms and legs.

Tingling: on vertex.

Tickling: in throat; in upper anterior part of larynx.

Trembling: of l. hand; of leg; through r. thigh.

Weak, sinking feeling: at stomach pit.

Itching: of head; of prepuce; in l. side of labia; of sore on r. leg.

" Tissues. ▮Enlarged glands after scarlatina; cold indurations, as found in scrofulous children.

▮Red, glistening appearance in ulcerations.

ⅠⅠNeuralgia and acute pains; rheumatism; gout; syphilitic sciatica; sexual debility.

▮Rickets; scrofula; diphtheria.

▮Sequelæ of diphtheria and syphilis.

" Skin. Sensation as if an insect was crawling on shoulders and neck, occasionally on hands.

▮Herpetic eruption in both axillæ, with light brownish scab, extremely painful when washing; eruption most in r. axilla, and in both instances appeared day previous to pain in labiæ, which was followed by a discharge of blood from vagina.

ⅠⅠOn face, hands, neck and chest, bright scarlet eruption, exactly like scarlatina. θDiphtheria.

▮Throat full of large foul, grey yellow patches; deglutition especially painful after sleep and from swallowing fruits (acid); lumpy sensation felt in middle of throat; unrest, delirium with undefined fears; considerable bright red, fine eruption on face and chest; itching with dry skin. θScarlatina.

ⅠⅠBright scarlet redness on chest and around neck; next day all over body except legs, which were, however, covered that night; skin in large patches assumed dark red color bordering on purple, as seen in malignant cases, while whole body seemed swollen. θDiphtheria.

ⅠⅠDiphtheria with or following scarlatina.

ⅠⅠIchthyosis, with branlike desquamation of skin.

▮Shining, glazed and red appearance of ulcers on shin and wrist. θSyphilis.

▮Very small blotches like fleabites. θDiphtheria.

▮Small blotches on chest, wrists and r. knee.

ⅠⅠSeveral boils on l. side. θSick headaches.

ⅠⅠCrusts on skin, under which greyish yellow matter formed and was squeezed out.

" Stages of Life, Constitution. From eight patients, seven were spare and dark, the eighth blonde.

Child, æt. 8 months, drooping and ailing since day before, grew < through night; diphtheria.

Girl, æt. 26 months; rickets.

Child, æt. 4; diphtheria.

Girl, æt. 4; diphtheria.

M. Y., æt. 5; diphtheria.

Girl, æt. 7, slender, tall, bony, with enlarged cervical lymphatics and tonsils; had diphtheritic croup six years ago.

Boy, æt. 9, three days before had spent several hours on ice skating, also had been exposed to some fatal cases of diphtheria; diphtheria.

Boy, æt. 12; convalescent from diphtheria.

Girl, æt. 13; diphtheria.

Girl, æt. 15; diphtheria.

Girl, æt. 18; affection of stomach.

Man, æt. 20, chancre which was cauterized; syphilis.

Man, æt. 22; acute neuralgia.

Young man, brother died of diphtheria; sore throat.

Young woman; nervous affection.

Woman, æt. 28, dark hair and eyes, full habit, has sore throat before menses, sometimes begins on one side, again on the other, has had it for several years, ever since she had diphtheria; diphtheritic sore throat.

Miss Z. G., æt. 28, tall, slender; parenchymatous metritis.

Woman, after exposure to draft; acute rheumatism.

Woman, æt. 40, strong, healthy, dark, now nursing a nine months' boy.

Woman, æt. 50, suffers after each attack of quinsy; acute rheumatism.

Man, æt. 50, had syphilis twenty-five years ago, first discovered a small sore at entrance to urethra, for two months rapidly growing <; syphilitic ulceration of penis.

Woman, æt. 90; sensation of film before eyes.

Relations. * " Acts best in single dose; if repeated, should be given at exact intervals." (Nichols.)

Memory weak: affects only what she has read (*Laches., Natr. mur., Staphis.*); forgetful, in writing uses too many words or not right ones (*Bovista, Graphit., Hepar, Laches., Lycop., Natr. carb., Natr. mur., Nux vom., Sepia*); absentminded (*Anac., Caustic., Conium, Dulcam., Laches., Natr. mur., Sepia*); cannot speak correctly half the time (*Calc. ostr., China, Graphit., Hepar, Laches., Lycop., Natr. carb., Natr. mur., Nux vom., Sepia*); substitutes name of object seen for that which is thought (*Amm. carb., Calc. carb., Sepia, Sulphur*); very restless, cannot concentrate her thoughts or mind to read; wants to leave everything as soon as it is commenced (*Nux vom., Silicea, Sulphur*); crying, fearing she was contracting consumption (*Calc. ostr., Paullin., Sepia*); exalted feeling of sensorium (*Platinum*).

---

* The names of corresponding remedies were, with a few exceptions, added by Lippe for Swan's Materia Medica.

Weak feeling in head, feeling as if a headache was coming on (*Ambra, Iodum, Phosphor., Stramon., Thuja*).

On going into cold wind felt a terrible pain in forehead
as if it would split open, > on going into warm room
(*Aurum, Nux vom., Rhus tox.*).

Headache < by noise or talking, > by keeping quiet;
confused feeling in head (*Calc. ostr.*).

Must have light, yet is intolerant of sunlight; diphtheria
(*Acon., Amm. mur., Bellad., Calc. ac., Calc. ostr., Gelsem.,
Ruta, Stramon.*).

Difficulty in distinguishing objects; in reading, letters run
together; after severe diphtheria (*Natr. mur.*).

Acrid coryza (*Aurum triph., Nitr. ac.*).

Soreness and scabbing of nostrils (*Kali bich., Thuja*).

Lips dry and peeling off (*Natr. mur.*).

Gums ulcerated, bleeding; teeth loose (*Iodum, Kali carb ,
Lycop., Mercur., Natr. mur., Phosphor., Staphis., Zincum*).

Throat: sensitive to touch externally (*Laches.*); < by
empty swallowing (*Ignat.*).

Breasts sensitive: to pressure (*Calc. ostr., Murex*); to deep
pressure (*Mercur.*); as if full of very hard lumps, very
painful when going up or down stairs (*Bellad., Calc. ostr.,
Carbo an., Lycop., Nitr. ac., Phosphor.*); soreness and enlargement (*Bellad., Bryon., Calc. ostr.*).

Sore throat commencing on l. tonsil (*Laches.*).

Small round or irregular, grey white ulcers on tonsils and
fauces (*Merc. jod.*).

Coarse shreds of membrane in throat; diphtheria (*Kali
bich.*); discharges of diphtheritic matter from vulva
and rectum (*Apis*).

Empty, weak feeling in stomach pit (*Digit., Ignat., Petrol.,
Sepia*); pain as from a stone or undigested food in
stomach pit (*Kali bich.*).

Pain in r. ovarian region (*Apis, Lycop., Pallad.*).

Sensation as if breath would leave her when lying down;
has to jump up and stir around (*Grind. robusta*).

Cramps in feet (*Lycop., Petrol., Silicea, Sulphur*).

Sciatica (*Curare, Graphit., Gnaphal., Kali bich., Iris vers.,
Laches., Phytol., Tellur.*).

Intense fever in morning, with perspiration (*Eupat. perf.*).

When walking, seems to be walking on air; when lying,
does not seem to touch bed (*Asar., China, Coffea, Natr.
mur., Nux vom., Opium, Rhus tox., Spigel., Stramon., Thuja*).

Dreams of going on a journey (*Lac. deflor., Laches., Sanguin., Silica*).

Icthyosis, with branlike desquamation of skin (after
Sulphur. and *Psorin.* had failed).

LAC VACCINUM DEFLORATUM.

Cow's milk skimmed.

The idea of potentizing skimmed milk originated with Swan upon reading Doukin's Skim Milk Treatment for Diabetes and Bright's Disease. The first proving was made by a lady in New York, in whose case the headache with nausea and constipation were strongly marked. A subsequent, more extensive proving was made under Swan by Dr. Laura Morgan. See Swan's Mat. Med. of Nosodes and Morbific Products, arranged by Berridge.

With but few exceptions the symptoms in the following arrangement have received clinical verification.

CLINICAL AUTHORITIES.—*Headache,* Farrington, Farrington's Clinical Mat. Med., p. 28; Laura Morgan, Boardman, Org., vol. 2, p. 257; Hahn. Mo., vol. 10, p. 220; *Periodical sick headache,* Morgan, T. H. M. Soc. Pa., 1881, p. 105; *Hemicrania,* Hahn. Mo., vol. 10, p. 220; *Chronic constipation* Schley, Swan, Hahn. Mo., vol. 10, p. 321; Knerr, MSS.; *Fainting spells,* Laura Morgan, Org., vol. 2, p. 256.

^{1} **Mind.** Loss of memory; listlessness and disinclination for either bodily or mental exertion.

▮Depression of spirits; don't care to live; question as to quietest and most certain way of hastening one's death.

During conversation, headache and depression of spirits >.

▮Depression with crying and palpitation. *θ*Fainting spells.

▮Imagines that all her friends will die and that she must go to a convent. *θ*Fainting spells.

▮Does not want to see or talk to any one.

Can remember what has been read only by a strong effort of will.

Vacillation of mind.

Great despondency on account of the disease, is sure he is going to die in twenty-four hours.

Has no fear of death but is sure he is going to die.

^{2} **Sensorium.** ▮Head light, with throbbing in temples.

▮Vertigo : on moving head from pillow ; < lying down and especially turning while lying, obliging to sit up.

Head feels heavy with marked tendency to fall to r. side.

▮Faintness and nausea when stepping upon floor in morning.

▮At first a sharp pain at apex of heart, as though a knife was cutting up and down ; this lasts a few seconds and is followed by strange feeling in head ; forehead feels extremely heavy, with dull sensation over eyes, and considerable throbbing, most marked on each side of head; rest of head feels very light; dimness of vision; can only distinguish light, not objects; at same time great loss of strength; cannot stand, but falls backwards, and remains entirely unconscious for two or three minutes; weakness passes off gradually, and is followed by crying, palpitation of heart and great depression of spirits; imagines that all her friends will soon die, and that she must go to a convent; she can produce an attack at any time by extending arms high above head, or by pressure around waist; spells come on at 7.30 P.M. θFainting spells.

³ **Inner Head.** ∎Pain first in forehead, then extending to occiput, very intense, distracting and unbearable; great photophobia, even to light of candle; deathly sickness all over, with nausea and vomiting, < by movement or sitting up; very chilly, and external heat does not >; frequent and profuse urination of very pale urine. θSick headache.

∎After light breakfast, pain in forehead, with nausea; very pale face, even lips looked white; vomiting of ingesta and afterwards of mucus and bitter water; deathly sick feeling in pit of stomach, < rising up in bed; profuse urination every half hour; urine colorless as water; great thirst; intense throbbing pain in vertex. θHeadache.

∎After injury subject to distress in head; severe pain in forehead just above eyes; breath offensive; appetite poor, nausea; at times sleeps for hours during attack; great distress across back; urine dark and thick.

∎Nausea, and sometimes vomiting, which >; pain in forehead as if head would burst, with blindness; pain is > by bandaging head tightly; < by light and noise; constipation, stools large; hands and feet cold. θHemicrania.

∎Periodical pain in forehead, as if head would burst, accompanied by violent efforts to vomit, and more rarely vomiting; hands and feet cold; diarrhœa alternating with constipation, the latter predominating; loss of appetite; smell or thought of food causes nausea; tongue moist, coated white; thirstlessness; always < at menstrual period; menses scanty and accompanied with colic. θHeadache.

∎Attacks come every eight days; during attack can neither eat nor drink, nor endure light or noise, does not even like to speak; great prostration, < during menstruation; when pains subside, inflammation of tonsils appears; tongue white and no relish for food. θHeadache.

❚❚Throbbing frontal headache, nausea, vomiting and obstinate constipation; especially in anæmic women.

❚Severe frontal headache; nausea and sometimes vomiting upon rising in morning, or from recumbent position at any time, or upon moving; great constipation; constant chilliness even when near fire; urine profuse and watery, or scanty and high colored; intense pain throughout whole spinal column; excessive thirst for large quantities; great depression of spirits; sudden prostration of strength at 5 P.M.; skin color of red rose, with swelling of face, neck, arms and body, generally in morning and during day and evening. θHeadache.

❚Severe pain over eyes, with intense throbbing in both temples; eyes feel as if full of little stones; eyeballs intensely painful, and on shutting eyes, pressure of lids increases pain; edges of lids feel contracted, and convey sensation as of a narrow band drawn tightly across eyeball; pain over l. hip; constipation and profuse urination during paroxysm. θHeadache.

❚Dimness of vision, as of cloud before eyes; profuse urination; full feeling in head; slight nausea at pit of stomach; face pale; feet cold; coldness in back.

❚Pain commencing in and above inner end of r. eyebrow; before rising in morning; soon after rising pain passed into eyeball; < until afternoon, at which time it became unbearable; < by walking and particularly by sitting down, though done carefully, also by heat radiated from fire or stooping, > on pressure; pressure on temples disclosed strong pulsation of artery; pain ceased entirely at sunset and did not return till next day.

❚Intense pain at point of exit of supraorbital nerve, diffused thence over forehead; attack commences with chill, quickened pulse, flushed face and discharges of wind from stomach.

❚Pains so severe that she would bury her eyes in her hands and press them into pillow. θSick headache.

❚Severe headache for years; severe pain over eyes; intense throbbing in temples.

❚General sore pain of head, produced by coughing.

❚Severe headache with a sensation as if top of her head was lifted off and was raised about five inches, and brains were coming out: head feels very hot and motion increases pain; face felt as if flesh was off bones and edges were separated and sticking out.

❚Pain first in forehead, extending through occiput, making her nearly frantic.

❚Intense headache in forehead and through head, < in vertex, afterward head felt bruised.

¡In morning nausea and sensation of a round ball full of pain in centre of forehead.

¡Throbbing in temples.

¡American sick headache, with gastric symptoms.

⁴ Outer Head. ¡Head feels large as if growing externally. Head heavy, falling to r. side.

¡¡General sore pain of head produced by coughing.

⁵ Sight and Eyes. ¡Dimness of vision; can only see lights, not objects; preceding headache.

¡Sensation as if eyes were full of little stones. θHeadache.

¡¡Great photophobia, even candle light unbearable.

Intense vertigo when opening eyes while lying, < when raising up; objects appeared to move swiftly from l. to r., at other times moving as if tossed up from below in every direction.

¡Great pain in eyes on first going into light, soon passed off; on closing eyes on account of light, pain was felt in eyeballs as if from pressure of lids.

¡Pain in and above eyes.

¡On closing eyelids painful pressure as if lids were short laterally, causing sensation of band pressing upon balls.

¡Upper eyelids feel very heavy; sleepy all day.

¡Pain in head, most marked over l. eye and in temple, extending into eyes, and causing profuse lachrymation.

⁷ Smell and Nose. ¡Painful pressure or tightness at root of nose. θCatarrh.

⁸ Upper Face. Deathly paleness of face.

¡Wasted, thin and excessively sallow, with dark stains beneath eyes.

¡Sallow complexion with eczematous eruption.

¡Flushes of heat in l. side of face.

¡Face, neck, arms and body generally flush color of a red rose, with swelling, but no itching or burning.

¡Sensation as if all flesh was off bones of face and edges were separated and sticking out.

¡¡Pimples on face and forehead. θIrregular menses.

¹⁰ Teeth and Gums. ¡Grinding of teeth when asleep, with pain in stomach and head with vomiting.

¹² Inner Mouth. ¡¡Mouth very dry.

¡Breath very offensive.

¡Mouth clammy and frothy, especially during conversation.

¹³ Throat. ¡Globus hystericus; sensation of a large ball rising from a point about lower end of sternum to upper end of œsophagus, causing distressing sense of suffocation.

¡Sore throat < when swallowing; slight, hacking cough.

¹⁴ Appetite, Thirst. Desires, Aversions. ¡Entire loss of appetite.

¡Great thirst for large quantities and often; intense thirst.

¹⁵**Eating and Drinking.** ▮Could not drink milk without its causing sick headache.

¹⁶**Hiccough, Belching, Nausea and Vomiting.** ▮Sour eructation.

❘❘Nausea in morning.

Nausea from a recumbent position at any time during day or evening, or upon moving or rising in morning.

▮Deathly nausea, cannot vomit, with groans and cries and great distress, great restlessness with sensation of coldness; although skin was hot, pulse was normal.

▮Nausea and vomiting and a sensation of deathly sickness, < from movement or rising up in bed.

▮Vomiting first of undigested food, intensely acid, then of bitter water and lastly of a brownish clot, which in water separated and looked like coffee grounds; no smell; bitter taste.

▮Incessant vomiting, which had no relation to her meals.

¹⁷**Scrobiculum and Stomach.** ▮Violent pain in pit of stomach, seldom lower, brought on by fatigue.

▮A good deal of wind and acid stomach, no tenderness.

▮❘Dyspepsia.

▮Bloating in epigastric region, with attacks of asthma; he could scarcely breathe; hard pressive pain at about fourth cervical vertebra.

¹⁸**Hypochondria.** ▮Cramps in epigastric region.

¹⁹**Abdomen.** ❘❘Abdomen sore and sensitive to touch.

▮Severe pain across umbilicus with headache.

▮Great fatigue from walking, on account of heaviness as of a stone in abdomen.

▮Constant pain in frontal region; nausea in morning, deathly paleness of face on rising in morning; aching pains in wrists and ankles; puffy swelling under malleoli; drawing pains, with heat, across lower abdomen and bearing down; frequent, scanty, pale urine; pressive bearing down in both ovarian regions; cannot bear pressure of arm or hand on abdomen; slight yellowish leucorrhœa; great lassitude and disinclination to exertion; depression of spirits; does not care to live; questions as to quickest and most certain mode of hastening one's death; great fatigue from walking, on account of heaviness, as of a stone in abdomen.

❘❘Drawing pain across lower part of abdomen, with heat and pressing, bearing down in pelvic region, both sides; cannot bear pressure of hand or arm on abdomen.

▮Flatulence.

▮Chronic gastro-enteritis, symptoms of chronic diarrhœa and vomiting.

²⁰**Stool and Rectum.** ▮Frontal headache; deathly sickness,

with or without vomiting; pale face in morning, also
lips and tips of fingers white; coldness over whole body.
θConstipation.

▮Is generally constipated, and when it is most persistent
very chilly; cannot get warm.

▮Frequent but ineffectual urging to stool.

▮▮Constipation: with chronic headache; most powerful purgatives were of no avail; fæces dry and hard; diarrhœa;
stool large and hard, passed with great straining, lacerating anus, extorting cries and passing considerable
blood; chronic.

I I Continual persistent constipation, > only by cathartics
and enemas, with violent attacks of sick headache, pain
first in forehead then extending to occiput, very intense,
distracting and unbearable; great photophobia, even to
light of a candle; deathly sickness all over, with nausea
and vomiting < by movement or sitting up; chilly,
and external heat does not relieve her; frequent and
profuse urination of very pale urine.

²¹ **Urinary Organs.**   ▮Frequent but scanty urination.

▮Profuse, pale urine.

▮▮Albuminuria.

▮Constant pain in region of kidneys, passing around each
side above hips to region of bladder, also downward
from sacral region to gluteal, and from thence down
back of thighs; pain burning, not > in any position, <
lying down.

▮Urine very dark and thick.

Urine very pale; cannot retain it.

I I Urine comes away drop by drop, or else gushes out with
a sensation of very hot water passing over parts; wetting bed at night.

²³ **Female Sexual Organs.**   ▮Pressive bearing down in ovarian region.

▮Drawing pain across uterine region, with heat and pressive bearing down in both ovarian regions; cannot bear
pressure of hand or arm on abdomen, intense distress in
lower part of abdomen during menstruation, not > by
any position; violent inflammation in ileo-cæcal region,
with intense pain, swelling, tenderness, fecal accumulation and violent vomiting.

▮Menses delayed a week with congestion of blood to head;
coldness of hands, nausea and vertigo; flow commenced
next morning after taking *Lac defl.*, scanty with pain in
back; sensation of weight and dragging in l. ovarian
region.

▮After putting hands in cold water sudden suppression
of menses; pains all over, especially in head.

| Irregular menstruation, sometimes very dark and scanty, sometimes colorless water.

| Slight yellowish leucorrhœa.

²⁴ Pregnancy. Parturition. Lactation. ▮Morning sickness during pregnancy; deathly sickness at stomach on waking; vertigo and waterbrash on rising; constipation.

| Decrease in size of breasts.

Has never failed to bring back the milk in from twelve to twenty-four hours.

▮Diminished secretion of milk.

²⁶ Respiration. ▮Asthma so that he could scarcely breathe, accompanied by bloating in epigastric region.

²⁷ Cough. | Short, dry cough, with difficult expectoration of a small lump of mucus, which > cough.

²⁸ Inner Chest and Lungs. ▮Soreness of chest with great pressure.

▮Tuberculous deposit in apices of both lungs.

²⁹ Heart, Pulse and Circulation. ▮Pressure around heart (not like grasping of *Cactus*), with dyspnœa and a feeling of certainty that he is going to die in 24 hours.

▮Sharp pain in apex of heart, as if a knife was cutting up and down; this preceded a heaviness of head, dulness over eyes, throbbing in temples and palpitation of heart.

▮Palpitation of heart and flushes of heat, especially in l. side of face and neck.

³¹ Neck and Back. ▮A symmetrical patch of herpetic eruption on each side of neck, itching and burning after scratching.

▮Hard, pressive pain at fourth cervical vertebra; chills creeping along back between scapulæ.

| Intense burning pain in small of back and sacrum, commencing in region of kidneys, passing around on both sides above hips into groins, also downward from renal region through gluteal region, down back part of thighs; pain, burning, and > by no position; lying down.

▮Constant pain in small of back.

³² Upper Limbs. | Ends of fingers icy cold, rest of hand warm.

³³ Lower Limbs. ▮Numbness and loss of sensation over outer and anterior surfaces of thighs.

▮Pains passing down under side of thighs to heels, and pains across top of feet as if bones were broken across instep; pains would come on as soon as she stepped upon floor in morning, upon which she would be faint and nauseated and would have to lie down.

▮Weakness and aching in ankles, puffiness.

▮Skin thickened at edges of feet.

³⁴ Limbs in General. | Cold hands or feet during headache.

| Aching pains in wrists and ankles.

³⁵ Rest. Position. Motion. No position >, burning pain in urinary region.

Lying down: vertigo $<$; severe frontal headache; burn-
ing pain in urinary region $<$.
Sitting up: sick headache $<$; deathly sick feeling in pit
of stomach $<$; nausea and vomiting.
Obliged to sit up: vertigo.
Sitting down: pain in eyeball $<$.
Cannot stand: falls backwards unconscious.
Motion: sick headache $<$; headache; pain in head $<$.
Disinclination to exertion.
Moving head from pillow: vertigo.
Turning while lying: vertigo $<$.
Rising: in morning, deathly paleness.
Extending arms high above head: produces fainting spells.
Stepping upon floor: faintness and nausea.
Walking: pain in eyeball $<$; great fatigue.

³⁶ Nerves. ||Great lassitude and disinclination to exertion.
|Great restlessness and extreme and protracted suffering
from loss of sleep at night.
|Feels completely tired out and exhausted, whether she
does anything or not; great fatigue from walking.
|Great loss of strength, commencing with a sharp, cutting
pain in apex of heart; forehead feels heavy, with a dull
sensation over eyes and throbbing, principally in temples, rest of head feels light.

³⁷ Sleep. ||Sleepy all day long.
Great restlessness, extreme and protracted suffering from
loss of sleep at night.

³⁸ Time. Morning: when stepping upon floor, nausea and faintness; nausea and vomiting; headache; before rising
pain in eyebrow; as of a round ball full of pain in centre
of forehead; deathly paleness.
During day: headache.
Afternoon: pain in eyebrow and eyeball $<$.
5 P.M.: sudden prostration of strength.
7.30 P.M.: fainting spells.
9 P.M.: hot fever.
Evening: headache.
Night: sleepless.

³⁹ Temperature and Weather. |Sensation as if cold air was
blowing on her, even while covered up warm.
External heat: does not $>$ chilliness; pain in eyeball $<$.
Cold water: putting hands in, sudden suppression of menses.

⁴⁰ Fever. ||Hot fever 9 P.M., continues until near morning,
wakes in profuse sweat, which stains linen yellow difficult to wash out
|Hectic fever; malignant typhoid.
|Sensation as if the sheets were damp.

⁴¹ Attacks, Periodicity. Periodical pain: in forehead.

Every half hour: profuse urination.
Sunset: pain in eyeball ceases.
Every eight days: attacks of sick headache.
Menstrual period: colic.

⁴³ Locality and Direction. Right: tendency to fall to side;
pain in and above inner end of eyebrow; head heavy,
falls to side.

Left: pain over hip; over eye; flashes of heat in side of
face; sensation of weight and dragging in ovarian region.

From l. to r.: objects appear to move.

⁴⁵ Sensations. As though a knife was cutting up and down
through heart; as if head would burst; eyes feel as if
full of little stones; sensation in lids as of a narrow band
drawn tightly across eyeball; as of a cloud before eyes;
as if top of head was lifted off; as if flesh was off bones
of face, and edges were separated and sticking out; as
of a ball of pain in centre of forehead; head as if
growing externally; objects appear as if tossed up from
below in every direction; pain in eyes as if from pressure of lids; as if eyelids were short laterally, causing sensation as of a band pressing upon balls; as of a large ball
rising from a point about lower end of sternum to upper
end of œsophagus; as of a stone in abdomen; as if bones
were broken across instep; as if sheets were damp; as if
cold air was blowing on her.

Pain: first in forehead, then in occiput; over l. hip; above
inner end of r. eyebrow; in eyeball; in stomach; in
region of kidney passing around each side above hips to
region of bladder, also downward from sacral region to
guteal, and from thence down back of thighs; in back;
all over; in small of back; down under side of thighs
to heels; across top of feet.

Distracting, unbearable pain: in forehead and occiput.

Intense pain: throughout spinal column; in eyeballs; at
point of exit of supraorbital nerve; in forehead and
through head.

Violent pain: in pit of stomach.

Severe pain: in forehead just above eyes; in head; across
umbilicus.

Sharp pain: at apex of heart.

Great pain: in eyes.

Intense distress: in lower part of abdomen.

Throbbing: in temples; in vertex.

Intense burning pain: in small of back and sacrum.

Burning pain: in urinary organs.

Cramps: in epigastric region.

Drawing pains with heat: across lower abdomen.

Aching pains: in wrists and ankles.

Sore pain: of head; 'in throat.

Hard, pressive pain: at about fourth cervical vertebra.

Painful pressure: at root of nose.

Constant pain: in frontal region.

Periodical pain: in forehead.

Soreness: of abdomen; of chest.

Pressive bearing down: in ovarian region; in pelvic region.

Pressure: around heart.

Heaviness: of head.

Heavy feeling: in forehead.

Dull sensation: over eyes.

Itching: of eruption on neck.

⁴⁴ Tissues. ▮Perverted and deficient nutrition.

▮▮Loss of weight.

▮Obesity.

▮▮Dropsy: from organic heart disease; from chronic liver complaint; far advanced Bright's disease; following intermittent fever.

▮▮Asthma; emphysema; pulmonary catarrh.

▮▮Obstinate neuralgia caused by derangement of abdominal organs, intestines and liver.

▮▮Fatty degeneration.

Diseases with faulty nutrition, in consequence of obscure subacute inflammation of stomach or intestines, followed by affections of the nervous centres.

⁴⁵ Touch. Passive Motion. Injuries. Touch: abdomen sensitive.

Pressure: around waist, produces fainting spells; pain in eyeball >; presses eyes into pillow with severe pain; cannot bear it on abdomen.

Bandaging head tightly: < pain.

After injury: subject to distress in head.

⁴⁶ Skin. ▮A symmetrical patch of herpetic eruption on each side of neck, itching and burning after scratching.

⁴⁷ Stages of Life, Constitution. Girl, æt. 13, dark hair, sick headache; sciatica.

Girl, æt. 17, light hair, blue eyes, one to three attacks every week, suffering three years; fainting spells.

Girl, æt. 18; irregular menstruation.

Woman, had been in habit of taking ten or twelve enemas every day, and often passed four or five weeks without action of bowels, suffering fifteen years; chronic consti-. pation.

Woman, small, slender, nervo-bilious, mother of four children, attacks came at least once a month, and for last two years every Saturday, suffering sixteen years; hemicrania.

Man æt. 22, musician, strong, active; chronic constipation.

Woman, æt. 29, tall, thin, mother of two children, light
hair and blue eyes, suffering from youth; headache.

Woman, æt. 30, nervo-sanguineous temperament, suffering
two years; headache.

Woman, æt. 32, small sized, mother of four children, suffering seven years; headache.

Woman, æt. 40, attacks two or three times a week, lasting
12 to 24 hours, during which she is unable to do anything; headache.

Woman, æt. 40, has been for several years subject to continual, persistent constipation, > only by cathartics and
enemas; violent sick headaches.

Man, æt. 49, at age of 21, fell from a roof and was carried
home insensible, since then subject to spells, which, as
he advanced in years, became more frequent, sometimes
occurring every week; headache.

Woman, æt. 71, very stout, suffering for some years;
headache.

⁴⁸ **Relations.** Compare *Lac can.*

LACHESIS.

The Surukuku Snake of South America.   *Ophidia.*

The first trituration, and first dilution in alcohol, of the snake poison, Trigo-nocephalus Lachesis, was made by Hering, on July 28th, 1828.

The first cases were published in the Archives, in 1835. In 1837 this remedy was introduced into our Materia Medica. See Effects of Snake Poison, by C. Hering, Denkschriften der Nordamerikanischen Akademie der homöopathischen Heilkunst, Allentown, Pa.

Provings by Hering, and under his direction by Stapf, Bute, Bauer, Behlert, Detwiller, Gross, Kummer, Reichhelm, Koenig, Wesselhoeft, Kehr, Koth, Matlack, De Young, Helfrich, Schmoele, and Lingen. Later provings were made by Robinson, Fellows (Fincke, not contained in Encyclopedia), Bartlett, Metcalf and Berridge. See Allen's Encyclopedia, vol. 5, p. 432.

CLINICAL AUTHORITIES.—*Maniacal jealousy*, Woost, Rück. Kl. Erf., vol. 5, p. 6; *Delirium tremens*, Hering, Rück. Kl. Erf., vol. 1, p. 143; *Melancholy*, Guernsey, Raue's Rec., 1871, p. 49; *Melancholia after confinement*, MSS.; *Mental disorder*, Berridge, Raue's Rec., 1872, p.51; Hom. Clin., vol. 4, p. 73; Wesselhoeft, Raue's Rec., 1871, p. 47; Smith, N. E. M. G., vol. 8, p. 314; Weber, Med. Inv., vol. 5, p. 34; Gross, Rück. Kl. Erf., vol. 1, p. 32; *Irritation of meninges of brain and spinal cord*, Pope, B. J. H., vol. 13, p. 479; *Brain irritation*, Nankivell, A. H. Rev., vol. 13, p. 360; *Inflammation of brain*, Lunzer, Rück. Kl. Erf., vol. 5, p. 44; *Sunstroke*, C. B. Knerr, MSS.; *Affection of brain*, Miller, Hom. Clin.,vol. 3, p. 97; *Encephaloma*, Jackson, Gilchrist's Surgery, p. 161, N. A. J. H., vol. 22, p. 363; *Vertigo*, J. C. Cummings,MSS.; *Headache* (4 cases), Neidhard, MSS.; C. H. Vilas, MSS.; Wesselhoeft, B. J. H.,vol. 22, p. 483; Sawyer, Am. Hom. Obs., vol. 2, p. 138 ; Pope, B. J. H., vol. 13, p. 478 ; *Megrim*, Tietze, Peters, Pope, Rück. Kl. Erf., vol. 5, p. 89 ; *Cephalalgia*, Raue's Rec., 1870, p. 287 ; *Supraorbital neuralgia*, Martin, Med. Inves, vol. 7, p. 594 ; *Asthenopia*, Norton's Ophth. Therap., p. 109 ; *Defective sight after diphtheria*, MSS. ; *Post-diphtheritic eye affection*, Martin, Org., vol. 2, p. 108 ; *Retinitis apoplectica*, Norton's Ophth. Therap., p. 109 ; *Inflammation of eye*, Rittenhouse, Trans. Hom. Med. Soc. Pa.,1873, p. 106 ; *Orbital cellulitis*, Allen, Norton's Ophthal. Therap., p. 108 ; *Pterygium*, Rittenhouse, Trans. Hom. Med. Soc. Pa., 1873, p. 107 ; *Partial deafness*, Martin, Raue's Rec., 1872, p. 81 ; *Affection of ear*, Martin, Hom. Clin., vol. 4, 149 ; Lippe, Rück. Kl. Erf., vol. 5, p. 159 ; *Epistaxis*, J. S. Linsley, MSS.; *Coryza*, MSS.; *Chronic nasal catarrh*, W. Story, MSS.; *Affections of nose*, Rosenberg, Rück. Kl. Erf., vol. 5, p. 173 ; *Neuralgia of face*, Bojanus, Raue's Rec., 1871, p. 179 ; Tietze,

NOTE.—A circular letter issued by Dr. Hering, in 1878, soliciting contributions of clinical matter, provings, etc., for a full collection of reports wherewith to celebrate the Fiftieth Anniversary of the introduction of Lachesis, was freely and generously responded to by numerous members of the profession, whose names appear in the list of Clinical Authorities, followed by the abbreviation MSS. The author did not live to finish his intended Monograph, but all that is essential and of guiding value in Lachesis is embodied in our arrangement.—EDS.

Rück. Kl. Erf., vol. 1, p. 425; *Swelling of face*, Duncan, Hom. Clin., vol. 1, p. 245; *Erysipelas of face*, Berridge, Times Retros., vol. 3, p. 30; *Parotitis*, Smith, Med. Inv., vol. 5, p. 106; *Bleeding of gums*, Leon, Rück. Kl. Erf., vol. 4, p. 666; *Glossomania*, Gross, B. J. H., vol. 12, p. 472; *Sore mouth of nursing women*, G. Pearson, MSS.; *Nursing sore mouth*, Raymond, Med. Inv., vol. 5, p. 72; *Affection of mouth after diphtheria*, MSS.; *Sore mouth and throat after scarlet fever*, Preston, Raue's Rec., 1870, p. 321; *Chronic irritability of fauces*, Wesselhoeft, B. J. H., vol. 22, p. 488; *Throat affection*, C. Hering, B. J. H., vol. 21, p. 370; *Affection of throat after diphtheria*, MSS.; *Inflammation of throat*, Raymond, Med. Inv., vol. 5, p. 72; *Angina*, Stow, Raue's Rec., 1870, p. 142; Berridge, Raue's Rec., 1870, p. 142; Fielitz, Jahr, Rück. Kl. Erf., vol. 1, p. 531; *Sore throat*, Blakely, Hom. Clin., vol. 1, p. 126; Boyce, Med. Inv., vol. 5, p. 6; (5 cases) Neidhard, MSS.; *Tonsillitis*, Hirschel, Rück. Kl. Erf., vol. 5, p. 242; Blakely, Raue's Rec., 1870, p. 141; Hom. Clin., vol. 1, p. 232; *Epidemic pharyngitis* (50 cases), Ward, Am. Hom. Obs., vol. 6, p. 226; *Chronic pharyngitis*, Miller, Raue's Rec., 1875, p. 246; *Diphtheria*, Guernsey, Oehme's Therap., p. 46; Allen, N. A. J. H., vol. 13, p. 99; Hale, Hom. Clin., vol. 1, p. 184; (3 cases) Hale, Oehme's Therap., p. 48; Goodno, Hom. Clin., vol. 3, p. 140; (2 cases) Goodno, Oehme's Therap., p. 49; (2 cases) Hirsch, Oehme's Therap., p. 46; (5 cases) Wesselhoeft, Oehme's Therap., pp. 47–48; Dunham, A. H. O., vol. 4, p. 111; Tietze, B. J. H., vol. 31, p. 124; Oehme, N. A. J. H., vol. 25, p. 68; T. S. Hoyne, MSS.; A. M. Piersons, MSS.; (3 cases) Piersons, Hah. Mo., vol. 10, p. 212; (8 cases) MSS.; Von Tunzelmann, Am. Hom. Rev., vol. 17, p. 741; C. W. Boyce, MSS.; Fellows, Am. Hom. Rev., vol. 5, p. 412; C. Pearson, MSS.; Rittenhouse, Raue's Rec., 1872, p. 103; Schmitt, Hom. Phys., vol. 4, p. 190; Beaumont, Org., vol., 3, p. 93; *Syphilitic phagedæna of fauces*, Hale, Raue's Rec., 1874, p. 109; *Spasmodic stricture of throat*, Bartlett, Rück. Kl. Erf., vol. 5, p. 242; *Foreign body in œsophagus*, Herzberger, B. J. H., vol. 36, p. 376; *Dyspepsia*, Hering, Rück. Kl. Erf., vol. 1, p. 586; *Affection of stomach*, Neidhard, MSS.; *Affection of liver*, Luther, Rück. Kl. Erf., vol. 5, p. 339; C. Neidhard, MSS.; *Affection of spleen*, C. Neidhard, MSS.; *Typhlitis*, Hering, Black, Rück. Kl. Erf., vol. 1, p. 725; *Peritonitis*, Wesselhoeft, B. J. H., vol. 22, p. 485; Bürkner, Rück. Kl. Erf., vol. 5, p. 669; *Tumor in l. groin*, H. C. Bartlett, MSS.; *Buboes*, Rück. Kl. Erf., vol. 5, p. 560; *Diarrhœa*, Gross, Rück. Kl. Erf., vol. 1, p. 837; C. Neidhard, MSS.; *Constipation*, Hering, Rück. Kl. Erf., vol. 1, p. 816; Smith, N. A. J. H., vol. 14, p. 176; *Croupous enteritis*, Gerson, Rück. Kl. Erf., vol. 5, p. 420; *Dysentery*, Boyce, Raue's Rec., 1874, p. 174; *Affection of anus and rectum*, Morgan, Am. Hom. Rev., vol. 4, p. 409; *Hemorrhoids*, C. Neidhard, MSS.; *Anal fistula*, Eggert, Raue's Rec., 1870, p. 219; Med. Inv., vol. 6, p. 143; *Strangury*, C. Neidhard, MSS.; *Ovaritis*, Conant, Times Retros., vol. 1, p. 93; *Sacculated ovarian disease*, Baer, Org., vol. 3, p. 103; *Ovarian tumor*, Dudgeon, Gilchrist's Surgery, p. 161, B. J. H., 1873, p. 183; *Uterine and ovarian tumors*; *Metritis*, J. C. Morgan, MSS.; *Chronic uterine catarrh*, Lindsay, Org., vol. 1, p. 471; *Leucorrhœa with sterility*, MSS.; *Puerperal convulsions*, Minton, Raue's Path., p. 902, Hom. Clin., vol. 1, p. 76; Colby, Raue's Rec., 1874, p. 247; G. B., N. E. M. G., vol. 11, p. 405; *Ovarian pain after confinement*, J. H. Patton, MSS.; *Phlegmasia alba dolens*, M., Allg. Hom. Ztg., vol. 108, p. 156; *Vitiated milk*, Rück. Kl. Erf., vol. 2, p. 412; *Aphonia*, Knickbocker, Raue's Rec., 1873, p. 88; *Affections of larynx*, Lobethal, Rück. Kl. Erf., vol. 3, p. 168; *Spasms of larynx*, Knickbocker, Raue's Rec., 1873, p. 89; *Spasm of glottis*, Smith, N. E. M. G., vol. 8, p. 310; *Croup*, Guernsey, Raue's Rec., 1871, p. 80; *Membranous croup*, Frost, Am. Hom. Rev., vol. 5, p. 491; *Bronchitis and aphonia*, Stow, Raue's Rec., 1874, p.

145; *Bronchial catarrh* (5 cases), Boyce, Am. Hom. Rev., vol. 4, p. 415; *Respiratory affections*, Hering, Rück. Kl. Erf., vol. 3, p. 18; *Dyspnœa*, Allg. Hom. Ztg., vol. 107, p. 157; *Asthma*, Hart, Raue's Rec., 1875, p. 118; Med. Inv., vol. 11, p. 225; Hering, Rück. Kl. Erf., vol. 3, p. 190; *Asthmatic cough*, Deck, B. J. H., vol. 31, p. 173; *Pains in chest*, C. Neidhard, MSS.; *Threatened paralysis of lungs*, Trinks, Rück. Kl. Erf., vol. 5, p. 762; *Chest affection*, Hering, B. J. H., vol. 2, p. 369; *Lung affection*, Hering, B. J. H., vol. 2, p. 377; Weber, Med. Inv., vol. 5, p. 33; Wurmb, Rück. Kl. Erf., vol. 5, p. 822; *Consumption*, Hering, Rück. Kl. Erf., vol. 3, p. 380; *Tuberculosis*, Wells, Hom. Clin., vol. 4, p. 121; Smith, N. E. M. G., vol. 8, p. 309; *Chronic pleuro-pneumonia*, C. Neidhard, MSS.; *Affection of heart*, Deck, B. J. H., vol. 31, p. 175; Hale, Org., vol. 2, p. 220; Stow, Raue's Rec., 1870, p. 197; *Cyanosis*, Von Tagen, Raue's Rec., 1871, p. 106; *Functional disease of heart*, Smith, N. E. M. G., vol. 8, p. 116; *Attacks of dyspnœa and palpitation*, Gerstel, Allg. Hom. Ztg., vol. 106, p. 99; *Affection of mammary gland*, Oehme, Rück. Kl. Erf., vol. 5, p. 648; *Mammary tumor*, Oehme, Rück. Kl. Erf., vol. 4, p. 304; *Abscess on l. side of neck, after scarlatina*, Wells, Am. H. Rev., vol. 4, p. 362; *Affection of spine*, Seward, Hom. Phys., vol. 3, p. 310; *Caries of dorsal spine*, Wesselhoeft, B. J. H., vol. 22, p. 481; *Phlegmonous inflammation of hand*, M., Allg. Hom. Ztg., vol. 108, p. 156; *Gangrene of hand*, Allen, Am. Hom. Rev., vol. 4, p. 558; *Affection of r. hand*, Hering, B. J. H., vol. 2, p. 374; *Whitlow*, Bell, Raue's Rec., 1870, p. 327; *Panaritium*, Kreuss, Stapf, Rück. Kl. Erf., vol. 3, p. 558; *Onychia*, Wood, Org., vol. 2, p. 106; *Contraction of psoas muscle after pelvic abscess*, Hale, Raue's Rec., 1874, p. 109; *Paralysis of legs and chest affection*, Wesselhoeft, B. J. H., vol. 22, p. 482; *Sciatica*, Miller, Raue's Rec., 1875, p. 246; Org., vol. 3, p. 357; *Affection of knee*, Fielitz, Rück. Kl. Erf., vol. 3, p. 587; *Varicose veins of knee*, Schüssler, Rück. Kl. Erf., vol. 5, p. 860; *Pain below knee*, J. H. Patton, MSS.; *Ulcer of leg*, J. C. Morgan, MSS.; *Ulcer, with paralysis of l. leg*, Baer, Org., vol. 3, p. 103; *Syphilitic ulcer on leg*, Hafen, Allg. Hom. Ztg., vol. 105, p. 108; *Gangrene of leg*, Allen, Am. Hom. Rev., vol. 4, p. 557; *Indolent ulcers on foot*, W. Story, MSS.; *Affection of second toe of r. foot*, B. J. H., vol. 2, p. 376; *Pain in joints*, Rück. Kl. Erf., vol. 5, p. 900; *Hysteria*, B. in D., Rück. Kl. Erf., vol. 2, p. 286; Bahrenberg, Allg. Hom. Ztg., vol. 101, p. 134; *Spasms in meningitis*, C. Neidhard, MSS.; *Uræmic convulsions*, Barrows, Times Retros., vol. 2, p. 14; *Convulsions* (3 cases), Finch, Hom. Clin., vol. 4, p. 30, Raue's Rec., 1871, p. 186; *Chorea*, Constantine Lippe, MSS.; *Epilepsy*, C. Mohr, MSS.; Tietze, Hering, Pulte, Rück. Kl. Erf., vol. 4, p. 577; (4 cases) Preston, Baker, Times Retros., vol. 1, p. 123; Friese, Raue's Rec., 1872, p. 228; *Tetanus*, Sircar, Raue's P., p. 890; Smith, Raue's Rec., 1874, p. 264; *Opisthotonos*, Oehme, Allg. Hom. Ztg., vol. 103, p. 207; *Catalepsy*, C. Mohr, MSS.; *Nervousness*, Deck, B. J. H., vol. 31, p. 174; *Nervous affection*, Bahrenberg, Org., vol. 3, p 90; *General breakdown after repeated attacks of pneumonia*, Kenyon, Am. Hom. Rev., vol. 5, p. 269; *Neuralgia*, Bojanus, Hom. Clin., vol. 3, p. 111; Howard, Org., vol. 3, p. 111; *Post-diphtheritic affection*, Martin, Org., vol. 2, p. 108; *Incipient paralysis; Sleeplessness*, C. Neidhard, MSS; *Intermittent fever*, Hering, Rück. Kl. Erf., vol. 4, p. 941; Lippe, Bernreuter, Times Retros., vol. 3, p. 30; *Intermittent, with ovarian abscess*, Linsley, MSS.; *Ague*, Walker, Dever, Jennings, Allen's Intermittent Fever, p. 160; C. Neidhard, MSS.; J. C. Morgan, MSS.; *Typhoid*, Mohr, Trans. Hom. Med. Soc. Pa., 1880, p. 208; Bojanus, Rück. Kl. Erf., vol. 4, p. 745; Boyce, Brewster, Miller, Raue's Rec., 1874, p. 284; Boyce, Med. Inv., vol. 5, p. 5; *Hydrophobia*, Hering, Rück. Kl. Erf., vol. 4, p. 624; Toothaker, Raue's Rec., 1874, p. 276; *Septicæmia, result of dissecting wound*, Dunham, Dunham's Lectures, vol. 2, p. 247; *Phlebitis*, Dunham, B. J. H., vol. 31, p. 124; (3 cases) Dunham, A. H. O., vol. 4, p. 110; *Rheumatism*, Linsley, Hom. Clin., vol. 1, p. 44; Smith, Raue's Rec., 1874, p. 254; *Hemorrhage in typhoid fever*, Guernsey, Hah. M., vol. 6, p. 175; *Erysipelas*, Gross, Kreuss, Rück. Kl. Erf., vol. 4, p. 143; Smith, Raue's Rec., 1874, p. 291; *Carbuncle*, Hering, Rück. Kl. Erf., vol. 4, p. 183; C. B. Knerr, MSS.; Dunham, A. H. O., vol. 4, p. 111; Berridge, Times Retros., vol. 3, p. 30; *Traumatic gangrene*, J. H. Patton, MSS.; (2 cases) Franklin, Hughes' Pharm., p. 493; B. J. H., vol. 27, p. 322; Simon, Rück. Kl. Erf., vol. 4, p. 1027; *Gangrene*, Hiatt, N. A. J. H., vol. 13, p. 493; J. C. Morgan, MSS., Gilchrist's Surg., p. 91; *Epidemic malignant pustule* (8 cases), Dunham, A. H. O., vol. 4, p. 110; B. J. H., vol. 31, p. 123; *Dropsy*, Wolf, Gross, Rück. Kl. Erf., vol. 4, p. 349; *Anasarca*, Frost, Am. Hom. Rev., vol. 5, p. 492; *Syphilis*, Hering, Rück. Kl. Erf., vol. 2, p. 123; Morgan, Am. H. Rev., vol. 4, p. 410; *Bedsores*, Strong, Raue's Rec., 1874, p. 285; *Measles*, Miller, Raue's Rec., 1873, p. 222, Raue's P., p. 1006; *Repercussion of measles*, Dunham, A. Hom. Rev., vol. 4, p. 32; *Malignant scarlatina*, Bringham, MSS.; *Scarlet fever*, P. P. Wells, MSS.; G. B. Saertelle, MSS.; Wells, N. A. J. H., vol. 24, p. 411; Gross, Lobethal, Rück. Kl. Erf., vol. 4, p. 53; Hughes, B. J. H., vol. 31, p. 125; Allen, Am. Hom. Rev., vol. 4, p. 556; *Skin affection*, Berridge, Hom. Phys., vol. 4, p. 288; *Eruption on arm and abdomen*, W. Story, MSS.; *Itch*, Hering, MSS., B. J. H., vol. 2, p. 375; *Eczema*, Scott, Hah. Mo., vol 1, p. 460; *Pustular eruption*, Wesselhoeft, B. J. H, vol. 22, p 486; Gross, Hering, Rück. Kl. Erf., vol. 4, p. 243; *Herpes zoster*, Elb, Allg. Hom. Ztg, vol. 110, p. 18; *Boils, abscesses*, J. H. Patton, MSS.; *Ulcers*, Griesselich, Gross, Rück. Kl. Erf., vol. 4, p. 284; *Indolent ulcers*, Smith, Gwynn, Raue's Rec., 1874, p. 295; Hall, Raue's Rec., 1873, p. 247; *Antidote to bee sting*, Boyce, Raue's Rec., 1870, p. 90; Baugh, Med. Inves., vol. 6, p. 54; *Antidote to Bufo*, Weber, Raue's Rec., 1870, p. 91; *Dog bite*, Linsley, MSS.; *Tarantula bite*, Hardenstein, Hom. Clin., vol. 4, p. 106; *Antidote to bite of rattlesnake*, Weber, Raue's Rec., 1870, p. 91.

¹ **Mind.** ▪Loss of consciousness.
▪▪Weakness of memory; makes mistakes in writing; confusion as to time.
▪Great dulness of mind with bodily weakness.   θTyphus.
▪Mind confused and wandering. θDiphtheria.
▪▪Quick comprehension; mental activity, with almost prophetical perception; ecstasy; a kind of trance.
▪No sooner does one idea occur to him, than a number of others follow in quick succession while he is writing.
▪Visions and delirious talk as soon as he shuts eyes; < noon till midnight.
▪Thinks: she is somebody else and in the hands of a stronger power; she is dead, and preparations are made for funeral, or that she is nearly dead and wishes some one would help her off; herself pursued by enemies, or fears medicine is poison; there are robbers in house and wants to jump out of window; herself under superhuman control; visions real; he will die.
▪Imagines he is followed by enemies who are trying to harm him; attempts to leave room as if frightened by visions behind him. θFistula.

❚❚Delirium at night, muttering, drowsy, red face; slow, difficult speech and dropped jaw.

❚Violent delirium especially after sleeping. θTyphoid.

❚Delirium; fears she will be damned.

❚Constant delirium which changes rapidly from one subject to another. θDiphtheria.

❚Delirium from overwatching, overfatigue; loss of fluids; excessive study.

❚❚Delirium tremens, attacks come most in afternoon, or after sleep; loquacious, jumps from subject to subject, cannot bear shirt or neckband to touch throat.

❚Most extraordinary loquacity, making speeches in very select phrases, but jumping off to most heterogeneous subjects; at same time proud, full of mistrust. θMania.

❚Religious monomania, fear of being damned.

❚❚One word often leads into midst of another story.

❚Insane jealousy.

❚His mind is disturbed before the attack. θEpilepsy.

❚After operation for fistula in ano, complained of his head, particularly pain in l. temple and occiput; aching pain in lumbar region; came home from work dizzy, faint and nauseated; talked incoherently, talked as it were in a strange language; since then quite without mind; will frequently cry and whine, then laugh in silliest manner; does not sleep at night; sleeps only a minute or two at a time during day; is often violent, only with difficulty can be kept in bed; endeavors to climb up bedpost; has an idiotic expression; articulation imperfect; tongue lolling about in mouth; eyes rolling vacantly; frequently rises, with great effort and awkwardness; body when standing bends toward l., must be supported; drags his feet in walking, direction of steps toward l.; entirely unable to feed himself; seems indifferent to food; imagines he is followed by enemies who are trying to harm him; attempts to leave room as if frightened by visions behind him. θMental disorder.

❚❚She is tempted to commit suicide. θMania.

❚❚Loquacity; much rapid talking; wants to talk all the time. θFevers.

❚Inclination to be communicative; vivid imagination; extremely impatient at tedious and dry things.

❚Is morbidly talkative and gives a rambling account of her ailments.

❚Jealousy, with frightful images, great tendency to mock, to satire and ridiculous ideas.

❚❚Exceptional loquacity with rapid change of subject; jumps abruptly from one idea to another.

❚Talks, sings or whistles constantly; makes odd motions with arm. θDiphtheria.

ııViolent laughing for one hour; dyspnœa.
ıUndertakes many things, perseveres in nothing.
ııDisinclined to his own proper work; complains of trifles.
ıAversion of women to marry.
πPerfect happiness and cheerfulness, followed by gradual
  fading of spirituality; want of self control; lascivious;
  felt as if she was clear animal right through, whilst all
  mental power was dormant; sensation as if in hands of
  stronger power, as if charmed, and as if she could not
  break the spell.
ıQuiet, sorrowful, lowness of spirits, > by sighing; repugnance to society and dislike to talk; solicitude about
  future, with disgust for life; inclination to doubt everything; mistrusts and misconstrues; indolence; aversion
  to every kind of labor and motion. θMelancholia.
ııFeels extremely sad, unhappy and distressed in mind on
  waking in morning.
ıSad; loathing of life; suspicious and peevish; moaning
  and complaining; skin shriveled and livid; nose, ears
  and forehead cold; as soon as he shuts his eyes he is
  delirious. θTraumatic delirium.
ıFainting fits with great and almost unconquerable sadness
  and gloom; dreads society; persistent constipation with
  sensation as though anus was closed.
ııGreat sadness and anxiety, < in morning on awaking.
ıWeak and unhappy, particularly in morning, when she
  feels, on awaking, friendless and forsaken; same symptoms if she awakens at night; appetite poor; constipated; feeling of constriction of anus; urine scanty and
  dark colored; has had domestic troubles. θMelancholia.
ıHopelessness.
ıDread of death, fears to go to bed; fears of being poisoned.
ıDiscouraged, loathing life. θMelancholy after confinement.
ıWeary of life, looks at everything from dark side; <
  morning, > through day; least noise disturbs sleep.
ıSatiety of life with longing for death.
ıShe is tormented by idea that her better principles might
  be overcome by irresistible desire to suicide. θMania.
ıVoluptuous, irritated state, fights it. θEpilepsy.
ıAmorousness; amativeness.
ııGreat sensitiveness and anxiety. θLiver complaint.
ıIrritability; ill humor; sensitive disposition.
ıPeevish, disposed to be morose or quarrelsome.
ıProud; jealous, suspicious; developing into mania.
ıMalice; thinks only of mischief.
ıSensitiveness, or general aggravation after mental exertion.
ıA girl, after excessive study, uses exalted language; exceedingly particular about language she uses, often cor-

recting herself after using a word, and substituting another of very similar meaning; talks about being under influence of a superior power. θMania.

❙Nightly attacks of anxiety; afraid of cholera, gets cramps in calves from fear; nausea, heavy feeling in abdomen, rolling in umbilical region.

❙❙Chronic complaints after long lasting grief or sorrow.

❙After domestic calamity; sleepless, or, when overcome by exhaustion, short naps disturbed by frightful dreams; springing up in bed with terror, and suffocation of chest and palpitation; irritability alternating with loquacious delirium; nightly hallucinations causing mental suffering; conscious of her state. θMental disturbance.

❙Mental derangement after vexation.

❙Ailments from fright, disappointed love or jealousy.

❙After a jealous quarrel, she put both hands to her chest and cried out "Oh! my heart!" then fell down and was in an asphyctic state for nearly twenty-four hours; no pulse could be felt, breathing hardly perceptible; lay on her back.

² **Sensorium.** ❙Left sided apoplexy, especially after mental emotions, or abuse of alcohol; blowing expiration, cannot bear neck touched.

❙Stupefaction or loss of consciousness, blue face and convulsive movements, tremor of extremities. θApoplexy.

❙Stupid state; complaining of pain and weight in head at school, on being brought home he generally lies dozing or waking for three or four hours; frequent waking at night; vomiting on alternate nights; face heavy, pupils slightly dilated, forehead hot, pulse 90; tongue clean; head pains through day. θIrritation of brain.

❙Vanishing of thought, with blackness before eyes, in paroxysms.

❙So giddy he could not stand; could not see letters, fell against wall; severe pains all over head.

❙❙Rush of blood to head: with heat in head; after alcohol; suppressed or irregular menses; climacteric period.

❙Vertigo with heaviness of head, dulness like lead in occiput. θTyphoid.

❙❙Dulness of cerebral function. θDiphtheria. θScarlatina.

❙Vertigo: early in morning; on waking; in evening; on looking up; on looking at any object closely; from walking in open air (at climaxis); from suppressed erysipelas; with pale face, migraine; momentary on closing eyes; with falling to l. side; before menses; on stooping; after lying down; on reaching up; with nausea, vomiting, headache; stupefying; as before apoplexy.

³ **Inner Head.** ▮Frontal headache; faint on rising.

▮In forehead: aching; with stitches; dull pain (angina faucium); pressing from without inward; violent headache when nasal discharge suddenly dries up.

▮Violent darting, stabbing pains, from upper part of forehead down to centre of head, as if knives were being thrust into brow; < least motion; violent pressure from above downwards. θHeadache.

▮Heavy pain in forehead extending to back and sometimes all over head, coming on at any time of day; pain in back part of hip and l. side, region of spleen, occasionally on r. side; abdomen sore, cannot bear least touch; costive; dull pain in legs.

▮Headache over eyes and in occiput, morning on rising.

▮Dull pain over and in eyes; nausea; pain top of head; giddiness on rising.

▮Pain over eyes, mostly l., with nausea. θSick headache.

▮▮Headache extending into nose.

▮Heat in forehead between attacks. θEpilepsy.

▮▮Throbbing pain in temple with heat in head. θMigraine.

▮Violent throbing pain in l. temple, particularly before menses.

▮Temporal nerves on one side painful, with throbbing in temples; heat in head; vertigo with paleness of face; pain in l. ovarian region; bloatedness of stomach.

▮Headache frightfully severe, brain feels as if it would burst skull, especially at temples; generally begins on rising in morning, seldom in afternoon; lying down > pain, but as soon as she raises head, pain is equally severe whether she sits or walks.

▮▮Pressing or bursting pains in temples, < from motion, pressure, stooping or lying down.

▮Severe, oppressive pain in one or the other temple, < on r. side; nausea; mouth clammy; cannot swallow the saliva; pain comes on at night and lasts till end of next day; usually > after vomiting; after eating, food rises in mouthfuls; frequent risings of frothy phlegm.

▮Drawing pain in l. temple with redness; soreness to least touch; fever; pulse full and quick.

▮Headache: pain from superciliary ridge to occipital protuberance, intolerable; could not sleep; slightly delirious; pupils dilated; pain intense; cold water externally > somewhat; at midnight, partly insensible; tongue stiff and protruding; speech incoherent, or saying same thing over and over; talks like a lunatic; idiotic look; does not comprehend what is said to him; whenever he rises staggers backwards; walks backwards until he comes in contact with wall, bed or table; takes hold of some furniture, and with greatest difficulty pulls himself forward; afraid of everybody, thinks everybody conspires to kill him; afraid of medicine, won't take any; partial paralysis on r. side.

∎Headache in l. frontal eminence, deep internally.

∎Left sided orbital neuralgia; lachrymation; previous to paroxysm rising of heat to head; during intervals a weak, nauseous feeling in abdomen.

∎Semilateral headache on r. side, creeping gradually towards l., until it goes around head; twitching in eyes when they are fixed upon an object; menses irregular, one week ahead of time; tardy digestion; constipation; frequent nausea; pain deep in orbit and over eyes, which are red and injected. θCephalalgia.

∎Every three or four days intense headache; pain throbbing and oppressive, chiefly in r. half of head, extending down same side of neck,which generally feels stiff and sore; pain < at catamenial period, which is attended with much aching across loins; menses dark and profuse, lasting eight to nine days.

∎One sided tensive headache, drawing from neck over head to eyes; vomiting; stiffness of neck; tenderness of scalp.

∎Headache on r. side, extending to neck and shoulders, with tension in muscles.

∎Tearing pain in whole l. side of head, from temple to collar bone; tears flow continually; pain without intermission; some nightly aggravations; > from warm applications; paralytic state of tongue; it inclined to affected side; could hardly speak; painful weariness of face, head and neck; tongue feels as if bound or tied up. θNeuralgia.

∎Cutting headache as if a part of r. side of head was cut off, < after rising or ascending; > from heat and after belching.

∎Hemicrania with giddiness, paleness of face, general sensation of stiffness and pain in l. side of abdomen.

∎Tearing on top of head from within outward; dizzy, face pale; faint, numb; face sunken, or bloated and red.

∎Pressure on top of head with hot throbbing of temples; constipation; any excitement causes headache; no catamenia for two months. θClimaxis.

∎Boring pain on vertex, nausea and vomiting. θItch.

∎∎Beating headache with heat, < on vertex and r. side, or over eyes; preceding a cold in head, with stiff neck.

∎Headache which had lasted six weeks; pain at first began in vertex, then extended over r. side of head and over face, with pricking as from needles in limbs of same side; < in afternoon.

❚Violent pressing, burning pain in top of head, from within outwards.

❚Burning vertex headache during menopause.

❚Boring and sticking on vertex.

❙❙Dull aching in sinciput.

❚Beating throbbing in vertex; with every movement.

❚❚Weight and pressure on vertex.

❚Congestion to head with other complaints.

❚Throbbing in head from least movement; red face.

❚Headache, with rush of blood to head.

❚Pressive headache, with nausea.

❙❙Dizzy, pressive headache; < on stooping.

❚Violent headache, with flickering before eyes.

❚❚Headache in sun, glimmering sight.

❚Headache preceding coryza.

❚Headache: catarrhal; congestive; from sunstroke; hysterical; rheumatic; menstrual; epileptic.

❚Terrible headache; nightly pain in limbs. θSyphilis.

❚Pain as if swollen in angle in front of styloid process, < from pressure.

❚Heaviness like lead in occiput; can scarcely raise it from pillow, in morning after waking, with vertigo.

❚Boring pain behind l. ear, with nausea and vomiting.

❚Feeling in back of head as if pressed asunder.

❚Numbness in occiput, with pain in forehead; on touching throat, darting from throat to occiput; chest feels dry.

❚❚Headache from occiput to eyes.

❚Headache every eight or ten days; toward evening pain in back of head, at first dull and gradually concentrating, acute boring behind l. ear, apparently at juncture of temporal, parietal and occipital bones; when boring pain reaches its height, generally towards morning, vomiting of food and slime; stitches in chest.

❚Soreness at vertex, gradually spread over r. side of head and face; same sensation, with pricking pains like pins and needles, in upper and lower extremities of same side; mouth very sore; cannot masticate food without great pain; after desire to micturate cannot retain urine; coughing produces flow of urine; < in afternoon, when soreness frequently changes to a sudden, darting pain in arm; drops things: slight vertigo.

❚Inflammatory conditions of brain; great vascular and nervous erethism.

' **Outer Head.** ❚Numbness and crawling on l. side of head, as in whole l. side.

❚Painful sensitiveness in l. temple from vertex down, and in l. half of face, when touched, or on moving muscles; sensation as if skin had been burnt by heat of sun.

▌Wants head closely wrapped up.
▌Tumors which perforate skull.
❘❘Sudden backward throwing of head. *θ*Epilepsy.
❘❘Bettered by shaking head.
▌Purplish swelling; delirious talk when closing eyes. *θ*Erysipelas of scalp.
▌▌Hair falls off, < during pregnancy; averse to sun.
❘❘Does not like hair touched; itching of scalp.
⁵ **Sight and Eyes.** ▌Oversensitive to light.
▌Flickering before eyes, as from threads, or rays of sun.
▌Flickering and jerking in r. eye, with congestion to head.
Flickering in peculiar angular zigzag figures, with headache.
▌Bright blue ring about light, filled with fiery rays.
❘❘Fog before eyes; in evening a bluish grey ring, about six inches in diameter, around light.
▌▌Dimness of vision: much black flickering before eyes, that seems very near; on waking.
▌▌Defective sight, after diphtheria.
❘❘Shortsightedness.
▌Unsteady look, eyes roll vacantly.
▌Eyes weak and dull, or distorted. *θ*Typhus.
▌Variety of pains and sensations in and around eyes, especially l.; very nervous; < thinking of eyes, using them, and waking in morning. *θ*Asthenopia.
▌Amblyopia, with lung or heart affections.
▌Hemorrhages into interior chamber, vitreous, retina and choroid.
❘❘Pupils at first contracted, then dilated. *θ*Fever.
▌Retinitis apoplectica; absorbs hemorrhage, controls inflammatory symptoms and diminishes tendency to retinal extravasation.
❘❘Phlyctenular keratitis, especially chronic recurrent; moderate redness of eye; photophobia.
▌Scrofulous keratitis with eruption on face, considerable photophobia and pains in eye and head, < in morning and after sleeping.
▌Ulcers on cornea; haziness.
▌Sharp, shooting pains from eyes to temples, top of head and occiput.
▌Stitches as from knives in eyes, coming from head.
▌Sticking drawing pain in r. eye, extending to vertex.
▌As if a thread was drawn from behind eye to eye.
▌Eyes feel as though they had been taken out and squeezed, and then put back again; pains < after sleep; wakens patient from sleep. *θ*Supraorbital neuralgia.
▌Pressure in orbits, with sensation of drawing from eyes to occiput.

▮▮Feels when throat is pressed, as if the eyes were forced out.

▮Stitching, burning and pressing pains in eyes.

▮▮Itching and burning of eyes.

▮Severe pains in and above eyes.

▮Intense and constant pain in l. eye, pain sharp and sticking, and sometimes extending to brow; uncertain, numb feeling on l. side of head; marked dimness of vision; terrific headache over eyes; wide awake in evening and very talkative; could not get to sleep until late, and when she did, would dream all the time; alternately dreaming and awakening; < after sleep, anxiously inquires why it is so; great prostration; seems exhausted mentally and physically; constantly laying aside bedclothes to get relief, they seemed to oppress her; seems as if she would die of exhaustion in morning; > in evening; intense pain in thigh, coming on after sleeping, and when gone, leaving a paralyzed feeling; confused feeling in head with vertigo.

▮▮Whites of eyes yellow. θJaundice.

▮Orbital cellulitis, following operation for strabismus; eye protruded; conjunctiva chemosed; purulent discharge; retina hazy and congested; point of tenotomy sloughing and a black spot in centre; < at night.

▮Pterygium.

▮Redness of eyes. θMania. θAngina faucium. θFevers.

▮Inflammation of eyes and lids, with pain in them.

▮Painful inflammation of l. eye, frequently recurring, characterized by a bundle of congested vessels extending from inner canthus toward cornea.

▮▮Eyes watery. θCatarrhal headache. θNeuralgia.

▮Fistula lachrymalis, accompanied by long standing eruption on face.

'Hearing and Ears. **▮▮**Sensitive to sounds; rushing and thundering in ears.

▮Painful beating, cracking, whizzing, drumming, with reverberation.

▮Whizzing as from insects in ears.

▮Ears feel as if closed from within. θAngina syphilitica.

▮Ears as if stuffed up.

▮Hardness of hearing, with dryness in ears, want of wax; numbness about ear and cheek.

▮After otorrhœa ear remained dry and obstructed, with almost entire deafness.

▮Diminished hearing.

▮Partial deafness, with dry wax in l. ear; noise in ear like tea kettle; sensation of numbness about ear and down l. cheek; sense of hunger every day at eleven.

▮Stoppage or stricture of Eustachian tube.

▮In evening, pain deep in l. ear; < from motion of temporal or masseter muscles; left in a few minutes and appeared just above l. external malleolus; < on stepping.

▮In night earache in r. ear, > by external warmth and lying on r. side.

▮Annoying pulsations in ear. θCarotid aneurism.

▮▮Tearing extending from zygoma into ear.

▮▮Pains in ears with sore throat.

▮▮Earwax too hard, pale. and insufficient; whitish, like chewed paper.

▮Polypus of ears.

▮▮Soreness and crusts around ears.

▮Threatened abscess of parotid gland. θTyphoid.

▮Ears excessively sensitive to wind.

⁷ **Smell and Nose.** ▮▮Nosebleed: dark; with amenorrhœa; before menses; typhus; blowing of blood, mostly in morning; trickling on blowing; from both nostrils; on swallowing, sensation as if tonsils were sore, like a wound, with stinging through ears.

▮Nasal, indistinct speech. θTyphoid.

▮▮Coryza preceded by headache; discharge watery, with red nostrils, herpes on lips.

▮Coryza preceded one or two days by a feeling of soreness, rawness and scraping in throat.

▮Scabs in nose; redness of point of nose.

▮Catarrh with sticking headache; stiffness of neck.

▮▮Swollen nasal mucous membrane; discharge of blood and pus. θCoryza.

▮Feeling of lump in throat; on swallowing, lump descends but immediately returns. θCoryza.

▮Mu.ous membrane of nose thickened, much sneezing; dry, stuffed feeling through front of head; gradually passes to fauces and chest; constant cough short and dry, with wheezing, face red and puffed, while eyes seemed almost pressed out. θHay asthma.

▮Many symptoms end with nasal catarrh.

▮Obstruction of nose, with buzzing in ears; headache; ill humor and inability to drink.

▮▮Complaints after suppressed coryza.

▮Undeveloped coryza with headache and mental worry.

▮Thick, yellow discharge in morning, sometimes streaked with blood, offensive; hawking; falling of mucus from posterior nares; l. side only; discharge of hard plug of mucus. θChronic nasal catarrh.

▮▮Pus and blood from nose.

▮Discharges offensive, sanious, corroding nostrils and lips.

▮Sudden discharge of pus and blood from nose, as from a

bursting abscess, seems to come from frontal cavities. θOzæna syphilitica.

❚❚Soreness of nostrils and lips.

❚Internal soreness of nose, and nose filled with scabs. θMercurio-syphilitic cases. θDrunkards.

❚Inflammation of nose with pimples and blisters.

❚Nose pointed, reddish, as if sore, and always some fluent coryza. θAngina syphilitica.

❚Red nose of drunkards.

❚Vesicular eruption about nose.

⁸ **Upper Face.** ❚Expression: of pain, with sopor; idiotic; epileptic; distorted; haggard.

❚Features distorted, face dark and much swollen, appeared almost in an apoplectic fit; had removed everything from his neck, saying he could bear nothing to touch it; could hardly breathe. θBee sting.

❚Haggard, face of unnatural color, cheeks yellow, with traces of red vessels visible and spots of circumscribed red; nose pointed and red, as if raw from a sore; nose always stuffed up.

❚Face pale: fainting; headache; before epileptic attack.

❚Blue circles around eyes.

❚Countenance deeply sallow. θScarlatina.

❚❚Yellow complexion, vermilion redness of cheeks, or small red bloodvessels shining through skin. θSyphilis.

❚Earthy, livid, cachectic complexion. θAbdominal troubles.

❚Bluish, purplish appearance of face, inability to bear anything around neck; cerebral symptoms. θScarlatina.

❚Face not red, but very livid and bluish. θPuerperal fever.

❚Blue face and lips. θEmphysema.

❚Livid face. θMetritis.

❚Face puffed. ❚Mania.

❚Red face, as in apoplexy; bloated, red, with headache, pains in limbs, stomach, etc.

❚❚Flushes of heat. θDrunkards. θClimacteric period. θConstipation. θSuppresed menstruation.

❚One cheek flushed, the other pale.

❚Severe pain commencing in r. inner canthus, and extending upwards and outwards in a semicircle, just above superciliary ridge; dull, heavy, and prevents him working; commences 9 A.M. and goes off in afternoon; skin extremely sensitive to touch. θNeuralgia.

❚Neuralgia, l. side, orbital; rising of heat to face before, and weak feeling in abdomen after attack.

❚Neuralgia of trigeminus; horrible; heat running up in head previous to attack; weak, nervous feeling in abdomen during intervals.

❚Tearing pain in whole l. side of head, from temple down

as far as collar bone, so severe as to cause tears to flow continually; < at night; articulation almost impossible; when tongue is put out it inclines to affected side; painful weariness of head, neck and face; tongue feels as if bound or tied up. θNeuralgia.

▮Sensation of warmth rising into head, followed by tearing pain beginning in forehead, but particularly affecting l. malar bone and parts under l. eye, and occasionally extending into eye, causing lachrymation; attack lasts several hours, then disappears for a day or two, and then returns without any cause; weak sensation in abdomen during free days.

▮Feeling of stiffness in malar bone from cervical glands.

▮▮Left side of face and lower jaw swollen, sensitive to touch.

.▮Cheeks swollen, skin tense, hot and crisp, as if it would crack. θPeritonitis.

▮Enormously swollen upper lip and nose; surface not changed from natural color; appearance that of puffiness, but hard to feel, much like swelling from a bee sting, or from a blow; vermilion border of lip a trifle more blue than natural; no pain or heat; menstruating.

▮Erysipelatous eruption beneath l. eye, which first itches at night; she was awakened with fright about trifles; in morning skin began to redden and swell, and became < after midday nap; next morning very thick and red, with incessant itching scarcely to be endured; whole lower lid swollen, red and itching.

▮Erysipelatous swelling of face; r. eye almost closed.

▮Erysipelas began close to l. side of nose, in a red, sore spot, then it became redder and extended up and down l. side of face; extends up as far as l. eye and is dusky; she feels languid.

▮Facial erysipelas, in a child a year old; inflammation partly involving scalp; on second or third day threatened metastasis to meninges; convulsive stiffening of child's penis.

▮Face swollen, bluish red or leaden hue; tongue dry, glossy, tremulous; < from noon until midnight. θErysipelas from a dissecting wound.

▮▮Erysipelas of face, with burning and itching, < after siesta; hammering headache.

▮Eruption in face followed by bluish spots.

▮Burning, swelling, redness and violent itching in face at night; later tetterlike cracks with oozing.

▮▮Facial herpes.

▮▮Itching in face.

⁹ **Lower Face.** ▮Drawing, tearing, throbbing, boring pain in jawbones.

❙On opening mouth, cracking in submaxillary joints and sensitive as if swollen.

❙Great difficulty in opening jaws. *θ*Angina faucium.

❙Lower jaw hangs down. *θ*Coma. *θ*Typhus.

❙Frothing at the mouth. *θ*Epilepsy.

❙Lips dry, black, cracked, bleeding. *θ*Diphtheria. *θ*Fevers.

❙Enormous swelling of lips.

❙Furuncular formation on lips, pain and erysipelatous areola; rapid and excessive loss of strength, patient being reduced from vigor to absolute prostration in twenty-four to thirty-six hours. *θ*Malignant pustule.

❙Mumps, particularly on l. side; enormously swollen, sensitive to least touch; least possible pressure causing severe pain; shrinks away when approached; can scarcely swallow; excessively peevish; throat sore internally; face red and swollen; eyes glassy and wild.

❙Threatened abscess of submaxillary gland. *θ*Typhoid.

❙❙Submaxillary and cervical glands swollen. *θ*Diphtheria.

❙❙Red suppurating blotches under jaw.

¹⁰ **Teeth and Gums.** ❙Teeth feel too long when biting them.

❙❙Raging, jerking, tearing, dull sticking in roots of lower teeth, through upper jaw to ear, periodic, after waking from sleep; soon after eating; from warm and cold drinks.

❙Boring, jerking, twitching, drawing, tearing, cutting, piercing, beating, pulsating pains in teeth.

❙❙Toothache: from eating; biting; something warm; drinking warm things or cold; during menstruation; when awaking; from getting wet; in the Spring; in Summer; > from external warmth; from cleaning teeth; with chilliness, heat, thirst; in persons who have taken too much mercury; with headache; with swelling of cheek; teeth too long, blunt.

❙Hollow teeth feel too long.

❙Pain in all decayed teeth during rush of blood to head.

❙Crumbling of teeth.

❙❙Gums swollen and spongy; easily bleeding.

❙Protruding gums, dark purple. *θ*Dentition.

❙Gums bluish, swollen, bleeding; aching < from warm drinks. *θ*Yellow fever.

❙❙Hemorrhage from gums.

¹¹ **Taste and Tongue.** ❙Sour taste; everything turns sour.

❙Slow, difficult speech, tongue heavy, cannot open mouth wide; cannot pronounce some words.

❙❙Worse from speaking.

❙Stammering; letters *s*, *b*, *t* and *w*.

❙Stammering in a child, æt. 4; in talking draws face awry; closes r. or both eyes, opens mouth wide or closes it.

ıStammering comes with second or third word or not in a
whole period; it seems *p*, *v* and *a* had the most influence.
∎∎Puts tongue out with difficulty; tongue trembles.
∎Difficulty of moving tongue, with impossibility of opening mouth wide.
∎Tongue: lolling about in mouth; swollen, coated white;
papillæ enlarged; dry, red, cracked at tip; red tip and
brown centre; mapped; sensation as if it was going to
peel; dry, black and stiff; tip cracked and bleeding; a
deep red color; a dry stripe in middle; anterior half red,
smooth and shining; black and bloody; sore on l. side,
with sticking here and there; tickling at root, exciting
cough; blistered about tip.
∎Blisters on inflamed tongue, change into ulcers, threatening suffocation; gangrene of tongue, on both edges.
∎Canker sores on tip of tongue; aphthæ.
∎Glossitis with titillation inducing cough.
∎Cancer of tongue.
¹² **Inner Mouth.** ∎∎Bad odor, stench, from mouth. *θ*Stomatitis.
∎Sensation on roof of mouth as if mucous membrane was
peeling off.
∎A bagging just in front of uvula, very soft, as if contain-
ing pus. *θ*After diphtheria.
∎Burning pain in mouth with swelling of lips and gums.
∎Dryness in mouth with thirst.
∎Dryness of mouth and throat, accompanied by continued
sensation in velum palati as if desquamation was about
to take place. *θ*Hysteria.
∎Much slime in mouth, with flakes of blood of disgusting
taste and smell.
∎∎Saliva abundant and tenacious. *θ*Scarlatina.
∎Constant salivation, which often interferes with speak-
ing; cough; expectoration; if the latter occurs after
dinner she frequently vomits her food.
∎Salivation with hawking and coughing. *θ*Syphilitic ulcers in throat.
∎Much slimy saliva, especially in back part of mouth.
∎Aphthous and denuded spots in skin and flesh of mouth,
preceded by burning pain and rawness.
∎Mouth very sore, parched and dry, and tongue somewhat
swollen and covered with blisters on each side.
∎Cannot swallow food after masticating it, because it rests
on back part of tongue and produces a thrilling pain
there. *θ*Cancrum oris.
∎Nursing sore mouth; swelling of tongue and lips, particularly lower lip; redness and burning sensation of
tongue and lips; redness and swelling of gums; at times,
dry, shining appearance of inflamed surface, at others

the parts were moist with increased secretion of saliva on lower lip, small white spots soon coalescing, and forming a continuous white patch; ulcers on sides of tongue; finally nausea and vomiting, followed by loose stools; loss of appetite; inability to take food from extreme sensitiveness of mouth and tongue, and distress at stomach after food had been taken; emaciation; debility; at times profuse perspiration; pale, sunken face.

‖Sore mouth in last stage of phthisis.

‖Syphilitic ulceration of mouth and throat.

[13] **Throat.** ‖Throat and neck sensitive to slightest touch or external pressure; everything about throat distresses, even the weight of the bedcovers.

‖If in evening on lying down anything touches throat or larynx, it seems as though he would suffocate and pain is much <.

‖Can endure nothing tight on throat; nausea is at times caused thereby.

∣Pain in throat on taking hold of it, extending even to nape of neck, with sticking always on swallowing, and scraping on swallowing bread, as if everything was raw; dryness of throat, without actual dryness of tongue.

‖Uvula elongated; fauces purplish, swollen, ulcerated.

∣Uvula elongated, constant inclination to hawk and scrape; hacking cough; purplish hue of fauces; tonsils but slightly enlarged; emaciation; face pale and haggard; sleep interrupted; appetite and strength impaired; feeling as if parts were swollen; some soreness on swallowing and a frequent sensation as if a small crumb was lodged in throat. θChronic irritability of fauces.

∣Soft palate, roof of mouth and tonsils much swollen and bright red. θAngina faucium.

∣Constant feeling as of something in throat to swallow.

‖Feeling of lump in throat; suffocative sensation; on swallowing, lump descends, but returns at once.

∣Sensation as of a lump in throat; awakes from sleep distressed and unhappy, as if from loss of breath. θHysteria.

∣Feeling of a ball in throat, or as if a button was stuck fast in pit of throat; not perceptible on swallowing food, but on attempting deglutition, and during this it seems to rise and sink, as if it was turned around; it always feels as if she could bring it up, but it will not come; must have whole neck bare.

∣ ∣Pain as if something lodged in r. side, stinging; lump moves towards stomach.

∣Spasmodic contraction of œsophagus.

∣Constant tickling in throat.

∣Something sticks in throat, causes a hemming, but will not loosen.

∎A great deal of phlegm in fauces, on opening mouth it forms big bubbles.

∎Much hawking up of mucus, which is excessively painful.

∎Fulness and soreness in throat. θTonsillitis.

∎Sensation of a painful contraction, as if tied, on attempting to eat. θAngina faucium.

∎∎Feeling as if a crumb of bread remained sticking in throat, obliging her to swallow, somewhat > by hawking.

∎Sensation in throat as if a morsel had remained sticking on swallowing.

∎Feeling of a ridge in both sides of throat; constant desire to swallow saliva; sides of throat externally tender.

∎Feeling like a snake in throat, soreness in l. side of throat, with choking like a ball; dryness < after eating; tickling and regurgitation of food; eructations of wind; stitch in r. side when walking; throat < by draught of air.

∎Spasmodic stricture on swallowing solids, causes a struggling—"goes the wrong way," gagging follows.

∎Throat feels ulcerated on swallowing.

∎∎Constant pain swallowing empty, not swallowing food.

∎∎Difficulty of swallowing saliva, not food.

∎∎Liquids cause more difficulty in swallowing than solids, they escape through nose.

∎∎Cannot swallow sweet or acrid things. θSyphilis.

∎Sensation of dryness in throat, with inclination to swallow.

∎Constant desire to swallow. θTonsillitis.

∎Much inclination to swallow, although it is very painful, with spasmodic contraction of throat; < on l. side and after sleep; cannot bear any pressure about neck.

∎Pain in throat, extending to ears; desire to swallow; < on deglutition; pharynx swollen, dark red.

∎Dryness in throat: without thirst, at night on waking; sticking as with a thousand needles that threatens to suffocate her; impedes swallowing.

∎Pain in small spot in throat at one side of larynx, somewhat posteriorly.

∎∎Throat and larynx painful on bending head backward.

∎On lying down, pain in top of throat.

∎Pain in l. side of throat, extending to tongue, jaw and into ear.

∎∎Pains in throat, in connection with those in ears.

∎Sensitiveness of throat as if sore, as after taking cold, with pain in l. side, < in evening.

∎Hawking of mucus, with rawness in throat, after a nap in daytime.

∎∎Much phlegm in fauces, with painful hawking.

∎Everything seems raw in throat.

▮Burning sensation of swelling; dryness in throat.

▮Constriction, dryness, stinging and great rawness of throat, especially of pharynx and larynx, with chills and rigors. θPharyngitis.

▮Mouth and throat get so dry that the act of trying to moisten them, after sleeping, will make patient scowl and cause tears to start. θTyphoid.

▮Sudden feeling as if a fishbone had stuck in throat, and some days after felt with increasing discomfort as if a sponge was hanging in throat; seemed to impede breathing, felt as if he could hawk it up, but attempt gave pain and did no good; felt as if there was a small, dry spot from which pain extended to ear; continual inclination to swallow, no pain on swallowing food but during empty deglutition and on applying external pressure; when he presses throat feels as if eyes would spring out of head, and externally as if he had got a blow on neck; between sternum and glottis a throbbing, choking sensation; throat > in morning, begins two or three hours after rising and continues till evening.

▮Feeling of obstruction in throat on swallowing, every other day, first on r. side; heat and smarting in l. throat, with hoarse voice, every day about 11 P.M.; < on waking in morning, goes off about 11 A.M.

▮Sore throat, with hoarseness, sensation like a lump in throat, inflammation very deep red; slight cough.

▮▮Right tonsil first affected, then left.

▮Pain, especially in r. side of throat, < by pressure, as if a thick substance was there, it feels very dry, no difficulty in swallowing solid food, but cannot easily swallow liquids, which get forced into nose on swallowing; pains < when she washes in morning and after sleeping in daytime; pain > in afternoon, at this time throat trouble becomes so prominent, without being painful, as to prevent speech.

▮Rawness and difficulty in swallowing, with sensation of spasmodic stricture about throat. θEpidemic pharyngitis and laryngitis.

▮Swallowing increases pain in ears or it sends pain into ears. θTonsillitis.

▮▮On attempting to swallow fluids pass through nose. θAngina faucium. θTonsillitis. θSyphilis.

▮Chills and nausea, followed by hot flushes and terrible choking, as though some one was pressing his windpipe between thumb and fingers. θPharyngitis.

▮Pain in head, < by light, noise and heat; eyes red and painful; great pain in back and limbs, did not permit her to lie, stand or sit quiet, must change position fre-

quently; fever, with dry mouth; sore throat on r. side,
with redness and swelling of r. tonsil, finally passing to
l. side; pain in limbs.

❚❚Soreness of throat, commencing on r. side and passing to
l., where it becomes fixed.

Boy, æt. 8; very sore throat, horrid pains all over head,
back and front, so giddy could not stand, had to be carried from school, could not see letters in his book, fell
against wall.

❚Pain in throat extends to ears, which feel stuffed.

❚Inflamed swelling l. side of throat, extending over ear,
threatening sphacelus.

❚Phlegmonous inflammation of throat.

❚Angina crouposa or nervosa with children or climacteric
women.

❚❚Chronic angina with periodic exacerbations.

❚Children spit much saliva with sore throat.

❚Empty swallowing is agonizing. θAngina.

❚Sore throat and mouth following scarlet fever; almost
total inability to swallow; fluids swallowed easier than
solids.

❚Feeling of large lump at back of throat; sometimes feels
as if some one grasped him by throat, causing feeling of
suffocation; nausea, retches as if to vomit up lump;
slight soreness of back of throat on swallowing saliva;
r. side of neck tender to touch; swallows saliva frequently, which makes lump seem to increase and rise
higher; feeling of pressure in middle of throat; must
clear throat before he can talk; all symptoms < on
waking in morning. θAngina.

Inability to swallow, liquids being returned through
nose; fauces bright red, tonsils much swollen; face pale;
small, hard and very frequent pulse; complete aphonia,
incessant effort to cry being heard only as a gasping
sound; great exhaustion, head hanging loosely backward, could hardly move a limb; mucous membrane of
throat extremely pale and covered with white shreds of
exudation; dysphagia, apparently paralytic.

❚After catching cold, inflammation and swelling of tonsils; velum palati and root of tongue inflamed; salivation and fetor oris; swallowing almost impossible, everything escaping through nose; can hardly speak;
sensation as if throat was filled with a lump threatening
suffocation; recumbent posture impossible; no sleep.

❚Angina, sudden in onset, appearing every year, causing
great pain and ending with suppuration of tonsils;
velum palati, uvula and posterior wall of pharynx red,
swollen and inflamed, protruding from both sides; constant desire to swallow, which is difficult.

∎Sensation of fulness and rawness in throat; frequent desire to swallow, which causes pain, extending deep into ear; fluids ejected through nose, with great fear of suffocation; gums, tonsils and uvula dark red and swollen, latter looking as if squeezed and crowded back ; large collection of mucus in mouth, which forms large bubbles when mouth is opened. θTonsillitis.

∎Fauces inflamed ; r. tonsil swollen ; l. tonsil first attacked. θTonsillitis.

∎Tonsils swollen, l. < with a tendency to r.; inability to swallow, threatening suffocation; or, on swallowing, pain shoots into l. ear; cannot bear anything to touch neck.

∎Swollen, congested tonsils, with yellow, small patches on each; great difficulty to swallow, with pain on l. side, shifting to r. and upwards to ear; heat and chills, alternating; commencing to get < at 4 P.M. θTonsillitis.

∎Left side; choking when drinking, fluids are driven out through nose; < in P.M., after sleep, from slightest touch; cannot bear bedclothes near neck. θQuinsy.*

∎∎Chronic enlargement of tonsils.

∎Sloughing ulcer in fauces, from an abscess in l. tonsil.

∎Numerous white spots on pale red surface in l. throat; ulcers on mucous membranes; both parotids much swollen, without much pain; pulse frequent and hard.

∎Right tonsil swollen; uvula elongated and clinging to r. tonsil ; between the two a yellowish white, part liquid exudation, with no especial tendency to formation of membrane ; fauces red; headache; fever; thirst; painful deglutition : enlarged submaxillary glands; distressing thirst. θDiphtheritis.

∎Pale, distressed face, blue rings around eyes; extreme prostration; speech and deglutition difficult; fauces pale red; white shreds of exudation on fauces and roof of mouth ; also ulcers with white edges distinct from exudation patches. θDiphtheritis.

∎Roof of mouth, tonsils and buccal cavity pale red; tough, yellow white membrane on l. tonsil.

∎∎Pain and soreness begin on l. side of throat. θTonsillitis. θDiphtheria.

∎Excessive tenderness of throat to external pressure. θTonsillitis. θDiphtheria.

∎∎Aggravation by hot drinks; liquids pain more than solids while swallowing.' θTonsillitis. θDiphtheria.

∎Face sickly, pale; dark rings around eyes; swallowing exceedingly painful; speaking difficult; weakness extraordinary; fauces pale red; white exudate on tonsils and

* In quinsy there is no remedy so often effective in breaking up the attack at its inception, nor in promoting resolution in its later stages.— C. Hering.

velum, looks like ulcers of mucous membrane with white edges; mind depressed. θDiphtheria.

▪Severe pain in forehead, changing to beating pain in vertex on assuming upright position; dizziness on fixing eyes on any spot on wall; severe pain in limbs, < about knees and elbows; flesh sore, < moving limbs; lassitude; nearly faints on rising; tenderness and pain in epigastrium; nausea, anorexia, tongue coated with yellow, dirty fur; unpleasant taste; tonsils swollen; patches of diphtheritic membrane half an inch wide, dirty grey color, on tonsils and extending down out of sight; began on l. side, which is most painful, < after sleeping or talking; skin at times hot and dry, at other times moist; pulse 90. θDiphtheria.

▪Constant delirium, changes rapidly from one subject to another; talks, sings, or whistles constantly; makes odd motions with r. arm, as if reaching for something; throat filled with membrane of dark color, which developed from l. to r.; no sleep for seventy-two hours, but during last twelve hours has occasionally fallen into a light sleep, which was followed by aggravation of all symptoms; badly smelling stools; urine high colored and of strong smell; body covered with bluish red eruption, round and elevated. θDiphtheria.

▪Inflammation and membrane beginning on l. side; external swelling of throat; unbearable fetor; besotted expression; temperature 104 to 105 degrees; pulse 140; epistaxis, several times a day, of venous blood; diarrhœa of blackish feces; could drink nothing hot; constant muttering delirium; discharge of yellowish mucus from nose, l. nostril first. θDiphtheria.

▪Sore throat, hurts to swallow, with difficulty in swallowing; fluid runs out through nose; dislike to have throat touched or examined; flushed face; quick pulse; breathing oppressed; membrane commences on l. tonsil and pharynx, extending to uvula and r. side. θDiphtheria.

▪Violent pain in throat, swollen tonsils, fever, heat; considerable exudate in choanæ; in sneezing a tough, skinny substance is blown out of nose. θDiphtheria.

▪Diphtheritic deposits first show themselves on l. tonsil, from there extending to r. side and then spreading further; neck is stiff, or external throat sore and quite tender to touch; patient coughs and feels < when awaking from sleep; expectoration very difficult and scanty; great loquacity, is only kept in check by hoarseness. θDiphtheria.

▪Throat greatly swollen internally and externally; discharge from nose and mouth of intensely fetid and excoriating fluid; fauces covered with diphtheritic membrane; pulse 110, small; extremities mottled and livid; swallowing almost impossible. *θ*Diphtheria.

∎Purplish appearance of mucous membrane of lips, buccal cavity and throat; diphtheritic spot as large as a pin head on l. tonsil; tongue pointed and purplish; pulse weak, 132; skin hot; urine scanty, dirty colored and containing albumen; bowels constipated; four days later submaxillary glands on both sides much swollen; running of acrid secretion from nose and mouth; diphtheritic stench; throat and even lips covered with thick, grey membranes. *θ*Diphtheria.

∎Diphtheria; membrane covering tonsils and posterior portion of throat; considerable pain on swallowing; pain < turning head, touching neck and on awaking from sleep; sleep disturbed by dryness of mouth and a feeling as if he would suffocate.

∎Tumefaction of throat slight and redness of mucous membrane hardly noticeable; diphtheritic deposits of two or three little patches hardly larger than a pin's head; prostration of strength quite alarming; pulse slow, feeble and compressed; a cold, clammy sweat frequently covered forehead and extremities: breath fetid; appetite gone; patient passed with alarming rapidity into a completely asthenic condition—sometimes prostration quite considerable before local evidence of disease could be detected. *θ*Epidemic diphtheria.

∎∎Diphtheritic patches in throat, spreading from l. to r.; fetid breath; < after sleep; great debility, feeble pulse; clammy sweat; headache and faintness.

∎Purple livid color of affected parts, with dull, dry appearance and little swelling, also pain out of all proportion to amount of inflammation. *θ*Diphtheria.

∎Throat rapidly sloughed and presented a bluish hue.

∎Girl, æt. 8, throat greatly swollen internally and externally; discharge from nose and mouth of an intensely fetid and excoriating fluid; fauces covered with diphtheritic membrane: pulse 110, very quick and small; extremities mottled and livid; swallowing nearly impossible; fetor almost overpowering. *θ*Diphtheria.

∎On l. side of throat several white exudate spots; mucous membrane pale red; parotids swollen; pulse frequent, hard; great apathy; somnolency, drooping eyelids.

∎Very difficult swallowing; complete aphonia; wheezing, hissing sound, in place of natural crying; excessive weakness; lets head hang; scarcely lifts limbs; fauces pale, covered with white exudate. *θ*Diphtheria.

∎Velum, tonsils and posterior wall of fauces pale red; on l. tonsil tough, yellowish white exudate. *θ*Diphtheria.

▮▮Peculiar hard ache all over, in head, back and legs; could not lie still, but constantly changed position. θDiphtheria.

▮Membranous deposit in choanæ; discharge of a skinny substance from nose when sneezing. θDiphtheria.

▮A greyish ulcerative crust appeared first on tonsils, spread over arch of amygdeli into posterior nares, sometimes downward into larynx, causing strangulation. θDiphtheria.

▮Tonsils swollen so that they almost meet, and covered with a tough, cheesy looking substance; feverish and very low. θDiphtheria.

▮Left tonsil one complete black slough, disease passing to r. side. θDiphtheria.

▮Pulse 130; skin hot and dry; face very red; drowsy; muttering delirium; greyish membrane developed from l. to r. θDiphtheria.

▮Subjective symptoms much more prominent than objective; complaints, especially swallowing, much more violent than one would suppose from extent of disease; sensation as of foreign body in throat, with stinging extending into ear; urging to swallow and desire to hawk up something, with attacks of choking; voice weak and hoarse; cough, causing pain in throat, was restrained, therefore it sounded short and suppressed. θDiphtheria.

▮Constitutional symptoms out of all proportion to local manifestations, prostration considerable even before any local evidences of disease could be detected. θDiphtheria.

▮Diphtheritic inflammation of throat; ulcers on tongue; suppuration of glands of neck; pleuritic, pericarditic and general dropsy in delayed desquamation, with great oppression; urine almost black; stools badly smelling; fever < in afternoon. θScarlatina.

▮Sensibility of affected parts increased and their motility essentially diminished. θDiphtheria.

▮After diphtheria speech disturbed, some words she could not articulate, because after a few minutes conversation a curtain seemed to fall down in front of her pharynx; teeth feel as if wedged; tongue feels scalded, cannot yawn because of sharp pain about root of tongue; if eating fast food stays in her throat; pain over eyes and sore feeling in eyeballs.

▮Ulcers in throat: < in wet weather; after mercury; from syphilis; extend into posterior nares; throat dry, awakens choking; soft palate full of cicatrices, with greenish yellow ulcers between; pains shooting; fetid breath.

▮Mercurial syphilis, with ulcerated sore throat, causing

a constant provocation to cough, with retching; painful deglutition; regurgitation of drink through nose; earthy, yellowish appearance of face, with small red bloodvessels shining through skin; coryza, nose sore; terrible headache; nightly pains in limbs. *θ*Syphilis.

·∎Syphilitic phagedæna of soft palate and fauces.

∎∎Gangrenous sore throat.

∎Secondary ulceration of throat, extending into posterior nares; obstruction of nose; offensive smell from mouth; stinging and shooting pains in ulcers; excessive dryness of throat, in spots; throat feels entirely "parched up" on waking; touching throat produces sensation of suffocation; sensitive to slightest movement of neck; symptoms somewhat > after eating. *θ*Syphilis.

¹⁴ **Appetite, Thirst. Desires, Aversions.** ∎Hunger, cannot wait for food.

∎At one time good appetite, at another none at all.

∎Constant thirst, with dry tongue and skin.

∎∎Great longing for drinks, but afraid to drink, as it brings on a discharge. *θ*Diarrhœa.

∎Thirst insatiable, with disgust for drink.

∎At 10 o'clock every night, with urgent and unquenchable thirst, dryness in throat and mouth, can scarcely breathe for thirst, must continually moisten mouth; drinking does no good and she dreads it; fever begins with rigor on going to bed, and the heat continues till about 4 A.M., with intervals of shivering; sweat toward morning; tearing pain in temples during hot stage, with burning heat in epigastrium; very sleepy day and night, but cannot sleep, except a little towards morning.

∎Desire: for oysters; for wine and spirituous liquors; for coffee, which agrees (dysmenorrhœa).

¹⁵ **Eating and Drinking.** Generally improved when eating.

∎After eating: gnawing in stomach >, but returns in a few hours. *θ*Cancer of stomach.

∎After eating: vertigo, languor, drowsiness; gagging and suffocating; dyspnœa; pressing, like a load in stomach; stomach puffed; eructations; diarrhœa; flashes of heat.

∎Craving hunger; > after eating; < after acid drinks; constipation; abdomen sensitive to weight of clothes; flushes of heat; flushes after eating, after mental or physical effort.

∎Better from eating fruit.

∎Fluids go down, but solids, even well chewed, cause a sensation of choking.

∎Complaints from wine or tobacco.

∎Worse from alcoholic drinks (except the snake bite).

¹⁶ **Hiccough, Belching, Nausea and Vomiting.** ∎Eructa-

tions: affording relief; amounting to vomiting; before
epilepsy; at every menstrual effort.
∎Everything sours; heartburn.
∣∣Always thirsty, but nausea after drinking.   θItch.
∎Nausea after drinking.
∣Nausea: want of appetite in forenoon; in attacks, weakness, even to syncope; dyspnœa, palpitation, cold sweat;
nosebleed (typhus); with great flow of saliva (cholera).
πSick stomach, with terrible retching, but no vomiting;
great fulness in head, with a confused, half conscious
feeling; flashing before eyes; numb feeling about head;
thinks she is going to die.
∎Vomiting: of bile or mucus; of food; in organic affections,
with hardening of abdominal viscera; of greenish matter; renewed by slightest motion (cholera); of blood
and pus.
¹⁷ **Scrobiculum and Stomach.**   ∎∎Pit of stomach sore to
touch.
∎Pressure in pit of stomach causes dull, stinging pain.
∎Tickling in pit of stomach causes tormenting cough.
∎Bloatedness of stomach, with belching of masses of wind.
∎Stomach bloated; no appetite; costiveness.
∣∣Violent pressure in stomach after eating, with feeling
of weakness in knees.
∎Stitching extending from stomach to chest.
∎Feeling as though something was gnawing in stomach,
though without pain; followed by gnawing in both
sides, extending across under ribs deep in abdomen.
∎Gnawing pressure > after eating, but returning as soon
as stomach is empty.   θCancer of stomach.
∎Cardialgia; body stiffened from pain, came on slowly and
passed off slowly; brought on by overwork.
∎At every menstrual effort cardialgia.
∎Appetite at one time good, at another poor, sometimes
such a gnawing that he can hardly wait for his meal;
after eating, vertigo, heaviness, lassitude, shortness of
breath and heaviness in stomach; smothered feeling in
chest, stomach full of wind, must belch much, with
relief; regurgitation of food; when he cannot belch becomes deathly sick; severe and annoying pressure in a
small spot between epigastrium and navel, which takes
away his breath, > by belching; during day several
attacks of nausea with shortness of breath, weakness
almost to loss of consciousness, palpitation of heart and
cold sweat; at night when in bed if least thing touches
mouth or nose respiration seems interfered with and
suffocation threatening; sleep disturbed by dreams, frequent waking; in morning heaviness and dejection;

constipation; pale and emaciated; face grey, pale yellow; after sitting, pain in thighs and stiffness of knees. *θ*Dyspepsia.

❚❚Dyspepsia, < as soon as he eats; costive; after mercury.
❚Cancer of stomach: gnawing pressure > after eating, returns in a few hours; sensiveness to contact, especially of clothes, with drunkards.

¹⁸ **Hypochondria.** ❚Acute pain in liver, extending towards stomach.

❚Inflammation and chronic obstruction of liver, sensitive to pressure or touch.

❚Catarrhal affection of liver.

❚Abscesses in liver; pain when coughing, as if ulcerated; excessively offensive stools, whether formed or not.

❚❚Liver complaints: at climaxis; after ague; pain as if something had lodged in r. side, with stinging.

❚Gallstones. (After *Calcar.*)

❚Nutmeg liver; cannot bear tight clothing, loosens jacket, arms molest; contractive tightness in region of liver.

❚❚Cannot bear any pressure about hypochondria.

❚Contractive feeling in region of liver.

❚❚Ulcerative pain about liver.

❚Pain as if from suppuration under ribs.

❚Fulness and heaviness in region of liver, and at same time pain in l. hypochondrium; coppery taste in mouth; hard morning cough.

❚Liver swollen and painful in anterior and superior aspect.

❚Sensation of coldness over whole body; fainting spells; pale, dirty yellow color of face; appearance of suffering; thick, yellow coating on tongue; dryness of mouth; great thirst; bitter taste; nausea; diarrhœa; great debility; nervous and despondent; great aversion to talking; climaxis. *θ*Bilious attacks.

❚Shooting pain in region of spleen, particularly on exercise by walking; skin brown near region of stomach; brown spots on hand; constipation.

¹⁹ **Abdomen.** ❚❚Painful distension, flatulence; can bear no pressure, the surface nerves are sensitive.

❚Abdomen distended and hard.

❚❚Is obliged to wear clothes, especially about stomach, very loose, they cause uneasiness; even in bed obliged to loosen and pull up nightdress to avoid pressure; dare not lay arm across abdomen on account of pressure.

❚Great sensitiveness to contact, especially to that of clothes. *θ*Cancer of stomach. *θ*Typhlitis. *θ*Metritis.

❚Sensitive over lower abdomen, can scarcely allow her clothes to touch her. *θ*Melancholy after confinement.

❚Distension of abdomen, with gurgling and rumbling in bowels before diarrhœa. *θ*Typhoid fever.

❚❙Abdomen distended, much annoyance from flatulence.

❙Bloated abdomen. *θ*Mania. *θ*Megrim. *θ*Epilepsy. *θ*Fevers.

❙Sensation of incarcerated flatus.

❙❙Feeling of emptiness in abdomen.

❙Pain as if something was lodging in r. side; stinging sensation; sensation as if a ball was rolling from that side towards stomach.

❙Squeamishness in abdomen, alternating with facial neuralgia.

❙At a small spot between navel and epigastrium a sense of unpleasant pressure, taking away breath, > by eructations, an hour after a meal.

❙Three months after weaning a six months old child menses had not returned; severe aching in small of back; every two or three days acute colicky pains low in abdomen, resembling labor pains, coming at various times of day; hard aching pain in uterus; sinking, fluttering feeling in epigastrium; stools loose; great sleepiness, constant desire to lie down, sleep in daytime < abdominal pains; milk very thin before weaning.

❙Tearing pain in abdomen. *θ*Dysmenorrhœa.

❙Cutting pain in r. side of abdomen throwing her into fainting fits; painful distension of abdomen; urging to urinate, but inability to do so except at long intervals.

❙Cramplike pains in abdomen, which feels hot. *θ*Dysentery.

❙Spasmodic colic, > by bending forward.

❙At times pains as if knife was thrust through abdomen.

❙Colic: stomach distended; incarceration of wind, belching relieves; pains change locality; sensitive to light pressure; with restlessness and fever.

❙Excessive griping, as though about to have diarrhœa.

❙Burning like fire in hypogastric and lumbar regions.

❙Coldness; thirst; abdomen very hot. *θ*Dysentery.

❙Abdomen hot and sensitive to touch; painful stiffness from loins down into thighs; scanty, turbid urine with reddish sediment; strangury; constipation; must lie on back with drawn up knees; especially in complications with typhilitis. *θ*Peritonitis.

❙Acute cutting, stinging pains, radiating from navel over upper portion of abdomen, excruciating from slightest touch as well as by motion, with tympanitic distension. *θ*Peritonitis.

❙Lies on back with knees drawn up; tenderness, pain and swelling in region of cæcum; pain extending from r. lumbar region through sacrum, through inguinal region and forepart of thigh, more especially when swelling is examined; urine scanty, high colored; strangury; bowels costive. *θ*Inflammation of cæcum.

❚Strangulated umbilical hernia; sloughing.

❚❚Tenderness in l. iliac region, intolerance of pressure.

❚Ileo-cæcal region very sensitive to touch; after great straining discharges a mass of croupous exudation. θChronic intestinal catarrh.

❚Threatened gangrene in strangulated hernia; skin covering hernial tumor mottled and dark; pain across abdomen; contractive sensation in abdomen; cutting, lacerating, burning pains; hernia exceedingly sensitive, will not admit handling.

❚For years violent pains over r. groin, drawing from ovary to uterus; pus passing with stool.

❚Violent pain of long standing in r. groin, extending either towards genital organs or upwards towards liver or chest.

❚Extreme nervous debility; great fear of death; hopeless of recovery; despair of salvation; desire to pick her fingers raw, or arms, or face, or pick threads from shawl, clothing, etc.; menses delayed, with general aggravation of symptoms; always < every four weeks for four or five days; fibrous tumor, size of orange, in l. groin.

❚Contraction of psoas muscle, drawing knee towards abdomen; hectic fever. θBubo.

❚Large hard swelling, with fistulous openings in inguinal region, extending towards abdomen; hectic fever. θBubo.

❚❚Long lasting, suppurating buboes of mercurio-syphilitic origin.

²⁰ **Stool and Rectum.** ❚Tormenting urging, but not to stool.

❚Wants to pass stool, but pain is so increased thereby, he must desist.

❚❚Fetid flatus.

❚❚Very offensive stools, whether formed or not.

❚Sensation as if feces ascended to chest. θPuerperal fever.

❚Stools: fetid; cadaverous smelling; frequent; corrosive; purulent; thin; pasty; bloody, watery; watery, light yellow, fecal; dark, chocolate colored; of decomposed blood, looking like charred straw; mixed blood and slime; < at night, after acids; during warm weather; thin, offensive; thin, slippery lumps; involuntary.

❚Sudden diarrhœa, with great urging, about midnight, thin, pasty, excessively offensive, ammoniacal.

❚Diarrhœa every evening for a week, preceded by transient pain in rectum, followed by throbbing as with little hammers, in anus.

❚Watery stools, with burning in anus, in evening.

❚Painless, brownish yellow diarrhœa, smelling like carrion; fluid mixed with small fragments of feces, like millet seeds; diarrhœa brought on by least quantity of food; had eighteen to twenty stools during night; tongue

red and dry; longs for drinks, but is afraid of aggravation it causes of the diarrhœa; sleep restless and full of
dreams; hands shriveled and cold; slight twitching
of hands; despondent; speech affected (sermo abdominalis); great emaciation and prostration, cannot sit up
in bed without assistance.

▮Great inclination for acids; discharges black and frothy;
sometimes vomiting of bile in morning.

▮Chronic diarrhœa, with gnawing and pressure in pit of
stomach. θSyphilis.

▮▮Diarrhœa: of mixed blood and slime in warm weather,
< by acid fruits; < at night and after sleep; with
frothy urine; a few days before or after catamenia, with
colic; during climaxis; of drunkards, with languor and
exhaustion, very excessive in hot weather and with large
hemorrhoidal tumors, which protrude after each pappy,
offensive stool, with constriction of sphincter and continued desire to evacuate.

▮Stool and urine involuntary. θFevers.

▮▮Hemorrhage from bowels; decomposed blood. θTyphus.

▮Flakes of decomposed blood, having form and appearance of perfectly charred wheat straw, in longer or
shorter flat pieces, portions more or less ground up.

▮Discharges have a penetrating, fetid smell and assume
a purulent character; great heat of abdomen. θSummer complaint.

▮Discharges chocolate colored, of a cadaverous smell; during evacuation burning in anus; cramplike pain in
abdomen; coldness; thirst; abdomen very hot; tongue
red and cracked at its point, or black and bloody.
θDysentery.

▮Could not protrude tongue, which caught on teeth; during a nap, restlessness, dyspnœa, distress and then stinking stool. θDysentery.

▮Dysentery; shivering without coldness.

▮Vomiting renewed by slightest motion, and nausea attended by great flow of saliva. θCholera.

▮Painful straining, with discharge of croupous exudate.

▮Pressive pains in umbilical region; violent gripes, with
contracted abdomen, or abdomen hard and tympanitic;
fetid stools. θEnteritis.

▮Chronic intestinal catarrh.

▮Soft stools of bright yellow color.

▮Alternate diarrhœa and constipation.

▮Costive, ineffectual urging; anus feels closed; stools
offensive.

▮Long lasting constipation with pressure in stomach and
unsatisfactory belching.

▮Stools: scanty, greyish, like potter's clay; hard like sheep dung; hard and difficult; frequent and hard; hard, scanty and insufficient.

▮Constipation with black tongue and lips. *θ*Scarlatina.

▮Constipation without other symptoms.

▮Feeling of unhappiness on awaking; sensation of constriction of anus. *θ*Constipation.

▮Absence of stool in persons suffering from hydrothorax.

▮Weight, fulness and pressure in bowels, with much flatulence. *θ*Chronic constipation.

▮Constipation, with ineffectual effort to evacuate.

▮Costiveness, with very hard stools, between catamenia; stool omitted twenty days. *θ*Angina syphilitica.

▮Stools in pieces, frequent, yellow, orange, sometimes tinged with blood. *θ*Gastric nervous fever.

▮Long lasting costiveness, with pressure in stomach and unsuccessful eructations.

▮Chronic constipation in a young lady, of ten years' standing, was obliged daily to use warm injections; weight, fulness and pressure in bowels, accompanied with a good deal of flatulency.

▮Fecal obstructions; intususception threatening sloughing.

▮No stool nor urine. *θ*Metritis. *θ*Puerperal fever.

▮Before stool: rumbling; ineffectual urging; constant and very painful pressure in rectum, without stool; constriction in rectum or sensation of plug in anus.

▮During stool: cramplike pain in abdomen; burning in anus; tenesmus; pain as if sphincter was torn with effort; tearing pains in rectum from below upward and backward, to point of producing eructations; feces remain at anus; aggravation of pains, so that it is necessary to cease all efforts.

▮After stool: burning at anus; tenesmus; protrusion of large hemorrhoïdal tumors, with constriction of anus and continued desire for stool.

▮Child always awakens in distress. *θ*Diarrhœa.

▮Stool lies in rectum, without urging.

▮Full feeling in rectum, and a sensation of little hammers beating. *θ*Fistula in ano. *θ*Climaxis.

▮Rectum prolapsed and tumefied.

▮Burning, cutting pains in rectum, < while standing morning till afternoon.

▮Constant and painful pressure in rectum, without stools.

▮Beating sensation in rectum; throbbing. *θ*Stricture of rectum.

▮Stitch in rectum or hemorrhoids when coughing or sneezing.

▮Uneven or tuberculated and indurated mass, surrounding and protruding from anus, through centre of this mass was an irregular, ragged and ulcerated fissure (the outlet from rectum), from which issued a sanious mucous discharge; stool almost impossible on account of obstruction and pain; soft and yielding tumors (hemorrhoidal) nearly filling rectum, as far as touch extended; constant throbbing with itching, shooting and burning in affected region; all symptoms < after sleep; had been diagnosticated as scirrhus of anus and rectum. θAffection of anus and rectum.

▮Piles for four years, came on first month of pregnancy; discharge of mucus, excoriating passage; sore, burning pain after every evacuation; very irritable nervous system; craving for pickles; acrid waterbrash.

▮▮Piles protruding or strangulated, or, with stitches upward at each cough or sneeze. θClimaxis. θDrunkards.

▮Hot, bleeding hemorrhoidal tumors.

▮Hemorrhoids: with scanty menses; in climacteric years.

▮Drawing pains from anus to umbilicus.

▮Spasmodic pains in anus internally, short time before and after stool.

▮Visible spasmodic tenesmus in paroxysms, from two to five minutes, extorting cries, passes blood and mucus.

▮Itching at anus, < after sleep.

▮Anus feels closed; sensation of a plug.

▮Painful constriction of anus, following prolapsus of rectum.

▮Fistulous abscess opened near anus.   θScarlatina.

³¹ Urinary Organs.   ▮Stitches in kidneys, extending downward and apparently through ureters.   θCystitis.

▮▮Pressure upon bladder; dull pain.

▮▮Feeling as of a ball rolling about in bladder or abdomen, when turning over.   θUterine displacement.   θCystitis.

▮Discharge of offensive mucus during micturition.   θCatarrh of bladder.

▮Ineffectual urging to urinate; burning when it does pass.

▮Urgent desire to urinate, with passage of much urine.

▮Frequent micturition, urine scanty, dark brown, turbid.

▮Violent burning when passing urine. θAnginasyphilitica.

▮Painful pressing and burning when making water.

▮Dribbling after urinating.

▮▮Constant sticking and cutting in forepart of urethra.

▮Urine of strong ammoniacal odor, involuntary; lying on back.   θGastric nervous fever.

▮High colored urine of strong smell. . θDiphtheria. θScarlatina.

▮Urine dark, with a brown, gravelly sediment, passing with a sharp, cutting pain.

▮▮Urine: almost black; frequent, foamy, dark.

▮Urine like coffee grounds. *θ*Scarlatina.
▮Urine dark or scanty, as in typhus. *θ*Diphtheria.
▮▮Black, scanty urine, with œdema, after scarlatina.
▮Urine red and hot. *θ*Angina faucium.
▮Scanty urine with red sediment. *θ*Typhlitis.
▮Urine heavily loaded with albumen.
▮Albuminuria with hydrothorax and dropsical enlarge-
ment of l. side and leg.
▮Strangury. *θ*Typhlitis.
▮▮No urine, no stool.
▮Urine almost suppressed. *θ*Scarlatina.

²² Male Sexual Organs. ▮Great excitement of sexual desire.
▮Epilepsy after suffering by lewdness, or morbid excite-
ment of sexual organs, onanism, frequent emissions of
semen, or jealousy.
▮Impotence.
▮Nocturnal emissions, with thrill of delight.
▮Excessive sexual desire, constant erections at night;
emissions, with profuse night sweats; cheerful disposition
and feeling of ease on awaking, succeeded by increased
mental concentration; semen has a pungent smell.
▮▮Sore pain in urethra, in forepart of penis.
▮Indurated foreskin, after chancres.
▮Mercurial syphilitic ulcers on penis.
▮Scrotum swollen to enormous size. *θ*Scarlatinal dropsy.
▮Sycotic ulcers, with bluish areolæ.
▮Paraphimosis when constriction causes gangrene, or
threatened gangrene, eruption on glans and mons
veneris.
▮▮Gangrene of glans.
▮Phagedenic chancres.
▮▮Buboes: with sore throat and headache; indurated or
with fistulous openings and hectic; after mercury; sup-
purating a long time.

²³ Female Sexual Organs. ▮Sexual desire excited to the highest pitch; perfectly insatiable; luxurious convulsive
thrills run all through her.
▮Tickling and jerking extending from thighs to genital
organs. *θ*Nymphomania.
▮▮Ovarian neuralgia, particularly l. side; tensive, pressing,
burning or stitching pains.
▮Frequent, troublesome, drawing pain in r. ovarian region,
from near hip bone down to os pubis, sometimes burning. *θ*Swelling of r. ovary.
▮Pain in r. ovarian region increasing more and more until relieved by a discharge of blood. *θ*Climaxis.
▮Terrible pain in r. ovarian region, with swelling.
▮Induration and suppuration of ovaries.

▮Right ovary size of a fist; 1½ inches thick, painful when pressed, attached to uterus by a string as thick as a finger.

▮Sharp, shooting pain in l. ovary; constipation; feels < in morning and after sleep. θOvaritis.

▮Tensive, pressing pains and stitches; inability to lie on r. side, on account of sensation as if something was rolling over to that side; swelling of ovary; suppuration; l. side. θOvaritis.

▮Painful, oblong swelling and induration in r. ovarian region, < by moral emotions, rapid movements, prolonged walks and overexertion. θUterine displacement.

▮Ovarian tumors; l. ovary first affected, tending to right.

▮▮Swelling, induration, tumors, neuralgia, suppuration, etc., of l. ovary.

▮Menses irregular, dark, dirty looking and offensive; looks like a pregnant woman at ninth month; abdomen hard, some parts more so than others; in l. ovarian region and directly under navel, extending up to stomach, very hard, as though fibrous, all other sections tense and more or less painful; at times dyspnœa and wheezing almost approaching suffocation; tongue red and glazed; appetite fickle; great thirst; scanty, high colored urine, with hæmatin and ten per cent. of albumen; constipation, with occasional discharge like horse dung in size, causing pain and weakness from which she would not recover for half a day or more; constant malaise. θSacculated ovarian disease.

▮Uterine and ovarian tumors, with profuse and prolonged menses; great sensitiveness of lower abdomen; severe, aching pain, anteriorly, in thighs, in branches of anterior crural nerve.

▮Uterine region feels swollen, will bear no contact, not even of clothing; bearing down pains.

▮Pains like a knife thrust into abdomen.

▮Uterus feels as if os was open.

πGenital parts much distended, swollen and red, everything seemed to be rolled out and mouth of womb open; nymphomania.

▮Laborlike pains as if everything would issue from vulva, followed by a slight discharge of blood.

▮Menstrual colic beginning in l. ovary.

▮▮Sensation as if pains from uterus and abdomen ascended towards chest.

▮Pain in uterine region as if swollen; displacement.

▮Violent, laborlike pressing from loins downwards during menses, which are scanty. θDisplacement.

▮▮Pains in uterine region, increase at times more and more till relieved by a flow of blood from vagina; after a few hours or days the same again, and so on.

▮▮Uterus does not bear contact and has to be relieved of all pressure; frequently lifts clothes, they cause an uneasiness in abdomen, no tenderness.

▮Womb enlarged, retroverted, hot and sensitive to touch; os open and sensitive; menses irregular; fundus found to be larger posteriorly.

▮Chronic metritis: with hypertrophy; menses too scanty and difficult; soreness about pelvic region. (Complemented by *Nitr. ac.*)

▮▮Congestion of womb with prolapsus.

▮Displacement in connection with or in consequence of change of life.

▮▮Prolapsus during climaxis, with flashes of heat, hot vertex; metrorrhagia and fainting; pain in l. hypogastric and ovarian region.

▮Chronic uterine catarrh, staining linen, rendering it stiff, accompanied by a severe pain in lumbar region. θSterility.

▮Uterine cancer, developing at climaxis, or as a consequence of change of life; pains increase rapidly, until relieved by profuse discharge of blood; violent pains, as if a knife was thrust through abdomen, which has to be relieved of all pressure.

▮▮Uterine hemorrhages of the menopause.

▮▮Menses: suppressed at regular time, but too short and feeble; scanty, with laborlike pressure from loins downwards; irregular; scanty, blood black; late, scanty and difficult; every two or three months, then profuse; reappearing during climaxis; blood lumpy, black or acrid.

▮Tenacious and acrid menstrual flow, with laborlike pains. θCancer of uterus.

▮Menorrhagia with chills at night, flashes of heat by day.

▮Amenorrhœa: the smaller the discharge the greater the pain; with vertigo, headache and bleeding from nose; with pain in stomach, chest and eructations at every menstrual time; swelling in region of l. ovary.

▮▮Persistent congestions at menopause.

▮Nosebleed and cardialgia instead of menses.

▮Strangulation of prolapsed vagina, parts deep purple.

▮Erectile tumors; hemorrhage vicarious; pain < until > by flow of blood; if bleeding returns, pain returns.

▮Fistula vagina; gangrene.

▮Before menses: desire for open air; vertigo; nosebleed; laborlike pains, < in l. ovarian region; bruised feeling in hips; > when flow begins; sudden attacks of cardialgia; oppression or spasms of chest; eructations; diarrhœa, with violent straining; colic, with sense of malaise; nervous distress; mucous sediment in urine; leucorrhœa three days before, discharge copious, smarting and slimy, stiffening linen and leaving a greenish stain; pain in back, with abdominal cramps and throbbing headache.

▮The day before catamenia irresistible desire to go in open air and run about. θDysmenorrhœa.

▮Menstrual colic on first day of catamenia.

▮Laborlike pains with catamenia.

▮▮During menses beating in head and burning in vertex; laborlike pains, as if everything was being pressed out, followed by a slight show; uterus feels as if os was open; violent pains first day in small of back and abdomen; tearing pain in abdomen; bruised feeling in hips; > as flow becomes free; violent cramps in bowels as if cut with knives; pressing pains from loins to privates; uterine pains running up; colic beginning in l. ovary; toothache < in proportion to diminution of flow; fainting in nervous women; cardialgia, oppression of chest and eructations; ovarian pain; discharge of blood or mucus from anus; epilepsy <.

▮Jealous disposition; craves coffee and feels > after drinking it; ulcers on legs with a purplish circumference. θDysmenorrhœa.

▮With menses a throbbing in rectum and violent pains; greatly troubled with wind; slime passes, sometimes blood as from an ulcer; pressure; feels as if a stricture was there.

▮Catamenia flow but one hour every day, on stopping, violent pains follow in region of l. ovary, alternating with gagging and vomituritio. θDysmenorrhœa.

▮Dysmenorrhœa of eighteen years' standing.

▮After menses: diarrhœa; common, acrid leucorrhœa; palpitation, with pain, as if heart was hanging by a thread, and every beat would tear it off.

▮Leucorrhœa: from three to eight days before menses; green or thick yellow; copious, smarting, stiffening linen, staining it greenish, milky.

▮Redness and swelling of parts, with mucous discharge.

▮Fungus hæmatoides on right mamma as large as a peony; blood poured out all over it as from a sponge.

▮For last four years stitching and cutting pains in l. breast, more or less severe, but always < before, during and after menses; at first pain limited to affected part, but finally extended to l. axilla, and thence down arm to hand; peculiar painful sensation of weakness and lameness in l. shoulder and arm, < using arm; occasionally l. mamma and arm become so painful that use of latter becomes impossible, and she is compelled to lie down;

on examination no visible swelling, but upon pressure with finger a three-lobed tumor, each lobe about as large as a pigeon's egg, can be detected lying about two inches above and somewhat to l. side of nipple; tumor movable and painful to pressure; examination causes pain which extends to shoulder and down arm, lasting 5–6 hours; shoulder and arm sensitive to pressure, the pain extending back into mamma; pale and emaciated; menses regular, lasting 3–4 days, with much pain on first day and day previous to their appearance; chronic fluor albus.

❙Breast has a bluish or purplish appearace; chills at night and flushes of heat by day.

❙Cancer having bluish or dark base, interspersed with black streaks of coagulated or decomposed blood.

❙Cancer of breast, with lancinating pains.

❙Scarlet, shining, herpetic eruption, under mammæ, < from scratching; odor offensive.

❙❙At menopause: flashes, hot vertex; metrorrhagia; fainting; uterine displacement; cancer; capillary circulation affected.

❙❙Suitable at beginning and close of menstruation.

"Pregnancy. Parturition. Lactation. ❙Persistent vomiting in pregnancy, occurring late in afternoon and evening.

❙Convulsions commenced on l. side, in face, and continued longer, and were more severe about neck and throat than elsewhere; sixty-five distinct convulsions. θPuerperal convulsions.

❙Violent convulsions in lower limbs, with coldness of feet, stretching backward of body, and screaming; puerperal.

❙From sunstroke two years previous to confinement had been ever since in bed; two hours after delivery convulsions; after twelve hours comatose, great heat in occipital and cervical regions; mouth dry; pulseless.

❙Face turgid; mouth filled with foam and blood; jaws convulsively set, tongue shockingly lacerated; pulse full and hard; respiration irregular; complete coma interrupted by frightful convulsions; sudden and forcible protrusion of tongue. θPuerperal convulsions.

❙Face livid, bluish; abdomen swollen; urinary and fecal evacuations suppressed; lochial discharge thin and fetid; unconsciousness with violent chills daily. θPuerperal peritonitis.

❙Lochial discharge thin, ichorous; tympanitis. θMetritis.

❙❙Phlegmasia alba dolens.

❙❙Pains in ovaries after confinement.

❙Sore mouth of nursing women, edges of tongue red and cracked, with smarting and aching pains.

❙Lancinating pains in mamma; pains down arm; breast bluish, with blackish streaks. *θ*Mastitis.

❙Breast has a bluish or purplish appearance; chills at night and flushes of heat by day.

❙Thin, blue milk discharging involuntarily; child does not want to nurse; after child has sucked awhile milk becomes natural in color.

❙Milk thin, blue; she awakens sad, despairing.

❙Mammæ swollen; nipples swollen, erect; painful to touch.

❙❙Extreme sensitiveness of nipples.

* Voice and Larynx. Trachea and Bronchia. ❙❙Loss of voice caused by paralysis or œdema of vocal cords.

❙❙Paralysis of vocal cords, particularly the left.

❙Unable to utter a loud word for a week; a spot tender to touch on anterior portion of neck. *θ*Menstrual irregularities.

❙Aphonia in phthisis; sputum tough and green.

❙Something hinders speech; hoarse; hawks constantly.

❙Hoarseness and cough; heart beat accelerated by quick motion or after drinking beer.

❙Hoarseness; rough, dry cough caused by scratching in larynx and trachea. *θ*Heart disease.

❙Increased hoarseness while speaking; voice will not come because something in larynx prevents it, which cannot be hawked loose, though mucus is brought up.

❙❙Hoarseness, rawness, dryness; larynx sensitive to touch.

❙Sensation as from a skin in larynx.

❙Feeling as of talons sticking into larynx, < by coughing.

❙❙Larynx sensitive to least touch, which causes suffocation; feeling of a lump in throat.

❙Larynx and whole throat painful to touch.

❙Great sensitiveness of larynx; hoarseness; a thick lump is felt in throat, as from accumulated mucus. *θ*Chronic bronchitis.

❙❙Feeling of a small lump in pit of throat, like a button; feels as if it might loosen, but does not.

❙Larynx and throat painful on bending head backward.

❙Pain in pit of throat extending to root of tongue and to hyoid bone, and to l. tragus, behind which it shoots out; painful to touch.

❙❙Feeling as if something was swollen in pit of throat and would suffocate him; it cannot be swallowed; soreness in throat.

❙Constriction, dryness, stinging and great rawness of throat, especially of pharynx and larynx, with chills and rigors. *θ*Epidemic pharyngitis.

❙Larynx swollen, sore, raw, scraping, somewhat also on pressing upon it; at same time is obliged to swallow.

∎Catarrh, with little secretion and much sensitiveness;
dry cough, coming from sense of tickling in larynx,
provoked by deep inspiration, speaking and pressure;
sense of fulness in trachea and painful aching in os
hyoides. θLaryngitis.

∎Chronic affections of larynx, where parts, without being
actually inflamed, are very sensitive; hoarseness; sensation as if a large mass of mucus had accumulated in
throat.

∎Impending croup during diphtheria; awakens suffocating, grasps throat; fears he is dying.

∎∎Croup < after sleep; seemingly sleeps into croupy spell.

∎Child seems as if it would choke while sleeping; breathes
> after waking. θCroup.

∎Awakened from sleep, apparently in a dying condition.
θMembranous croup.

∎Croup in children subject to inflammatory rheumatism.

∎Child arouses with a paroxysm of choking, almost loses
its breath, and sometimes goes into convulsions. θCroup.

∎Membranous croup, last stage; membrane coughed up
in pieces like a glove finger; very sore throat.

∎Membranous croup with diphtheritic sore throat, or
malignant scarlet fever; breath very offensive; glands
of neck swollen; soreness of neck to touch.

∎∎Suddenly something runs from neck to larynx, stopping
breathing, it awakens him at night. θSpasmus glottidis.

∎Constriction of larynx, attended with dryness of whole
throat and mouth, invariably after sleeping.

∎Nightly attacks of spasm of glottis after first sleep; suffocation and livid face; during day sensation of foreign
body in throat, with difficulty in swallowing.

∎Paroxysms recur as often as child gets into a sound sleep.
θLaryngismus stridulus.

πFrightful gasping or grasping at larynx, almost suffocated
at night in an attack; she thought she was dying from
inability to breathe; rolling from side to side in bed.

∎Sensation as if something was in trachea which might
be raised, comes partly up and then goes back again.

∎After attack of influenza dry, harassing, concussive cough;
< after sleep. θBronchial catarrh.

∎Mucous membrane of nose thickened; much sneezing;
dry, stuffed feeling through whole front part of head;
gradually passing to fauces and chest; constant dry,
short cough, night and day, sitting, lying or walking;
wheezing breathing; face red and puffed; eyes seem
almost pressed out. θBronchial catarrh.

∎Cough excited by even light pressure on larynx, or as
soon as he falls asleep, often with choking, as if suffoca-

tion was inevitable; after a long, dry and wheezing
paroxysm of cough there is suddenly a profuse expectoration of frothy, tenacious mucus, which gives great
relief. *θ*Chronic bronchitis.

▮Continued fever, < at night; pulse 150; respirations 70
per minute; red spot on one cheek, frequently changing
sides; l. lung impervious to air; constant cough, < at
night; later r. lung affected; uneasy and restless;
throws itself in all positions in efforts to breathe; face
dark; constant spasmodic cough with labored breathing; on falling asleep for a few moments throat became
so dry that a condition like croup came on, and all
suffering increased. *θ*Bronchial catarrh.

▮Can only breathe in upright position, and that with great
labor; thickening of mucous membrane seems to fill
lung completely; constant cough from titillations behind sternum, seemingly at bifurcation of trachea; no
expectoration, yet chest seems full of fluid when coughing. *θ*Bronchial catarrh.

▮Dry cough, squeaking râle and aphonia; external throat
sensitive to touch; soreness, tenderness, sensation of
weight in l. ovarian region; < after sleep; pale, scanty
menses, with loss of sexual instinct. *θ*Bronchitis.

▮Bronchial attacks in subjects of cyanosis and cardiac
disease.

** Respiration.**   ▮▮Constantly obliged to take a deep breath.

▮▮Desperate fits of suffocation, must sit up in bed; cutting
pain in abdomen.

▮Obliged to sit up and lean r. side against a pillowed
rocking chair that pain in l. chest with dyspnœa, might
be >; frequent small pulse; diminished strength of
heart's action; could not bear neck and waistbands
fastened.

▮Difficulty of breathing > when sitting bent forward; <
when talking and after eating.

▮Oppression and want of breath : < when walking and
after spiritous liquors; heart disease; at every menstrual
effort.

▮Shortness of breath and suffocative attacks caused by
touching larynx and < on moving arms.

▮▮The least thing coming near mouth or nose interferes
with breathing; lying in bed at night slightest covering
over mouth or nose produces suffocating dyspnœa.

▮In morning when sitting up quickly, breathing slow,
difficult, whistling. *θ*Asthma.

▮▮Oppression of chest during sleep.

▮Lays hand upon upper third of sternum and declares she
cannot get her breath below there.

❙Chest stuffed as it were; cannot lie down from a sense of suffocation and must open doors and windows to obtain air; a suffocating short cough, with scanty and difficult expectoration; head must always be high, and she generally rests it on her hand.

❙Great dyspnœa, < in afternoon and after sleep; l. side; badly smelling stools even if formed. θPneumonia.

❙❙Chest feels constricted.

❙❙Suddenly something runs from neck to larynx and interrupts breathing completely; it wakens at night. θSpasmus glottidis.

❙Cannot sleep, as soon as he falls asleep breathing is immediately interrupted. θAcute rheumatism.

❙Suffocating fits, waking from sleep with throwing arms about; cyanotic symptoms; swelling of liver; black urine. θHydrothorax.

❙Awakes with fear of suffocation in middle of night.

❙❙During heat as of orgasm of blood he is obliged to loosen clothes about neck; sensation as though they hindered circulation of blood, with a kind of suffocative feeling.

❙❙Asthma: < from covering mouth or nose, touching throat, moving arms, on awaking, after eating or talking; > sitting bent forward.

❙Sharp pain through lungs, great dyspnœa; < sitting erect, or lying down, > bending forward and throwing head back; feeling of intense constriction in all parts of chest, as if lungs were being pressed up into throat, causing extreme agony, so that she despaired of life; feeling as though a cord was tightly tied around neck; must loosen clothes at neck and epigastrium; at times sensation as though heart turned over and ceased beating for a moment, then commenced again with increased force; lung seems full of mucus, yet none can be raised; face almost purple during paroxysms.

❙❙Œdema pulmonum; emphysema.

❙❙Threatening paralysis of lungs, greatest difficulty in breathing, with long lasting attacks of suffocation.

❙Hay asthma.

❙Itching disappears, she is very short of breath and full of anxiety. θItch.

²⁷ **Cough.** ❙Constant dry, hacking cough. θOvaritis.

❙❙Dry, hacking cough, caused by touching throat or in morning after sleep.

❙Every contact with open air causes a violent tickling cough, accompanied by expectoration of mucus.

❙Fluttering, nervous, slight cough, apparently excited by a tickling in larynx.

❙Cough caused by pressure on larynx or by any covering

on throat; by a tickling in pit of throat and sternum; when falling asleep; from ulcers in throat.

❙Cough, with rawness of chest, difficult expectoration and pains in throat, head and larynx.

❙Constant titillation in throat inducing cough; constant hawking going on to empty retching, without nausea; seldom any expectoration, but when there is it is brought up with extreme difficulty and at risk of suffocation.

❙Crawling in ulcers, irritation to cough. θAngina syphilitica.

❙Short, gagging, very fatiguing cough from tickling in pit of throat, cannot get anything loose.

❙Frequent attacks of short cough from tickling in pit of stomach, dry during night; difficult, sometimes watery, salty mucus, which has to be swallowed again.

❙Cough: < during day; after sleeping; changes in temperature; alcoholic drinks; acids and sour drinks.

❙Short, superficial, tickling cough, very exhausting, sometimes causing vomiting; difficult expectoration of thin, tough mucus, or thick, roundish lumps; often coughs, hawks, spits, without bringing up anything; coughs only during day; cough in open air and after speaking, which seems to make everything dry; in damp weather and after eating fish; cough seems to originate in epigastrium, where it produces a tickling sensation and severe pain.

πSuperficial, nervous cough from tickling in larynx, at 9 P.M. until going to bed.

❙Cough after rising from a lying position.

❙Cough during sleep, without being conscious of it.

❙Bronchial cough, < after sleeping.

❙❙Cough after sleep; breath fetid; complete loss of appetite.

❙Dry cough, squeaking râle and aphonia; throat sensitive to touch; soreness, tenderness, sensation of weight in l. ovarian region; < after sleep; pale, scanty menses, with loss of sexual instinct. θBronchitis.

❙After influenza, dry, harassing, concussive cough; < after sleeping, lasting all Winter and following Spring.

❙After occasional attacks of hæmoptysis, dry, sore cough, < at night and in early morning, and also by reclining. θPhthisis pulmonalis.

❙❙Cough as if some fluid had gone into wrong passage.

❙With every cough feeling as of an ulcer in stomach.

❙Gagging, persistent cough, from tickling in throat, under sternum, or in stomach; < on falling asleep or during day, from change of temperature and alcoholic drinks.

❙Hard, racking cough and profuse expectoration. θHepatitis.

❙Child coughs in evening on lying down, afterwards during sleep, sometimes awakened thereby; faint and weak.

❙❙Cough most during day.

❙Cough excited by increased secretion of fluid in larynx.

❙Feels pretty well when she gets up; thinks she will be able to do a good day's work, until 11 A.M., when she becomes weak and faint; tongue sore across middle from side to side, and beats; throat seems to swell and beat; fits of coughing, expectoration of tenacious mucus; > after two o'clock; perspires at night, starts up suddenly with choking; cannot bear bonnet strings tied tight; no appetite; flatulence; to be costive; > out of doors and when moving about.

❙Coughing or sneezing causes stitching pains in affected parts. θCancer of uterus.

❙❙Sympathetic cough of cardiac affections.

❙During cough: tension in head; pains in epigastrium, abdomen and anus; burning in chest; ulcerative pain above and along ribs; stitches in chest; running of water from the mouth; vomiting; discharge of urine; pain in hemorrhoidal tumors.

❙Constant provocation to cough, with retching and gagging.

❙❙With every single cough a stitch in hemorrhoidal tumor.

❙Pain in anus when coughing or sneezing.

❙Cough with hoarseness.

❙Paroxysms of suffocating, spasmodic cough, with tickling in larynx.

❙Dyspnœa and cough, with slimy, blood streaked, very copious sputa. θGastric nervous fever.

❙❙Sharp pain through lungs with great dyspnœa; < sitting erect or lying down; > bending body forward and throwing head back; feeling of intense constriction in all parts of chest, as if lungs were pressed up into throat; constriction in throat as if cord was tied around, necessitating loosening of covering; sensation as if heart turned over and ceased beating for a while, after which pulsations increased in force. θSpasmodic asthma.

❙❙Must cough hard and long before he can raise.

❙After a long, wheezing cough, suddenly spits up profuse, frothy, tenacious mucus.

❙Spitting large quantities of ropy mucus. θDiphtheria.

❙Expectoration: scanty, difficult, watery, saltish; must be swallowed again; straining and vomiting.

* **Inner Chest and Lungs.** ❙Oppressive pain in chest, as if full of wind, > by eructation.

❙❙Full feeling of chest and a pushing pressing from within outward. θHeart disease.

❙Contraction of chest waking him after midnight, with slow, heavy, wheezing breathing, compelling him to sit up bent forward.

▮Pain in chest as from soreness; burning in chest.
▮Stitches in l. side of chest, with difficult breathing.
▮Stitching pain through r. side of chest. θHepatitis.
▮Chest feels as if stuffed; cannot lie down, from sense of
   suffocation; must open doors and windows to obtain
   air; suffocating, short cough, scanty and difficult expectoration; fever at 10 P.M., unquenchable thirst,
   dryness in throat and mouth, can scarcely breathe for
   thirst, must continually moisten mouth, drinking does
   no good, and she dreads it; fever begins with rigor on
   going to bed, heat continues till 4 A.M., with intervals
   of shivering; sweat towards morning; tearing pain in
   temples during hot stage, burning heat in epigastrium;
   sleepy, day and night, but cannot sleep, except a little
   towards morning; frequent micturition, urine scanty,
   dark brown and turbid; abdomen distended, flatulence;
   cannot bear anything upon abdomen; little appetite;
   frequent coryza; feeling of ball in throat, as if a button
   was fast stuck in pit of throat; not perceptible on
   swallowing food, but on attempting deglutition, and
   during this it seems to rise and sink, as if it was turned
   around, feels as if she could bring it up but it will not
   come; must have whole neck bare, cannot endure bedclothes, nor even tie cap strings. θChest affection.
▮Burning, stinging, like coals of fire from chest through to
   shoulders.
▮Hepatization, particularly of l. lung; great dyspnœa on
   awaking. θPneumonia.
▮Pulse very quick, wiry, excited and strong; frequent
   chills and fever; no appetite; constipation; sputa as if
   mixed with brickdust; discouraged, homesick and despairing; covers his head with bedclothes, and sighs and
   laughs by turns, and always thinks there is something
   wrong. θPneumonia.
▮▮Threatened paralysis of lungs with great dyspnœa and
   long lasting suffocative paroxysms. θPneumonia.
▮Dropsy of chest; awakens suffocating; liver swollen;
   scanty, dark urine; palpitation. θAfter scarlatina.
▮▮Sibilant râles.
▮Chronic pleuro pneumonia; hepatization; difficulty of
   breathing; dyspnœa particularly on r. side.
▮Measles, followed by whooping cough, inflammation of
   lungs, bloody expectoration, high fever and terrible
   coughing spells; intense capillary bronchitis; pulse
   135; dry crepitation over both lungs, somewhat veiled
   by co-existing coarse bronchial râles; finally suppuration
   of both lungs supervened, with following symptoms;
   great emaciation, cadaverous appearance, eyes sunken

and glassy, rattling in bronchi, expectoration of cream
colored pus, hectic flush, pulse rapid, cannot be counted
correctly, picking and boring l. nostril, until it is raw
and bleeding; lips parched and dry, tongue dry, dark
brown coating at root, tip red; trembling of tongue
when attempting to protrude it; cannot put out tongue,
it sticks to front teeth; sordes on teeth; great prostration; can bear nothing about throat; plaintive moaning; after every coughing spell such exhaustion it seems
she will die.

▮Useful when tubercles follow pneumonia.

▮Woman, æt. 26, tall and slender, tuberculous tendency of
family; cough for more than two months; frequent, dry,
short and sharp, or harsh sound; loss of appetite and
strength; emaciation; prominent clavicles; no respiratory murmur in posterior superior half of l. lung.

▮Afternoon fever, chills and flushes alternating; pulse, 112;
copious night sweat wakes him from first sleep; violent
titillating cough, sensitiveness of larynx; difficult expectoration, in hard lumps, of offensive taste, sometimes
salty; burning deep in chest, pleuritic pains, < from
coughing; morning cough, vomiting; dulness in l. infraclavicular region, sensitiveness to touch; shortness of
breathing, a sense of constriction of chest. θTuberculosis.

▮Difficult expectoration of offensive, purulent sputa, with
straining even to vomiting. θTuberculosis.

²⁹ **Heart, Pulse and Circulation.** ▮▮Heart feels as if too
large for containing cavity.

▮Feeling of constriction about heart.

▮▮Cramplike pain in præcordial region, causing palpitation, with anxiety.

▮Great pain in heart.

▮Palpitation: with numbness of arm; choking from slightest exertion; > by sitting down or lying on r. side;
with fainting and anxiety; chronic with young girls.

▮Irregularity of beats of heart.

▮She feels beating of heart, with weakness, to sinking.

▮Palpitation after exertion or sudden excitement > by
lying down; feels sick and faint; his face becomes white,
but on lying down symptoms pass off in two minutes;
for some time has been unable to lie on l. side because
it caused pain at heart or dull oppression; lying on r.
side weight of l. arm is painful; fulness at heart, as if
pressing against side or had not free play. θHeart disease.

▮Wakes from a troubled sleep of a few moments with a
violent shock in præcordia and a sensation of suffocative
constriction of chest; extreme distress for breath; face
livid and covered with warm sweat; visible palpitation of

heart; heart seems to stand still and then start with a
tremendous bound, followed by rapid tremor; pulse irregular, intermissions growing more protracted. θFunc-
tional disturbance of heart.

▮Restless, trembling; anxiety about heart; hasty speech;
suffocation on lying down; weight on chest; heart feels
constricted. θRheumatism of heart.

▮Restless and trembling; hasty talking; great oppression;
anguish about heart in rheumatism; irregularity in
beats of heart. θPericarditis.

▮Tremulous irritability of heart after scarlatina or fevers.

▮Constant dyspnœa; sense of suffocation in chest and cardiac region, uninfluenced by position, exercise, etc.;
pulse 160, feeble, small and occasionally intermittent;
heart's action ditto; a mouthful of food or drink causes
distress, burning and pain till vomited; believes she
will not recover, but without anxiety. θHeart affection.

▮Obliged to sit up and lean r. side against pillowed chair,
that pain in l. chest, with dyspnœa, might be >; frequent small pulse; could not bear neck and waistbands
fastened. θHeart disease.

▮Hypertrophy of l. ventricle, with sensation as if heart
was too large for its containing space.

▮Suffocative attacks on touching larynx or moving chest;
fainting and anxiety from slightest motion of child;
purple color of skin; coldness of extremities. θCyanosis.

▮Pericarditis, or endocarditis, after scarlatina or diphtheria.

▮Favors resorption of exudate in pericarditis.

▮Weight in chest with anxiety; spasmodic pain in heart,
palpitation, feels constricted; sensation as if heart intermitted a single beat, produces slight cough which seems
to re-establish circulation; shortness of breath after
every motion, especially of hands; great weariness; inability to lie down on account of a suffocating sense of
fulness in chest, necessity of removing all pressure from
neck and chest and gasping for breath, when > of this
lies on l. side with head high; most adapted to cases
where fibrin is deposited on surfaces of heart, valves or
investing membrane. θRheumatism of heart.

▮Dilatation of r. ventricle.

▮▮Woman, æt. 50, fleshy; dilatation of l. ventricle, aorta
and carotid; when quiet she could lie down and sleep for
an hour or two; when excited must sit by open window;
bronchiæ are readily affected by cold; lungs fill up;
could only breathe in upright position with great labor;
constant cough from titillation behind sternum, at bifurcation; no expectoration, yet chest seems full of fluid.

▮▮Ebullitions in chest.

❙❙Cyanosis neonatorum.

❙Surface of body mottled; every effort to lift or move babe would cause it to cry out with pain; child's breathing after a crying spell so labored as to almost amount to asphyxia; extremities and feet cold; face and limbs puffed. *θ*Cyanosis.

❙Pulse: small, weak and accelerated; unequal; intermittent; alternately full and small; weak, slow, small.

❙❙Pulse weak and empty. *θ*Infiltration on back.

❙Induration of veins and surrounding cellular substance.

❙Atheromatous condition of arteries in old people.

❙Capillaries fill quite slowly after pressure on skin. *θ*Scarlatina.

³⁰ Outer Chest. ❙Blueness of skin.

Sensation of heat like from a hot stove on outer chest.

❙❙Burning pain as if in flesh of chest, two or three inches below l. nipple.

❙Swelling from above clavicle down to below pectoralis major, smooth and elastic, not painful, not red.

³¹ Neck and Back. ❙Blueness of external throat from distension of veins.

❙❙Intolerance of tight neckbands.

❙Pain in nape of neck to distraction. *θ*Werlhoff's disease.

❙❙Stiff neck, moves jaw with difficulty; tearing from nape of neck up either side, to top of head.

❙Nape of neck painful to touch, and stiff.

❙❙Stiffness of neck, on r. side, sore to touch, giddiness with choking in throat.

❙Nape of neck sensitive to external pressure.

❙Stiffness of nape of neck, with catarrh.

❙Swelling entirely on l. side; smooth, livid appearance; suffocative sensations produced by touching neck or swelling. *θ*Bronchocele.

❙Glands of throat and neck badly swollen. *θ*Scarlatina.

❙Swelling on l. side of neck from angle of jaw downward to near clavicle, suppurated and abscess was discharged with lancet; after this patient declined and became much exhausted in strength; face pale, of dirty, dingy hue, with puffy aspect; appetite nil; restlessness day and night; constant hot, dry skin; extremely peevish and whining; abscess formed a large cavity from which there was sloughing of cellular tissue; no sign of healthy granulations; discharge foul and copious; pulse 140 and small; could not eat solid food on account of soreness of neck; extremely sensitive to all motions of head; profuse hemorrhage from abscess, at least a pint of blood; great prostration, refused food, discharges more foul, pulse rapid and feeble; constant leakage of dark colored blood from sore. θAfter scarlatina.

∎Abscess near l. clavicle, another on l. side of neck. θAfter scarlatina.

Stitches in upper part of back, or along spine from below upward, or in whole back and in nape of neck, with stinging in r. arm and sensation as if it had gone to sleep, with itching on arms, hips and lower limbs.

∎From cervical vertebræ down to lumbar, whole r. side of back, width of three or four inches, much swollen, elastic, painless to pressure: dull pains intolerable after exertion, has to lie down in a kind of tetanic state. θInfiltration of cellular tissue.

∎Myelitis.

∎Pain in back, with great restlessness, with yawning and stretching of arms and legs; weariness, as from too great exertion, with awkward, tottering gait, with jerks, taking away breath or going into abdomen; small, painful spot, low down in back.

∎Intolerable drawing in small of back and down into legs, especially noticed in ischia, frequently in evening; drawing extending from small of back up back; drawing extending from back to hips, with urging to urinate.

∎∎Pain in small of back: as if lame and weak; intermittent fever; palpitation; dyspnœa; constipation; dysmenorrhœa.

∎Aching pain in lumbar region. θFistula.

∎Stiffness in sacrum, bending or beginning motion, extending to hip joint and thigh as if sinews were too short.

∎Continual pain in sacrum and coccyx.

∎Pain in os coccygis, when sitting down, feeling as if sitting on something sharp.

∎Continual pain in os sacrum and coccyx; drawing pain, as if sprained, in small of back, preventing motion; agonizing pain when rising from a seat. θCoccygodynia.

∎Tenderness in whole spine, most in neck, below occiput; headache in occiput and forehead; on turning or moving head pain in spine of neck into brain; pressure of finger on spine of neck sends pain to brain; pressure on dorsal spine sends pain to stomach; cannot bear to be raised up, and cannot raise herself in bed because of severe pain; little sleep. θAffection of spine.

∎Girl, æt. 5 years, since two years of age affected with caries of dorsal vertebræ resulting in deformed chest, leaving child feeble; lost control of both legs; toes moved sometimes involuntarily; she coughs some during day, but particularly at night on going to bed; much thirst; pain in spine, lies only on back; much

wheezing and rattling of mucus; fever and thirst at
night; respiration feeble and difficult, with blueness of
face; each coughing fit produced sweating; expectoration impossible; sleep much interrupted.

▮Boils half an inch in diameter near spine, with violent
burning, throbbing pain.

▮▮Carbuncle in back of neck, purple or gangrenous.

Upper Limbs.   ▮▮Pain in r. shoulder joint with headache.

▮Lameness in l. shoulder.

▮Soreness of r. shoulder, < when lying on it. θHepatitis.

▮Left shoulder and arm weak and lame, < lying on arm.

▮Painful feeling of weakness and lameness in l. shoulder
and arm, < by using arm; shoulder and arm sensitive
to touch. θTumor in l. mamma.

▮▮Axillary glands swollen, painless, purplish.

▮Garlic-like smell of sweat in axillæ.

▮Left arm nearly double its size, from elastic cellular infiltration.

▮Arms so weak that she is unable to raise them.

▮Makes odd motions with r. arm as if reaching for some
object. θDiphtheria.

▮Tetters on arms and hands.

▮Brown spots on elbow joint.

▮Wrists very painful and swollen; could not study by day
or sleep at night, for burning pain. θAfter bee stings
on both wrists.

▮Left hand and arm numb while pain and redness in foot
disappeared; pain and redness returned to foot, and
hand and arm were well. θRheumatism complicated
with epilepsy.

▮Pain in wrist joints as if sprained.

▮Twitching of hands. θDiarrhœa.

▮Tingling and pricking in l. hand; hands go to sleep.

▮Trembling of hands. θDrunkards.

▮The hands are cold as if dead.

▮Swelling of hands.

▮Phlegmonous inflammation of hand with great swelling
and tendency to extend up arm.

▮Dark blue, blackish, hard swelling of back of hand and
fingers, icy cold with a burning feeling, sensitive to
touch in attacks every day, come suddenly, disappear
slowly; rubbing upwards hastens disappearance; after
touching ice.

▮Livid swelling of back of r. hand and fingers; began with
severe itching and "creeping;" hand becomes blue and
gradually darker, mottled, very hard; cold, but seems to
him burning hot; sensitive to pressure; burning and
pricking in finger ends; heat of stove > pain, but <

creeping sensation; throbbing pain at outside of wrist; sharp pain extending to elbow; spasmodic pain in elbow, when carrying arm in a sling; pain in one small spot under shoulder, pricking and burning in hand as it slowly goes away.

▮A laborer had been working among lumber three days before and thought he must have been poisoned; hand commenced swelling two days ago until it was three times its size; very red, pits on pressure, between first and second knuckle, opening as large as a three cent piece, looking like dirty soft soap; around this and along first three knuckles skin bluish black and inflated by gas; skin under black skin looked rotten, separated on opening first and second fingers, showing same soapy appearance, hand burnt (deep in) terribly; pain in red streaks that ran up from wrist; constant thirst; pulse not rapid, but soft.

▮Thumbs bend inwards. θEpilepsy.

▮Rheumatic swelling of index finger and wrist.

▮▮Panaritium, bluish swelling; stinging, pricking pains intense; erysipelas; necrosis, with fistulous openings; assumes purplish hue, becomes gangrenous.

▮Finger much swollen, looks bluish, has fistulous openings from which bony splinters have been discharged, three months in this state, during which time woman twice suffered difficulty in swallowing. θSore finger from bite of a drunken man, cauterized.

▮Pricking in extremities of fingers. θPanaritium.

▮Whitlow with necrosis of tendon, and much discoloration.

▮Right index finger atrophied; fetid sanious discharge from beneath nail; integument about root of nail tawny brown, bordering upon purple in parts. θOnychia.

▮Warts and excrescences on hands and fingers.

▮▮Numbness of finger tips (morning).

▮Cold, sweaty hands.

▮▮Bluish, mottled appearance of hands.

▮▮Panaritium, pricking, tingling, more than stinging; blue far around.

▮Felons, with proud flesh.

[33] **Lower Limbs.** ▮Painful stiffness from loins down to sacrum and thighs.

▮Contraction of psoas muscle, after abscess.

▮Coxalgia, < 3 P.M. and after sleep.

▮▮Bruised feeling in hips. θDysmenorrhœa.

▮Sciatica for five days, with intolerable shooting pains, extending from l. hip down to foot, followed by sensation of intense heat as from a hot iron in parts affected,

and afterwards by perspiration and general prostration;
pains extorted cries, < after sleeping.
∎Feet and legs œdematous, r. leg <; pale face; tongue
yellow; sclerotic yellow; r. sided sciatica at night,
awaking him; pains come suddenly and disappear
gradually.
∎Pain constantly changing locality, now in head, now in
teeth, now in sciatic nerve, attended with nervousness,
palpitation of heart; burning like fire in hypogastrium,
lumbar region and behind sternum. θSciatica.
∎Pain in thighs, as if swollen, in back part.
∎∎Gressus gallinaceus.
∎Weakness, especially of legs.
∎Uneasiness in lower limbs.
∎∎Feeling of weakness in knees after eating, with pressure
in stomach.
∎∎Feeling as from a sprain in r. knee.
∎Stinging tearing in knees, with swelling.
∎∎Aching in knees on waking in morning.
∎Sensation as if hot air was going through knee joints,
which were shaky.
∎Left knee feels as if sprained.
∎Swelling of knees, tension in bend, difficulty in stretching.
∎∎Pain in legs and stiffness in knees after sitting.
∎Near l. knee joint a bunch of varicose veins size of a fist;
veins as thick as a thumb and hard as a rope.
∎Contraction of hamstrings, after popliteal abscess.
∎Synovial fluid dried up; pain in knee day and night.
∎On external side of knee bluish redness. θErysipelas of leg.
∎∎Much pain of an aching kind, in shin bones only.
∎A half painful sensation of a sore place immediately be-
low lower edge of patella of l. leg, this trifling thing
almost driving him wild; great distress of mind, as if
some terrible evil was impending, the evil dreaded
being in some way connected with the pain, but how,
he could not tell.
∎Pains as if burnt in different places on tibia, at first itching, but after rubbing there appeared rather sensitive
spots as large as a quarter dollar, with dark blue red
margins and dry scurf.
∎Caries of tibia.
∎Erysipelas with pustules; leg swollen bluish red, discharged matter from several holes, presenting appearance of a large carbuncle, with itching.
∎Erysipelas of leg; restless, could not sleep, least movement or touch on leg almost throwing child into convulsions; very angry appearance, dark blue spots on
upper part just below knee, rest of limb of a dark, glossy
redness.

▮Ulcer on r. leg, with varicose swelling, after a fall.

▮Leg below knee terribly swollen, black and spotted. θRattlesnake bite on toe.

▮▮Phlegmasia alba dolens.

▮Hard red patch, with scabs on calf of l. leg; tender; thin, yellow fluid discharge from under scabs; itching, especially in cold weather.

▮Legs, from knees to end of big toes, covered with scales, circular or elliptic, raised and free on circumference, attached in centre and of horny consistence, resting on a purple bluish colored base; < every Spring; itching and burning, especially during warm weather, and when heated, or when warm in bed. θEczema.

▮▮Flat ulcers: with thin, offensive discharge and bluish areolæ; become erysipelatous from motion.

▮Ulcers of legs; bottom of ulcers uneven and dirty; discharge thin, odor offensive.

▮After scratching legs at night until raw, rapid suppuration, followed by a large, dirty looking, painful ulcer.

▮After running nail into foot, for which a salve was given, small ulcer where nail had pierced, soon followed by others, until whole plantar surface was covered; very little moisture from ulcers, which soon began to dry up, forming a thick, dry scale which covered sole of foot, in some places being a half inch thick.

▮Had been using washes of sulphate of copper, sulphate of zinc, sugar of lead, etc., for a year; ulcer at last dried up and patient was discharged as cured; on taking cold, a few weeks after, her entire foot and ankle broke out into small ulcers, resembling original sore; great pain in ulcers, itching of feet and ankles, almost unbearable; leg < after sleep and > from warmth.

▮▮Chronic indolent ulcers of legs, flat with purple skin; many small sores around main ulcer, which has an uneven bottom, burning and bleeding, even when lightly touched; ichorous, offensive discharge.

▮Virulent phagedenic ulcers.

▮▮Black, gangrenous ulcers and wounds on legs.

▮Chronic ulcers of lower extremities (probably of syphilitic origin) in which discharge ceased; extremity œdematous and hard, slightly red, swelling extending up along course of principal veins; great and sudden prostration of strength; low, muttering delirium and general typhoid symptoms. θPhlebitis.

▮Lacerating, jerking, rheumatic pains in legs as soon as he falls asleep; irregular action of heart and valvular murmur from rheumatic metastasis; deadly pallor of face. θRheumatism.

❙Uneasiness in lower limbs.

❙❙Trembling of legs.

❙Convulsions particularly violent in lower limbs, coldness of feet, stretching backward of body and crying out.

❙❙Swelling of l. leg and foot.

❙Rose red swelling of ankles. *θ*Erysipelas.

❙Injured ankles; severe contusions and lacerations; gangrene; bluish purple vesicles covering a dirty looking ash grey ground.

❙Woman, æt. 40, who had not menstruated for one year, sprained her foot; after exercise ankle greatly swollen, erysipelatous to knee; sticking pain in ankle when walking; upper part of foot covered with dark lentil shaped pimples.

❙Pain in second toe of r. foot; by evening livid swelling to knee, more painful when he walked; pain in both knees; cannot stretch out foot; toe painful on pressure.

❙Foot like marble from varicose swellings.

❙Swelling of feet, < after walking. *θ*During pregnancy.

❙Icy coldness of feet; cold before epileptic attack.

❙Tingling in toes.

❙❙Gangrenous ulcers on legs and toes; rhagades of toes.

❙Proud flesh about ingrown toenails or in old wounds·stinging; purplish appearance.

❙Inflammation and suppuration of old chilblains.

❙Rheumatic swelling of index finger and wrist joint; rheumatic pains in knees, stinging, tearing and sense of swelling; swelling of knees with tension in bends of knees, difficulty in stretching limb and pain of thigh (posteriorly) as if swollen; bluish red swellings; pains < after sleeping; after profuse sweats l. side most affected; or the affection commences on r. and goes over to l.; arthritic contractions of limbs after abuse of mercury and quinine. *θ*Rheumatism.

³⁴ **Limbs in General.** ❙❙Erysipelas of legs or arms; surface bluish, swelling glossy, impending gangrene.

❙Rheumatism, with swelling of wrists and ankles.

❙Three years ago, after great mental emotion, sudden cessation of menstruation, since then, headache, toothache, pain in joints, sciatica; for last year erratic pains in joints, particularly in morning on awaking; nervous irritability, palpitation, burning as from fire in hypogastrium, loins and behind sternum; transient flushes of heat in face, without sweat; loss of appetite; white coated tongue; pressure in stomach; constipation; several dry, painless varices in anus.

❙Acute or chronic rheumatism, recurring every year.

❙❙Bluish swelling of joints, after sprains.

❚❚Dark bluish swelling of cellular tissue, on hands, arms, legs, very sensitive; impending gangrene.
❚Boils on thighs and fingers.
❚❚Nightly burning in palms and soles.
❚Limbs stiff, straight or curved, after abuse of mercury.
❚Arm and leg paretic; crawling as if asleep. θInfiltration on back.

³⁵ **Rest. Position. Motion.** Lying down: vertigo; pain in head >; pressing or bursting pains in temples; anything touches throat seems as if he would suffocate, pain much <; pain in top of throat; constant coughing; slightest covering over nose and mouth produce suffocating dyspnœa; pain in lungs <; stiffness in sacrum.
Lying on r. side: > earache in r. ear; palpitation >; weight of l. arm on l. side is painful; as if something was rolling to that side of abdomen.
Cannot lie on l. side: causes pain at heart.
When lying on r. shoulder: pain <.
Lying on l side, with head high: > suffocating.
Lying on l. arm: shoulder and arm weak and lame.
Lying on back: involuntary urine; pain in spine; mouth open; must lie on back with knees drawn up, peritonitis, typhlitis.
Constant desire to lie down: acute pain in abdomen.
Must lie down: pain in back intolerable.
Cannot stand, has to lie down: child loses consciousness.
Lying with body and limbs doubled up: during chill.
Recumbent position impossible: from sense of suffocation; inflammation and swelling of tonsils.
Cannot lie, stand or sit quiet: pain in back and limbs.
Rising from lying position: cough.
Must change position frequently on account of pain in back and limbs.
Head always must be high: generally resting on hand.
Sitting: causes pain in thighs and stiffness at knees; constant cough; difficult breathing; pain in lungs and dyspnœa <; palpitation >; pain in coccygis; pain in legs; stiffness in knees.
Assuming upright position: pains in head change to beating in vertex.
Can only breathe in upright position.
Could not sit up without assistance.
When sitting bent forward: difficulty of breathing >; contraction of chest >.
Bending forward: spasmodic colic >; stiffness in sacrum.
Bending head backward: throat and larynx painful.
Bending and throwing head back: pain in lungs >.
On reaching up: vertigo.

Stooping: vertigo; pressing, bursting pains in temples; dizzy; pressive headache <.

Standing: body bends towards l.; cutting pains in rectum <.

Could not stand: vertigo.

Stretching backwards of body: during convulsions.

Cannot stretch out foot: pain in knee.

Rising: faint; pain in top of head and giddiness; staggers backwards; pulls himself forward with greatest difficulty; cutting headache <.

Rising from seat: agonizing pain in small of back.

Cannot raise herself up in bed: because of severe pain.

Could scarcely raise head from pillow.

Unable to raise arms: on account of weakness.

Cannot use arm: on account of pain in l. mamma; compelled to lie down.

Using arm: pain <; shortness of breath and suffocative attacks <; weakness and lameness in l. shoulder and arm.

Raising head: pain in head <.

Turning head: pain in throat <; pain in spine of neck into groin.

Bettered by shaking head.

Turning over: feeling as of a ball rolling about in bladder or abdomen.

Rolling from side to side in bed: suffocating attacks; from hour to hour.

Makes odd motions with r. arm.

Throws arms about: in suffocating fits.

Throws herself in all positions: to get breath.

Sudden backward throwing of head.

Motion: aversion to every kind; pain in head <; pressing or bursting pains in temples; beating in head; of temporal and masseter muscles < pain in ear; of limbs; flesh sore; slightest, renews vomiting; causes excruciating pain in abdomen; rapid, pain in r. ovary<; causes heart beat; symptoms of chest >; causes suffocative attacks; stiffness in sacrum.

Every movement: throbbing in head; causes fainting and anxiety; of hands, causes shortness of breath; of leg, almost throws girl into convulsions; flat ulcers become erysipelatous.

Cannot move: nervous aches all over.

Cannot stand or move legs: except an involuntary drawing up of toes.

Difficulty of moving tongue: with impossibility of opening mouth wide.

Stepping: < pain in ear.

Walking: drags his feet; vertigo; backwards; stitch in r.
side; shooting in region of spleen; constant cough; oppression and want of breath <; sticking pain in ankle;
swelling of knee painful; feels like falling forwards; before chill became blind and giddy.

Overexertion: pain in r. ovary <.

³⁶ **Nerves.** ❚Nervous irritability; restlessness; jerking.

❚Restless tossing, moaning; children with sore throat.

❚❚Nervous exaltation; hysteria.

❚❚Trembling in whole body, thinks she will faint or sink
down from weakness.

❚Trembling of limbs and internally, with fever and faintness, evenings. θTyphoid.

❚Nervous aches all over; hysterical spells of trembling;
cannot move, work or sleep; dark forebodings of future;
any news, excitement, or a harsh word makes <; <
after sleep. θNervous affection.

❚Cramps in chest and abdomen; with crying and loud
complaining; dryness in mouth and throat; sensation
as if epithelium was peeling off gums. θHysteria.

❚Child now and then loses consciousness and sight for a
second, turns and twists eyes like one who fights with
sleep; closing lids, sinking of head all in a moment;
cannot stand, has to lie down.

❚Crawls upon floor, laughs and is very cross by turns;
attacks last from half an hour to an hour; child acts
strangely, will not play with other children; exhibits
no love for mother; seems to hate her mother and
friends, hides; runs away from strangers, looks at them
through her fingers; bites and spits at other children;
six years ago was frightened by a snake.

❚Spasms of legs.

❚Convulsions, particularly violent in lower limbs; coldness
of feet; stretching backwards of body and crying out.

❚Convulsions and other spasms, with violent shrieks.

❚Severe pains in back of head; violent convulsions, requiring several strong persons to prevent her from injuring
herself; attempts to pull hair out of back part of head.

❚Unconscious; hands clenched; l. hand, l. foot and r. eyelids in constant motion; painless abscess on inside of r.
wrist, one inch in diameter.

❚Delirium and convulsions from night watching, over-
fatigue and solicitude.

❚Sudden and forcible protrusion and retraction of tongue.

❚After having ears pierced, chorea; < l. side; l. side of
body in continual motion; cross, irritable; throws away
anything she has in her hands at time; ears sore and
ulcerated where they had been pierced; finally motion

very violent, partial paralysis of l. side; could hold nothing in hand; when walking frequent stumbling and dragging of l. foot; unnaturally loquacious; < after sleep.

‖Great depression of spirits and apprehension of death; neck stiff and sensitive to touch; blue spots or blisters on skin; epistaxis; hemorrhage from bowels, of decomposed blood; great prostration. θChorea.

‖Epilepsy: from onanism or otherwise connected with sexual function after great lewdness, jealousy, fluor albus, or seminal emissions; during catamenia; during climacteric period; during sleep.

‖Epileptic convulsions; eyeballs turned upward; cries falling down unconsciously, foam at mouth, sudden and forcible protrusion of tongue; hands clenched; limbs twitching; deep sleep.

‖Creeping sensation beginning at back of neck, moving slowly down spinal column. θEpilepsy.

‖Before attack: cold feet; palpitation of heart; bloating of abdomen; belching; heaviness of head; vertigo; headache; paleness of face. θEpilepsy.

‖Headache and congestions of blood to head; before attack absentminded, confused; throws head back, froth at mouth, clenches hands, throws arms and legs about; between attacks, severe vertigo; constant headache; sensation of heat in forehead; trembling of limbs, < l. side; curious dreams at night. θEpilepsy.

‖Striking about with hands and feet. θEpilepsy.

‖One week after frostbitten toe which had ulcerated, rigors; shooting pains in back; opisthotonus, in twenty-four hours trismus; remission midnight till noon; after midnight profuse sweat and agitated sleep; throat sensitive to contact, swallowing painful. θTetanus.

‖Peculiar tetanic look, half closed eyes and stiffness of neck; partial lockjaw; rigidity and pain in muscles of back; after cutting off two outer phalanges of third r. toe, by being run over by a carriage wheel; soft parts of toe look gangrenous nine days after accident.

‖Stitches in cardiac region, in paroxysms, three or four times a day; hacking cough with blood spitting; pains take away his breath while they last, but cease suddenly; cough during day and after lying down, none in the night; raises blood in morning; opisthotonus with loss of consciousness only for a moment; trismus with constriction of throat, pulls and tears at throat; several paroxysms in quick succession.

‖Hydrophobia.

‖Climaxis; menses irregular; blood scanty, dark, fluid, and sometimes lumpy; for a year past frequent cataleptic attacks, preceded by cold, stiff feeling of upper lip, as if she had a moustache of ice. *θ*Catalepsy.

❚Feeling of weariness; languor; exhaustion as from warm weather; inclination to lie down, especially after eating.

❚Great weakness in back, extending into limbs.

❚❚Great physical and mental exhaustion, constantly sinks down from weakness; < in morning.

❚❚Weakness of whole body, in morning on rising, especially in arms and feet.

❚Weakness in morning in sleep; on waking general sick feeling, vertigo, feeling of lead in occiput, can scarcely raise head from pillow; all joints seem sprained.

❚Feeling as though body was overwhelmed by a disintegrating tendency, with sinking of all forces.

❚❚Trembling all over; exhausted, faint.

❚❚Fainting, with pain in heart, nausea, pale face, vertigo.

❚❚Muscular prostration. *θ*Diphtheria. *θ*Scarlatina.

❚Heaviness and dulness in head, particularly in occiput; sensation of heat in head; hands numb; heaviness < from motion, > sitting still; if head is placed ever so high, she thinks it too low; drowsiness in afternoon every other day; starting on falling asleep; heat in head and arms at night, with weakness in epigastrium; sleeps little, and fulness and heaviness in head are < in morning; restlessness, driving from place to place; symptoms change place; now more in l. arm, now in foot, which is cold as ice; every cold gives her a sore throat; swelling and stiffness, painful when swallowing and to touch; now and then a sudden stitch in region of heart, which makes her weak; hemorrhoidal tumors, very painful during stool; frequent urging; menses too late and profuse, with throbbing headache.

❚No sleep until after midnight; great despondency and sadness, weakness of memory; headache in sun, with glimmering of eyes; swollen and easily bleeding gums; sore throat, with sensation of fulness, or as of a plug in throat; tonsils enlarged; constant dryness of throat; frequent entire loss of voice; burning pain in region of l. ovary, menstruation irregular; corrosive leucorrhœa for ten days after menstruation; everything sours in stomach, heartburn incessantly; pressing, burning pain in top of head, from within outward; dry, hacking cough; palpitation; constipation; cold limbs below elbows and knees. *θ*General breakdown after repeated attacks of pneumonia.

❚Menstruation irregular; suppressed for eight months; swelled abdomen; restless, nervous, morbidly talkative complaining, yet giving a very rambling account; no

sleep for three nights, partly owing to nervous restlessness, partly to what she calls shivering and shaking fits
which come over her; for some time sleep broken, followed by headache and despondency; least worry and
excitement puts her into heat and fever; urine scanty,
high colored, offensive, passed with much pain; bowels
inclined to be loose; nervous and discouraged after
eating; nausea and load at stomach; dress unfast-
ened and quite loose at upper part of chest, says she,
cannot bear it tight, nor can she bear things tight
around her waist; faintness and hunger about 11 A.M.
*θ*General prostration after childbearing.

▪Suddenly eyesight nearly gone; speech disturbed, after
a few minutes conversation a curtain seemed to fall
down in front of pharynx; teeth feel as if wedged;
tongue feels scalded; cannot yawn because of sharp
pain about root of tongue; when eating fast, food stays
in throat; pain over eyes and sore feeling in eyeballs;
has to read and sew with glasses of an octogenarian;
bagging just in front of uvula, which is very soft and
feels like pus; at apex of bag a whitish prominence, as
if an abscess was about to discharge. *θ*Post diphtheritic affection.

▪Lying with body and limbs doubled up; nose, ears and
forehead very cold; giddiness and blindness; skin
shriveled, cold, livid; pulse thready, dying away;
rapid gaping, incessant sighing; blue rings around eyes;
increasing stupor. *θ*Shock from injuries.

▪▪Awkward gait; l. side weak.

▪▪Gressus gallinaceus.

▪Left side of body numb, cold; abdomen and feet also
cold; sparks before eyes; on walking feels like falling
forward, pain from top of head downwards. *θ*Incipient
paralysis.

▪Progressive locomotor ataxy.

▪Palsies depending on apopleptic condition of brain, exhaustion or extremes of temperature.

▪▪Body when standing bends towards l., must be supported;
drags feet in walking, direction of steps towards left.

▪▪Paralysis: left sided; after apoplexy, or cerebral exhaustion; painful.

▪Child, muttering delirium; yellowish red, dry, tremulous tongue; moderate thirst; pulse 70; rational for a
little time when awake, then subsides into delirium;
paralysis of motory nerves of l. limbs.

▪After exposure entire paralysis of both legs, cannot stand,
or move legs with exception of an occasional involuntary drawing up of toes; cough < during night and on

going to bed; thirst during meals, drinks much at a
time; pain in spine, lies only on back at night; finally
cough more severe and accompanied by fever and thirst;
respiration feeble, difficult, with blueness of face; each
coughing turn produced perspiration; expectoration impossible; sleep interrupted.

²⁷ **Sleep.** ▮Great drowsiness.

▮Sleepiness without being able to sleep.

▮▮As soon as he falls asleep the breathing stops.

▮▮When falling asleep is awakened by tickling cough.

▮Could not sleep on account of strangulation. θScarlatina. ·

▮▮Sleepy and weak after dinner.

▮Persistent sleeplessness.

▮▮In evening very wide awake and talkative; lively as
soon as the gas is lit.

▮Sleepless: from anxiety; especially before midnight, with
talkativeness; on account of internal restlessness; abdomen and chest seem swollen; restless and nervous,
burning in soles of feet, stinging all over.

▮Afraid to go to sleep for fear he will die before he wakes.

▮Tossing about, moaning, during sleep; children.

▮Restless sleep, with dreams and frequent waking.

▮Awakens at night and cannot sleep again.

▮▮Troubles come on during sleep, and patient wakes in
distress or pain; cough, asthma or spasm.

▮Awoke in a fright about something trifling.

▮▮On waking: vertigo; dry, hacking cough; all symptoms
worse.

▮▮Not refreshed after a good sleep. θHeart disease.

▮Restless sleep, with many dreams and frequent waking.

▮Constant dreaming, frequent waking, and again dozing
and dreams, in morning is heavy and out of sorts.

▮▮Amorous dreams.

²⁸ **Time.** Morning: unhappy and distressed in mind; great
sadness; heaviness and dejection; vertigo; on rising,
headache over eyes; heaviness in occiput; vomiting of
food and slime; epistaxis; thick, yellow discharge from
nose; on awakening eyes <; pains in eye and head <;
as if she would die of exhaustion; blowing of blood; skin
began to redden and swell; throat >; hard cough;
vomiting of bile; pain in rectum < till afternoon; ovaritis <; difficult breathing; numbness of finger tips;
aching in knees; feels bruised.

9 A.M.: neuralgia in face begins.

Forenoon: want of appetite.

Noon till midnight: visions and delirious talk<; swollen
face; erysipelas <.

Day: sleeps a minute or two at a time; symptoms >; head

pains; short, dry cough; after a nap, hawking of mucus and rawness in throat; after sleeping, pains in throat <; very sleepy but cannot sleep; several attacks of nausea, with shortness of breath; sleep < pains in abdomen; flushes of heat; sensation of foreign body in throat; constant cough; cough <; restlessness; pain in knee; talks too much; itching in paroxysms.

Afternoon: attacks of delirium tremens; headache <; soreness of vertex changes to darting; facial neuralgia goes off; tonsillitis <; fever <; dyspnœa <; violent chill; intermittent fever, < 2 P.M.

3 P.M.: coxalgia >.

Evening: vertigo; pain in back of head; bluish grey ring before eyes; wide awake and talkative; feels nearly well; pain deep in l. ear; if anything touches throat, seems as though he would suffocate; pain much <; sensitiveness of throat <; watery stools with burning; cough on lying down; drawing in back and legs; trembling of limbs; violent chill; heat in hands and feet; burning in palms and soles.

9 P.M. until going to bed: nervous cough.

Night: loquacity; delirium; does not sleep; pain comes on and lasts till end of next day; short, dry cough; tearing pain in side of head <; orbital cellulitis <; earache in r. ear; eruption beneath eye itches; itching on face; dryness in throat; comatose; very sleepy, but cannot sleep till towards morning; least touch on mouth and nose causes threatened suffocation; stools bloody and slimy; eighteen or twenty stools; constant erections; menorrhagia with chills; something runs from neck to larynx, stops breathing and awakes him; almost suffocated; constant cough; fever <; awakens with fear of suffocation; dry cough; perspires very much; restlessness; fever and thirst; pain in wrists; sciatica in r. leg; pain in knee; constant dreaming; chills; burning in palms and soles; heat as from orgasm of blood; itching intense; burning in ulcers.

Before midnight: sleepless.

Midnight: became insensible; sudden diarrhœa; wakened by contraction of chest.

After midnight: no sleep.

*° **Temperature and Weather.** Worse during Spring and Summer, or from extremes of temperature; < from the sun's rays.

Open air: vertigo, from walking; desire for, before menses; causes violent, tickling cough; symptoms >; after scarlet fever swelling of whole body; must open doors and windows; during suffocating attacks.

Draft of air: throat <.

· Must sit by open window: heart disease.

In sun: headache.

Heat: headache; ulcers >.

Warm weather: diarrhœa <; legs burn and itch.

Warm room: chill abates.

Warmth of bed: itching of legs <; cannot keep limbs quiet.

External warmth: desire for; toothache >; pains in head >; earache >; wants head closely wrapped up.·

Hot drinks: throat symptoms <; cause toothache; bleeding of gums <.

' Heat of stove: pain in hands >; creeping sensation <.

Change of temperature: cough <.

Damp weather: cough <.

Wet weather: ulcers in throat <.

Getting wet: causes toothache.

Exposed all day to cold, wet weather, at night comatose.

Washing: pains in throat <.

Cold water: headache >; burning in ulcer >.

Cold or warm drinks: cause toothache.

Cold weather: itching of scabs on calves of legs.

Complaints in damp, warm Spring weather.

⁴⁰**Fever.** ❙Shivering without coldness. θDysentery.

❙Cold shudders ascending.

ⅠⅠSingle paroxysms of shivering.

ⅠⅠIcy coldness of feet.

❙Cold feet, with oppression of chest.

❙Numbing coldness.

❙Violent chill in evening, chattering of teeth and feeling as in trismus.

ⅠⅠChill in afternoon, pains in limbs, pleuritic stitches, oppression of chest and convulsive movements.

Chill runs from hollow of back upwards over shoulders, nape of neck, back of head as far as vertex, with a sensation as if drawn at base, goose flesh on parts affected.

❙Chill: commencing in small of back; runs up back to head; beginning across back and shoulders; > in warm room; desires external warmth.

❙Shaking chills in several attacks daily, the almost unconscious woman is thrown about in bed. θPuerperal fever.

ⅠⅠShaking chill for two hours. θErysipelas of leg.

❙Unconscious; livid face; shaking chills; skin hot or cool. θMetritis.

❙Rigors, nausea, subsequent fever. θEpidemic laryngitis.

❙Wants to be near fire and lie down; heat makes him feel >, but chill continues.

❙❙Child must be held firmly to > pain in head and chest
and prevent shaking; feels > if held or pressed down.

❙After icy cold calves, shaking chill with warm sweat;
then strumming through limbs, intermingled with
flushes of heat.

❙Chill and heat alternate and change place.

❙Chills at night, flushes of heat by day.   θMenorrhagia.

❙❙Shivering during heat.

❙Heat, particularly on hands and feet, in evening.

❙❙Burning in palms and soles, evening and night.

❙❙Heat at night, as from orgasm of blood; throat sensitive.

❙Internal sensation of heat, with cold feet.

❙Dry, burning skin.

❙Heat: with violent headache; livid complexion; oppression of chest; deep breathing and sleep; great loquacity.

❙Great inclination to sweat.

❙Sweat: profuse, with most complaints; cold, stains yellow; brownish yellow; bloody, staining red; between
paroxysms of fever; at night; affords relief.

❙Sweat about neck after first nap.   θPhthisis.

❙❙Strong smelling perspiration in axilla, like garlic.

❙Intermittent fever; severe pain and soreness on pressure
in region of spleen, shooting to breast or l. side of neck.

❙Intermittent fever recurs every Spring, or after suppression in previous Fall by quinine; < in afternoon, 2
P.M.; face red, headache, feet cold; talking during hot
stage; excessive burning and rending pain during
relapse into bilious intermittent after quinine.

❙Intermittent fever in Spring or begining of Summer.

❙Intermittent fever for eight years, suppressed by large
doses of quinine in Summer, to return every Spring;
complexion when fever was present a grey, ash color.

❙Chills for six months in Summer and Fall, suppressed
with blue mass and quinine, returned following May;
convulsions during chill.

❙Sinking chills annually, in August, for nine years, has
always been dosed heavily with morphine, brandy and
quinine to prevent "fatal third chill;" drenched in
sweat for many days after each attack, takes months to
recuperate; fever always tertian.

❙Restlessness; pain in lumbar region; constipation;
tongue coated thick, brown, furrowed and tending to
dryness; soreness across bowels; chill comes on at 2.30
P.M.; body drawn up in a heap; tip of nose and ears
cold and icy; forehead cold; skin shriveled and livid;
pulse filiform, dying away; rapid yawning, incessant
sighing; dark areola around eyes, fast becoming darker
as she sinks into stupor.   θTertian ague.

▮Intermittent fifth day after confinement; chills daily,
with great violence, for a week (sewer gas in house);
inflammation of l. ovary; shuddering; prostration; at
end of fourth week discharge of pus and blood through
abdominal wall.

▮▮Typhus: delirium; tongue red or black, dry or in fissures, especially on tip; trembles when put out, or tip
remains under lower teeth or lip.

▮Stools, with sediment of flakes of decomposed blood, having appearance and form of perfectly charred wheat
straw, in longer or shorter flat pieces, together with
portions more or less ground up; violent epistaxis in
morning. θTyphoid.

▮After prolonged quiet; loquacious mood; talks day
and night, if not to those in room, to imaginary persons; jumping from subject to subject; desire to lie in
bed with clothing away from neck. θTyphoid.

▮Great prostration daily increasing, until twenty-three
days had passed without any crisis; complete delirium
with muttering, and complete prostration; the only
position was upon back; if placed on side rolled at
once upon back; tongue dry, black and cracked;
patient evidently sinking. θTyphoid.

▮On ninth day, profuse, sour sweat without relief; delirium; headache; eyes strongly injected, gaze unsteady;
loss of consciousness; constant unintelligible mumbling;
pulse hard, small, 120–140; tongue dry, black, cracked
and bleeding, can be protruded only with great difficulty, then trembles; lips cracked, black, bloody;
unquenchable thirst; hardness of hearing; abdomen
soft, but in all places painful; stools (lumpy) crum-
bling frequent, yellow, orange colored, or tinged with
blood; urine suppressed; profuse sweats; finally, involuntary escape of stool and strongly smelling ammoniacal urine; will lie only upon back; dyspnœa and
cough with copious expectoration of blood streaked
mucus. θTyphoid.

▮Case had run into fifth week, became thoroughly dyscra-
sic, death seemed imminent from asthma. θTyphoid.

▮Typhoid fever, third week, with delirium; tongue dry,
black, cracked; throat dry and cracked; unable to put
tongue out.

▮Muttering delirium; yellowish red, dry, tremulous
tongue; moderate thirst; pulse 70; rational for a little
time when awake, then subsides into delirium; paralysis of motory nerves of limbs. θTyphoid.

▮Exposed all day to cold, wet weather; at night comatose; high fever; tongue dry, red at tip, soon becoming

brown in centre; pupils contracted, then dilated; vomiting of greenish water; restless from colic, requiring three attendants to keep him on bed; continually throws off bedcovers; unconscious of external impressions; pulse about 120, four beats to one respiration; involuntary stools and micturition.

▮Fever < in afternoon, sweat without alleviation; symptoms < after sleep; loss of consciousness; muttering; stupor; sunken countenance; dropping of lower jaw; dry, red or black tongue, cracked on tip and bleeding; in attempt to protrude it, it trembles, or tip remains under lower teeth and does not come out; dry lips, cracked and bleeding; stools very offensive, whether formed or loose; dyspnœa and cough, with slimy, bloody expectoration. θTyphus.

▮▮Yellow fever: delirium at night; loquacious, disposed to quarrel; slow, difficult speech; drowsy; rush of blood to head; red face; yellow conjunctiva; yellow or purplish tint of skin; blood dark, non-coaguable; small wounds bleed much; perspiration stains yellow; lips dry, cracked and bleeding; tongue heavy, trembling, dry and red, cracked at tip; tip red, centre brown; difficult speech; sour eructations; heartburn; nausea after drinking; vomiting, with palpitation; dyspnœa; anxiety about heart; cannot lie on l. side; irregular weak pulse; urine almost black; persistent sleeplessness; fainting; trembling all over; sudden flushes of heat; sensitiveness about neck and pit of stomach against any pressure; < when waking; > after nourishment.

▮Blood dark and does not coagulate. θYellow fever.

▮Cellulitis, particularly of rectum and anus, with burning and blue color of skin. θYellow fever.

⁴¹ **Attacks, Periodicity.** Periodic: raging through upper jaw to ear; exacerbations with chronic angina.

Attacks: of weakness, even to syncope; of sensitiveness to touch in hands; of itching.

After every evacuation: sore, burning pain.

Alternate: heat and chills; squeamishness and facial neuralgia; diarrhœa and constipation.

After few minutes conversation: a curtain seems to fall down in front of pharynx.

At long intervals: urination.

For one hour: violent laughing.

For one hour every day: catamenial flow.

For two hours: shaking chill.

A few hours after eating: gnawing in stomach.

Every few hours or days: flow of blood from vagina.

For several hours: tearing pain in head then disappears for a day or two.

For five or six hours: pain in arm and shoulder.

Several times a day: epistaxis of venous blood; most violent shaking chill.

4 A.M.: heat continues from bedtime.

10 A.M.: fever.

Until 11 A.M.: feels well, then faint and weak.

Afternoon: delirium tremens; vomiting; fever.

Evening: persistent vomiting.

2.30 P.M.: chill.

Nightly attacks: of anxiety; hallucinations; pain in limbs; at 10 o'clock dryness of throat and thirst; of spasm of glottis; burning in palms and soles; burning in ulcers.

Towards morning: sweat.

First day of menses and day previous to appearance: pain.

Every day at 11 A.M.: hunger; throat >; violent chills.

Every day at 11 P.M.: heat and smarting in l. throat.

Alternate nights: vomiting.

Every other day: feeling of obstruction in throat on swallowing; chill ascending back.

On second or third day: threatened metastasis to meninges.

Every two or three days: acute colicky pains.

For three nights: no sleep.

Three days before menses: leucorrhœa.

Every three or four days: intense headache.

From three to eight days before menses: green, thick yellow leucorrhœa.

For five days: sciatica.

On ninth day: profuse sour sweat without relief.

Every eight or ten days: headache.

For ten days after menstruation: leucorrhœa.

For twenty days: no stool.

Twenty-three days passed without crisis: typhoid.

For many days, after each attack of chill: sweat.

Third week: typhoid fever with delirium.

The day before catamenia: great desire to go in open air.

Every four weeks, for four or five days, nervous debility <.

For several weeks: partial deafness.

Every two or three months: menses late.

For three months: fistulous opening in fingers, during this time she suffered twice with difficulty in swallowing.

At every menstrual effort: eructations amounting to vomiting; cardialgia; oppression of chest.

For eight months: no menstruation.

Lasting all Winter and Spring: cough.

In the Spring: toothache; diarrhœa.

In the Summer: toothache.

Every Spring: lower extremities covered with scales <; intermittent fever, or after suppression in previous Fall, by quinine; eruption.

Every Fall: eruption.

Every year: angina; acute or chronic rheumatism; in August, for nine years, sinking chills.

For one year: no menstruation.

Sunstroke two years previous to confinement, in bed ever since; two hours after delivery convulsions.

After twelve hours comatose.

Three years ago: after great mental emotion, sudden cessation of menstruation; erratic pains in joints.

For four years: piles; stitching, cutting pains in l. breast.

For eight years: intermittent fever.

For ten years: constipation.

Eighteen years' standing: dysmenorrhœa.

For last twenty years: eruption on l. forearm and on l. lower abdomen.

For years: violent pains over l. groin; succession of carbuncles.

⁴² **Locality and Direction.** Right: pain in side; oppressive pain < on side; partial paralysis; semi-lateral headache; as if part of side of head was cut off; soreness of vertex to side of head; pricking pain in limbs; severe pain commencing in inner canthus, extending to superciliary ridge; jerking in eye; sticking, drawing pain in eye; pain in ear > lying on side; pain as if something was lodged in side of throat; stitch in side; feeling of obstruction in throat; pain in side of throat; tonsil swollen; uvula clinging to tonsil; makes odd motions with arm; as if something was lodged in side; as of a ball rolling from side to stomach; tearing in abdomen; cutting in side of abdomen; pain from lumbar region through sacrum; violent pain over groin; swelling of ovary; pain in ovarian region; ovary size of a fist; induration in ovarian region; fungus hæmatoides on mamma; lung affected; must lean to side to > pain in chest; stitching pain through side of chest; dyspnœa <; lying on r. side weight of l. arm is painful; dilatation of ventricle; stiffness of neck on side; stinging in arm; side of back swollen; pain in shoulder joint; soreness of shoulder; makes odd motions with arm; livid swelling of back of hand and fingers; index finger atrophied; leg œdematous; sciatica in leg; knee as if sprained; ulcer on leg; pain in second toe of foot; stitching pain in side of chest; thick patches of exanthem on side from spine to sternum; immense carbuncle side of spine; rheumatism commences.

Left: pain in temple; body bends toward direction of steps; apoplexy on side; falling to side from vertigo; pain in side; pain over eye; drawing pain in temple; headache in frontal eminence; neuralgia on side; tearing pain in whole side of head; pain behind ear; numbness and crawling on side of head; painful sensitiveness in temple and in half of face; discharge from nose; pain in eye; orbital neuralgia; tearing pain in head; tongue inclined to side; tearing pain in malar bone and parts under eye; side of face and lower jaw swollen; uncertain numb feeling in head; painful inflammation of eye; dry wax in ear; sensation of numbness down cheek; pain deep in ear; erysipelatous eruption beneath eye; erysipelas began close to side of nose extending up and down side of face up as far as eye; tongue sore on side; soreness in side of throat; heat and smarting side of throat; inflamed swelling side of throat; tonsil swollen; pain shoots from tonsil to ear; abscess in tonsil; numerous white spots on pale red surface in throat; yellow white membrane on tonsil; pain and soreness begin on side of throat; inflammation and membrane beginning on side; diphtheritic spot as large as a pinhead on tonsil; side of throat several white exudate spots; tonsil one complete black slough; pain in hypochondrium; pain in side of abdomen; tenderness in iliac region; fibrous tumor in groin; dropsical enlargement of side and leg; pain in ovarian region; ovarian neuralgia; swelling, induration and other anomalies of ovary; sharp, shooting pain in ovary; suppuration in ovary; enlargement of ovary; ovarian region hard; menstrual colic beginning in ovary; pains in breast; pain in axilla; painful weakness and lameness in shoulder and arm; convulsions on side of face; pain in tragus; lung impervious to air; soreness, tenderness and sensation of weight in ovarian region; stitches in side of chest; dyspnœa; hepatization of lung; constant picking and boring of nostrils; no respiratory murmur in posterior superior half of lung; dulness in infraclavicular region; lying on side causes pain at heart; weight of arm on side is painful; hypertrophy of ventricle; lying on side with head high > suffocating; burning pain below nipple; swelling on neck; abscess near clavicle; abscess on side of neck; lameness in shoulder; weakness of arm and shoulder; arm nearly double its size; tingling and pricking in hand; shooting from hip to foot; knee as if sprained; near knee joint a bunch of varicose veins; sore place below lower edge of patella; hard red patch with scabs on calf of leg; flat

ulcers on leg; swelling of leg and foot; rheumatism <
side; side weak; side of body numb and cold; paralysis
of motory nerves of limb; severe pain shooting up side
of neck; veins in whole side of thorax up to throat
much dilated; eruption on forearm and side of abdomen;
index finger quadrupled in size; hand and forearm
much swollen; side partially paralyzed; granular swelling on side of throat; parotid enormously swollen; flat
open ulcers on leg; paralysis of leg; sensation absent in
arm; side of pharynx sore.
First r. then l.: semilateral headache; tonsils affected.
From above downwards: violent pressure in head; stitches
in kidneys; pressure from loins; pain from top of head.
From below upward: stitches in spine.
From below upward and backward: tearing pain in rectum.
From without inward: pressing in head.
From within outward: tearing on top of head; violent
pressing, burning pain in top of head; puffing pressure
in chest; cardiac pressure.
From l. to r.: pain in throat; diphtheria developed; discharge from nose; legs œdematous; erysipelas spreads;
ulceration in throat; ovarian tumors; rheumatic pain.
Changes locality: rheumatic pains; sciatica.
Sensations. Sensation as if she was somebody else; as if
frightened by visions behind him; as if knives were
being thrust into brow; as if brain would burst skull;
tongue as if bound or tied up; as if a part of r. side of
head was cut off; as if swollen in angle in front of
styloid process; back of head as if pressed asunder; as
if skin had been burnt by heat of sun; flickering before
eyes as from threads; stitches as from knives in eyes;
as if a thread was drawn from behind to eye; eyes as if
they had been taken out, squeezed, and then put back
again; as if eyes were forced out, when throat is pressed;
whizzing as from insects in ears; ears as if closed from
within; as if had moustache of ice; ears as if stuffed
up; as if tonsils were sore like a wound; as if sore;
skin as if it would crack; submaxillary joints as if
swollen; teeth as if too long; as if tongue was going
to peel; as if mucous membrane was peeling off; as
if desquamation was about to take place in velum
palati; as though he would suffocate; as if everything was raw in throat; as if parts of throat were
swollen; as if a small crumb was lodged in throat; as
of something in throat to swallow; as if lump, ball or
button in throat; distressed as if from loss of breath;
as if something was lodged in r. side of throat; throat
as if tied; feeling like a snake in throat; choking like

a ball; throat as if ulcerated; sticking as of a thousand
needles in throat; as if two lumps as large as fists came
together in throat; throat as if sore; throat as if raw;
as if fishbone had stuck in throat; as if a sponge was
hanging in throat; as if he could hawk it up; as if there
was a small dry spot from which pain extended to ear;
as if he had had a blow on neck; as if a thick substance
was in throat; feeling of large lump at back of throat;
as if some one grasped him by throat; retches as if
to vomit up lump; uvula looked as if squeezed and
crowded back; as though some one was pressing windpipe between thumb and fingers; odd motions with r.
arm as if reaching for something; teeth feel as if wedged;
tongue feels as if scalded; pain in liver as if ulcerated;
as if something had lodged in r. side; as if a ball was
rolling from r. side to stomach; as if a knife was
thrust through abdomen; griping as though about to
have diarrhœa; as if feces ascended to chest; throbbing as with little hammers in anus; as if from suppuration under ribs; arms feel as if closed; as of plug in
anus; as if sphincter was torn with effort; as of a ball
rolling about in bladder or abdomen; uterine region as
if swollen; as if a knife was thrust into abdomen;
uterus feels as if os was open; as if everything would
issue from vulva; as if pains from uterus and abdomen
ascended toward chest; as if everything was being
pressed out; as if bowels were cut with knives; as if a
stricture was in rectum; as if heart was hanging by a
thread, and every beat would tear it off; as of a skin in
larynx; as of talons sticking into larynx; as of a small
lump in pit of throat, like a button; as if a large mass
of mucus had accumulated in throat; choking as if suffocation was inevitable; as if something was in trachea
which might be raised; chest as if stuffed; as though
clothes hindered circulation; as if lungs were being
pressed into throat; as though a cord was tightly tied
around neck; as though heart turned over and ceased
beating for a moment; as if some fluid had gone into
wrong passage; as though there was an ulcer in stomach; as if lungs were pressed up into throat; as if chest
was full of wind; chest as if sore; like coals of fire from
chest through to shoulders; as if heart was too large for
cavity; as if heart was pressing against side or had not
free play; as if heart intermitted a single beat; heat as
from a hot stove on outer chest; burning as if in flesh of
chest; as if r. arm had gone to sleep; back as if lame and
weak; as if sinews in sacrum were too short; as if sitting
on something sharp; small of back as if sprained; wrists

as if sprained; hands cold as if dead; as of a hot iron from hip to foot; thighs as if swollen; as of a sprain in r. knee; as if hot air was going through knee joints; l. knee as if sprained; as if burnt in different places on tibia; burning as from fire in hypogastrium, loins and sternum; crawling as if asleep in arm and leg; as if epithelium was peeling off gums; as of a plug in throat; teeth feel as if wedged; tongue feels as if scalded; head as if drawn at base; skin around carbuncle as if too short; as if flesh was being torn from bones.

Pain: in l. temple and occiput; in forehead; in back part of hip and l. side; region of spleen; over eyes; top of head; in l. ovarian region; from superciliary ridge to occipital protuberance; deep in orbit of eyes; in l. side of abdomen; in back of head; in eye; deep in l. ear; in ears; in limbs; in stomach; in throat to nape of neck; on swallowing; in small spot in throat at one side of larynx; in top of throat; in l. side of throat extending to tongue, jaw and ear; in epigastrium; as though something was gnawing in stomach; in liver; in l. hypochondrium; in abdomen; in region of cæcum; from r. lumbar region through sacrum and inguinal region and forepart of thigh; in rectum; in r. ovarian region; in uterine region; in hypogastric region; in stomach; from l. breast to axilla down arm to hand; down arms; in pit of throat to root of tongue and to hyoid bone and to l. tragus, behind which it shoots out; in l. chest; pain in hemorrhoidal tumors; in chest; in heart; in nape of neck to distraction; in small of back; in coccygis; in os sacrum; in spine; in r. shoulder joint; in wrists; in wrist joints; in one small spot under shoulder; in red streak that ran up from wrist; changing locality, now in head, now in teeth, now in sciatic nerve; in thighs; in legs; in knee; in a sore place below lower edge of patella; in second toe of r. foot; in joints.

Sensitiveness of internal and external parts.

Intolerable colic.

Tension: from neck to eyelids; and thread, along arms and legs; in external parts.

Ulcerative pain: in internal parts.

Burning as from fire: in hypogastric region; in loins; behind sternum.

Agonizing pain: in back when rising from seat.

Intense pain: in head; down neck; in l. eye; in thigh; in arm and hand.

Violent pain: in head; in throat; over r. groin, extending either to genital organs or to liver and chest.

Severe pain: all over head; in and above eyes; from inner canthus upward and outward in a semicircle just above superciliary ridge in forehead; in limbs; in lumbar region; in epigastrium.

Terrible pain: in head; over eyes; in r. ovarian region.

Acute pain: in liver and towards stomach.

Great pains: in back and limbs; in heart; in ulcers on foot.

Anguish: about heart.

Horrid pains: all over head.

Sharp pain: at root of tongue; through lungs; extending from wrist to elbow.

Raging: in roots of lower teeth.

Violent, darting, stabbing pains: from upper part of forehead down to centre of head.

Lancinating pains: in breasts.

Lacerating pain: in legs.

Cutting, lacerating, burning pains: in abdomen.

Acute cutting, stinging pains: radiating from navel over upper portion of abdomen.

Cutting: in head; in teeth; in r. side of abdomen; in rectum; in abdomen; in l. breast.

Sharp, cutting. pains; when passing water.

Tearing pain: in temples; in whole l. side of head from temple to collar bone; in top of head; from zygoma into ear; in forehead and l. malar bone and under l. eye; in jawbones; in roots of lower teeth; in temples; in abdomen; in rectum; from nape of neck up either side to top of head; in knees.

Sharp, shooting pains: from eyes to temple; in l. ovary.

Shooting pain: into l. ear; in throat; in region of spleen; in rectum; from l. hip down to foot.

Piercing pains: in teeth.

Sticking cutting: in forepart of urethra.

Sticking: on vertex; in head; in ankle.

Stitching pain: in eyes; from stomach to chest; through r. side of chest; in back.

Stitches: in forehead; in chest; in eyes; in r. side; in rectum; in kidneys, downward and apparently through ureters; in ovary; in hemorrhoidal tumors, with cough; in l. side of chest; in upper part of back; in whole back.

Painful beating: in ears; in rectum.

Bursting pain: in temples.

Beating pain: in head; in vertex; in teeth.

Ulcerative pain: about liver; above and along ribs.

Boring: on vertex; behind l. ear; in jawbones; in teeth.

Pleuritic pains: in chest.

Throbbing pain: in temple; in vertex: in head; in jawbones; at outside of wrists.

Darting: from throat to occiput; in arm.
Hammering: in head.
Pulsating pains: in teeth.
Thrilling pain: at root of tongue.
Neuralgia: l. side orbital; horrible of trigeminus; in face; ovarian.
Rheumatic pains: in head; in legs; in knees.
Aching pain: in lumbar region; in forehead; in l. frontal eminence; r. side of head gradually going to l.; across loins; from occiput to eyes; in r. ear; in small of back; in thighs anteriorly; in branches of anterior crural nerve; in os hyoides; in knees; in shin bones.
Hard aching: all over; in head; back and legs; in uterus.
Dull aching: in sinciput.
Violent laborlike pressing from groins downward.
Acute colicky pains: low in abdomen.
Excessive griping: in abdomen.
Laborlike pains: in uterus.
Bearing down pains: in uterine region.
Gnawing: in stomach; in sides and deep into abdomen.
Cramps: in abdomen; in chest.
Cramplike pains: in abdomen; in præcordial region.
Menstrual colic: beginning in l. ovary.
Spasmodic colic.
Sensation of incarcerated flatus.
Sticking, drawing pain: in r. eye; in l. eye; in throat.
Dull sticking: in roots of lower teeth.
Stinging, burning pains: in panaritium.
Burning stinging: of skin.
Burning, throbbing pain: in boils on spine.
Burning pain: in top of head; in vertex; in eyes; in mouth; in rectum; in l. ovary; in wrists.
Burning heat: in epigastrium; in hypogastric and lumbar regions; from hip to foot; behind sternum.
Stinging: through ears; in throat; in r. side; in r. arm; in tips of fingers; in knees; all over.
Sore pain: in urethra; in forepart of penis.
Smarting: in l. throat.
Burning: in vertex; of eyes; of erysipelas in face; of face; of tongue and lips; of swelling of throat; in anus; in rectum; when urinating; in chest; in icy cold hands; in finger ends; in hands; terrible deep in hand; of eczema on legs; in palms and soles.
Pricking pain: in upper and lower extremities.
Dull, stinging pain: in stomach.
Heat: in forehead; in l. throat; in occipital and cervical regions.
Heavy pain: in forehead to back and all over head.

Dull pain: in forehead; in legs; over and in eyes; in bladder.

Pressing pains: in eyes; in umbilical region; in l. ovary; from loins to privates.

Tensive pain: from neck over head to eyes; in l. ovary.

Drawing pain: in l. temple; from eyes to occiput; in jawbones; in teeth; from anus to umbilicus; in ovarian region; intolerable in small of back and down into legs; up back; from back to hips.

Spasmodic pains: in anus internally; in heart; in elbow.

Throbbing: in anus; in rectum.

Soreness: of neck; at vertex; of mouth; in throat; of nostrils and lips; of internal nose; of internal throat; in l. side of throat; of external throat; about pelvic region; of larynx; of r. shoulder.

Soreness: in region of spleen; across bowels.

Sore feeling: in eyeballs.

Scraping: in throat.

Rawness: of throat.

Bruised feeling: in hips.

Painful pressure: in rectum; when making water.

Gnawing pressure: in stomach.

Laborlike pressure: from loins downwards.

Violent pressure: on top of head; in stomach.

Pressure: in orbits; in stomach; severe in a small spot between epigastrium and navel; in bowels; upon bladder.

Oppressive pain: in one or other temple; in chest.

Painful contraction: in throat.

Painful sensitiveness: in l. temple, from vertex down and in l. side of face.

Great sensitiveness: of lower abdomen.

Tenderness: of scalp; in l. iliac region; in epigastrium; in whole spine; of body.

Peculiar painful sensation of weakness and lameness: in l. shoulder and arm.

Distress: at stomach.

Painful weariness: of face, neck and head.

Extraordinary weakness: diphtheria.

Weak feeling: in abdomen; in knees; in l. shoulder and arm; in legs.

Sinking, fluttering feeling: in epigastrium.

Uneasiness: in lower limbs.

Contractive tightness: in region of liver; in abdomen.

Throbbing, choking sensation: in throat.

Choking sensation: in throat.

Suffocative sensation: in throat.

Dry, stuffed feeling: through whole front of head.

Stuffed feeling: in ears.

Feeling of obstruction: in throat.'
Smothered feeling: in chest.
Strumming: through limbs.
Twitching: in eyes; of hands.
Jerking: in r. eye; in lower teeth; in teeth; from thighs to genitals; in legs.
Trembling: in whole body; of limbs and internally; of tongue.
Pricking: in l. hand; in finger ends; in extremities of fingers.
Crawling: on l. side.
Titillation: behind sternum.
Tickling: after blowing nose; at root of tongue; in throat; in pit of stomach; from thighs to genital organs; in larynx; in pit of throat and sternum.
Tingling; in l. hand; in toes.
Dryness: of mouth; of throat.
Weight: in head; on vertex; in bowels; in l. ovarian region; on chest.
Heaviness: of head; in occiput; in stomach; in region of liver.
Confused feeling: in head.
Full feeling: of chest.
Fulness: in throat; in head; in region of liver; in bowels; in trachea; at heart.
Dull oppression: in breathing.
Oppression: of chest.
Constriction: of anus; in rectum; of throat; of chest; about heart.
Dulness: in occiput; in l. infraclavicular region.
Paralyzed feeling: in thigh after pain has gone.
Lameness: in l. shoulder.
Numbness: in occiput; of l. side; about ear and cheek; of arm.
Numb feeling: on l. side of head; about head.
Stiffness: of neck; in malar bone; of knees; painful from loins down into thighs; in sacrum; in knees.
Emptiness: of stomach.
Coldness: over whole body; of limbs; of upper lip.
Itching pain: in l. ovary.
Itching: of scalp; of eyes; of eruption under eyes; of lower lid; of facial erysipelas; of face; of rectum; of anus; on arms, hips and lower limbs; in hands; in different places on tibia; of eczema on legs; of feet and ankles; of pustules in palms of hands; in internal parts.
" Tissues. Emaciation, with muscular relaxation; skin and muscles lax.
 Great tenderness of all flesh; it is exceedingly difficult to

handle the child at all; the least touch seems to hurt it, and to leave a deeper blueness, like a bruise.

❚❚Hemorrhages, blood dark, incoagulable; typhoid.

❚❚Affections produced by blood poisoning; pyæmia.

❚Venous stasis with a direct paralytic-like affection of medulla spinalis combined with general anæmia.

❚❚Bluish color of affected parts; cyanosis.

❚Small wounds bleed much.

❚Purpura. θScorbutic purpura.

❚Inflammation of internal organs with suppuration.

❚Veins on whole l. thorax up to throat much dilated.

❚Menopausia troubles, especially when capillary circulation is affected.

❚❚Dropsy; from liver, spleen and heart disease; after scarlatina; urine black, legs œdematous, first l. then r.

❚❚Cellulitis, with burning and blue color of skin.

❚❚Ulcers sensitive to touch; ichorous, offensive discharge; many small pimples surround them; areolæ purple; > from warmth.

❚❚Gangrene, or carbuncles from blood poisoning.

❚Malignant local inflammations, with secondary blood infection and nervous prostration.

❚Circumscribed gangrene; idiopathic and traumatic; of tongue; of foot.

❚❚Suppuration, particularly in internal parts.

❚Traumatic gangrene, restores vitality to parts apparently dead and induces renewed circulation without sloughing.

❚❚Malignant pustule.

❚❚Sphacelus.

❚❚Gangrena senilis.

❚Melanosis, colloid and encephaloid cancer; violent burning, gangrenous spots.

❚Ulcers and wounds bleed readily and profusely.

" **Touch. Passive Motion. Injuries.** Touch: cannot bear shirt or neckband on throat; can scarcely bear clothes to touch lower abdominal region; temple sore; on throat causes darting; face sensitive; lower jaw sensitive; throat swollen and sensitive; pit of stomach sore; liver sensitive; stomach sensitive; slightest, causes excruciating pain in abdomen; ileo-cæcal region sensitive; uterine region sensitive; womb sensitive; nipple sore; a spot on anterior portion of neck tender; larynx sensitive; pit of throat painful; neck sore; on larynx causes suffocative attacks; on throat causes cough; infraclavicular region sensitive; nape of neck painful; shoulder and arm sensitive; hands sensitive; ulcers on legs bleed and burn; ulcers sensitive; produces black and bluish spots.

Taking hold of throat causes nausea.

Cannot bear bonnet strings tied tight.

Does not like hair touched.

Hernia will not admit handling.

Pressure: bursting pains in temples; pain in front of styloid process $<$; on throat causes sensation as if eyes were forced out; on throat causes severe pain; pain in r. ovary; tumor in breast painful; larynx sore; cough $<$; on larynx causes cough; capillaries fill quite slowly; nape of neck sensitive; of finger on spine of neck sends pain to brain; on dorsal spine sends pain to stomach; swelling on hand sensitive; toe painful.

Cannot bear pressure: about neck, hypochondria, abdomen, stomach and l. iliac region.

Abdomen sensitive to weight of clothes.

Uterus does not bear contact and has to be relieved of all pressure; frequently lifts clothes, they cause uneasiness.

Feels $>$ if held firmly or pressed down.

After scratching at night on calf: an ulcer.

When effort is made to lift or move babe it cries out.

Shock from injuries.

After a fall: ulcer on r. leg, with varicose swelling.

After running nail into foot: small ulcer.

∎Gangrene of hand, ten days after a bullet wound in hand.

∎Wound in hand from explosion of a pistol; fifth day gangrene.

∎Hydrophobia.

∎From dissecting wound in finger that member very much swollen, hand and forearm much swollen and œdematous; a hard red line extended from wrist to axilla; axillary glands swollen; arm and hand intensely painful; whole l. side partially paralyzed; extreme prostration; low muttering delirium at night; marked aggravation on waking; abscesses formed under deep fibrous tissues of finger and hand.

∎Dog bite (seven cases); in two adult males who used alcoholic drinks there were shudderings and flushes of heat at intervals of a few weeks for two years.

∎After compound fracture of leg six or eight gangrenous spots, as large as a dime, and each point marked by a black blister which broke and revealed circular spots of gangrene; livid appearance of skin; delirium on closing eyes; $<$ after sleep. θGangrene.

Compound comminuted leg fracture, terminating in gangrene and threatening speedy destruction of limb.

∎Gangrene of finger which had been mashed; on fourth day after injury shooting pains from finger to wrist and up arm; on fifth day fetid odor and some grey

blisters indicated gangrene; next day line of demarcation formed entirely around finger; patient restless, cheerful beyond reason; by twelfth day all traces of gangrene
had disappeared; no tissue lost by sloughing.

A man a week ago was struck by corner of a heavy box on
inner surface of leg and cutting down into calf; leg much
inflamed; leeches were applied; severe chill; since chill
nothing has remained on his stomach; severe pains set
〳 in, whole of wound and two leech bites gangrenous;
very severe headache; breath very fetid; sleepless, his
shining eyes constantly in motion; tongue trembling;
pulse 110, small and irregular.

❙Elderly lady was bitten by a pet cat through ball of
thumb; whole hand and arm swollen and painful;
thumb suppurated and for months resisted all efforts
to heal.   *θ*Carbuncle.

❙Bedsores in typhoid fever; ulcers red and inflamed, with
black edges.

❙Small wounds bleed much.

❙Old chronic flat ulcers on lower limbs, with discolored
areolæ.

" Skin.   ❙Itching over whole body, burning; yellow or purplish blisters; scabies.

❙Itching intense, almost driving to distraction, mostly at
night, but also by paroxysms in daytime; often changing to a severe, burning stinging sensation.   *θ*Pustular
eruption.

❙Skin dry and burning.   *θ*Diphtheritis.   *θ*Scarlatina.

❙Jaundice.   *θ*Hepatitis.   *θ*Typhoid.

❙❙Red lumps and tubercles.

❙❙Rash all over; small smooth spots size of a needle point.

❙❙Yellow, red and copper colored spots.

❙Ecchymosis; purple or black spots.

❙❙Purpura hæmorrhagia.

❙Bluish black swellings; dark blue blisters.

❙Body covered with bluish red eruption, round and elevated.   *θ*Diphtheria.

❙Child, æt. 1, had gums lanced, bled five days, finally flow
arrested, but child became cachectic and dropsical;
black and blue spots appeared all over him; least touch
or pressure produced them; much < after sleeping; extreme deathly paleness.

❙❙Small reddish spots on face, neck and arms.

❙Miliary eruption; rash appears slowly or turns livid or
black; comatose.

❙High fever; stitching pain on r. side of chest and back;
thick patches of exanthema on r. side, from spine
to sternum, and from fifth to ninth ribs; at first erup-

tion vesicular, then pustular; whole surface of skin
occupied by eruption, very red and swollen, especially
intense around margin of each patch; high fever, adynamic in character, slight morning remission; on fifth
day pains in back unbearable; several groups of pustules near spine have a hemorrhagic appearance,
gradually spread from one group to another until it
reached axillary line; sufferings of patient almost unendurable; will take no food except a small quantity of
soup and wine; great prostration from loss of sleep,
from pain. θHerpes zoster after external application
of *Rhus tox.*

ıFor last twenty years, eruption on l. forearm and on l.
lower abdomen; eruption begins as a small boil which
disappears, leaving a dry, scaly, itching eruption; then
other boils appear successively, all going through same
process; this goes on until most space between elbow
and wrist, and a space as large as palm of hand on lower
abdomen is covered with itching dry eruption; > for
a few weeks, when little boil reappears and same process
is gone over.

ııOld reddish herpes, with thick scurf in region of whis-
kers; reappearance of suppressed herpes in face.

ıPale, chlorotic, emaciated; blackish or bluish blisters
with sanious, fetid contents. θHerpetic ulcers.

ıVesicles large, usually of yellow color first, and then turning dark with much pain; vesicles break and leave an
excoriated surface, which burns when touched; eruptions every Spring and Fall; < from acids. θHerpes.

ııVesicular eruption, with a red crown.

ııRed spots, with vesicles on fingers and thighs.

ııEruption of yellow or purplish blisters.

ııBullæ dark from bloody serum within. θPemphigus.

ııGangrenous blisters.

ıNew pustules and at same time many of older ulcers and
scabs surrounded by blue halo; veins of legs enlarged
from pregnancy, unusually blue and knotty, almost appearance of incipient gangrene; itching, burning and
stinging pains.

ıPustules size of pea to five cent piece, on back, legs and
particularly about ankles; isolated pustules, rapidly
filled with sero-purulent matter and surrounded by an
inflamed halo came in small crops; these pustules soon
dried into hard, dry scabs easily knocked off, leaving
red moist surfaces sensitive to contact with atmosphere
or bedclothes.

ıConfluent smooth, round, white pustules of size of a mustard seed in palms of hands; they contained a white
fluid and itched intolerably.

▮Index finger of l. hand quadrupled in size; hand and forearm much swollen and œdematous, a hard red line extending from wrist to axilla; axillary glands swollen; arm and hand intensely painful; whole l. side partially paralyzed; extreme prostration, causing disease to be at first mistaken for typhus, low muttering delirium at night; marked aggravation of suffering and prostration on awaking from sleep; abscesses forming under deep fibrous tissues of finger and hand. θSepticæmia, result of dissecting wound.

▮Swelling assumes a purplish hue, and patient commences to be delirious as soon as he closes his eyes; bloated red face, attended by heat; coldness of extremities; tendency to faint, with numbness; swelling of part is not great, but firm; suppuration occurs in spots, does not discharge, but dries up into cheesy mass, which is revealed by skin covering it drying up and peeling off; sometimes bullæ containing dark colored serum. θErysipelas.

▮Erysipelas contracted while dissecting; has been sick a week; face swollen, bluish red, or leaden hue; tongue dry, glossy, tremulous; < from weight of clothes, from noon until midnight.

▮▮Dark red, very large and thick swelling, soft as dough when touched.

▮▮Varicose veins ulcerate.

▮Bedsores in typhoid fever; ulcers red and inflamed, with black edges.

▮Furuncular formation, generally upon lower lip, attended with severe pain and frequently surrounded by erysipelatous areola; rapid and excessive loss of strength, reduced from vigor to absolute prostration within twenty-four hours. θEpidemic malignant pustule.

▮Bluish color of pustule, and red streaks along lymphatic vessels. θMalignant pustule.

▮Immense carbuncle, six inches in diameter, appeared in dorsal region to r. of spine, attended with rigors, nocturnal sweat, fever and prostration. θAfter bite of a cat.

▮Dark redness around sore, which discharges dark, bloody pus; tension of skin around carbuncle, as if too short; nightly burning in ulcer, obliging one to rise and wash it with cold water. θAnthrax.

▮Black and blue spots; ecchymoses all over body; least touch or pressure produces them; tenderness of body; deathly paleness of face; < after sleep. θAnasarca.

▮After scarlet fever, upon going out into air before desquamation had occurred, swelling up of whole body, scrotum as large as child's head, urine diminished, respiration oppressed; on l. side of throat glandular swelling, extending up behind ear.

∎Inflammation slow; skin over dead cellular tissue little disposed to ulcerate, and when finally perforated in three or four places, discharge scanty, thin, sometimes bloody; great prostration. θCarbuncle.

∎Man, had suffered for several years from a succession of carbuncles and indolent boils; lately four successive carbuncles, none of which ran a complete course; after each of these carbuncles patient's health deteriorated, until, after last, took to bed, with hectic fever; an abscess deep in adductor muscles of thigh being opened, discharged about a quart of pus; formation and discharge of pus continued profuse; patient rapidly growing feeble, with severe hectic; loss of appetite; great local suffering. θCarbuncle (seven weeks afterwards remnants of four carbuncles inflamed, abscesses formed and sloughs were discharged; abscesses occurring in inverse order of original appearance of carbuncle).

∎Purplish color of affected part; erysipelas spreads from l. to r. θErysipelas neonatorum.

∎∎Marked swelling and redness of throat, with difficulty of swallowing, elevated papillæ on tongue, severe pain in head, flushed and turgid appearance of face, great restlessness, eruption of miliary character, or when it fails to come to the surface. θScarlet fever.

∎∎Sore throat and great difficulty in swallowing; fever; pulse 120, quick and small; throat sore to touch externally; as yet no eruption. θScarlet fever.

∎Pleuritic, pericarditic and general dropsy in delayed desquamation, with great prostration. θScarlatina.

∎Scarlet fever and scarlet eruptions, with swelling of cervical glands, black lips and reddish tongue.

∎∎Throat symptoms assume a virulent character; signs of blood poisoning and prostration. θScarlatina.

∎Lies on back with open mouth; l. parotid enormously swollen; tongue dry and loaded with drying, offensive mucus, extending back upon pharynx, obstructing passage of throat; nose stopped with bloody mucus, having dried down, thoroughly impacting both nasal passages, high up; eyes turned back; could not be aroused in least from most profound stupor; pulse compressible and small. θMalignant scarlatina.

∎Cankerous ulcers spread from mouth to near chin, with sanious discharges from nostrils and throat; constantly recurring spasms of almost entire muscular system; vibratory movements in spasms, short and tremulous. θScarlatina.

▮▮Scarlatina maligna, advanced stages, typhoid states, threatening gangrene; destructive decomposition of both fluids and solids.

▮Boy, æt. 9, had scarlet fever under allopathic treatment, survived swelling on l. side of neck followed, which suppurated, abscess opened with lancet, afterwards boy declined in flesh, strength and appetite; much exhausted; face pale, dirty, dingy; puffy, no appetite; restless, hot, dry skin; peevish and whining; abscess discharging foul and copious pus; very sensitive to all motions of head; a large cavity, no appearance of healthy granulations; pulse 140 and small; motions of jaw in masticating solid food could not be borne.

▮Alternate delirium and stupor; irrational, slow muttering delirium; pulse soft, wavy, quick; calor mordax; respiration attended by moaning; rapid, whistling; occasional single cough; grasping at throat, as if to tear away clothing from it; pupils widely dilated; urine scanty, constipation; countenance cadaverous; breath putrescent. θRepercussion of measles.

▮Girl, æt. 9, had, during previous winter, scarlatina very severely; it left her delicate and deaf; was exposed to measles; six days after, rash appeared with a copious discharge from ears; two days later, discharge suddenly ceased and rash disappeared; immediately became feeble and prostrate; wild, muttering delirium; great thirst, drinking little at a time; singularly biting heat of skin next day; pulse soft, wavy; hardly to be counted; calor mordax; moaning respiration, rapid, whistling; occasionally a single cough with a moan after each cough, and a grasping at throat, as if to tear away clothing from it; pupils widely dilated; no stool for two days; urine scanty and seldom passed; countenance cadaverous; breath putrescent.

▮Livid eruption; countenance almost black; tongue coated dark brown, sordes on teeth, inability to protrude tongue. θMeasles.

▮▮Black measles.

▮Itching on whole body, hands and feet; after burning pains there appeared vesicles, with much itching, throbbing, heat, there formed a diffuse, red swelling, some vesicles as large as a nut, at first filled with water, but afterwards containing pus; a good deal of inflammation about parts; some pustules dark blue, with burning, throbbing pain in swelling, as if flesh was being torn from bones; pains attack head, teeth, breast, back; severe, burning pain in head, causing sense of sickness and nausea; throbbing in head at every movement; stu-

pefied sleep after attacks; pains < at night; constant
thirst but drinking makes her sick; sometimes itching
goes off, then she is short of breath and full of
anxiety. θItch.

∎After scratching at night on calf, an ulcer size of a dollar,
discolored, very painful.

∎Peculiar bluish red or livid appearance of ulcers.

∎Malignant ulcers; bleed readily; discharge bad smelling
ichor; deep, filthy suppuration; gangrenous; indolent,
with blue color.

∎Flat open ulcers on l. leg, with erysipelas.

∎∎Ulcers, surrounded by pimples, vesicles and smaller
ulcers.

∎Areola of ulcer assumes a bluish color. θSycosis.

∎Ulcer dried up by washes; on taking cold a few weeks
after her entire foot and ankle broke out into small
ulcers, resembling original sore; great pain in ulcers;
itching of feet and ankles, almost unbearable; leg <
after sleep and > from warmth. θIndolent ulcer.

∎Chronic indolent ulcers of legs, flat, with purple skin;
many small sores around main ulcer, which has an uneven bottom, burning and bleeding, even when lightly
touched; ichorous, offensive discharge.

∎Ulcers small and scattered about upon neck and face.

∎Skin around ulcers and wounds is yellow, green, lead
colored, bluish red or black.

∎Superficial ulcers, foul at bottom, with red crowns.

∎Brownish red areola about ulcer became blackish blue.

∎Flat ulcers with a bluish white base.

∎Spreading, superficial, shallow ulcer; paralysis of l. leg.

∎Burning in ulcers at night.

∎Chronic indolent ulcers, with an uneven bluish bottom
and offensive odor.

∎Painful ulcers, sometimes with proud flesh.

∎Pain in old cicatrices of ulcers; old red scars reopen.

∎Spongeous ulcerations of syphilitic origin.

∎Cancerous ulceration, putrefaction, flesh falls off piecemeal.

∎∎Boy, æt. 10, large sore on centre of forehead, covered
with a hard black scab, tissue around hard and inflamed; puffy swelling extended down on both sides of
neck, which was much swollen, as were his lips; on
taking a swallow of water grasped throat and evinced
greatest pain; face very red but mottled white; ears burning hot to touch yet pulse but 85, irregular and softish;
picked at hair continually; every few minutes twitching of arms; throat swollen and red; next morning tonsils covered with dirty white membrane; in evening
abundant scarlet rash; bleeding of dark blood from
nose and mouth.

ǀǀChronic ulcers of legs (probably of syphilitic origin); discharge ceased, extremity œdematous; a hard, slightly red swelling, extending up course of principal veins; great and sudden prostration; low muttering delirium, general typhoid symptoms. θSecondary phlebitis.

ǀǀCarbuncles, with purple surroundings and many small boils around them; must rise at night and bathe to allay burning; also when suppuration is tardy and systemic weakness obtains; cannot bear bandages.

ǀMalignant furuncles, very painful, turn blue and spread.

ǀǀSore spots become fungoid, dark red to brownish, with whitish spots; burning on wiping.

ǀǀFungus hæmatoides.

ǀSpots yellow, green, red, lead and copper colored, pale, livid; hard and pale swelling; ulcers surrounded by nodes and vesicles; muscles fall off in shreds from bone; loss of sensation; toes fall off. θLeprosy.

ǀǀSensation absent in l. arm; toes fall off; l. side of pharynx sore, with suppurating ulcers; menstruation alternately profuse and absent. θLeprosy.

ǀǀBedsores, with black edges.

ǀScars redden, hurt, break open and bleed.

ǀWarts.

[47] **Stages of Life, Constitution.** ǀAffections of meagre, weak, melancholy persons, or of those who are chlorotic, with sickly complexion; women at climacteric period, with frequent metrorrhagia and hot flushes, burning vertex, headaches, pain in back, or hot flushes by day and cold flashes by night, insomnia, < in afternoon, evening and after sleep; throat diseases commence on l. side—rheumatism on right.

ǀǀBetter adapted to thin and emaciated than to fat persons; or adapted to those who have been changed both mentally and physically by their illness.

ǀSuits people with a vivid imagination.

ǀMelancholic or choleric temperament, with phlegmatic constitution; with dark eyes and disposition to lowness of spirits and indolence.

ǀBilious temperament.

ǀǀWomen of choleric temperament, freckles and red hair.

ǀDark eyes, disposed to sluggishness and indolence.

ǀǀClimacteric ailments; hemorrhoids, hemorrhages, hot flushes, burning vertex headaches; especially after cessation of flow.

ǀWomen who have not recovered from change of life, "have never felt well since that time."

ǀDrunkards; headaches, hemorrhoids; prone to erysipelatoid inflammations.

▮Erysipelas of old people.

▮After onanism. θEpilepsy.

▮People injured by mercurial treatment.

▮▮In all syphilitic mercurial diseases. θTertiary syphilis.

Infant, æt. 2 months; cyanosis.

Girl, infant, æt. 6 months; malignant erysipelas.

Girl, æt. 9 months; diphtheria.

Child, æt. 9 months, scrofulous; diphtheria.

Boy, æt. 1, scrofulous, apparently healthy, had incisors lanced, obstinate hemorrhage ensued, which was finally stopped by perchloride of iron; anasarca.

Child, æt. 21 months, light complexion, blue eyes; bronchial catarrh.

Boy, æt. 2; membranous croup.

Girl, æt. 3, blonde, spare built.

Child, æt. 3; typhoid fever.

Girl, æt. 4, light hair, blue eyes, slight build; suppuration of lungs.

Boy, æt. 4; diphtheria.

Boy, æt. 5, attends school, previous good health, suffering six weeks; brain irritation.

Girl, æt. 5, dark straight hair and blue eyes, when two years old had caries of dorsal vertebræ; paralysis of legs and chest affection.

Boy, æt. 5, in good health and spirits, has abscess on wrist; convulsions.

Girl, æt. 6; diphtheria.

Boy, æt. 6, epileptic, with thick head, pale, bloated look, delicate constitution, suffering fourteen days; diphtheria.

Child, after being frostbitten; tetanus.

Boy; post-diphtheritic eye affection.

Boy, sick five days; diphtheria.

Girl, after excessive study; mental disorder.

Girl, æt. 6; ague.

Girl, æt. 6; diphtheria.

Boy, æt. 8, suffering five days; diphtheria.

Boy, æt. 8, cold contracted in wet weather; bronchial catarrh.

Girl, æt. 8; diphtheria.

Boy, æt. 8; diphtheria.

Boy, æt. 8; affection of throat.

Boy, æt. 8, scrofulous; scarlatina.

Girl, æt. 8, light red hair, nervous and sensitive, bright and cheerful when well, after having ears pierced; chorea.

Girl, æt. 9, a few months ago had scarlatina, which left her delicate and deaf, nine days ago exposed to measles, two days ago rash appeared along with copious discharge from ears, now rash and discharge both disappear; repercussion of measles.

Girl, æt. 9, frightened when three years old by snake; affection of mind.

Boy, æt 9, fair skin, dark eyes, short stature, well developed, healthy; after scarlatina abscess on l. side of neck.

Boy, æt. 9, pale, weakly, subject to epileptiform spasms; diphtheritis.

Girl, æt. 9; diphtheria.

Girl, æt. 10; pharyngitis.

Boy, æt. 10, suffering from scarlatina, upon going out before desquamation; dropsy.

Boy, æt. 10; scarlatina.

Boy, æt. 10, highly nervous temperament, psoric taint; scarlet fever.

Girl, æt. 10; diphtheria.

Boy, æt. 12; affection of knee.

Girl, æt. 12, healthy looking, suffering eight days; affection of throat.

Girl, æt. 13; typhoid fever.

Boy, æt. 14; tonsillitis.

Boy, æt. 16, strong and active, red hair, dark eyes, freckled complexion; peritonitis.

Girl, æt. 16, light complexion; typhoid.

Girl, æt. 16; tonsillitis.

Boy, æt. 17, subject to inflammation of throat; angina.

Girl, æt. 18, governess, robust constitution, suffering a week without perceptible cause; neuralgia.

Girl, æt. 18; diphtheria.

Girl, æt. 20, blonde, slim, mild disposition; erysipelas.

Weakly girl, æt. 20; diarrhœa.

Girl, æt. 20, bilious temperament, full habit, from sitting on stool and practicing at piano, suffering four years; affection of spine.

Woman, æt. 20, after giving birth to child which died on fourth day of erysipelas; peritonitis.

Girl, æt. 20, blonde, thin, mild temperament; erysipelas on leg and foot.

Woman, æt. 20, strong; angina.

Young man, tall, active, dark hair and eyes; diphtheria.

Young man, scrofulous, weak, has had for several years eczema on arms and leg ulcers; tonsillitis.

Young lady, bilious lymphatic temperament, suffering ten years; constipation.

Young woman, delicate, nervous temperament; diphtheria.

Young woman, married, refined sensibilities; mental disturbance.

Young man; phthisical habit, had been coughing two months; pulmonary tuberculosis.

Young man, weakened by disease and medicine and further by fracture of clavicle; affection of r. hand.

Strong young man; affection of second toe of r. foot.

Young man, after excessive study; glossomania.

Young man, phthisical habit, emaciated, six months ago
had pneumonia ; lung affection.

Young, robust sea captain, previously suffered from abscess
of throat; affection of throat.

Girl, æt. 20, after taking purgative medicine for some
digestive troubles; diarrhœa.

Man, æt. 21, scrofulous; angina.

Man, æt. 22; pharyngitis.

Man, æt. 22, physician, result of wound incurred during
post mortem examination of a case of puerperal peritonitis; septicæmia.

Man, æt. 23; pneumonia.

Girl, æt. 23; epilepsy.

Woman, æt. 23, slender build, premature labor; puerperal
convulsions.

Woman, æt. 24, multipara, small, fair, nervous, sanguine
temperament; puerperal convulsions.

Man, æt. 24, wears glasses; asthenopia.

Woman, æt. 24, brunette; facial neuralgia.

Man, æt. 25, medium height, fair complexion, muscular,
and accustomed to outdoor exercise; chronic irritability
of fauces.

Girl, æt. 26; diphtheria.

Man, æt. 28, small, brown hair, during childhood frequent
convulsions, after being cured of caries; epilepsy.

Woman, æt. 28, sunstroke two years previous to confinement, from which she had ever since been confined to
bed; puerperal convulsions.

Woman, æt. 28, suffering several weeks; partial deafness.

Man, æt. 29, suffering since fourteenth year; epilepsy.

Woman, æt. 30, medium height, dark complexion, black
hair, subject to swelling of glands and morbid discharges
from mucous membranes, had three abortions, now in
eighth month of pregnancy; pustular eruption.

Woman, æt. 30; chronic affection of larynx.

Woman, æt. 30, brunette, nursing 5 months; thin milk.

Woman, æt. 30, married, weak constitution, tuberculous
tendency; tumor in breast.

Man, æt. 30, another 23; fever.

Man, æt. 30, laborer, after injury : gangrene of leg.

Woman, æt. 30, single; pharyngitis.

Married woman, æt. 30, tuberculous, weakly constitution,
somewhat emaciated and pale, skin dry; since ten years
no child; tumor in l. mamma.

Woman, æt. 31, unmarried, suffering for many years; headache.

Woman, æt. 32, married, after night watching; convulsions.

Woman, æt. 32, brunette, choleric temperament; mania.

Man, æt. 32, sanguine nervous temperament; ague.

Countess V., æt. 33, after rubbing a mixture of *Rhus tox.* and alcohol upon abdomen for a strain of uterine ligament; herpes zoster.

Man, editor; typhoid fever.

Man, plethoric, tendency to hydrothorax; periodic asthma.

Man, after mercurial treatment; syphilis.

Lady, worn out with solicitude and care of a sick friend, had delirium followed by convulsions.

Woman, æt. 40, one year without catamenia; erysipelas on foot joint.

Woman, slender form, menstrual irregularities; aphonia.

Woman, married; effects of domestic troubles; melancholy.

Woman, weakly, sensitive mind, during climacteric, after grief at death of husband and loss of fortune; affection of throat.

Woman, after taking charge of child with itch; itch.

Woman, married many years, but never pregnant; chronic uterine catarrh. (Afterwards bore a child.)

Woman, post diphtheritic affection.

Woman, subject Spring and Fall to acute pneumonia; had been treated for many years allopathically; ovaritis.

Woman, wasted, slim, pale; ulcers on legs.

Woman, æt. 35, sickly and weak, slim, strong bones, bilious constitution, mild temper; infiltration on the back.

Man, æt. 35, pharyngitis.

Man, æt. 35; diphtheria.

Man, æt. 39, dark complexioned, emaciated, eight weeks ago operation for fistula in ano, suffering four weeks; mental disorder.

Woman, æt. 40, single, large and fleshy, subject to attacks of catarrh for fifteen years; bronchial catarrh.

Woman, æt. 40, suffering 20 years; hysteria.

Man, æt. 40; gangrene of hand.

Man, æt. 40, after receiving wound on head by falling off horse; gangrene of wound.

Woman, æt. 40, has not menstruated for one year; erysipelas.

Woman, æt. 40, tall, slender, pale; ulcers on legs.

Woman, æt. 40; indolent ulcer.

Man, æt. 40, phthisical; ulcers on legs.

Man, æt. 40; bee sting.

Woman, æt. 42, mother of two children, sanguine bilious temperament; asthma.

Woman, æt. 42, sanguine bilious temperament; asthma.

Woman, æt. 43, married; irritation of meninges of brain and spinal cord.

Woman, æt. 43; ulcers on leg.

Lady, æt. 43, slim, large, cachectic, scrofulous; intestinal croup.

Woman, widow, æt. 43; catalepsy during climaxis.

Woman, æt. 45, full habit, nervous, light hair, blue eyes, lively disposition, suffering for years; headache.

Married woman, æt. 45; chronic nasal catarrh.

Woman, æt. 48, 18 months after climaxis, catamenia had been copious, very dark, had been subject to congestion towards head and chest; swelling of r. ovary.

Woman, æt. 48, bilious, nervous temperament, has for many years, every Spring and Fall, had acute pneumonia, for which she was salivated, bled, blistered and purged; general breakdown.

Woman, æt. 49, seamstress, for three years; cephalalgia.

Woman, climacteric period; anal fistula.

Man, æt. 45, suffering three weeks; spasm of glottis.

Man, æt. 45, full habit and bilious temperament; functional disturbance of heart.

Man, æt. 48, subject to follicular pharyngitis; pharyngitis.

Man, æt. 49, light complexioned, suffering five days; sciatica.

Woman, æt. 50, just passed critical period, suffering six months; affection of anus and rectum.

Woman, æt. 50; itch.

Woman, æt. 50; chronic affection of larynx.

Woman, æt. 50; foreign body in œsophagus.

Woman, æt. 50, phlegmatic, sanguine temperament, small stature, father and brother died of heart disease; attacks of dyspnœa and palpitation of heart.

Woman, æt. 50, large and fleshy, at critical period, had suffered several years with dilatation of l. ventricle, aorta and carotid artery; bronchial catarrh.

Woman, æt. 51, after sudden suppression of menses by a mental emotion; rheumatism of vagus.

Woman, æt. 52, married, leuco-phlegmatic, very fat, suffering for twenty years; eruption on arm and abdomen.

Woman, æt. 52; sacculated ovarian disease.

Woman, æt. 53, plethoric, robust, choleric; ulcer on leg.

Woman, æt. 56, passing through climacteric period; affection of liver.

Man, æt. 57, nervous bilious temperament, dark hair and skin, suffering thirty-five years; eczema.

Man, æt. 60, married, subject five years to occasional attacks of severe pains in back of head; convulsions.

Man, æt. 60, strong, well built, full chest, blue eyes, suffering since he was six years old; headache.

Elderly woman, thin and cachectic; phthisis pulmonalis.

Lady, æt. 60, tall, dark, leathery skin, feeble, thin, nervo-
bilious, fond of good living; tertian ague.

Man, æt. 60, strong, well built, blue eyes; headache.

Woman, æt. 65, stout, fleshy, for many years periodical
attacks from hepatic apostema.

Woman, æt. 69; ulcers on legs.

Woman, æt. 70, suffering six months; bronchial catarrh.

Woman, æt. 76, suffering a long time from suffocative
cough; chest affection.

Man, æt. 80; vertigo.

Man, æt. 86; sciatica.

⁴⁸ **Relations.** Antidoted by: Radiate heat outwardly, alcohol
inwardly; salt. The dilutions are antidoted by: *Alum.*,
Arsen., *Bellad.*, *Coccul.*, *Coffea*, *Hepar*, *Mercur.*, *Nitr. ac.*,
Nux vom., *Phos. ac.*, according to effects.

It antidotes: effects of *Bufo*, *Crotal.*, *Rhus tox.*

Compatible: *Acon.*, *Arsen.*, *Bellad.*, *Bromum*, *Carbo veg.*,
Cinchona, *Hepar*, *Hyosc.*, *Kali bich.*, *Lac canin.*, *Lycop.*,
Mercur., *Nitr. ac.*, *Nux vom.*, *Oleand.*, *Phosphor.*, *Pulsat.*,
Silica, *Sulphur*, *Tarent.*

Incompatible: *Acet. ac.*

Complementary: *Hepar*, *Lycop.*, *Nitr. ac.*

Compare: *Crotal.*, *Naja trip.*, *Elaps. cor.* and *Bothrops can.*,
in their general effects on the blood and nervous system;
Sulphur and *Lycop.* in aphasia; *Theridion* and *Moschus*,
vertigo < closing eyes, sun headaches; *Arsen.*, *Hydr. ac.*,
Lauroc., *Digit.* and *Veratr.*, fainting from cardiac weakness; *Kali carb*, heart hangs by a thread; *Glonoin*, *Bellad.*, *Camphor*, *Natr. carb.*, and *Therid.*, effects from heat
of the sun; *Stramon.*, *Agaric.*, *Mephitis*, *Act. rac.* and
Paris quad., loquacity; *Opium*, *Hyosc.*, *Arnica*, *Alum.*,
Lycop., *Rhus tox.*, typhoid fever; *Mercur.*, *Cinchona*, *Pulsat.*, *Bryon.*, *Gelsem.*, catarrhal and rheumatic headache; *Silica*, desire to have head wrapped up; *Crotal.*,
Phosphor. and *Arnica* in retinal apoplexy; *Crotal.* and
Elaps, otorrhœa; *Apis*, *Arsen.*, and *Kali carb.*, œdema of
face; *Cicut.*, dyspnœa from spasm; *Apis*, *Rhus tox.* and
Euphorb., erysipelas, herpes, etc.; *Phytol.*, sore throat,
debility, etc.; *Lac can.*, *Crotal.* and *Naja*, diphtheria;
Cinchona, *Carbo veg.*, *Hepar*, *Kreos.*, *Kali bich.*, *Nux vom.*
and *Lycop.*, dyspepsias and abdominal diseases; *Colchic.*
and *Elaps*, cold feeling in stomach; *Bellad.*, *Caustic.*,
Natr. mur., *Nitr. ac.*, *Ignat.*, *Kali bich.*, *Opium*, *Plumbum*,
Mezer. and *Coccul.*, constriction of anus, anal tenesmus
and dysentery; *Anacard.*, sensation of plug in rectum;

Hepar, Asaf., Lycop., Mur. ac., Silica, Sulph. ac. and
Arsen., ulcerations; *Apis, Arg. met., Platin., Murex, Pallad.,
Lycop.,* and *Graphit.,* ovarian and uterine diseases;
Crotal., Helleb., Digit., Tereb., Apis and *Colchic.,* vesical
and renal affections, with hæmaturia; *Calc. ostr.,* gall
stones; *Phosphor.* and *Thuja* fungus hæmatoides; *Natr.
mur.* and *Ledum,* effects of bee sting; *Lact. ac.,* fulness
of throat and constriction; *Tarent. cuben.,* painful carbuncles.

CPSIA information can be obtained
at www.ICGtesting.com
Printed in the USA
LVHW060558260323
742530LV00050B/519